Essentials of
Pharmacotherapeutics

Essentials of
Pharmacotherapeutics

B. V. S. Lakshmi

M.Pharm., Ph.D.

Professor and HOD, Dept. of Pharmacology,
HOD, M.Sc. Clinical Research,
School of Allied and Healthcare Sciences,
Malla Reddy University, Secunderabad.

M. Sudhakar

M.Pharm., Ph.D.

Professor and Principal,
Malla Reddy College of Pharmacy,
(Affliated to Osmania University),
Maisammaguda, Secunderabad.

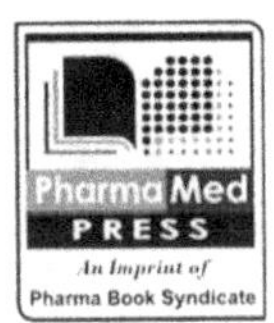

PharmaMed Press

An imprint of BSP Books Pvt. Ltd.

4-4-309/316, Giriraj Lane,
Sultan Bazar, Hyderabad - 500 095.

Essentials of Pharmacotherapeutics

by B. V. S. Lakshmi and M. Sudhakar

Published by

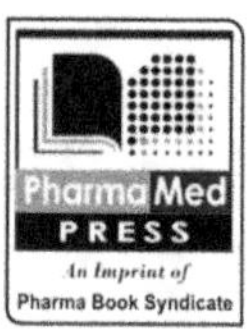

PharmaMed Press

An imprint of BSP Books Pvt. Ltd.

4-4-309/316, Giriraj Lane, Sultan Bazar, Hyderabad - 500 095.

Phone: 040-23445688 Fax: 91+40-23445611

E-mail: info@pharmamedpress.com

www.pharmamedpress.com/pharmamedpress.net

ISBN: 978-93-90211-76-0 (Hardback)

PREFACE

It is matter of great rejoice to write the preface of the first edition "Essentials of Pharmacotherapeutics".

Pharmacotherapeutics is a connecting bridge between pathophysiology, pharmacology and applications of drugs in the clinical field. Adequate insight of Pathophysiology will be helpful for better understanding of pharmacology.

This book will be useful from the academic point of view, especially for pharmacy students. We have tried to give maximum recent and updated information and also made a sincere effort to create a perfect mixture of a reference and examination oriented book. The highlight of the book is the incorporation of case studies of different topics at the end of each chapter.

Keeping this in view, it is our endeavour to provide a comprehensive text of therapeutics through lucid language covering diagrams, flowcharts and tables wherever necessary.

Although we have tried to give the best valuable information, however, continuous research, clinical examinations, individual sensitivity may show change in effectiveness of therapy and hence treatment of any nature should not be substituted by our book. We hope that the book shall cater to the needs of students and faculty in understanding the fundamentals of pharmacotherapy of diseases.

We will be grateful to all the readers who finally judge the quality of this book and feedback for the same is welcomed.

-Authors

CONTENTS

Section X: Oncology

Section XI: Infectious Diseases

Section XII: Gastrointestinal Disorders

Section XIII: Hematological Disorders

Section XIV: Neurological Disorders

Section XV: Psychiatric Disorders

ABBREVIATIONS

AB	:	Amyloid B
ACD	:	Atopic Contact dermatitis
ACEIs	:	ACE Inhibitors
ACR	:	American College of Rheumatology
AD	:	Alzheimer's Disease
AED	:	Anti-epileptic Drugs
AIDS	:	Acquired Immunodefiency syndrome
AKI	:	Acute Kidney Injury
ALT	:	Alanine transaminase
AMPA	:	α-amino -3-hydroxy-5-methyl-4-isoxazolepropionic acid
ARF	:	Acute Renal Failure
ARB	:	Angiotensin Receptor Blockers
AST	:	Aspartate Aminotransferase
BDZ	:	Benzodiazepines
BID	:	bis in die, twice a day
BRCA 1	:	Breast Cancer gene 1
Ba SO$_4$	:	Barium Sulphate
BUN	:	Blood Urea Nitrogen
CABG	:	Coronary Artery Bypass Grafting
CAD	:	Coronary Artery Disease
CBC	:	Complete Blood Count
CBT	:	Cognitive Behavioral Therapy
CBV	:	Coxsackie B Virus
CD20	:	Cluster of differentiate 20
CGMP	:	Cyclic Guanosine Mono Phosphate
CHD	:	Congestive Heart Disease
CHE	:	Cholesterol Esters

CHF	:	Congestive Heart Failure
Chy	:	Chylomicrons
CKD	:	Chronic Kidney Disease
CNS	:	Central Nervous System
COPD	:	Chronic Obstructive Pulmonology Disease
COX-2	:	Cycloxygenase-2
CRP	:	C-reactive protein
CRTZ	:	Chemo Receptor Trigger Zone
CSF	:	Cerebrospinal Fluid
CT scan	:	Computed Tomography Scan
DA	:	Dopamine
DM	:	Diabetes Mellitus
DMARDS	:	Disease Modifying Anti-Rheumatic Drugs
DNA	:	Deoxy Ribonucleic Acid
DOT	:	Daily Observation Therapy
DSM	:	Diagnostic & statistical Manual for Mental Disorders
ECG	:	Electrocardiography
EEG	:	Electroencephalography
ESR	:	Erythrocyte Sedimentation Rate
ESRD	:	End Stage Renal Disease
FAB	:	French American British
FAB	:	Fragment Antigen – Binding
FDA	:	Food and Drug Administration
FENa	:	Fractional Excretion of Sodium
G	:	Gram
GABA	:	Gama-aminobutyric Acid
GFR	:	Glomerular filtration rate
GIT	:	Gastrointestinal Tract
Glu	:	Glutamine Acid
GTP	:	Guanosine Triphosphate
Hb	:	Hemoglobin
HER	:	Human Epidermal Growth Factor Receptor

HGPRT	:	Hypoxanthine Guanine Phosphoribosyl Transferase
HLA	:	Human Leukocyte Antigen
HPF	:	High Power Field
HSV	:	Herpes Simplex Virus
5HT	:	5 Hydroxy Tryptamine
ICD	:	Irritant Contact dermatitis
ICD	:	International classification of Disease
INR	:	Indian rupee
IOP	:	Intraocular Pressure
LMWH	:	Low Molecular Weight Heparin
Mg/dL	:	Milligram/deciliter
MHC	:	Major Histocompatibility Complex
MI	:	Myocardial Infarction
MOA	:	Mechanism of Action
MRI	:	Magnetic Resonance Imaging
MSME	:	Mini Mental Status Exam
MTX	:	Methotrexate
NE	:	Norepinephrine
NKD Q1	:	National Kidney Dialysis Outcomes and Quality Initiative
NMDA	:	N-methyl – D – Aspartate
NO	:	Nitric Oxide
NSAIDs	:	Non-Steroidal Anti-inflammatory Drugs
NSTEMI	:	Non ST Segment Elevated Myocardial Infarction
OD	:	Once a Day
OTC	:	Over the Counter
PCAG	:	Primary Closure Angle Glaucoma
PCI	:	Percutaneous Coronary Intervention
PET	:	Positron emission tomography
POAG	:	Primary Open Angle Glaucoma
PTCA	:	Percutaneous Transluminal Coronary Angioplasty
QID	:	Quarterly in a Day
QOL	:	Quality of Life

RAAS	:	Renin Angiotensin Aldosterone System
RNA	:	Ribonucleic Acid
RRT	:	Renal Replacement Therapy
SCr	:	Serum Creatinine
SPECT	:	Single –photon emission computed tomography
SSRIS	:	Selective Serotonin Receptor Inhibitors
STEMI	:	ST Segment Elevated Myocardial Infarction
TCA	:	Tricyclic Anti-Depressants
TEE	:	Tran esophageal echocardiogram
TGs	:	Triglycerides
TID	:	Three Times a Day
TMT	:	Treadmill Test
TNF	:	Tumor Necrosis Factor
TNFi	:	Tumor Necrosis Factor Inhibitors
TTE	:	Transthoracic Echocardiogram
TPA	:	Tissue Plasminogen Activator
RPA	:	Recombinant Plasminogen Activator
UV	:	Ultraviolet
UFH	:	Unfractionated Heparin
U/L	:	Units/Litre
UVA	:	Ultraviolet A light
UVB	:	Ultraviolent B light

CHAPTER - 1

Hyperlipidaemia

Introduction to Hyperlipidaemia

Hyperlipidaemia is abnormally elevated levels of any or all lipids or lipoproteins in the blood. It is the most common form of dyslipidaemia. Hyperlipidaemia are divided into primary and secondary subtypes. Primary hyperlipidaemia is usually due to genetic causes while secondary hyperlipidaemia arises due to other underlying causes such as diabetes.

Lipids are biological molecules which are not dissolved in water but can be dissolved in organic solvents. In the body, lipoproteins/lipids are present in the intestines, liver and/or intestines and liver.

Lipoproteins: These are large globular particles that contain an oily core of nonpolar lipid (cholesteryl esters of triglycerides) surrounded by a polar coat of phospholipids free (i.e. unesterified) cholesterol and apoproteins. There are five classes of lipoproteins that differ from one another in size, density and properties of triglycerides and cholesterol.

Lipoproteins are of five types:

- Chylomicrons
- Very lowdensity lipoprotein (VLDL)
- Intermediate density lipoprotein (IDL)
- Low density lipoprotein (LDL)
- High density lipoprotein (HDL)

Chylomicrons

These are the largest particles both in size as well as in density, and its concentration is directly correlated with dietary triglyceride contents.

VLDL: Very low-density lipoproteins are smaller particles carrying lesser triglyceride contents than chylomicrons, and are secreted from the liver. VLDL carries cholesterol from the liver to organ and tissues in the body. They are formed from the combination of cholesterol and triglycerides.

IDL: VLDL particles after degradation by lipase enzyme in the capillaries of adipose tissue and muscle give rise to intermediate density lipoprotein.

LDL: Low-density lipoproteins are synthesised partly in intestinal cycle and partly after lipolysis of VLDL. It is directly correlated to Congestive Heart Disease (CHD).

HDL: HDL is commonly referred as good cholesterol. High-density lipoproteins are synthesised in the liver. It carries cholesterol and other lipids from tissues back to the liver for degradation. HDL plays an antiatherogenic role.

Lipoprotein Metabolism and Transport [1]

Dietary lipids are absorbed in the intestine with the help of bile acids. Chylomicrons (Chy) are formed and passed into lacteals—reach blood stream via thoracic duct. During their passage through capillaries, the endothelium bound lipoprotein lipase hydrolyses the TGs into fatty acids which pass into muscle cells to be utilized as energy source and in fat cells to be reconverted into TGs and stored. The remaining part—chylomicron remnant (Chy. rem.) containing mainly Cholesterol Esters (CHE) and little TG is engulfed by liver cells, which have receptors for the surface apoproteins of Chy. rem., and digested. Free Cholesterol (CH) that is liberated is either stored in liver cells after reesterification or incorporated into a different lipoprotein and released in blood or excreted in bile as CH/bile acids. Liver secretes very low density lipoproteins (VLDL) containing mainly TG and some CHE into blood. VLDL is acted upon by endothelial lipoprotein lipase in the same way as on Chy and the fatty acids pass into adipose tissue and muscle; the remnant called intermediate density lipoprotein (IDL) now contains more CHE than TG. About half of the IDL is taken back by the liver cells by attachment to another receptor (LDL receptor), while the rest loses the remaining TGs gradually and becomes low density lipoprotein (LDL) containing only CHE. The LDL circulates in plasma for a long time; its uptake into liver and other tissues is dependent on the need for CH. The rate of LDL uptake is regulated by the rate of LDL receptor synthesis in a particular tissue.

The CHE of LDL is deesterified and used mainly for cell membrane formation. The CH released into blood from degradation of membranes is rapidLy incorporated in high density lipoproteins (HDL), esterified with the help of an enzyme lecithin: cholesterol acyltransferase (LCAT) and transferred back to VLDL or IDL, completing the cycle. The excess lipoproteins in plasma are phagocytosed by macrophages for disposal. When too much of lipoproteins have to be degraded in this manner, CH is deposited in atheromas (in arterial walls) and xanthomas (in skin and tendons). Raised levels of VLDL, IDL and LDL (rarely Chy and Chy. rem. also) are atherogenic, while HDL may be protective, because HDL facilitates removal of CH from tissues

Epidemiology

In India, more than 10 Million people per year are suffering with hyperlipidaemia. The most prone people are diabetic and Coronary Artery Disease (CAD) patients. Hyperlipidemia disease has afflicted humankind since antiquity. In 2002, coronay heart Epidemiological evidence strongly supported the positive correlation between blood lipids, hyperlipidemia and its complications, mainly CHD. This relationship has been shown between and within cultures. While fats play a vital role in the body's metabolic processes, high blood levels of fats increase the risk of coronary heart disease (CHD). Cardiovascular diseases, especially coronary heart disease (CHD), are epidemic in India. According to American Heart Association, the Centres for Disease Control and Prevention, the National Institutes of Health and other government sources, cardiovascular disease is the leading global cause of death, accounting for more than 17.3 million deaths per year, a number that is expected to grow to more than 23.6 million by 2030.

Etiology

- Genetics
- **Diet and Obesity:** Food choices paly a role in high cholesterol. Obesity increases the amount of LDL cholestrol the liver makes. It also decreases clearance of LDL cholesterol form the blood. Inflammation throughout the body is a common complication of obesity. This constant inflammation decreases the body's response to changes in dietary fat intake. Insulin resistance is also common in obesity. It causes changes in the enzymes the body needs to hnadLe cholesterol normally.
- **Diabetes Mellitus:** The predominant abnormality of fat metabolism in diabetes is hypertriglyceridemia due to an increase of triglyceride-carrying lipoproteins, the chylomicrons and the very-low-density lipoproteins. VLDL and chylomicrons, which transport endogenous and exogenous triglycerides, are broken down by lipoprotein lipases. In insulin deficiency, the activity of the lipoprotein lipases is decreased, and this is one of the most common **causes of** hyperlipidemia in poorly controlled diabetes in type 1 and type 2. These patients also have decreased HDL cholesterol levels.
- **Smoking:** Hyperlipidemia and smoking are linked by an intricate network of multiple relations. The concentration of high-density lipoprotein (HDL) cholesterol is lower in heavy smokers, and the concentrations of triglycerides and cholesterol are higher. Due to this waxy plaques build up in the arteries.
- **Alcoholism:** Drinking alcohol raises the triglycerides and cholesterol in the blood. If triglyceride levels become too high, they can build up in the liver, causing fatty liver disease. The liver can't work as well as it should and can't remove cholesterol from blood, so cholesterol levels begin to rise.
- **Glucocorticoids:** Triglycerides are significantly increased in patient who took different time of glucocorticoids. Short term use is having less effect when compared to long term use.
- **Drugs like β-blockers:** Suppression of beta-adrenergic activity leads to unopposed alpha-adrenergic stimulation. In turn, alpha-adrenergic stimulation leads to a decrease in peripheral lipoprotein lipase activity and a subsequent reduction in catabolism of very low-density lipoprotein and triglycerides
- **Hypothyroid:** Body needs thyroid hormones to make cholesterol and to get rid of the cholesterol it does not need. When thyroid hormone levels are low, the body does not break down and remove LDL cholesterol as effficiently as usual. LDL cholesterol can then build up in the blood.
- **Lack of physical activity:** Lipoprotein metabolism is altered, so increased levels of LDL and decresased HDL cholesterol levels.

Types of Hyperlipidaemias based on causing factor:

1. **Primary Hyperlipidaemia** - Primary hyperlipidaemia is often genetic. It is a result of a defect or mutation in lipoproteins. These changes result in problems with accumulation of lipids in the body. It includes –

   (a) **Familial combined hyperlipidaemia:** It occurs as a history of familial hyperlipidaemia. It is mainly caused due to high levels of VLDL. When there is an increase in the synthesis of VLDL and LDL results in increase in triglycerides. This type is mainly seen in teenagers.

   People suffering with this type are more prone to get CAD which can lead to sudden heart attacks.

   (b) **Familial hypercholesterolaemia:** It occurs due to increase in the total cholesterol. The LDL is increased 2-3 times than the normal level. Signs of cholesterol deposition are seen in the form of
   - ✓ Corneal arcus: Deposition of lipids in cornea
   - ✓ Tendon xanthomas: yellowish papules in tendons

   (c) **Familial hyperlipoproteinaemia:** This type is mainly seen due to the accumulation of chylomicrons and VLDL. Due to the failure of clearance of Apo E in hepatic system, there is an increase in triglycerides and cholesterol.

   Signs and Symptoms:
   - ✓ Tubo eruptive xantomas: yellowish raised nodules on skin; mainly elbows and knees.
   - ✓ Palmar striae: yellowish raised streaks on palms

   (d) **Familial lipoprotein lipase deficiency**: Failure of lipolysis leads to accumulation of chylomicrons in plasma. Lipoprotein lipase deficiency will lead to hypertriglyceridaemia and chylomicronaemia. This type is mainly seen in children.

   Signs and Symptoms:
   - ✓ Abdominal pain
   - ✓ Spleenomegaly
   - ✓ Acute pancreatitis
   - ✓ Deposition of lipids in the eye

Table 1.1 Common forms of primary hyperlipidemia.

	Lipoprotein abnormality	Drug therapy
Familial hypercholesterolemia	↑↑LDL	Lovastatin
Familial defective apolipoprotein B	↑↑LDL	None
Polygenic hypercholesterolemia	↑LDL	Lovastatin
Familial lipoprotein lipase deficiency	↑Chylomicrons	Nicotinic acid
Familial hypertriglyceridemia	↑VLDL	Gemfibrozil
Familial combined hyperlipidemia	↑VLDL, ↑LDL, ↓HDL	Nicotinic acid, clofibrate
Familial dysbetalipoproteinemia	↑Chylomicrons, ↑LDL, ↓IDL, ↓HDL	Gemfibrozil

2. **Secondary hyperlipoproteinaemia:**

Acquired (Secondary) hyperlipidemia – Acquired hyperlipidemia (secondary dyslipo-proteinemias) results from underlying disorders and lead to alterations in plasma lipid and lipoprotein metabolism. This type of hyperlipidemia may mimic primary forms of hyperlipidemia and can have similar consequences. They may result in increased risk of premature atherosclerosis, pancreatitis and other complications of the chylomicronemia syndrome. The most common causes of acquired hyperlipidemia are given below.

- Diabetes Mellitus
- Use of drugs such as diuretics, β-blockers and estrogens.
- Alcohol consumption.
- Some rare endocrine disorders and metabolic disorders.
- Hypothyroidism
- Renal failure
- Nephrotic syndrome

Table 1.2 Common forms of secondary hyperlipidemia.

	Lipid abnormalities	Lipoprotein abnormalities
Diabetes mellitus	↑TG	↑VLDL, ↓HDL
Nephrotic syndrome	↑Chol	↑LDL
Uremia	↑TG	↑VLDL, ↓HDL
Hypothyroidism	↑Chol	↑LDL
Obstructive liver disease	↑Chol	↑Lp(a)
Alcoholism	↑TG	↑VLDL
Oral contraceptive	↑TG	↑VLDL, ↓HDL
β-Adrenergic blocking agents	↑TG	↑VLDL, ↓HDL
Isotretinoin	↑TG	↑VLDL

Complications of Hyperlipidaemia

I. **Atherosclerosis:** It is a common disorder and occurs when fat, cholesterol and calcium deposits in the arterial linings. This deposition results in the formation of fibrous plaques. A plaque normally consists of three components: 1) atheroma which is a fatty, soft, yellowish nodular mass located in the centre of a larger plaque that consists of macrophages, which are cells that play a role in immunity; 2) a layer of cholesterol crystals; and, 3) calcified outer layer. Atherosclerosis is the leading cause of cardiovascular disease.

II. **Coronary Artery Disease (CAD):** Atherosclerosis is the major cause of CAD. It is characterised by the narrowing of the arteries that supply blood to the myocardium and results in limiting blood flow and insufficient amounts of oxygen to meet the needs of the heart. The narrowing may progress to the extent that the heart muscle would sustain damage due to lack of blood supply. Elevated lipid profile is correlated to the development of coronary atherosclerosis.

III.   **Myocardial Infarction (MI):** MI is a condition which occurs when blood and oxygen supplies to the cardiac arteries are partially or completely blocked, resulting in damage or death of heart cells. The blockage is usually due to the formation of a clot in an artery. This condition is commonly known as heart attack. The studies show that one-fourth of survivors of myocardial infarction were hyperlipidemic.

IV.   **Angina Pectoris:** Angina is not a disease but a symptom of an underlying heart condition. It is characterised by chest pain, discomfort or a squeezing pressure. Angina occurs as a result of a reduction or a lack of blood supply to a part or the entire heart muscle. Poor blood circulation is usually due to CHD when partial or complete obstruction of the coronary arteries is present.

V.   **Ischemic stroke or Cerebrovascular Accident (CVA):** It occurs when blood circulation in part of the brain is blocked or diminished. When blood supply, which carries oxygen, glucose, and other nutrients, is disrupted, brain cells die and become dysfunctional. Usually, strokes occur due to blockage of an artery by a blood clot or a piece of atherosclerotic plaque that breaks loose in a small vessel within the brain. Clinical trials revealed that lowering of LDL and total cholesterol by 15% significantly reduced the risk of first stroke.

Formation of Choleslterol

Fats and carbohydrates are digested and absorbed in the deodenum and opens in the small intestine. Small intestine has Na^+ and glucose transporters and glucose will be reabsorbed in the blood. Liver also receives glucose. With the help of glycolysis process, glucose in converted into pyruvate and enters into acetyl CoA. This acetyl CoA is converted into cholesterol.

Table 1.3 Normal levels for a lipid profile.

Lipids	Desirable value	Borderline	High risk
Cholesterol	Less than 200 mg/dL	200-239 mg/dL	240 mg/dL
Triglycerides	Less than 140 mg/dL	150-199 mg/dL	200-499 mg/dL
HDL cholesterol	60 mg/dL	40-50 mg/dL	Less than 40 mg/dL
LDL cholesterol	60-130 mg/dL	130-159 mg/dL	160-189 mg/dL
Cholesterol/HDL ratio	4.0	5.0	6.0

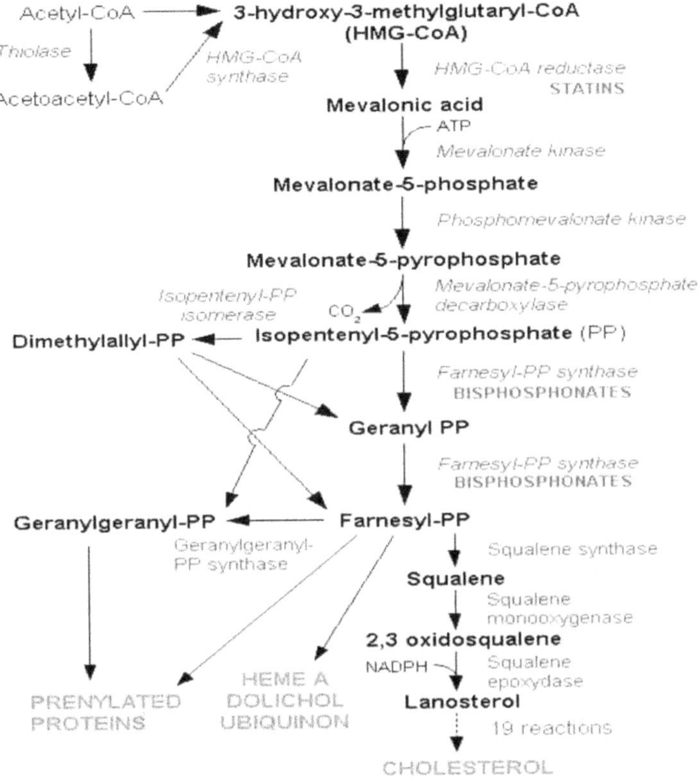

Fig. 1.1 Synthesis of Cholesterol.

Pathophysiology

Risk factors for hyperlipidaemia are HTN, DM, obesity, smoking, stress and genetic factors. Due to increase in cholesterol, accumulation of cholesterol from VLDL and LDL takes place. Free radicals oxidize the LDL. LDL is oxidized in the endothelial cells and released. Monocyte adhesion molecule (initial step for development of atherosclerotic plaque) attaches to oxidized LDL. Circulating monocytes attaches to endothelial surface. These trap the monocytes in endothelium and release chemoattractants (a substance which attracts motile cells). Monocytes are squeezed into the endothelium and converted to macrophages which contain LDL receptors. Ingestion of the excess VLDL and LDL particles, accumulatation in blood vessels by VLDL receptors. This process continues and forms foam cells. This leads to formation of raised lesions on blood vessels and forms fatty streaks. It further leads to atherosclerotic plaque, endothelium damage, vasoconstriction and initial Ischemic symptoms. Initially the plaque contains large lipids which were made from foam cells. During the plaque growth, macrophages, endothelial cells and smooth muscles get activated releases growth factor which leads to smooth muscle cell proliferation (plaque) and gets hardened by collagen coronary artery remodeling resulting in sudden MI and death.

Clinical Manifestation and Features

Signs and Symptoms

- ✓ Most patients are asymptomatic for many years.
- ✓ Symptomatic patients may complain of chest pain, pain, palpitations, sweating, anxiety, shortness of breath, abdominal pain, loss of consiousness or difficulty with speech or movement.
- ✓ Depending on the lipoprotein abnormality, signs on physical examination may include cutaneous xantomas, peripheral polyneuropathy, high blood pressure and increased body mass index or waist size.

Diagnosis Algorithm [2]

Check the fasting lipid profile (FLP) (atleast 2 times)

1. If LDL-C $\geq$ 250mg/dL: Request a specialist.
2. If $130 \leq$ LDL ≤ 250 mg/dL: Secondary cause exclusion; risk evaluation and CHILD (Cardiovascular Health Integrated Lifestyle Diet) for 6 months + Lifestyle modification should be followed. After the followup of 6 months if LDL-C is less than 130 mg/dL-continue CHILD and FLP should be done every 1 year.
3. If LDL-C 130-189 mg/dL; the patient has no family history and no risk factors-follow CHILD and FLP testing should be repeated every 6 months.
4.   (i) If LDL-C $\geq$ 190 mg/dL1
     (ii) If LDL-C 160-189 mg/dL; the patient has family history, > 1 high risk factor or $\geq$ moderate risk factors
     (iii) If the patient has a) LDL-C 130-159 mg/dL b) ≥ 2 high risk factors c) 1 high risk factor or ≥ 2 moderate risk factors or clinical cardiovascular disease
   - ➢   Statin treatment should be initiated.
5. If TG $\geq$ 500mg/dL: Request a specialist.
6. If $130 \leq$ TG < 500 mg/dL: CHILD for 6 months + lifestyle modification with weight loss.
7.   (i) If TG < 130 mg/dL: Continue CHILD –TG. Check FLP every 1 Year.
     (ii) If TG 130-199 mg/dL: Follow CHILD-TG and reinforce weight loss. Increase fish intake. FLP after 6 months
     (iii) If TG $\geq$ 200-499 mg/dL: If non-HDL-C $\geq$ 145mg/dL –consider omega-3 fatty acids.
1. Know the complete history of the patient.
2. Check if there are any cardiovascular risks.
3. Serum lipid tests to check - total cholesterol, VLDL, LDL, HDL
4. According to NCEP ATP –III guidelines
   - ✓ Total cholesterol < 200mg/dL $\rightarrow$ desirable
                                           200-239mg/dL $\rightarrow$ boderline high
                                           $\geq$240mg/dL $\rightarrow$ high risk

- ✓ LDL cholesterol
  - < 100mg/dL → optimal
  - 100-129mg/dL → normal or above optimal
  - 130-159mg/dL → boderline high
  - 160-189mg/dL → high
  - ≥190mg/dL → very high
- ✓ HDL cholesterol
  - <40mg/dL → low
  - ≥60mg/dL → high
- ✓ Triglycerides
  - <150mg/dL → normal
  - 150-199mg/dL → borderline high
  - 200-499mg/dL → high
  - ≥ 500mg/dL → very high

REVISED NCEP ATP III VS ACC/AHA ATP IV GUIDELINES

National Cholesterol Education Program (NCEP) Adult Treatment Panel (ATP) Guidelines

NCEP ATP III

1. Risk categories: 3 main risk catgories- CHD/CHD risk equivalent (DM, clinical CHD, symptomatic CAD, PAD)
2. + risk factors & 10-yr risk ≤ 20%
   0-1risk factors & 10-yr risk < 10%
3. Treatment targets: LDL-C primary target <100mg/dL
   < 130mg/dL (< 100 if risk 10-20%)
   <160mg/dL
4. Treatment recommendations: statin (or bile acid sequesterants or nicotinic acid) to achieve LDL-C goal
5. Risk factor counting
6. Treat to LDL goal
7. Address NON-HDL target

NCEP ATP IV

1. **Risk categories:** 4 statin benefit groups: clinical ASCVD; primary LDL-C elevations ≥190mg/dL; DM without clinical ASCVD; No DM/CVD with 10-yr ASCVD risk ≥7.5%
2. **Treatment targets:** Intensity of statin therapy; High intensity statin therapy (LDL-C reduction ≥ 50%) is recommended for most patients in 4 statin benefit groups
3. **Treatment recommendations:** Maximally tolerated statin first-line to reduce risk of ASCVD events
4. **There is no target**
5. **The intensity of statin therapy is the focus of treatment**

Summary

Although there are similarities between ATP III and American College of Cardiology (ACC/AHA) guidelines, the two are fundamentally different. In contrast, the ATP III panel made use of all types of relevant science. It emphasized Randomised Control Trials (RCTs), but where appropriate, used epidemiological data, genetic and metabolic studies, and various in vivo and in vitro investigations to flesh out the guidelines. Evidence statements based on various types of scientific data were developed to stand behind recommendations. ATP III is the summation of several decades of research on the relation of atherogenic lipoproteins to ASCVD. It is based on the concept that lowering atherogenic lipoproteins will prevent ASCVD. ACC/AHA guidelines under the influence of an Institute of Medicine (IOM) paradigm are transformed into statin treatment instructions. They give lip service to lifestyle intervention but are embarrassed by a lack of RCTs to underpin lifestyle recommendations. They further can be questioned because they make risk assessment based on older data that may not be suitable for the current US population. Since the ACC/AHA guidelines depend entirely on RCTs, they should not be considered to be comprehensive cholesterol guidelines. Therefore, if using these guidelines, the physician must rely on a heavy dose of clinical judgment. ATP III is still useful for guiding the physician's clinical judgment.

Pharmacological Therapy

Classification of Drugs

1. **HMG Co-A reduactase inhibitors:** Lovastatin 20-8-mg/Provastatin 20-40mg/ Simvastatin 20-80mg
   Fluvastatin   20-80 mg/Atorvastatin 10-80 mg
2. Bile acid sequestrants: Cholestyramine 4-16g/colestipol 5-20g/Colesevelam 2.6-3.8g
3. Nicotinic acid: Immediate release (Crystalline) nicotinic acid 1-5-3g
4. **Fibric acids:** Gemfibrozil   600mg bid/Fenofibrate 200 mg
   Clofibrate 1000mg bid

Management

Non-Pharmacological Treatment

✓ Change lifestyle modification and sedentary lifestyle.
✓ Dietary modifications like reduce salt intake and salt rich food.
✓ Weight reduction by physical activities, yoga etc.,
✓ Alcohol and smoking cessation.

Pharmacological Treatment

HMG CoA Reductase Inhibitors

Statins inhibit 3-hydroxy-3-methylglutaryl coenzyme A (HMG CoA) reductase, inturrupting conversion of HMG-CoA to mevalonate, the rate limiting step in cholesterol biosynthesis. When used as monotherapy, statins are the most potent cholesterol and LDL lowering agents. Constipation occurs in fewer than 10% of patients taking statins. Other adverse effects include elevated serum aminotransferase levels (primarily alanine aminotransferase), elevated creatine kinase levels, myopathy, and rarely rhabdomyolysis.

> E.g.,: Atorvastatin 10-80mg
> Rosuvastatin 5-40mg
> Simvastatin 10-20mg

Fibric Acids

Fibrate monotherapy is effective in reducing VLDL. Plasma HDL levels may rise 10-15% or more by fibrates. GI complaints occur in 3% to 5% of patients, rash in 2%, dizziness in 2.4%, and transient elevations in transaminase levels and alkaline phosphatase in 4.5% and 1.3%, respectively.

> E.g.,: Gemfibrozil 600mg-1.5gm, fenofibrate 200mg, clofibrate 1000mg bid

Ezetimibe

Ezetimibe interferes with the absorption of cholesterol from the brush border of the intestines. It is approved for monotherapy and for use with statins. The dose is <u>10 mg once daily</u>, given with or without food. When given alone, it results in 18% reduction in LDL cholesterol. When given with a statin, it lowers LDL by an additional 12% to 20%.

Bile Acid Resins (BARs)

The primary action of BARs is to bind bile acids in the intestinal lumen, with a concurrent interruption of enterohepatic circulation of bile acids, which decreases the bile acid pool size and stimulates hepatic synthesis of bile acids from cholesterol. It helps in depletion of hepatic pool of cholesterol which results in an increase in cholesterol biosynthesis and an increase in the LDL on liver which increases the HDL levels.

> Side effects may include Gastro Intestinal (GI) irritation, epigastric fullness, nausea.

> E.g.,: Cholestyramine 8gm TID Cholestepin hydrochloride 10gm BD

Niacin

It decreases the synthesis of VLDL which inturn leads to decrease in the synthesis of LDL and increase in the HDL. Niacin also increases HDL by reducing its catabolism. The principal use of niacin is for mixed hyperlipidemia or as a second-line agent in combination therapy for hypercholesterolemia. It is a first-line agent or alternative for the treatment of hypertriglyceridemia and diabetic dyslipidemia.

Side effects: pruritis (itching), Elevated liver function tests, hyperuricemia, and hyperglycemia, hepatitis is more common with sustained-release preparations.

Contraindications: Liver disease, gout and diabetes.

Dose – 0.5mg to 1gm TID

E.g., Niaspan 1-2gm OD

Fish Oil Supplements

Diets high in omega-3-polyunsaturated fatty acids, reduces the cholesterol, triglycerides, LDL and VLDL and may elevate HDL cholesterol. It may be most useful in patients with hypertriglyceridemia. E.g., Lovaza 4gm/day as 4 times [1gm,1gm,1gm,1gm]. This product lowers triglycerides by 14-30% and raises HDL by 10%.

Algorithm [3, 4, 5]

Primary prevention: Assess the ASCVD (Atherosclerotic cardiovascular disease) risk in each age group and emphasize adherence to healthy Lifestyle

1. **Based on age**
   (a) If age group is 0-19 yrs-then lifestyle modifications are advised to prevent or reduce ASCVD risk. Diagnosis of Familial hypercholesterolemia is to be done based on that a statin is advised.
   (b) If age group is 20-39 yrs: Estimate lifetime risk and encourage lifestyle modifications to reduce ASCVD risk. Statin therapy can be considered if family history is present.
   (c) If age group is 40-75 yrs and LDL-C>70-190 mg/dL without diabetes mellitus, then 10-year risk has to be estimated.
      (i) If risk is <5%-considered as "Low risk": emphasize on lifestyle modification to reduce risk.
      (ii) If risk is 5% --< 7.5%, considered as "Borderline risk": moderate-intensity statin therapy to be initiated.
      (iii) If risk is ≥ 7.5%-<20%, considered as "Intermediate risk": if risk estimate + risk enhancers favor statin, initiate moderate –intensity statin to reduce LDL-C by 30%- 49%.
      (iv) If risk is ≥ 20%: considered as "High risk": Initiate statin to reduce LDL-C ≥50%.
2. (a) If LDL-C ≥ 190mg/dL: Directly high-intensity statin has to be initiated
   (b) If the patient has diabetes mellitus and age between 40-75 yrs: Moderate –intensity statin has to be initiated
   (c) If age >75yrs: clinical assessment to be done and risk discussion is encouraged.

3. **Adults with chronic kidney disease:** Starting moderate-intensity statin alone or in combination with ezetimibe can be useful

4. **Adults with chronic inflammatory disorders and HIV:** In adults age 40–75 with LDL-C 70–189 mg/dL with a 10-year ASCVD risk of over 5%, discuss moderate- or high-intensity statin therapy

5. **Women:** History of premature menopause (before age 40) or history of pregnancy-related disorders (hypertension, pre-eclampsia, gestational diabetes, small-for-gestational-age infants, and preterm deliveries) are risk-enhancing factors and should influence lifestyle and pharmacologic therapy decisions

ASCVD Risk enhancers:

1. Family history of premature ASCVD
2. Persistently elevated LDL-C $\geq$ 160mg/ dL
3. Chronic kidney disease
4. Metabolic syndrome
5. Pre-eclampsia
6. Inflammatory diseases (esp-R. Arthritis, psoriasis, HIV)

Secondary Prevention: Atherosclerotic Disease [6, 7]

High-intensity statin therapy is recommended for all patients with atherosclerotic cardiovascular disease, including acute coronary syndromes, myocardial infarction, stable or unstable angina, or with a history of coronary or other arterial revascularization, stroke, transient ischemic attack, or peripheral artery disease including aortic aneurysm, all of atherosclerotic origin.

(a) If the patient subgroup is at very high risk: If low-density lipoprotein cholesterol (LDL- C) levels are $\geq$ 70 mg/dL with the maximal tolerated statin therapy, it is reasonable to add ezetimibe

   If LDL-C level is $\geq$ 70 mg/dL on maximal tolerated statin and ezetimibe, it is reasonable to add a PCSK9 inhibitor

(b) If the patient subgroup is not at very high risk

   Age $\leq$ 75: Goal is LDL-C reduction by 50%

   Use moderate-intensity statins if high- intensity statins are not tolerated

   If LDL-C $\geq$ 70 mg/dL on high-intensity statins, it is reasonable to add ezetimibe

   Age > 75: Starting or continuing either moderate- or high-intensity statins is reasonable

NCEP ATP III Major Risk Factors That Modify LDL-C Goals

Positive Risk Factors ($\uparrow$Risk)

Age: Male $\geq$45 yr

Female: $\geq$55 yr

Family history of a premature CHD (definite MI or sudden death before 55 yr in father or other male first-degree relative or before 65 yr in mother or other female first-degree relative)

Current cigarette smoking

Hypertension ($\geq$140/90 mm Hg or on antihypertensive drugs)

Low HDL-C (<40mg/dL)

Negative Risk Factor ($\downarrow$Risk, protective)

Intensity of statin therapy:

1. High intensity and target reduction in LDL by $\geq$ 50%
   Atorvastatin   40-80mg
   Rosuvastatin   20-40mg
2. Moderate intensity and target reduction in LDL by 30-50%

Atorvastatin	10-20mg	Rosuvastatin	5-10mg	Simvastatin	20-40mg
Pravastatin	40-80mg	Fluvastatin XL	80mg	Pitavastatin	2-4 mg

3. Low intensity and target reduction in LDL by < 30%

Simvastatin	10mg	Pravastatin	10-20mg	Lovastatin	20mg
Fluvastatin	20-40mg	Pitavastatin	1 mg		

Statin-Associated Side Effects (SASE)

1. **Statin-associated muscle symptoms (SAMS):**
   (a) Myalgias (CK normal)-infrequent
   (b) Myositis/myopathy (CK > ULN) with concerning symptoms or objective weakness-Rare
   (c) Rhabdomyolysis (CK >10× ULN + renal injury) Rare HMG CoA Reductase
   (d) Statin-associated autoimmune myopathy (HMGCR antibodies, incomplete resolution) Rare
2. **Liver:** Transaminase elevation 3× ULN- infrequent
3. **Central nervous system:** Memory/cognition-rare

NCEP ATP III and AHA/ACC LDL-C Goals and Cutpoints for Therapeutic Lifestyle Changes (TLC) and Drug Therapy

1. If the Risk Category is CHD or CHD risk equivalents (10-year risk >20%), then the
   (a) LDL- C reduction target goal is to achieve < 100 mg/dL of LDL-C (reasonable goal is <70mg/dL)
   (b) If LDL-C is >100mg/dL therapeutic lifestyle changes to be initiated
   (c) If LDL-C is >100mg/dL drug therapy has to be initiated.
2. If the Risk Category is: 2+ risk factors and 10-year risk is 10% to 20% then,
   (a) LDL-C reduction target goal is <130mg/dL (reasonable goal is <100mg/dL)
   (b) If LDL-C is >130mg/dL Therapeutic Lifestyle Changes to be initiated
   (c) If LDL-C is >130mg/dL (100-129mg/dL) drug therapy has to be initiated.

3. If the Risk Category is: 2+ risk factors and 10-year risk is <10% then,
    (a) LDL-C reduction target goal is <130mg/dL
    (b) If LDL-C is >130mg/dL Therapeutic Lifestyle Changes to be initiated
    (c) If LDL-C is >160mg/dL drug therapy has to be initiated.
4. If the Risk Category is: <2 risk factors
    (a) LDL-C reduction target goal is <160mg/dL
    (b) If LDL-C is >160mg/dL Therapeutic Lifestyle Changes to be initiated
    (C) If LDL-C is 190mg/dL (160-189mg/dL) LDL-C lowering drug therapy is optional.

Treatment Algorithm/Therapy for Hypertriglyceridemia

1. Borderline high triglyceride level (150-199mg per dL)   or
2. High triglyceride level (200 to 499mg per dL)   or
3. Very high triglyceride level (500mg per dL)

Then initiate therapeutic lifestyle changes, optimize glycemic control in patients with diabetes, screen for metabolic syndrome, and search for secondary or acquired causes.

(i) If the patient is at or near LDL-C goal- consider adding a fibrate, niacin, or fish oil to achieve the non-HDL-C goal. Consider statins for moderate to high risk patients for myopathy.
  ➤ If the patient is not near LDL-C goal-then add a statin, increase or switch statins until patient is at or near the LDL-C goal.

ii) If the triglyceride level is higher than 1000mg per dL—Initiate a very low-fat diet (15% or less of calorie intake) and aggressive body weight redction.
  ➤ Observe and follow up. If now the triglyceride level is 500mg per dL or lower- then work on reaching LDL-C goal.
  ➤ If triglyceride level is not below 500mg per dL –then add a fibrate or niacin. Consider adding a fish oil to reach LDL-C goal.

Drug Induced Hyperlipidemia [8, 9, 10]

Table 1.4 Drugs That May Cause Dyslipidemias.

	LDL Cholesterol	Triglycerides	HDL Cholesterol
Cardiovascular /Endocrine			
Amiodarone	↑Variable	↔	↔
β-Blockers***	↔	↑10-40%	↓5-20%
Loop diuretics	↑5-10%	↑5-10%	↔
	LDL Cholesterol	**Triglycerides**	**HDL Cholesterol**
Thiazide diuretics . (high dose)	↑5-10%	↑5-15%	↔
Sodium-glucose co-transporter 2 (SGLT2) inhibitors	↑3-8%	↔↓	↑Variable

Contd…

	LDL Cholesterol	Triglycerides	HDL Cholesterol
Steroid Hormones/Anabolic Steroids			
Estrogen	↓7-20%	↑40%	↑5-20%
Select progestins	↑Variable	↓Variable	↓15-40%
Selective Estrogen Receptor Modulators	↓10-20%	↑0-30*	↔
Danazol	↑10-40%	↔	↓50%
Anabolic steroids	↑20%	↔	↓20-70%
Corticosteroids	↑Variable	↑Variable	↔
Antiviral Therapy			
Protease inhibitors	↑15-30%	↑15-200%	↔
Direct Acting Antivirals	↑12-27%	↔	↑14-20%
Immunosuppressants			
Cyclosporine and tacrolimus	↑0-50%	↑0-70%	↑0-90%
Corticosteroids	↑Variable	↑Variable	↔
Centrally Acting Medications			
First Generation antipsychotics	↔	↑22%	↓20%
Second Generation antipsychotics	↔	↑20-50%	↔
Anticonvulsants	↑Variable	↔	↑Variable
Other Medications			
Retinoids	↑15%	↑35-100%	↔**
Growth Hormone	↑10-25%	↔	↔↑7%
ABBREVIATIONS: LDL, low-density lipoprotein; HDL, high-density lipoprotein. *Raloxifene has not been shown to increase Triglyceride levels, while reported increases of up to 30% have been reported with use of tamoxifen**Data remains conflicting and some evidence shows a decrease, no effect, or increase***Varies based on individual drug			

Several medications and medication classes have been reported to affect the lipid profile. Risk factors include elevated lipid levels at baseline and high cardiovascular (CV) risk patients. This should be considered when evaluating patients with elevated levels of total cholesterol (TC), low-density lipoproteins cholesterol (LDL-C), non-high-density lipoprotein cholesterol (Non-HDL-C), triglycerides (TG) and reductions in high-density lipoprotein cholesterol (HDL-C). Cardiovascular medications, antipsychotics, anticonvulsants, hormones and certain immunosuppressives are just some of the more commonly known medications to have a negative impact on lipid levels. In some cases, this is a class effect and in others it might depend on dose and specific drug.

Case Study of Hyperlipidemia

Summary

A 46 years old male patient was admitted in hospital with the chief complaints of positive Tread Mill Test (TMT), for cardiac risk assessment. Past medical history includes hypertension and DM. Past medication history include T.telma-H 40mg OD, T.AZULIX – MF 2mg MF OD. Weight: 95.3kg, Height: 175cm. Blood pressure:140/80 mmHG; Pulse rate: 84/min; CVS:S1 S2 normal.

Lab Reports:

Hb:15.8 g/dL; PCV:45.8; RBC:4.98millions; WBC: 6800thousands; PLATELETS:2.43lakhs

Serum creatinine:0.9 mg/dL, Blood sugar:201 mg/dL; Total cholestral:240 mg/dL

LDL cholesterol :155 mg/dL; Triglycerides:180 mg/dL; HDL:32 mg/dL

Coronary angiogram: mild CAD

Final diagnosis: Based on subjective and objective data, patient was diagnosed with **hyperlipidemia, mild CAD**, type 2 diabetes mellitus , HTN.

Treatment:

Start medication:

INJ. Hydrocortisone 100mg IV STAT

INJ. Fentanyl 50mg IV STAT

INJ. Heparin 5000IU IV STAT

Drug Chart:

T.ROZALET	10/75 mg	OD
T.TELMA	40mg	OD
T.AZULIX	2mg	BBF OD

Drug Indications:

Drug name	Generic name	Indication
ROZALET	Rosuvastatin+clopidogrel	Lower the cholesterol levels and reduce the risk of narrowing arteries.
TELMA – H	Telmisartan+hydrochlorthiazide	Treatment of HTN
AZULIX-MF	Glimipiride+metformin hydrochloride	Lowers blood glucose levels.

Discharge Medication

Cap.roseday-CV (Rosuvastatin+Clopidogrel) 10mg/75mg OD {after dinner}

T. Telma – H (Telmisartan+hydrochlorthiazide) 40mg OD

T. Azulix (Glimepiride) 2mg OD BBF

T. Taxim – O (Cefixime) 200mg BD 3 days.

Drug Drug Interactions

Hydrochlorthiazide +glimepiride	Minor interaction	Hydrochlorothiazide decreases the effect of glimepiride by phrmacodynamic antagonism
Hydrochlothiazide +metformin	Minor interaction	Hydrochlothiazide will increase the level or effect of metformin by basic drug competition for renal tubular clearance

Assignment

1. **What are the laboratory test values indicating hyperlipidemia:**
   Total cholestral: 240 mg/dL.(normal: <200 mg/dL)
   LDL Cholesteral: 155 mg/dL(normal <100 mg)
   HDL: 32 mg/dL (normal -40-60 mg/dL)
   Triglycerides: 180 mg/dL (normal<150 mg/dL)

   Severity:

   Total cholesterol: high
   LDL cholesterol: borderline high
   HDL: low, major risk factor for heart disease.

2. **What are the risk factors for cardiovascular disease:**
   Modified risk factors: Type 2 diabetes, High blood pressure, High cholesterol, Obesity, Over weight
   Non modified risk factors: age; -male gender: men have greater risk of cardiovascular disease, -heredity.

3. **What is the CAD risk categorisation and target LDL goal**

Risk category	Risk factors	LDL
High risk	>2 factors (DM,HTN,obesity)	<100 mg/dL

4. **Write the pharmacological goals of treatment:**
   - reduction of cardiovascular events, relief of symptoms of Cardiovascular Artery Disease (CAD)
   - reduction of cholesterol levels, controlling blood glucose levels
   - in case of HTN, lower the blood pressure

5. **Write the non pharmacological treatment goals:**
   - controlling the amount of salt in the diet, -Lose excess weight
   - reduce stress, -procedures: coronary artery bypass surgery, angioplasty.

6. **Write the non pharmacological therapy to maintain total cholesterol level:**

   - reduce the amount of saturated fat in diet, losing weight, -eating plenty of fruits and vegetables, garlic and fish oil, exercise, smoking cessation.

7. **What are the pharmacotherapeutic options for hyperlipidemia and Cardiovascular Disease (CAD)**
   Antiplatelet therapy: clopidogrel 75 mg PO/Day
   Beta blockers: Atenolol: 25-50 mg/day
   Statins: rosuvastatin: 10-20 mg OD
   ACE inhibitors: captopril: initial 25 mg PO
   Calcium channel blockers: amlodipine: 5mg/day PO initially

8. **What are the Life Style Modifications**
   - The goal of life style change is to prevent further build up of plaque and decrease damage to blood vessels.

   Dietary Changes: Avoid saturated fat, full fat dairy products, low salt diet.

   - exercise regularly, reduce excess weight, decrease or discontinue alcohol consumption.
   - control blood glucose levels, Maintain normal blood pressure, stress management
   - cardiac rehabilitation, use medication regularly, adhere to treatment plan.

9. **What drug monitoring parameters are necessary for evaluating the efficacy and safety of the patient?**
   - Rosuvastatin- cretinine, liver enzyme abnormalities, creatine kinase are monitored periodically.
   - Clopidogrel-monitor platelet function
   - Telmisartan-monitor BP, electrolytes.
   - Glimepiride- monitors blood glucose levels.
   - Metformin- monitors hemoglobin and renal function.

10. **Write the patient counselling measures:**
    - **High blood pressure:** Makes heart work harder, damages blood vessels and also cause greater plaque buildup, To control blood pressure, Maintain a healthy body weight
    - Take mediation as prescribed, Follow health nutrition plan, Practice stress management
    - **High blood cholesterol:** High levels of LDL can damage artery walls. HDL cholesterol is good, Healthy body weight, Take medication
    - **Diabetes:** It can lead to changes in the circulatory system these changes may cause damage to heart. Eat regular meals; -eat breakfast; -limit sugars, regular soft drinks.

Nutrition Plan

Include vegetables and fruits at each meal, Choose healthy oil, Eat fresh food, Choose low fat dairy products, Use garlic in food, Consult doctor if any complications are seen, Patients are often concerned about anti platelet agents due to potential for bleeding and may discontinue these agents.

Garlic: Garlic showed a significant reduction in total cholesterol level in some studies. Raw garlic is more beneficial than the cooked form in reducing blood lipid and glucose levels. Garlic has a beneficial effect on blood lipid and glucose.

Fish Oil: Oily fish such as salmon, sardines contain two important fatty acids called docosahexaenoic acid and eicosapentanoic acid. Eating a diet that include one or two serving of oily fish per week can lower triglycerides and reduce the risk of CAD.

References

1. Hong Choi et al., High-Density Lipoproteins: Biology, Epidemiology, and Clinical Management. The Canadian journal of cardiology. 2016; 33 (3): 141-150.
2. Eun-Jung Rhee et al., 2018 Guidelines for the management of dyslipidemia. The Korean Journal of Internal Medicine. 2017; 34(4):723-771.
3. Sunil kumar kots et al., Metabolic pancreatitis: Etiopathogenesis and management. Indian Journal of Endocrinology and Metabolism / Sep-Oct 2013 / Vol 17 | Issue 5. 799-805.
4. Ahmed SM, Clasen MD, Donnelly MD. Managment of dyslipidemia in adults. Am Family Physician 1998;57:1-16.
5. Chait A, Brunzell JD. Acquired hyperlipidemia (secondary dyslipoproteinemias). Endocrinol Metab Clin North Am 1990; 19:259-78.
6. Gao W, He HW, Zhao H, Xiao-Qing Lian XQ, Wang YS, Zhu J, et al. Plasama levels of lipometabolism related miR-122 and miR-370 are increased in patients with hyperlipidemia and associated with coronary artery disease. Lipids Health Dis2012;11:55.
7. Stone NJ. Secondary causes of hyperlipidemia. Med Clin North Am 1994;78:117-41.
8. Sundaram M, Yao Z. Recent progress in understanding protein and lipid factors affecting hepatic VLDL assembly and secretion. Nutr Metab 2010;27:35.
9. Wouters K, Shiri-Sverdlov R, Van Gorp PJ, Van Bilsen M, Hofker MH. Understanding hyperlipidemia and atherosclerosis: Lessons from genetically modified apoe and ldlr mice. Clin Chem Lab Med 2005;43:470-9.
10. Megan Herink. Medication Induced Changes in Lipid and Lipoproteins. Endotext. 2018.

CHAPTER - 2

Angina Pectoris

Introduction to Angina Pectoris

Angina pectoris is a clinical syndrome of ischaemic heart disease caused due to the imbalance between the myocardial oxygen supply and myocardial oxygen demand. It is characterised by paroxysmal pain in the substernal or precordial region of the chest; discomfort or pressure usually in the chest caused by a temporarily inadequate blood supply to the heart muscle. Often the pain radiates to the left arm, neck, jaw. Its more common in men than in women.

Types of Angina

There are 3 types:-

   (i)   Stable (or) typical Angina (exertional angina, classical angina)
   (ii) Prinzmetal's /variant Angina (Vasospastic Angina)
   (iii) Unstable (or) Crescendo Angina (angina at rest)

Stable (Or) Typical Angina

- This is the most common pattern.
- It is characterised by attacks of pain following physical exertion or emotional excitement and is relieved by rest
- The pathogenesis of the condition lies in chronic stenosing coronary atherosclerosis that cannot perfuse the myocardium adequately when the work load on the heart increases. During the attacks, there is depression of ST segment in the ECG due to poor perfusion of the subendocardial region but there's no elevation of enzymes in the blood as there is no irreversible myocardial injury

Prinz Metal's/Variant Angina

- This pattern of angina is characterised by pain at rest and has no exact relationship with physical activity

- Its's exact pathogenesis is not known
- It may occur due to sudden vasospasm of a coronary trunk induced by coronary atherosclerosis, or due to the release of humoral vasoconstriction by mast cells in the coronary adventitial
- ECG shows ST segment elevation due to transmural ischaemia
- These patients respond well to vasodilators like nitro-glycerine

Unstable or Crescendo Angina

- Also referred to as 'Pre- infarction angina' (or) acute coronary insufficiency, this is the most serious pattern of angina
- It's characterised by more frequent onset of pain of prolonged duration and occurring often at rest. It's an indication of an impending acute myocardial infraction
- Unstable angina and acute Myocardial Infarction (MI) can be distinguished by ST segment changes of ECG:
- Acute MI is characterised by ST segment elevation while unstable angina may have non ST segment elevation MI.
- Multiple factors are involved in the pathogenesis of unstable angina like,
  - ➢ Stenosing coronary atherosclerosis
  - ➢ Complicated coronary plagues (e.g.,: superimposed thrombosis, haemorrhage, rupture, ulceration etc)
  - ➢ Platelet thrombi over atherosclerotic plagues and vasospasm of Coronary Artery (CA)
- Often the lesions lie in a branch of the major coronary trunk so that collaterals prevent infarction.

Acute Myocardial Infacrtion

- Acute MI is the most important and feared consequence of coronary artery disease. Many patients may die within the first few hours of onset.

Epidemiology

- Its prevalence is higher in men than in women and it increases sharply with age- between 65 to 74 years; the proportions are about 14% for men and 8% for women.
- Present estimates are that angina affects 8,365,000 people in the united states- 4,070,000 men and 4,295,000 women aged 20 or older
- 50% of patients with CHD have stable angina pectoris as their first clinical presentation
- Chronic stable angina pectoris affects around 2-4% of the population in western countries
- Data suggests that more than 1.3 million people in the UK are lining angina (approx. 775,000 men and 560,000 women)

Etiology

- Angina is caused by reduced blood flow to your heart muscle (ischemia) when the blood flowing doesn't carry enough O2
- Coronary Artery Disease (CAD)
  - ➢ It's the most common cause of reduced blood flow to the heart muscle
- HTN, coronary artery spasm, aortic stenosis
- Atherosclerosis
  - ➢ The coronary arteries become narrowed by fatty deposits called plaques
- Cardiomyopathy
  - ➢ It is a disease of the heart muscle. It isn't a single condition, but a group of conditions that effect the structure of the heart and reduce its ability to pump blood around the body
  - ➢ It can effect anyone at any age
  - ➢ It can effect the shape, size and thickness of the heart muscle walls
- Narrowing of arteries due to the accumulation of fats, cholesterol, calcium and other substances
- Blood clots can also block arteries and reduce the flow of O_2 rich blood to the heart

Risk Factors

- Tobacco use: Chewing tobacco, smoking and long-term exposure to smoke damage the interior walls of arteries, including the arteries to the heart allowing deposits of cholesterol to collect and blocks blood flow
- Diabetes:
  - ➢ It increases the risk of CAD, which leads to angina and heart attacks by speeding up atherosclerosis
- High Blood Pressure:
  - ➢ High BP damages arteries by accelerating hardening of the arteries
- High blood cholesterol or triglyceride levels
- Family history of heart disease
- Older age
  - ➢ Men older than 45 years
  - ➢ Women older than 55 years have a greater risk than younger adults
- Obesity: Raises the risk of angina and heart disease because its associated with high blood cholesterol levels
- Lack of exercise
- Stress:
  - ➢ Too much stress or anger also can raise blood pressure. Surges of hormones produced during stress can narrow the arteries and worsen angina

Pathophysiology

Stable angina

> Atherosclerosis leads to decreased blood vessel lumen diameter. Decreased volume of blood is supplied to the heart. So there is decreased myocardial blood supply.

> Due to increased physical activity or stress there is increased heart rate and contractility and decreased time in diastole. So decreased filling takes place. As a result there is increased myocardial oxygen demand.

> **Myocardial ischemia results from imbalance between blood supply and oxygen demand.**

> This is called as stable angina. Myocardial ischemia causes cells to switch from aerobic to anaerobic metabolism.

> Ischemic changes may activate sensory pain fibres in myocardium, so the person experiences chest pain, pressure or discomfort, pain radiates to left arm.

> Because of myocardial ischemia there is predominant increase in vagal tone and person has nausea, hypotension, bradycardia.

Unstable angina

> In Atherosclerosis (Primary cause) if there is coronary arterial atherosclerotic plaque rupture or erosion, there is platelet aggregation and thrombus formation. Hence partial occlusion of the involved artery. This causes decreased myocardial blood supply to different organs.

> Secondary causes: Coronary artery vasospasm/coronary embolism/increased blood viscosity (ploycythemia, thrombocytopenia)/spontaneous coronary artery dissection/ congenital anamolies/increased myocardial Oxygen (O_2) demand like tachycardia, shock, anemai, exertion, stress.

> Due to the above secondary causes there is increased Myocardial O_2 demand.

> Myocardial ischemia results from imbalalnce between blood supply and oxygen demand which is called as unstable angina pectoris.

> Myocardial ischemia causes cells to switch from aerobic to anaerobic metabolism. As a consequence of this

  (a) Impaired myocardial relaxation- results in increased diastolic pressure so increased pulmonary pressure, so causes dyspnoea.

  (b) Cardiac sensory fibres mix with somatic sensory fibres and enter the spinal cord nerve roots, causing pain which radiates to shoulder, left arm, lower jaw, neck, abdomen, upper back.

  (c) Non-transmural or subendocardial ischemia causing ST depression.

  (d) Inferior wall ischemia-stimuales vagal tone- cuasing hypotension, nausea, syncope.

Clinical Manifestation and Features

Signs and Symptoms [1]

- Retrosternal chest discomfort (pain behind sternum) with symptoms like pressure, heaviness, sequences, burning choking sensation lasts in the chest for more than a few minutes
- Pain extending beyond from the chest to shoulder, arm back, or even to teeth and jaw
- Nausea, vomiting, sweating, fatigue, pain, chest tightness
- Pain while eating, exposure to cold or emotional stress. Pain lasts for 1-5 mins
- Signs of abnormal lipid metabolism
- During the episode of angina, symptoms like SOB, nausea, fatigue, dizziness, sweating and anxiety are seen

Angina in Women

- Women's angina symptoms can be different from the classic angina symptoms. Women also may experience
  - Nausea
  - SOB
  - Abdominal pain
  - Discomfort in neck, jaw, or back
  - Stabbing pain instead of chest pressure

Diagnosis with Algorithm [2]

Collaboration Management

- Assessment:
  - History / Clinical manifestations/ Cardiovascular assessment
  - Laboratory assessment / Troponin I and T/ CK- MB
- CT scan: to detect that Ca^{+2} in the coronary arteries if the plaque has Ca^{+2}
- Radiographic assessment
  - ECG: to check the electrophysiology of the heart
  - Angiogram:-to check or to detect the no of blocked valves
  - Echo cardiogram: heart ultrasound examination which shows the structural abnormalities of the heart
  - STRESS TEST: tread mill test to check the heart rate
  - NUCLEAR STRESS TEST: injecting a radioactive substance into the veins by using a specialized camera to obtain the images of the heart during rest and immediately after stress test
  - Cardiac Catheterization
- To prevent oedema for parts with H/O angina, MI or CHF
- To determine if there's any coronary heart disease which leads to heart failure

Laboratory Tests [3]

- Haemoglobin, fasting glucose and fasting lipid panel, high-sensitivity C-reactive protein (HSCRP); homocysteine level, evidence of chlamydia infection and elevations in lipoprotein, fibrinogen and plasminogen activator inhibitor may be helpful. Cardiac enzymes are normal in stable angina.
- Troponin T or I, myoglobin and creatine kinase myocardial band (CK-MB) may be elevated in unstable angina

  - Lipoprotein values:

LDL cholesterol- very low   (<70 mg/dL)

Low (70-99mg/dL)

High (100-129 mg/dL)

Very high (≥130 mg/dL)

The largest proportion of patients have: LDLC ≥130mg/dL (32.6%)

LDLC- 100-129 mg/dL (32.1%)

LDLC-70-90mg/dL (24.9%)

LDLC-<70 mg/dL (10.4%)

Classification OF DRUGS

1. Nitrates

   (a) *Short acting:* Glyceryl trinitrate (GTN, Nitroglycerine)
   (b) *Long acting*: Isosorbide dinitrate (short acting by sublingual route), Isosorbide mononitrate, Erythrityl tetranitrate, Pentaerythritol tetranitrate
2. β *Blockers* Propranolol, Metoprolol, Atenolol and others.
3. *Calcium channel blockers*
   (a) *Phenyl alkylamine:* Verapamil
   (b) *Benzothiazepine:* Diltiazem
   (c) Dihydropyridines: Nifedipine, Felodipine, Amlodipine, Nitrendipine, Nimodipine, Lacidipine, Lercanidipine, Benidipine
4. Potassium channel opener Nicorandil
5. Others Dipyridamole, Trimetazidine, Ranolazine, Ivabradine, Oxyphedrine

Clinical Classification

A. Used to abort or terminate attack GTN, Isosorbide dinitrate (sublingually).
B. Used for chronic prophylaxis All other drugs.

Management

Goals of Treatment

- To prolong life, Minimize infarct size, Reverse ischemia, Reduce cardiac work
- Prevent and treat complications
- Initial Treatment
- Rapid triage OMI (oxygen, monitor and I/V line)
- Check vital signs and O_2 saturation
- ECG within 10 minutes and repeat ECG
- Blood sample for enzymes, CBC, and lipotropic

Non- Pharmacological Therapy

- Primary prevention through modification of risk factors should reduce prevalence of CHD. Secondary intervention is effective in reducing subsequent morbidity and mortality
- Risk factors of CHD can be classified into alterable and unalterable. Unalterable risk factors include gender, age, family, history or genetics, environmental influences and to some extent, DM.
- Alterable risk factors include smoking, HTN, Hyperlipidaemia, Obesity, sedentary lifestyle, hyperuricemia, psychological factors such as stress and use of drugs that may be detrimental (e.g.,: progestins, corticosterol, calcineium inhibitors)

Treatment (Pharmacological)

1. **Nitrates:** Vasodilators

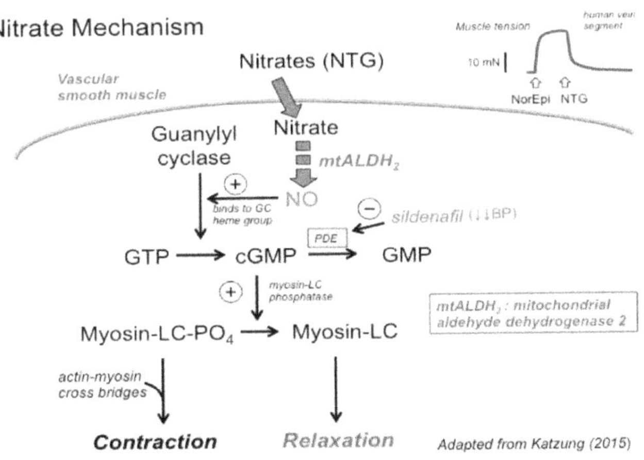

Fig. 2.1 Mechanism of action of nitrates.

Source: Katzung BG (2015): Vasodilators & the treatment of angina pectoris (Chapter 12). In: *Basic and Clinical Pharmacology. 13e.* Katzung BG, Masters SB, Trevor AJ (Editors). McGraw-Hill / Lange.

Mechanism of Nitrates: Organic nitrates have the chemical structure RNO_2. The nitro group is reduced to form NO in by a mitochondrial enzyme (aldehyde dehydrogenase-2). Free nitrite is released, which is converted to Nitric Oxide (NO). NO activates guanylyl cyclase (GC) by interacting with its heme group. Activated GC converts GTP to cGMP. cGMP activates a phosphatase which dephosphorylates myosin light chains, resulting in decreased interaction between actin & myosin filaments, and relaxation. cGMP is normally short lived due to metabolism by intracellular phosphodiesterase (PDE). Drugs such as sildenafil can inhibit PDE, resulting in a potentially dangerous intensification of the vaso-relaxant effect of nitrates.

Uses of Nitrates in Angina

- Although nitrates dilate both peripheral capacitance and resistance vessels, the effect on venous capacitance vessels predominates even in low doses
- Dilation on capacitance vessels leads to pooling of blood in veins and to a diminished venous return to the heart (decreased preload). Therefore ventricular end diastolic pressure is reduced.
- The benefit of decreasing preload is reduction in oxygen demand, which makes these drugs useful in classical angina.
- At high concentrations, nitrates also relax arteriolar smooth muscle, which leads to a decrease in the total peripheral resistance and a decrease in aortic resistance to left ventricular ejection (decrease in afterload).
- Nitrates benefit patients with variant angina by relaxing smooth muscle of the epicardial coronary arteries and relieving coronary artery spasm.
- Nitroglycerine is the main stay of therapy for relieving acute coronary vasospasm because of its rapid onset of action.

(a) Short acting
- Nitro-glycerine
  Dose: IV (6mcg/min)
  Oral [2.5-9 mg; TID daily]
  Sublingual/Lingual [0.3mg]

(b) Long acting
- Isosorbide Dinitrate: It is short acting by sublingual route
  Dose: 5mcg/min to 20mcg/min TID [IV infusion if needed]
- Isosorbide mononitrate
  Dose: 20Mg: OD or BID
- Erythritol tetranitrate
  Dose: 5-10 Mg: TID
- Pentaerythritol tetranitrate
  Dose: 10-20 mg : TID

Adverse effects: Hypertension (HTN), bradycardia, heart block, bronchospasm, fatigue, malaise, depression.

Table 2.1 Nitrates: Routes of Administration, Dosages, and Frequency of Dosing.

Nitrates	Routes of Administration	Dosages	Frequency
Nitroglycerin	Sublingual tablet	0.15–0.6 mg	As needed
(Glyceryl trinitrate)	Sublingual spray	0.4 mg	As needed
	Intravenous	5–400 µg/min	As needed
	Sublingual tablet	0.3–0.6 mg	As needed
BID	Ointment (topical) 2%	0.5–2 in (7.5–30 mg)	As needed
	Patch	1 Patch (2.5–15 mg)	2 × daily
Isosorbide mononitrate	Sublingual/oral tablet	10–40 mg	2 × daily
	Sustained release	30–120 mg	1 × daily
	Sustained release	5–20 mg	2 × daily
Isosorbide dinitrate	Sublingual/oral tablet	2.5–10 mg	Every 2–3 h
	Sustained release tablet	5–40 mg	2–3 × daily
	Sustained release tablet	40–160 mg	2 × daily
Pentaerythrityl tetranitrate	Sublingual tablet	5–10 mg	As needed
	Oral tablet	10 mg	3 × daily

2. **β – Blockers:** General MOA: β–Blockers act by reducing cardiac work and O_2 consumption as a consequence of decreased heart rate, inotropic state (force of contraction) and mean BP. β-Blockers limit increase in cardiac work that occurs during exercise or anxiety by antiadrenergic action on heart

- Atenolol
  Dose: 500mg
  Frequency: Once Daily (OD)
  Side effects: constipation, dizziness, dry mouth, confusion, depression, insomnia.
  Contraindications: Sinus bradycardia, severe COPD, Psoriasis, pregnancy, anaphylactic shock.
- Labetolol
  Dose: 100mg
  Frequency: BID
  Side effects: Dizziness, upset stomach, fatigue, stuffy nose, tingling scalp or skin
  Contraindications: Severe bradycardia, cardiogenic shock, severe hypotension
- Metaprolol
  Dose: 400mg
  Frequency: OD
  Sides effects: nausea, vomiting, dry mouth fatigue, dizziness, depression, bloating

Contraindications: severe bradycardia, sick sinus syndrome, advanced Atrio Ventricular (AV) block, diabetes

- Propanolol
  Dose: 3.125mg
  Frequency: BID
  Side effects: Itching, cold hands or feet, dry or peeling skin, hallucinations, muscle cramps
  Contraindications: Sinus bradycardia, sinus shock, bronchial asthma, in patients with known hypersensitivity to propranolol hydrochloride
- Bisoprolol
  Dose: 1.25mg
  Side effects: dry mouth, nausea, vomiting, stomach pain, increased urination, stuffy nose, insomnia, anxiety
  Contraindications: depression, cerebrovascular disease, hyperthyroidism, Diabetes Mellitus (DM)
- Nadolol
  Dose: initial 40mg/day and increase gradually [160- 240mg]
  Side effects: fainting, blurred vision, fever, chills, sore throat, chest pain or discomfort, irregular, heartbeat, sudden weight gain
  Contraindications: diabetes, myasthenia gravis, partial heart block, asthma

3. **Calcium channel blockers:** General MOA: Their direct action include vasodilation of system arterioles and coronary arteries leading to reduced arterial pressure and coronary vascular resistance, as well as depression of myocardial contractility and conduction velocity of Sinoatrial (SA) and Alrioventricular (AV) nodes.
   - They in short dilate the arteries, reduce BP and reduce the force of contraction of heart.

Antianginal action:

- Improvement in the coronary blood flow
- Decrease in then oxygen demand of the heart due to reduction in systemic vascular resistance (vasodilation) and BP (afterload)
- Verapamil in addition, reduces the heartrate. As a group, these drugs can be used in anginal patients with Chronic Obstructive Pulmonary Disease (COPD) in whom beta blockers are contraindicated.

(a) Phenyl Alkylamine:

   Verapamil

   Dose: 15mg   Frequency: BiD

   Side effects: dizziness, constipation, nausea, slow heartbeat, headache, fatigue, skin rash

   Contraindication: complete heart block, myasthenia gravis, severe HF, liver problems, kidney disease.

(b) Benzothiazepine:
Dilitazem: Dose: 3omg   Frequency: QID
Side effects: dizziness, weakness, nausea, upset stomach, sore throat
Contraindications: sick sinus syndrome, hypotension (BP<90mmHg systolic) asthma, liver problem, kidney disease with reduced kidney function

(c) Dihydropyridines:
- Nifedipine: Dose: 10mg Frequency: BID
  Side effects: mild dizziness, weakness, headache, heart burn, nausea, muscle cramps, tremors, cough, wheezing, sore throat, stuffy nose
  Contraindications: porphyria, severe HF, abnormally low BP, liver problems, kidney disease
- Amlodipine: Dose: 5-10mg   Frequency: OD
  Side effects: headache, oedema of ankles or feet, dizziness, fatigue, nausea, abdominal or stomach pain
  Contraindications:-severely low BP patients, liver disease, hypersensitivity to amlodipine
- Nicardipine: Dose: 20mg   Frequency: (Three times in a day) TID
  Side effects: Dizziness, light headedness, swollen ankles, headache
  Contraindications:-liver problems, abnormally low BP
- Lacidipine: Dose: 4mg Frequency: OD
- Nimodipine: Dose: 30-60mg   Frequency: 4-6 hourly for 3 weeks

Table 2.2 Calcium Channel Blockers used for Ischemic Heart Disease [4].

Generic name (Trade name)	Usual Daily Dosage (mg)	Peak Response (hr)	Duration of Response (hr)	Common Side Effects
Dihydropyridines				
Amlodipine	5–10 QID	6–12	24	Headache, flushing, edema
Felodipine	2.5 QID	2–5		
Nifedipine	30–90 QID	4–6		
Nifedipine	10–30 TID	0.1	4–6	Headache, hypotension, dizziness, flushing, edema
Nicardipine	20–40 TID	0.5–2	8	
Non-Dihydropyridines				
Diltiazem	60–120 tid	2.5–4	8	Hypotension, bradycardia, dizziness, flushing, edema
Diltiazem	240–280 qd	10	24	
Verapamil	80–120 TID	6–8	8	
Verapamil SR	120–240 BID	5	12–24	

4. **Potassium Channel Openers:** General MOA: They open ATP activated K+ channels in Smooth Muscle. Their most prominent action is hyperpolarization and relaxation of vascular as well as visceral SM which ultimately lowers BP
   - NICORANDIL
     Dose: 5-20mg
     Frequency: BID
     Side effects: yellowing of skin, nausea, vomiting, fatigue
     Contraindications: cardiogenic shock, Left Ventricular (LV) failure
5. **Antiplatelet Drugs:**
   - Prevent thrombus formation by inhibiting platelet aggregation.
   - In patients with aspirin intolerance, clopidogrel is given
   - Clopidogrel is also used in combination with aspirin after stunt placement
     - Aspirin
       Dose: 75mg daily
       Side effects: vomiting, stomach pain, heartburn, nausea, swelling of eyes, lips and face, hoarseness
       Contraindications: inadequate vitamin K, Gout, anaemia, haemophilia, decreased platelets, alcoholism, peptic ulcer, liver problems, pregnancy
     - Dipyridamole
       Dose: 25-100mg
       Frequency: TID
       Side effects: dizziness, vomiting's, diarrhoea, upset stomach, headache
       Contraindications: liver problems, bronchospasm, abnormally low BP
     - Clopidogrel
       Dose: 75mg/day for up to 12 months
   - Concomitant therapy with Aspirin
     Aspirin: (75-325 mg QID) + Clopidogrel

Table 2.3 Characteristics of Antiplatelet Drugs.

Drug	Site of Action	Time to Peak Action	Half-life	Typical Dose Administered	Route/ Dosing Interval
Aspirin	Inhibition of CO_X enzyme	1-2 hours	15-20 min	In Europe loading does 300 mg, Maintenance dose 75 mg	Oral OD
Clopidogrel	Thienopyridine prodrug irreversibly binds to the $P2Y_{12}$ receptor	45 min	6 hours	Loading dose 300 – 600 mg, Maintenance dose 75 mg	Oral OD
Prasugrel	Thienopyridine prodrug irreversibly binds to the PZY_{12} receptor	30 min	7 hours	Loading dose 60 mg, Maintenance dose 10 mg	Oral OD

Contd...

Drug	Site of Action	Time to Peak Action	Half-life	Typical Dose Administered	Route/ Dosing Interval
Ticagrelor	Cyclopentyl-triazolopyrimidine drug, reversibly binds to $P2Y_{12}$ receptor	1.5 hours	7 hours	Loading dose 180 mg, Maintenance dose 90 mg	Oral OD
Cangrelor	Adenosine triphosphate analogue, reversibly binds to $P2Y_{12}$ receptor	2 min	3-6 min	Bolus 30 mcg/kg injection then 4 mdg/kg/min infusion	Intravenous one time treatment
Abciximab	Glycoprotein IIb/IIIa receptor inhibitor	30 min	30 min	Bolus 0.25 mg/kg injection then 0.125 mcg/kg/min infusion	Intrevenous One time treatment

Table showing pharmacological properties of the antiplatelet drugs discussed in the review. BD = twice daily; COX = Cyclooxygenase; OD = Once daily; QDS = four times daily.

Source: Ridker PM; JUPITER Study Group. Rosuvastatin in the primary prevention of cardiovascular disease among patients with low levels of low-density lipoprotein cholesterol and elevated high-sensitivity C-reactive protein: rationale and design of the JUPITER trial. Circulation *2003; **108:2292**–7.*

6. **Cytoprotective drugs:**
   - TRIMETAZIDINE
     Dose: 20mg
     Frequency: TID
     MOA:
   - It acts through non-haemodynamic mechanism
   - It protects the myocardium from the harmful effects of ischaemia by preventing the mechanism of unsaturated fatty acids by lipid peroxidation and inhibiting superoxide cytotoxicity
   - It also inhibits free radical formation and intracellular acidosis
   - It doesn't show direct effects on the Cardiovascular System (CVS) but is known to reduce attacks of angina and increase the exercise capacity when used along with other antianginal drugs
     Side effects: gastric burning, dizziness, fatigue, muscle cramps
     Contraindications: Parkinsonism, tremors, severe renal impairment
   - Ranotazine
     Dose: 500 mg BD and increase to 100mg BD daily
   - Reduces Ca^{+2} overload in ischaemic myocytes through inhibition of late sodium current
     Side effects: dizziness, headache, constipation, nausea

7. **Ace inhibitors:**
   - They inhibit the Renin-Angiotensin Aldosterone System (RAAS) mechanism

- Dilate the blood vessels and reduce Blood Pressure (BP)
  - Ramipril
    Dose: 2.5-5mg
    Frequency: OD
  - Captopril
    Dose: 12.5-15mg
    Frequency: BD or TID
  - Enalapril
    Dose: 5-40mg
    Frequency: OD or BD

Approach for prevention and management of stable angina

Therapies to prevent episodes of angina: First line: Offer a β blocker such as bosiprolol 5-10mg daily. Aim for heart rate between 50-60 bets per minute.

1. If β blocker is contraindicated or not tolerated consider a rate controlling calcium channel blocker (Diltiazam or Verapamil).

   (i) If rate controlling calcium channel blocker is contraindicated or not tolerated consider a dihydropyridine calcium channel blocker (Amlodipine). If symptoms are not satisfactorily cotrolled condsider adding a long acting nitrate-Nocorandil, Ivabradine or Ranolazone.

   (ii) If symptoms are not satisfactorily controlled consider adding a long acting nitrate - Nicorandil, Ranolazine.

2. If additional anti-anginal therapy is required, add a dihydropyridine calcium channel blocker (Amlodipine 5-10 mg daily). If dihydropyridine calcium channel blocker is contraindicated or not tolerated consider adding a long acting nitrate- Nocorandil, Ivabradine or Ranolazone.

3. If both β blocker and calcium channel blocker are contraindicated or not tolereated consider monotherapy with: a) Nocorandil b) Ivabradine c) Ranolazone.

- If symptoms are not adequately controlled, consider referral for revascularisation, an additional anti-anginal may be added while awaiting cardiology review.

Medical Treatment of Unstable Angina and Acute Non-ST-Elevation Myocardial Infarction

If the patient is diagnosed with crescendo angina (unstable angina) and non-Q wave myocardial infarction

   (i) The patient has continuing symptoms even after bed rest and medical therapy; he is a candidate for cardiac catheterisation and coronary arteriography. But medical therapy is advised for those without significant artery disease or unsuitable anatomy for Percutaneous Transluminal coronary angioplasty (PTCA) or coronary artery bypass grafting (CABG). If the patient is eligible then either a) PTCA and/or stenting b) CABG is adviced.

(ii) Aymptomatic patients after bed rest and after institution of medical therapy. Low level of exercise or other stress test with perfusion or functional imaging is adviced.

   (a) Medical therapy adviced for those patients without angina, ECG change or reversible perfusion or functional abnormality with low or moderate levels of effort or stress.

(iii) Patients with angina ≥ 1 mm ST segment deviation from a normal baseline, or reversible perfusion defect or elevation with chronic ECG monitoring, the candidate is eligible for cardiac catheterisation and coronary arteriography. But medical therapy is advised for those without significant artery disease or unsuitable anatomy for Percutaneous Transluminal coronary angioplasty (PTCA) or coronary artery bypass grafting (CABG). If the patient is eligible then either a) PTCA and/or stenting b) CABG is adviced.

Case Study of Unstable Angina/Hypertensive Emergency

Summary

A 59 years male patient was admitted in cardiology department with chief complaints of chest pain with chest discomfort epigastric pain and upper back ache. He has past medical history of CAD angina TVD. Surgical history: CABG (2007). On the day of admission his BP was 190/110 mmHg.

Diagnosis: The patient was diagnosed with unstable angina with hypertensive emergency.

Progress Chart

Day 1: Investigations are Complete Blood Pressure (CBP) blood sugar levels

Day 2: Echocardiogram (ECHO) revealed. Report: post Coronary Artery Bypass Grafting (CABG) status concentric Left Ventricular Hypertrophy (LVH) no Left Ventricular Regional Wall Motion Abnormalities (LVRWMA) good Left Ventricular (LV) systolic function grade 1 LV diastolic dysfunction. No PAH\PE\LV clot intact septate. Few laboratory investigations revealed mild leucocytosis. Patient was on clopidogrel. Patient is systematically better. By the end of the day chest pain decreased no Shortness of Breath (SOB).

Day 3: left vertebral artery stenosis\right common internal artery occluded, so he was prescribed with heparin stat dose

Assignment-Unstable Angina

1. What is the initial treatment for an unstable angina patient?

Pharmacologic management of patients with Unstable Angina (UA)/Non-ST Elevated Myocardial Infarction (NSTEMI).2,11 ECG, electrocardiogram.

- Administer aspirin (162-325 mg, non-enteric coated). Select initial treatment strategy: Conservative Vs invasive.

    (a) Conservative strategy: Initiate a second antiplatelet agent (Clopidogrel or Ticagrelor) with a loading dose followed by a daily mainatenance dose. Or initiate anticoagulation with unfractionated heparin or enoxaparin or fondaparinux.

    (b) Invasive strategy: Initiate a second antiplatelet agent (Clopidogrel or Ticagrelor, prasugrel with or without an IV GP IIb/IIIa inhibitor. A loading dose of a P2Y12 receptor inhibitor is recommended in patients for whom Percuatneous intervention is planned followed by a maintenance dose. Or initiate anticoagulation with unfractionated heparin or enoxaparin, fondaparinux or bivaluridin.

- Consider the need for acute anti-ischemic and analgesic therapies. i) Supplemental oxygen ii) Nitroglycerin iii) IV morphine sulfate iv) beta blocker v) ACE inhibitor or ARB vi) statin.

- Consider the following medications for long term management: i) Aspirin 75-162 mg indefinitely ii) P2Y 12 receptor inhibitor for upto 12 months iii) statin shoul be initiated regardless of LDL or dietary modifications iv) Beta blocker v) ACE inhibitor or ARB v) aldosterone antagonist.

Source: Jneid H, Anderson JL, Wright RS, et al. 2012 ACCF/AHA focused update of the guideline for the management of unstable angina/non-ST segment myocardial infarction (updating the 2007 guideline and replacing the 2011 focused update): A report of the American College of Cardiology Foundation/ American Heart Association Task Force on Practice Guidelines J Am Coll Cardiol. 2012;60:645– 681.

2. What is thrombolysis in MI (TIMI) RISK SCORE FOR UNSTABLE ANGINA \NON st elevation MI?

Thrombolyis in MI score (TIMI Score) is used to determine the likelihood of ishaemic events or mortality in patients with unstable angina or ST segmental elevation MI (NSTEMI)

Each of the criteria includes one point for TIMI scoring

*age $\geq$ = 65 years

*Three or more risk factors for coronary artery disease (CAD)

(Family history of CAD, HTN, hypercholestremia diabetes mellitus tobacco use)

Known CAD (stenosis >50%

Aspirin use in the past 7 days

Severe angina ($\geq$ = episodes in 24 hrs)

ST deviation $\geq$ = 0.5 mm

Elevated cardiac level

Score	Risk of death \death\MI \urgent revascularization by day 14
0-1	5%
2	8%
3	13%
4	20%
5	26%
0-7	41%

3. What are the modifications used in the management of unstable angina?

Unstable angina may require patients may take nothing orally if stress testing or an invasive procedure is anticipated otherwise a diet low in cholesterol and saturated fat is recommended *sodium restriction should be instituted for patients with heart failure or HTN.

4. What are AHA recommendations for aspirin use in initial antiplatelet/anticoagulant therapy?

(i)   Medical therapy without stent group: Non–enteric coated, chewable aspirin (75 to 162 mg) indefinitely & Clopidogrel 75mg/d for atleast 1 month and ideally upto 1 year. If he has indication for anticoagulation-add warfarin.

(ii) Bare metal stent group: Aspirin (162 to 325mg) for atleast 1month then 75 to 162mg/d indefinitely & Clopidogrel 75mg/d for atleast 1 month and ideally upto 1 year. If he has indication for anticoagulation-add warfarin.

(iii) Drug eluting stent group: Aspirin (162 to 325mg) for atleast 3-6 months then 75 to 162mg/d indefinitely & Clopidogrel 75mg/d for atleast 1 month and ideally upto 1 year. If he has indication for anticoagulation-add warfarin.

(Source: ACC/AHA 2007 Guidelines for the Management of Patients with Unstable Angina/Non–ST-Elevation Myocardial Infarction).

Hypertensive Emergencies

1. What is Hypertensive emergency and urgency?

It is high blood pressure with potentially life threatening symptoms and signs indicative of acute impairment of one or more organ systems (brain, eyes, heart, aorta or kidneys)

Hypertensive urgency: Having systolic BP over 180 mmHg or

Diastolic BP over 110 mmHg

2. What neurological end organ damage can occur in hypertensive emergency?

It indicates hypertensive encephalopathy, cerebral vascular accident, sub arachnid hemorrhage or intracranial hemorrhage

3. What are the most common clinical manifestations of Hypertension emergency?

Cerebral infraction Cerebrovascular Accident (CVA); Pulmonary Edema; Hypertensive encephalopathy

Congestive heart failure; Other clinical presentation include: intracranial hemorrhage, aortic dissection, eclampsia, acute myocardial infarction, Retinal and renal involvement

4. Which symptoms of hypertensive emergency indicate end organ damage?

Specific symptoms that suggest end organ dysfunction are:
Chest pain - indicates myocardial ischemia
Back pain - indicates aortic dissection
Dyspnea: indicates pulmonary edema or congestive heart failure
Bleeding - (brain) indicates stroke
Eclampsia - occurs during pregnancy

5. Why is sodium nitroprusside used to treat hypertensive emergencies?

Sodium nitroprusside binds to oxyhaemogoobin to release cyanide, methaemoglobin, nitric oxide leads to activation of granylyl cyclase. In the presence of nitric oxide this causes increased intracellular production of cGMP which activates protein kinase G activates phosphatases Inactivates myosin light chain kinase. Myosin light chains are involved in muscle contractions. The end result is vascular smooth muscle relaxation which allows vessels to dilate.

6. What are the treatment guidelines for hypertensive emergencies associated with pheochromocytoma?

Table 2.4 Parenteral drugs for treatment of hypertensive emergency.

Drug	Dose	Onset of action	Adverse effects
Diuretics Furosemide	20-40 mg i.v. injection in 1-2 min. repeated and higher doses with renal insufficiency	5-15 min	Volume depletion, hypokalemia

Vasodilators
  Sodium
  nitroprusside
	0.25-10 µg/kg/min as i.v. infusion	Within 30 sec	Nausea, vomiting, tachycardia, thiocyante and cyanide intoxication

Nitroglycerin	5-100 µg/min as i.v. infusion	2-5 min	Headache, vomiting, methemoglobinemia, tolereance with prolonged use
Nicardipine	0.5-6 µg/kg/min as i.v. infusion	5-10 min	Headache, flushing tachycardia, local phlebitis
Hydralazine	10-20 mg i.v. injection	10-20 min	Headache, flushing, tachycardia, worsening of angina
Sympatholytics			
Labetalol	20-80 mg i.v. injection every 10 min; 2 mg/min as i.v. infusion	5-10 min	Nausea, vomiting, bronchospasm, heart block orthostatic hypotension
Phetolamine	1-10 mg i.v. injection then 0.5-2 mg/min as i.v. infusion	1-2 min	Headache, flushing, tachycardia

7. Which medications are used to treat Acute Coronary Syndrome (ACS) in a patient with hypertensive emergencies[5]?

For acute coronary syndrome beta blockers and nitroglycerin are the preferred drugs

Treatment indicated if the the Sysstolic (SBP) is above 160mmHg or Diabefilic Blood Pressure (DBP) is over 100mmHg

Reduce the BP by 20 percent to 30 percent of baseline

Note: Nitrates administered in the presence of phosphodiesterase type 5(PDE-5) inhibitors may induce profound hypertension

Contraindications: Thrombolytics if the BP is above 185/100 mmHg

8. Which medications are used to treat Hypertension with the following conditions-

(a) With pregnancy: Hydralazine, labetolol and nicardipine are preferred
(b) With intracerebral hemorrhage: labetolol, Nicardipine, Esmolol
     Contraindications: Nitroprusside and Hydralazine
(c) Acute ischemic stroke: labetolol And Nicardipine
(d) Subarachnoid hemorrhage: Nicardipine, labetolol and Esmolol
     Avoid Nitroprusside and Hydralazine
     Maintain the SBP below 160mmHg until the aneurysm is treated or cerebral vasospasm occurs
(e) Acute heart failure: IV Nitroglycerin or Sublingual Nitroglycerin and IV enalaprilate
     Treat with vasodilator (in addition to diuretics) for SBP of 140mmHg

References

1. Arnett DK, Blumenthal RS, Albert MA, et al.
2. Aronow WS. Treatment of hypertensive emergencies. *Ann Transl Med.* 2017 May. 5 (suppl 1):S5.
3. Whelton PK, Carey RM, Aronow WS, et al. 2017 ACC/AHA/AAPA/ABC /ACPM/AGS/APhA/ASH/ASPC/NMA/PCNA Guideline for the Prevention, Detection, Evaluation, and Management of High Blood Pressure in Adults: A Report of the American College of Cardiology/American Heart Association Task Force on Clinical Practice Guidelines. *Hypertension.* 2017 Nov 13.
4. Marhefka GD. Acute hypertension: hypertensive urgency and hypertensive emergency. *Consultant.* March 2016. 56(3):222-32
5. Aggarwal M, Khan IA. Hypertensive crisis: hypertensive emergencies and urgencies. *Cardiol Clin.* 2006 Feb. 24(1):135-46.

CHAPTER - 3

Electrophysiology of Heart

Introduction

Definition

Electrophysiology of heart is the science of elucidating, diagnosing and treating the electrical activity of heart. The term is usually used to describe study of such phenomena by invasive catheter recording of spontaneous activity as well as cardiac response to program electrical stimulation.

- An inherent and rhythmical electrical activity is the reason for the heartbeat. The source of electrical activity is the network of specialized cardiac muscle fibre called auto rhythmic fibres because they are self excitable.
- These auto rhythmic fibres repeatedLy generate action potential than trigger heart contraction; they continue to stimulate the heart even after it is removed from the body.
- During embryonic development only 1% of cardiac muscle fibres become auto rhythmic fibres. These rare fibres have two important functions [1].
  1. They act as pacemaker setting the rhythm of electrical excitation that causes contraction of heart.
  2. They form the conduction system, a network of specialised cardiac muscle fibres that provide a path of each cycle of cardiac excitation to progress through the cardiac conduction system.
- Cardiac excitation normally begins in the Sinoatrial (SA) node located in the right atria wall just inferior to the opening of the superior vena cava Sinoatrial (SA) node cells do not have a stable resting potential rather they repeatedLy depolarize to the threshold spontaneously.

This spontaneous depolarization is a pace maker potential when the pace maker potential reaches threshold it triggers an action potential. Each action potential from the Sinoatrial (SA) node propagates throughout both atria via gap junction in the intercalated disc of atrial muscle fibre following the action potential the atria contract.

Electrical Conduction System of Heart (Electrophysiology)

Action Potential [2]: It is defined as the change in the electrical potential associated with the passage of an impulse along the membrane of a muscle cell or nerve.

Depolarization: Unlike auto rhythmic fibres contractile fibres have a stable resting membrane potential that is a close to -90 mV. When a contractile fibres brought to threshold by an action potential from neighbouring fibers its voltage-gated Na^+ channels open which allows the inflow of Na^+ because the cytosol of contractile fibres is electrically more negative than interstitial fluid. Inflow of Na^+ down the electro chemical gradient produces a rapid depolarization within a few milliseconds, the Na^+ channels automatically inactive and Na+ inflow decreases.

Plateau Phase: A period of maintained depolarization it is due to the opening of voltage gated slow calcium channels in the sarcolemma. When these channels open calcium ions move from interstitial fluid into the cytosol. The increased calcium concentration in the cytosol ultimately triggers contraction. Several voltage gated K+ channels are also found to take part in plateau phase where outflow of K+ takes place therefore depolarization is sustained during the plateau phase where calcium inflow is balanced by K+ outflow. It lasts for about 0.25secs and then membrane potential of contractile fibres is close to the OmV.

Repolarization: It is due to the closure of calcium channels and there is K+ outflow when additional voltage gated channels open. Outflow of K+ restores the -ve resting potential

- By conducting long atrial muscle fibres the action potential reaches the AV node located in the spectrum between the 2 atria, just anterior to the opening of the coronary sinus.
- From the Atrio Ventricular (AV) node the action potential enters the AV bundLes this is also known as bundLe of HIS. These bundLes extend through the intra ventricular spectrum toward the apex of the heart.
- Finally the large diameter purkinje fibre rapidLy conduct the action potential from the apex of the heart upwards to the remainder of the ventricular myocardium then the ventricles contract, pushing the blood upwards towards the semi lunar valves.

On their own auto rhythmic fibres in the SA node would initiate and activate action potential every 0.6 secs or 100 times per minute. This rate is faster than that of any other auto rhythmic fibres because action potential from the SA node is carried through the conduction system and it stimulates other areas before those other areas are able to generate an action potential on their own at a slower rate. The SA node acts as the normal pace maker of the heart. Nerve impulses from the autonomic nervous system and blood borne hormones modify the timing and strength of each heartbeat.

Eg: Acetyl choline (Ach) released by the parasympathetic division of the Autonomic Nervous System (ANS) slows SA node pacing to about 75 action potential per min or 1 for every 0.8 secs.

Hyperpolarization: It is defined as the change in the cell membrane potential that makes it more negative. It is the opposite of depolarization it inhibits action potential by increasing the stimulus required to move the membrane potential to the action potential threshold.

Resting Phase: It is a negative potential generated in the cytosol. Where the K^+ channels open, outflow of K^+ takes place and Na^+ channels gets closed.

Refractory period: It is defined as the time interval during which a second contraction cannot be triggered. It lasts longer than the contraction itself as a result another contraction cannot begin another relaxation takes place. Contraction cannot occur in cardiac muscle. Their pumping function depends on altering contraction and relaxation.

Artificial Pacemaker [3]: If the SA node becomes damaged or diseased the slower AV node can pick up the pace making task rate of spontaneous depolarization is 40 to 60 times per min. If the activity of the both nodes is suppressed the heart beat can be maintained by auto rhythmic fibres in the ventricles the AV bundLe a bundLe branch or purkinje fibres however the pacing rate is so slow (20-35) beats per minute that blood flow to the brain is inadequate. When this condition occurs, normal heart rhythms can be restored and maintained by surgical implanting and artificial pace maker.

It is a device that sends out small electrical currents to stimulate the heart to contract a pace maker consists of battery and impulse is generated and it is usually implanted beneath the skin just inferior to the clavicle. The pace maker is connected to one or two flexible wires that are threaded to the superior vena cava and then passed into the right atrium and ventricles. New pacemakers referred to an activity adjusted pacemaker, automatically fasten the heart beat during exercise.

Electrocardiogram: The ECG is used to access cardiac rhythm and conduction. It provides information about chamber size and is the main test used to access for myocardial ischemia and infraction.

- The basis and ECG recording is that the electrical depolarization of myocardial tissue produces a small dipole current which can be detected by electrode pairs on the body surface.
- To produce an ECG these signals are amplified and either printed or displayed on a monitor. During sinus rhythm, the SA node trigger atrial depolarization, producing a P wave.
- Depolarization proceeds slowly through the AV node which is too small to produce a depolarization wave detectable from the body surface.
- This bundLe of this bundLe branches and purkinje system are then activated initiating ventricular mycordial depolarization which produces the QRS complex. The muscle mass of the ventricles is much larger than that of atria so the QRS complex is larger than the P-wave.
- The interval between the onset of the P-wave and the onset of the QRS complex is termed the PR interval and largely reflects the duration of the AV nodal conduction.
- Injury to the left or right bundLe branch delays ventricular depolarization, widening the QRS complex selective injury of one of the left fascicles affects the electrical axis.
- Repolarization is a slower process that spreads from the epicardium to the endocardium. Atrial repolarization does not cause a detectable signal but ventricular repolarization

produces the T-wave. The QT interval represents the total duration of ventricular depolarization and repolarization.

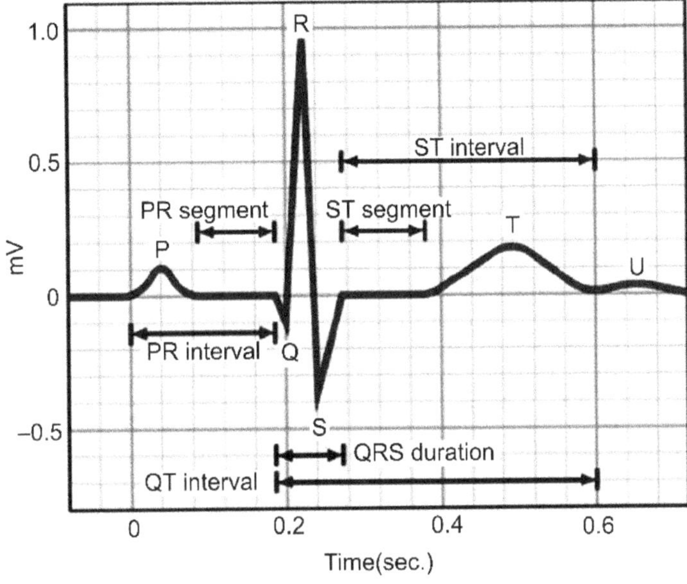

Fig. 3.1 Electrocardiogram.

Source: Shuo-tsung chen et al., Hiding Patients Confidential Datainthe ECG Signal viaa Transform-Domain Quantization Scheme. Journal of Medical Systems. 2014; 38(6):54.

- P-wave indicates SA node atrial depolarization.
- PR-interval-time required for the impulse to leave SA node travel through atria, AV node and reach purkinji fibres.
- QRS-complex-represents ventricular depolarization discharge of Ca^{+2} and Na^+ ions from the ventricles.
- T-wave-later phase of ventricular repolarization.
- QT-interval-time between onset of vertricular depolarization and end of ventricular repolarization.
- Phase 0-cellular depolarization i.e., ions of Na^+ will enter into cells.
- Phase1-also called small and rapid repolarization due to transient efflux of Potassium ion by opening of K^+ channels.
- **Phase-2**: Predominantly due to inward calcium current (Ica^{+2}) by opening of L-type of voltage operated calcium channels and also due to continuous leak of K+ ion outside cell.
- **Phase-3**: Due to activation of delayed rectifier K current through opening of K^+ channels. This is also known as repolarization phase send corresponds with the QT or heart rate corrected QT interval (QTc) of ECG.

- **Phase-4**: It is isoelectric in PF and ventricular fibers but is unstable in automatic pacemaker cells. There is spontaneous depolarization (also called as diastolic depolarization) so that once threshold potential is achieved and a subsequent depolarization and action potential is generated. There is movement of calcium along with sodium to generate this pacemaker current in SA node.

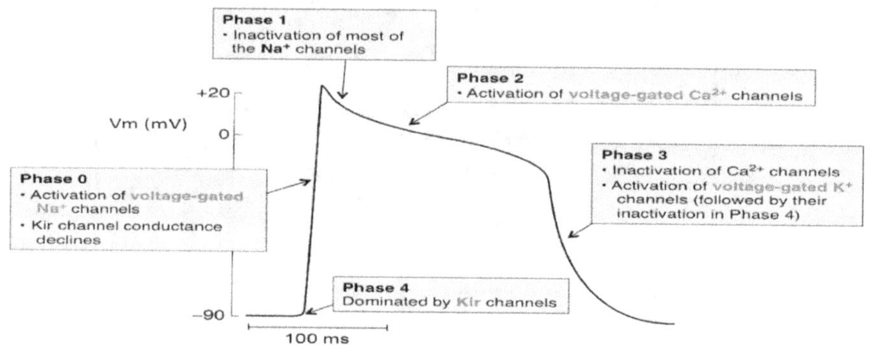

Fig. 3.2 Phases of an action potential in a vertricular cardiac muscle cell.

Source: Rudy Y (2008). "Molecular basis of cardiac action potential repolarization". *Annals of the New York Academy of Sciences*. 1123 (1): 113–8.

Electrophysiology of Arrhythmia

The genisis of arrhythmias [4]: Cardiac rhythm disturbances are the result of altered impulse generation (automaticity), altered impulse propagation (conductivity), or both the factors acting together. The factors which precipitate arrhythmias include myocardial ischemia with hypoxia and pH and electrolyte abnormalities: excessive stretch: excessive discharge of endogenous catecholamines; excessive sensitivity to autonomic regulators; and excessive exposure to drugs like digitalis and other potentially cardio toxic substances.

1. **Automaticity defect (ectopic impulse generation):** Normally the sinoatrial (SA) node, the pace maker, has the highest degree of automaticity, and is responsible for normal sinus rhythm. This spontaneous electrical activity of the SA node is independent of the CNS control, but is affected both by sympathetic (accelerator) and parasympathetic (slowing) activity of the ANS. Under certain circumstances, due to drugs or pathological changes, when the SA node is suppressed as in some bradyarrhythmias, other specialized conduction tissue with automatic properties takes up the role of the pacemaker. Thus, specialised atrial fibres, atrioventricular nodal tissue, the bundLe of his or the purkinje fibres developed an enhanced automatically when the SA pacemaker fails. Such a site is known as the ectopic focus, and the cells exhibit an increased tendency to depolarize during diastole. Arrhythmias due to increased automatically in subsidiary or latent pacemakers result from myocardial ischaemia or damage, hypopotassaemia or digitalis intoxication. Circulating catecholamines also increase automatically and induce

arrhythmias. Automaticity in ectopic foci may be enhanced, causing various automatic or re- entrant tachyarrhythmias. Alterations in the rate of impulse generation may occur even when the SA node is the dominant pacemaker, causing sinus irregularities.

Electrophysiologically, normally the phase 4 slope of cardiac cells other than the SA node is lesser than the SA nodal cells. Under certain conditions, the purkinje fibres or other conduction tissue cells may develop a much steeper phase 4 slope and take over an ectopic phase 4 function. Common arrhythmias due to ectopic automatically include premature ventricular beats, ventricular tachycardias, and ventricular escape rhythms. Nearly all antiarrhythmic drugs (except bretylium) depress ectopic automatically but decreasing the slope of phase 4 depolarization. In addition to this, quinidine, procanamide and propanonol also increase the threshold voltage for fibre activation. Lidocaine and phenytoin do not share the later property.

2. **Triggered activity:** It is an important cause of tachyarrhythmias and is seen in the form of afterdepolarizations. These are of two types:

    (a) **Early after depolarizations (EADs):** Occur at *slower heart rates* during phase 3 down slope of Action Potential (AP) and are precipitated by hypokalemia. They prolong APD and QT interval and can be blocked by shortening of Action Potential Duration (APD) (Magnesium & electrical overdrive). Torsades de pointes (TDP) are due to EADs.

    (b) **Delayed after depolazations (DADs):** These occur at the end of phase-3 or during phase –4, are caused by digitalis overdose, catecholamines and ischemia. These usually occur at *faster heart rates*. The common denominator is Ca++ overload, which cause oscillations in phase-4. One of the oscillations may achieve threshold limit and thus is conducted as premature depolarization.

3. **Conductivity Defect (Altered Impulse Conduction) [5]:** Some arrhythmias may be attributed to a defective transmission of the cardiac action potential. In myocardial ischemic or hypoxic states any region of the heart may transmit impulses slowly or acts as conduction block. Simple slowing in the rate of ventricular contraction follows AV blockade or bundLe branch block. More complex arrhythmias like paroxysmal atrial tachycardia, AV nodal tachycardias and many ventrical tachycardias are probably the result of retrograde transmission or re-entry mechanism. When the velocity of the propagating action potential is slowed, the likelihood of the conduction block increases, and the phenomenon of re-entry operates. For re-entry to occur, the conduction block must be unidirectional. In the time needed for re-entrant conduction, repolarization of the normal purkinji tissue occurs and the ventricular cell can be reactivated, giving a premature ventricular beat single re-entry impulses produce ventricular premature beats. A continuing self-sustaining re-entrant loop (circus movement) would lead to a ventricular tachycardia. Electrphysiologically, the conduction velocity and the effective refractory period are the important determining factors, whether or not a re-entrant arrhythmia is perpetuated.

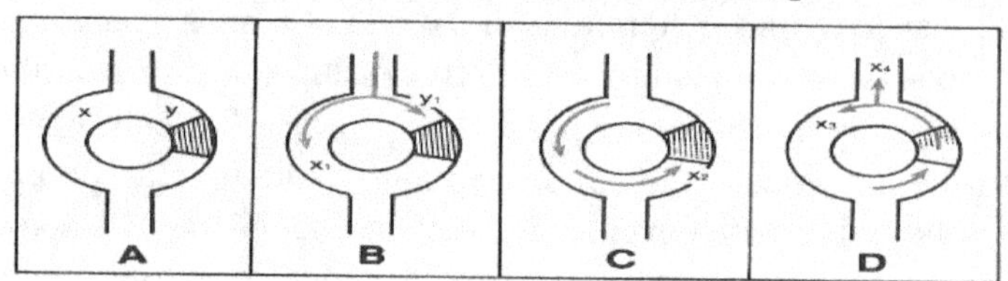

Fig. 3.3 Reentry phenomenon.

Source: Exerpted from pp 567-574 of Grauer K, Cavallaro D: ACLS: Comprehensive Review (Vol. 2) - 3rd Edition, Mosby Lifeline, St. Louis - 1993.

General Mechanism of Action of Antiarrhythmic Drugs

Drugs slow automaticity: Automaticity is reduced by:

1. Elevation of threshold potential- Quinidine, propranolol, verapamil (less negative) diltiazem, potassium 1
2. Reducing Resting Membrane Potential (RMP) (More negative)- Adenosine, lidocaine, phenytoin
3. Prolonging APD Effective Regractory Period (ERP) - Quinidine, amiodarone (Class Ia & III)
4. Reducing slope of phase-4. - Class IV drugs, propranolol

Drugs reduce after depolarizations: EADs and DADs are inhibited by:

1. Inhibiting upstroke of AP (Na^+ or Ca^{++} currents in fast and slow fibers respectively)-Verapamil and phenytoin inhibit DADs.
2. Shortening of APD-Isoprenaline inhibits EADs -Magnesium acts by blocking triggered beats and reduce EADs induced heterogeneity in ventricular cells.

Drugs affect conduction and reentry by:

1. Slowing anterograde (upside down) conduction in AV node: Digoxin, propranolol and verapamil. Paroxysmal supraventricular tachycardia (PSVT) is terminated in this way. Rate reduction in atrial fibrillation also occurs by this mechanism.
2. Prolongation of refractoriness (& thus retrograde or downside-up conduction) in accessory pathways by Na^+ channel block. Example is use of Class-Ia drugs to terminate PSVT in Wolf-Parkinson-White (WPW) syndrome.
3. Converting unidirectional block into bi-directional block by facilitating conduction in slow conducting pathway. Lidocaine blocks extrasystoles in myocardial infarction by this mechanism. Facilitated conduction through AV node by phenytoin makes it a useful drug in digoxin induced atrial tachycardia with varying AV nodal block.
4. Reduction in the dispersion (variablility) of refractoriness by lengethening of ERP also blocks reentry by quinidine

Case Study of Supra Ventricular Tachycardia

Summary

A 38year old male patient was admitted into hospital with complaints of lower retro sternal chest pain and chest discomfort since 1hour and palpitations with sweating. Patient had no history of any cardiac disorder. Patient's Complete Blood Picture (CBP) showed normal values, ECG shows complex tachycardia.

Diagnosis: Based on the above investigations the person was diagnosed with supra ventricular tachycardia.

Treatment given:

Tab dilzem-diltiazem	30mg	TID
Tab Pantocid-pantaprazole	40mg	OD
Tab Clonotril-clonazeapm	0.25mg	HS
Cap Atorfil- IV-atorvastatin	10mg	OD
InjCordarone-amiodarone	150mg	STAT
Inj adenosine-adenosine	6mg	STAT
Inj Pan -pantaprazole	40mg	STAT
InjZofer-ondansetron	8mg	STAT

Daily Progress: On day one the patient was identified with supra ventricular tachycardia (narrow complex) . He was given with adenosine injection of 6mg. On day two no palpitations and chest pain was seen.

Patient Counselling

1. Eat a healthy diet low in salt and fats. Rich in fruits and vegetables
2. Exercise regularly.
3. Maintain a healthy diet.
4. Control blood pressure and cholesterol levels.
5. Reduce alcohol intake
6. Maintain follow up of medications regulaRly.

Assignment

1. What is Supra Ventricular Tachycardia (SVT)?

It is defined as tachycardia (arterial or ventricular rates greater than 100bpm at rest) mechanism involves tissue from bundLe of His or above.

These SVTs include:

- Inappropriate sinus tachycardia
- Atrial Tachycardia AT (including focal and multifocal AT)
- Macro re-entrant AT
- Junctional tachycardia
- AV nodal Reentry Tachycardia (AVNRT) and various forms of accessory pathways.

2. What are the types of SVT?

- Physiological tachycardia: sinus tachycardia.
- Atrial tachyarrythimias: inappropriate sinus tachycardia (IST), Sinus nodal re-entrant tachycardia (SNRT), Ectopic atrial tachycardia, multifocal atrial tachycardia (MAT), Atrial flutter, Atrial fibrillation
- Atrio –ventricular tachyarrhythmias: Atrio-ventricular nodal re-entrant tachycardia (AVNRT), Non-peroxyzomaljunctional tachycardia (NPJT), Junctional ectopic tachycardia.

3. What is Atrial Fibrillation (AF)? What Cardiovascular (CVS) risk factors promote it?

A supraventricular tachycardia resulting from uncoordinated electrical activity causing a mechanical malfunction of the atrial heart muscle.

Risk factors: Hypertension (HTN), Ischemic Heart Disease (IHD), dilated cardiomyopathy, cardiac tumors, pulmonary embolism, hyperthyroidism, obesity, obstructive sleep etc.

4. What are the clinical presentations of AF?

Chest pain, dizziness, fatigue, inability to exercise or weakness, palpitations, Shortness of Breadth (SOB), light headedness, confusion.

5. What is the role of Transthoracic Echocardiography (TTE) and Trans Esophageal Echocardiography (TEE) in diagnosis of AF?

TTE is helpful for :

- Evaluate valvular heart disease
- Atrial and ventricular chamber and valve dimensions can be evaluate .
- To estimate ventricular function and thrombi.
- To estimate pulmonary systolic pressures and pericardial diseases.

TEE: Evaluate for atrial thrombus and to guide cardio version.

6. What is the risk of stroke associated with AF?

The rate of ischaemic stroke in patients with non rheumatic AF average 5%/year is between 2-7 times the rate of stroke in patients with AF. The attribual risk of stroke from AF is 1.5% (50-59 years,)

7. What is the efficacy of anticoagulation with warfarin to decrease stroke associated with AF?

Clinical trials demonstrated that it reduces the risk of stroke by 50-80%

Rivaroxaban, edoxaban have proven effective to warfarin to prevent stroke and thromboembolism. Warfarin is superior to clopidogrel or a combination of clopidogrel and aspirin in prevention of embolic risk patients.

8. What is the long term goal of anticoagulants in AF and which are approved?

The goal is to reduce the risk of thromboembolism. Patients in AF have a risk of stroke or peripheral embolism that is approximately 5 times that of individuals in sinus rhythm. Currently approved drugs include warfarin, debigatran, rivaroxaban, apixadan, edoxaban

9. How safe is clopidogrel and aspirin in patients with AF?

The American College of Chest Physicians (ACCP) 9 guidelines

In patients with low risk: no anti-thrombotic therapy

In patients with intermediate risk: Oral Anti-coagulant therapy- Aspirin + clopidogrel

In patients with high risk: Oral Anti-coagulant therapy- Aspirin + clopidogrel

Dabigatran 150mg BID

10. What are the common medications in atrioventricular nodalreentral tachycardia?

Medication include:

- Adenosine first line agent 6mg/2ml IV
- Digitalis 0.1mg/ml IV
- CCB: Diltiazem 120mg, verapamil 2.5mg/ml
- Beta blockers: Esmolol 2g/100ml, Atenolol 25mg, Metoprolol 1mg/ml IV

References

1. Rode DM. Antiarrhythmic drugs (chapter 34). In Goodman and Gilman's The pharmacological basis of therapeutics, 11th Ed, New Delhi, McGraw-Hill,2006, pp899-932.

2. Dimarco JP, Gersh BJ, Opie LH: Antiarrhythmic Drugs and strategies (chapter-8). In Opie LH and Gersh BJ editors-drugs for the heart, 6th ed, New Delhi, Elsevier, 2005, pp 218-274.

3. Sharma HL & Sharma KK. Drug therapy of cardiac arrhythmias (chapter 23) In Principles of Pharmacology, 1st Ed, Hyderabad, Paras Publishers,2007, pp297-313.

4. Tripathy KD. Antiarrhythmic drugs (chapter 36), In essentials of medical pharmacology, 5th Ed, New Delhi, Jaypee,2003, pp 472-485.

5. Klein AL, Grimm RA, Murray RD, et al, for the Assessment of Cardioversion Using Transesophageal Echocardiography Investigators. Use of transesophageal echocardiography to guide cardioversion in patients with atrial fibrillation. *N Engl J Med.* 2001 May 10. 344 (19):1411-20.

CHAPTER - 4

Myocardial Infarction

Introduction to Myocardial Infarction

Myocardial infarction is the irreversible death of the heart muscle due to prolonged lack of oxygen supply or ischaemia.

It is commonly known as a heart attack. The word, 'myocardium' refers to the heart muscle, while the word, 'infarct/infarction' has Latin origins and means to plug up or cram. It usually means death of a tissue.

MI and angina pectoris are usually mistaken as one another, but the difference is that the heart tissue undergoes necrosis in MI. This does not happen in angina pectoris, often times angina is considered as a warning sign of an impending heart attack.

Epidemiology

It is a very common cardiovascular disorder. More than 1.5 million cases are seen in India every year. Women typically experience heart attack with atypical or no symptoms.

Men are more prone to heart attacks. (Twice as much as women)

In 2015, there were 15.9 million recorded cases. Of which 4 million were NSTEMI (Non-ST segment elevated Myocardial Infarction) and the others were STEMI. (ST segment elevated Myocardial Infarction)

It is one of the world's expensive conditions to treat.

STEMI is more common than the other types of MI.

Risk Factors and Etiology

Non-Modifiable Risk Factors

- Old age more than 40yrs.
- Family history: can be inherited from parents to children.
- Gender: myocardial infarction is 3 times more in men than women.

Modifiable Risk Factors

- **Smoking:** It can damge the walls of arteries because of toxic substances in cigarette anf leads to atherosclerosis. There is narrowing and thickening of arterial walls Myocardial Infarction (MI).
- **Hypertension:** Our arteries are designed to pump blood at a certain pressure. If that pressure is exceeded, the walls of the arteries will be damaged. Injury to endothelial lining and atherosclerosis takes place. Narrowing and thickened arterial walls. Risk of MI.
- **Diabetes mellitus:** It inceases the rate of atherosclerotic progression and adversely affects the lipid profile.
- **Dyslipidaemia:** Narrowing of blood vessels due to high cholesterol levels or lipids.
- **Lack of physical activity:** improper lipid metabolism. LDL level increases. Starts accumulating in blood vessels Myocardial Infarction (MI).
- **CAD is the primary cause:** It is the accumulation of plaques in the coronary arteries that lead to blockage which subsequently leads to ischaemia and necrosis.
- **Obesity:** More lipids are produced. LDL level increases and leads to atherosclerosis and risk of MI.
- **Chronic alcoholism:** Increased oxidative stress and accumulation of free radicals and cause lipd peroxidation.
- **High stress levels:** Release stress hoemones like adrenaline, NA and cortisol. There is increase in heart rate and elevated blood pressure. It causes damage over time to all blood vessel. The damage increases the risk of plaque buildup in coronary arteries or can even cause a rupture of plaque. This leads to MI
- Drugs like oral contraceptives, NSAID's, cocaine and amphetamines. (Drug induced MI)
- Endometriosis in women.
- Exposure to gases like nitrogen dioxide, carbon dioxide and Sulphur dioxide.
- Bacteria. (An example is Helicobacter pylori)
- Genetics. (Chromosome 9 changes)
- Thyroid storm caused by severe untreated hyperthyroidism characterized by high BP, fever and heart failure.
- Plaque rupture.
- Ventricular hypertrophy.
- Coronary spasms and clots.
- MI may occur as a late consequence of the blood vessel inflammatory disease, Kawasaki disease due to the formation of coronary artery aneurysms.

Pathophysiology

There is formation of clots and plaques. The risk factors and causes of MI, lead to abnormally high lipid levels. The gradual buildup of cholesterol and fibrous tissue leads to the formation of plaques in the blood vessels. It is known as atherosclerosis. Due to this formation of plaques, inflammatory cells especially macrophages move into the affected vessel walls. Over time they become thicker with the products of cholesterol (LDL mostly) and they lead to the formation of foam cells. The foam cells die eventually and there is formation of a Cholesterol core. Further stimulation of inflammatory response to stabilize the plaque, as cholesterol crystals cause injuries to the vessel walls. The plaque now calcifies; it may even ulcerate in some cases. There is Clot or thrombus formation. The clot/plaque ruptures usually in the vessels of the heart due to increased injury and inflammation, vasoconstriction and platelet activation. Also, activation of extrinsic coagulation cascade occurs as a result of exposure of blood to thrombogenic lipid core. Blockage of the vessels occur where there is rupture. This blocks the flow of blood and oxygen and leads to prolonged ischaemia in the heart. Necrosis due to ischaemia occurs. This leads to the death of some parts of the heart tissue i.e. myocardial infarction.

Clinical Manifestation and Features [1]

Signs and Symptoms

- Angina or chest pain that is often described as a sensation of tightness and squeezing.
- Retrosternal chest discomfort.
- Pain radiating from the jaws to the shoulders, neck and forelimbs usually on the left side of the body. A distinctive feature is that the pain persists even on change of position.
- Sweating/ Nausea/ Shortness of breath/ Vomiting/ Fainting.
- Fatigue and malaise/ Heartburn/ Indigestion.
- Other less common symptoms are light headedness, palpitations, change in the heart rate and blood pressure. These are known as the atypical symptoms and are seen in women and 30% of the patients.
- 5% of the people have silent MI, that means that they have no significant discoverable symptoms at all.

Complications of Myocardial Infarction

1. Impaired contractility: As a result of this it causes
   (a) Venticular thrombus leading to stroke (Embolism)
   (b) Hypertension—so decreased coronary perfusion. Resulting in increased ischemia. Ultimately leads to cardiogenic shock.
   (c) Congestive heart failure.
2. Tissue necrosis: Because of necrosis there will be papillary muscle infarction → mitral regurgitation → congestive heart failure.
3. Tissue necrosis also causes ventriculat rupture and causes cardiac tamponade.
4. Electrical instability so leading to arrhythmias.
5. Pericardial inflammation leading to pericarditis.

Types of MI: MI is usually classified into two types:

- STEMI that stands for ST segment elevated MI.
  An attack of MI is considered STEMI when the ECG shows ST segment elevation in two

or more relate leads irrespective of the time. And Q wave progression is seen. The segment is elevated due to the complete interruption of regional myocardial blood flow. This is 25-40% of MI's. It's the most dangerous type and this leads to a lot of deaths.

- NSTEMI that stands for non-ST segment elevated MI.
  In NSTEMI, the ST segment is depressed, the T wave is inverted and new Q waves are formed. This type is rare and less severe. In this type the coronary artery is not completely blocked that is why it is easier to treat and is less dangerous.

In 2012, an international consensus classified MI into the following types:

- ➢ Spontaneous MI related to plaque erosion, rupture, fissuring and detection.
- ➢ MI related to ischaemia due an increased demand or a decreased supply. (examples are coronary artery spasm, coronary embolisms, anemias, fluctuations in the BP, arrhythmias.)
- ➢ Sudden unexpected cardiac death where MI is detected after an autopsy of the body before the appearance of cardiac biomarkers in the blood.
- ➢ MI associated with Percutaneoius Coronary Intervention (PCI) and stent thrombosis.
- ➢ CABG associated MI.
- ➢ MI that is associated with spontaneous coronary artery dissection in young and fit women.

Diagnosis with Algorithm [2, 3, 4]

- Symptoms of ischemia can be detected by physical examination and blood tests.
- The blood tests include the levels of adenosine, thrombin, myocardial bands, troponin and myocardial creatinine kinase. All of these are biomarkers and their levels increase in the case of MI.
- ECG is performed. It is used to detect what kind of MI the patient suffers from.
- If the patient has STEMI the changes in the ECG are:
- The ST segment is elevated, Q wave progression.
- If the patient has NSTEMI the changes in ECG are:
- The ST segment is depressed and the T wave is inverted and new Q waves are observed.
- If the ECG detects STEMI, reperfusion is initiated immediately and if NSTEMI is detected a stress test is performed for further diagnosis of risk. (Low risk, moderate risk, high risk). The NSTEMI treatment is started.
- An echocardiogram is performed. In a STEMI the coronary artery is completely blocked and in NSTEMI it is partially blocked.
- Stress test. It is a test that measures the heart's ability to respond to external stress in a controlled clinical environment. The stress response is induced by exercise or intravenous pharmacological stimulation. If there is high risk CABG is performed.
- Angiography.
- Autopsy.

Management

Short-term Goals of Therapy

1. Early restoration of blood flow to the infarct-related artery to prevent infarct expansion (in the case of MI) or prevent complete occlusion and MI Unstable Augina (UA),
2. Prevention of complications and death,
3. Prevention of coronary artery reocclusion,
4. Relief of ischemic chest discomfort, and
5. Maintenance of normoglycemia.

Nonpharmacologic Therapy

- For patients with ST Segement Elevated Acute Company Syndrome (STE) ACS, either fibrinolysis or primary PCI (with either balloon angioplasty or stent placement) is the treatment of choice for reestablishing coronary artery blood flow when the patient presents within 3 hours of symptom onset. Primary PCI may be associated with a lower mortality rate than fibrinolysis, possibly because PCI opens more than 90% of coronary arteries compared with less than 60% opened with fibrinolytics.
- In patients with Non ST Segement Elevated Acute Coronary Syndrome (NSTE) ACS, clinical practice guidelines recommend either PCI or coronary artery bypass grafting revascularization as an early treatment for high-risk patients, and that such an approach also be considered for moderate-risk patients.

Role of Pharmacological Therapy with Algorithm

1. **Immediate adjunctive treatment**
    - **(i)** Nitrates: Decrease anginal symptoms by inducing coronary vasodilation and improving myocardial O_2 supply, and by decreasing myocardial O_2 demand by decreasing preload through venodilatation
    - **(ii)** Beta blockers: Decrease myocardial O_2 demand by decreasing heart rate and contractility; in addition, also contribute to electrical stability
    - **(iii)** Calcium channel blockers: Decrease myocardial O_2 demand by decreasing heart rate and contractility, decreasing wall stress via decreased blood pressure, and decreasing preload via venodilatation
    - **(iv)** Morphine: Reduces myocardial oxygen demands by decreasing chest pain and anxiety
    - **(v)** Oxygen: Improves oxygen supply in patients with hypoxemia
2. **Antiplatelet therapy**
    - **(i)** Aspirin: Prevents further thrombus formation by inhibiting platelet synthesis of thromboxane A_2, an important mediator of platelet activation

(ii) Clopidogrel (or other ADP receptor blockers): Inhibit ADP-mediated activation of platelets, thereby preventing expansion of the existing thrombus; have superior outcomes when used in combination with Aspirin

(iii) GP IIb/IIIa inhibitors: Potent antiplatelet agents that block the final common pathway of platelet aggregation; often used in patients undergoing PCI as they are very effective in reducing cardiac events in these patients.

3. **Anticoagulant therapy**

   (i) Unfractionated heparin (UFH) or low molecular weight heparin (LMWH): UFH an LMWH, which preferentially bind to antithrombin III and factor Xa, respectively, slow thrombin formation and impede clot development

4. **Fibrinolysis**

   (i) Recombinant Tissue-type Plasminogen Activators (tPA) Recombinant Plasminogen Activators (rPA): Transform the inactive precursor plasminogen into the active protease plasmin, which lyses fibrin clots, thereby accelerating lysis of the occlusive intracoronary thrombus and restoring blood flow

5. **Primary percutaneous coronary intervention (PCI)**

   (i) Plain old balloon angioplasty (POBA): Inflation of a balloon within a stenosed coronary artery mechanically dilates the affected vessel to restore blood flow, both by compressing the atherosclerotic plaque and stretching the underlying media

   (ii) Bare metal stents: Mechanically maintain the patency of coronary arteries occluded by atherosclerotic plaques

   (iii) Drug-eluting stents: In addition to maintaining patency, these stents release antiproliferative agents such as sirolimus or paclitaxel, which prevent neointimal proliferation (migration of smooth muscle cells and production of extracellular matrix), thereby decreasing the rate of in-stent restenosis

6. **Surgical revascularization**

   (i) Coronary artery bypass graft (CABG): Restores coronary blood flow by using a healthy patent artery to bridge circulation around an occlusive lesion within an atherosclerotic coronary vessel

Pharmacologic Management of Patients with ST-Elevated Myocardial Infarction (STEMI)

If the patient is suspected with STEMI based on clinical symptome, history, cardiac biomarkers and ECG- immediately aspirin shoud be administered (162-325mg, non-enteric coated). Then treatment strategy should be selected based on time of presentation from symptoms onset and hospital capabilities.

(a) Diagnostic angiogram can be performed. Either PCI or CABG can be done. Later loading dose of second antiplatelet agents and patient to be continued on $P2Y_{12}$ receptor inhibitor. For the long term management of the patient the following medications are to be indicated

(i) Aspirin 75-162 mg to be continued indefinetely

(ii) P2Y12 receptor inhibitor to be continued for upto 12 months

(iii) Statin (regrdLess of LDL or dietary modification)

(iv) Beta blockers

(v) ACE-inhibitors or ARBs or aldosterone antagonists

(b) Directly the patient can be treated with fibrinolytic therapy without PCI or CABG

(i) Either tenecteplase (or) reteplase (or) Alteplase can be initiated

(ii) Clopidogrel can be givan for atleast 14 days upto 1 year

(iii) Anti-coagulant (heparin, enoxaparin or found a parinox) can be given atleast 2 days upto 8 days.

(iv) Later mediacations to be continued for long term management as indicated above.

Pharmacologic Management of Patients with

Unstable Angina (UA)/Non-ST Elevated Myocardial Infarction (NSTEMI)

If the patient is suspected with UA or NSTEMI based on clinical symptom, history, cardiac biomarkers and ECG.

(i) Consider need for acute anti-ischemic and analgesic therapies in the patient. Immediately supplemental oxygen has to be initiated. Followed by Nitroglycerine, IV morphine sulaphate to relieve pain can be given. A beta blocker or ACE inhibitor can be started. The patient also has to be put on statin. The patient to be put on observation. The following medication can be considered for long term management:

(a) aspirin (75-162mg to be continued indefinitely

(b) P2Y12 receptor inhibitor to be continued for upto 12 months

(c) Statin to be initiated regardLess of LDL or dietary modifications

(d) Beta blocker or ACE inhibitor or ARBs OR Aldosterone antagonist

(ii) Administer aspirin (162-325mg, non-enteric coated). Then select initial treatment strategy- either Conservative strategy OR Invasive strategy.

(a) Conservative strategy: a second antiplatelet agent to be initiated- clopidogrel or ticagrlor with a loading dose followed by a daily maintenance dose or Iinitiate anticoagulation with UFH or enoxaparin or foundaparinox

(b) Invasive starategy: a second antiplatelet agent (Clopidogrel, ticagrelor, prasugrel with or without an IV GP IIb/IIIa inhibitor) has to be initiated. A loading dose of a P2Y12 receptor inhibitor is recommended in patients for whom PCI is planned followed by a maintenance dose. Anticoagulation with UFH or enoxaparin or foundaparinox has to be initiated.

Early Pharmacotherapy for ST-Segment Elevation Acute Coronary Syndrome

1. Intranasal oxygen (if oxygen saturation is less than 90%);
2. Nitroglycerin (NTG): IV Nitroglycerin is indicated in the first 48 hrs after STEMI for treatment of persistent ischemia, or hypertension of oral or topical nitrates are useful beyond the first 48 hrs after STEMI for treatment od angina
3. An ACE inhibitor to be given who can tolerate or Angiotensin Receptor Blocker (ARB) should be administred to STEMI patients who are intolerant to ACE inhibitors OR long term aldosterone blockade should be prescribed for post-STEMI patients without significant renal dysfunction.
4. Anti-platelet drugs: Aspirin 162-325 mg given on day 1of STEMI; a clopidogrel who are unable to take aspirin.
    (a) a β-blocker;
5. Anti-thrombotics: IV unfractionated heparin (UFH) (bolus of 60U/kg, maximum 4000I IV; initial infusion 12U/kg per hour, maximum 1000u/H) or Low Molecular Weight Heparin (LMWH) to be used in patients after STEMI who are at high risk for systemic emboli; or enoxaparin
6. Fibrinolysis in eligible candidates.

If the candidate is eligible for CABG surgery: Anti-coagulant therapy is to be discontinued for surgery or Antiplatelet therapy with aspirin as soon as possible without cessation for surgery or $P2Y_{12}$ antagonist as sson as possible, but shoud be discontinued for surgery.

Fibrinolytic Therapy [5,6]

A fibrinolytic agent is indicated in patients with STE ACS presenting within 12 hours of the onset of chest discomfort who have at least 1 mm of STE in two or more continuous ECG leads or a new left bundLe-branch block.

Absolute contraindications to fibrinolytic therapy include:

1. active internal bleeding;
2. previous Intra Cranial Hemorrirage (ICH) at any time;
3. ischemic stroke within 3 months;
4. known intracranial neoplasm;
5. known structural vascular lesion;
6. suspected aortic dissection; and
7. significant closed head or facial trauma within 3 months. Primary PCI is preferred in these situations

Alteplase: 15-mg IV bolus followed by 0.75-mg/kg infusion (maximum 50 mg) over 30 minutes, followed by 0.5-mg/kg infusion (maximum 35mg) over 60 minutes (maximum dose 100 mg).

✓ **Reteplase:** 10 units IV over 2 minutes, followed 30 minutes later with another 10 units IV over 2 minutes.

✓ **Tenecteplase:** A single IV bolus dose given over 5 seconds based on patient weight: 30 mg if <60 kg; 35 mg if 60 to 69.9 kg; 40 mg if 70 to 79.9 kg; 45 mg if 80 to 89.9 kg; and 50 mg if 90 kg or greater.

✓ **Streptokinase:** 1.5 million units in 50 mL of normal saline or 5% dextrose in water IV over 60 minutes.

Aspirin

- **Aspirin** should be administered to all patients without contraindications within the first 24 hours of hospital admission. It provides an additional mortality in patients with ST Segement Elevated Acute Coronary Syndrome (STE ACS) when given with fibrinolytic therapy. Non–enteric-coated aspirin, 162 to 325 mg, should be chewed and swallowed as soon as possible after the onset of symptoms.
- A daily maintenance dose of 75 to 162 mg is recommended thereafter and should be continued indefinitely.
- Low-dose aspirin is associated with a reduced risk of major bleeding, particularly GI bleeding.

Platelet P2Y 12 Inhibitors

- **Clopidogrel:** 300- to 600-mg loading dose is given on the first hospital day, followed by a maintenance dose of 75 mg daily. It should be continued indefinitely.
- **Prasugrel:** 60mg oral loading dose followed by 10mg orally once daily.

Glycoprotein IIb/IIIa Receptor Inhibitors [7]

- They block the final pathway of platelet aggregation, namely cross-linking of platelets by fibrinogen bridges between the GPIIb and IIa receptors on the platelet surface.
- **Abciximab** is a first-line GP IIb/IIIa inhibitor for patients undergoing primary PCI who have not received fibrinolytics. It should not be administered to STE ACS patients who will not be undergoing PCI.
- The dose of abciximab is 0.25 mg/kg IV bolus given 10 to 60 minutes before the start of PCI, followed by 0.125 mcg/kg/min (maximum 10 mcg/min) for 12 hours.
- Bleeding is the most common significant adverse effect.

Anticoagulants

- **UFH** is a first-line anticoagulant for STE ACS, both for medical therapy and PCI.
- For STE ACS, the dose of UFH is 60 units/kg IV bolus (maximum 4,000 units) followed by a continuous IV infusion of 12 units/kg/hour (maximum 1,000 units/hour).

- Enoxaparin dose is 1mg/kg subcutaneous every 12 hours or 24 hours.
- Foundaparinox dose is 2.5mg IV bolus followed by 2.5mg SC once daly

Nitrates

- Immediately upon presentation, one Sublingual Nitroglycerin (SL NTG) tablet should be administered every 5 minutes for up to three doses to relieve chest pain and myocardial ischemia.
- The usual dose is 5 to 10 mcg/min by continuous infusion, titrated up to 200 mcg/min until relief of symptoms or limiting side effects (e.g., headache or hypotension). Treatment should be continued for approximately 24 hours after ischemia is relieved.
- The most significant adverse effects of nitrates are tachycardia, flushing, headache, and hypotension.

β-Adrenergic Blockers

- If there are no contraindications, a β-blocker should be administered early in the care of patients with STE ACS (within the first 24 hours) and continued indefinitely.
- **Metoprolol**: 5 mg by slow (over 1 to 2 minutes) IV bolus, repeated every 5 minutes for a total initial dose of 15 mg. If a conservative regimen is desired, initial doses can be reduced to 1 to 2 mg. This is followed in 15 to 30 minutes by 25 to 50 mg orally every 6 hours.
- **Propranolol**: 0.5 to 1 mg slow IV push, followed in 1 to 2 hours by 40 to 80 mg orally every 6 to 8 hours.
- **Atenolol**: 5 mg IV dose, followed 5 minutes later by a second 5-mg IV dose; then 50 to 100 mg orally every day beginning 1 to 2 hours after the IV dose.
- The most serious side effects early in Acute Coronary Syndrome (ACS) are hypotension, bradycardia, and heart block

Calcium Channel Blockers

- Are preferred in patients who have Contraindicatiosn (CI) to β-**Adrenergic Blockers**
- Diltiazam: 120mg to 360mg sustained release orally once daily
- Verapamil: 180 to 480 mg sustained release orally once daily
- Amlodipine : 5 to 10 mg orally once daily.

Early Pharmacotherapy for Non–ST-Segment

Elevation Acute Coronary Syndrome [8]

According to Amercian College of Cardiology/American Heart Association (ACC/AHA) practice guidelines, early pharmacotherapy should include:

1. **Intranasal oxygen** (if oxygen saturation is <90%);
2. Sub Lingual (SL) **NTG** (IV therapy for selected patients);

3. **Aspirin**;
4. An oral **β-blocker** (IV therapy optional); and
5. An **anticoagulant Unfractionated Heparin (UFH), Low Molecular Weight Heparin (LMWH) [enoxaparin], fondaparinux, or bivalirudin). Morphine** is also administered to patients with refractory angina.

Secondary Prevention Following MI

Desired Outcome

The long-term goals after MI are to:

1. Control modifiable coronary heart disease (CHD) risk factors;
2. Prevent development of systolic heart failure;
3. Prevent recurrent MI and stroke; and
4. Prevent death, including sudden cardiac death.

Pharmacotherapy

General Approach

- Pharmacotherapy that has been proven to decrease mortality, heart failure, reinfarction, or stroke should be started before hospital discharge for secondary prevention.
- The ST Elevated or Non ST Elecvated Acute Coronary Syndrome (ACC/AHA) guidelines suggest that after MI from either STE or NSTE ACS, patients should receive indefinite treatment with **aspirin**, a **β-blocker**, and an **ACE inhibitor**.
- All patients should receive Sublingual (SL**) NTG** or **lingual spray** and instructions for use in case of recurrent ischemic chest discomfort.
- **Clopidogrel** should be considered for most patients, but the duration of therapy is individualized according to the type of ACS and whether the patient is treated medically or undergoes stent implantation.
- All patients should receive annual **influenza vaccination**.
- Selected patients also should be treated with long-term **warfarin** anticoagulation.
- For all ACS patients, treatment and control of modifiable risk factors such as hypertension, dyslipidemia, and diabetes mellitus are essential.

Case Study of Posterior MI

Summary

A 41years male Patient was admitted in cardiology department with complaints of ongoing right sided chest pain, retrosternal pain with burning sensation of 4 hours duration. He also has history of burning sensation in chest on and off since last 2 days. Mild Shortness of Breath

(SOB) present. Vitals were checked. Blood Pressure (BP) was high (210/130mmHg). Heart rate – 120 beats/min. The patient was admitted. Investigations were carried out. Blood picture was normal. ECG showed Sinus Tachycardia, (ST) ↓, 2vol v6I, Augumented Vector Left (avl)-MAI. 2D ECHO showed –mild Left Ventrcular (LV) dysfunction.

Diagnosis: The patient was assessed as posterior MI, MILD LV dysfunction, Killips class-I: Normal.

Therapy was started with loading doses of:

   Tab Aspirin - 150mg 2tabs

   Tab Brilinta - ticagrelor 90mg 2tabs

   Tab Storvas - atorvastatain 80mg stat

   Inj. Lasix - furosemide 20mg iv

   Inj. Pantocid - panataprazole 40mg iv

   Inj. NTG - nitroglycerin 5mg/min

Planned for Emergency CAG, Primary PTCA

Radiological Report: Coronary Angiogram (CAG) - two vessel disease. Left Anterior Descending Artery (LAD) - long segment 80% stenosis. Left Circumflex Artery (LCX) proximal total occlusion with thrombosis distally. Then primary Percutaneous Transluminal Coronary Angioplasty (PTCA) sent to Left Circumflex Artery (LCX) major oxy performed timi 3 flow restored. Good result was STENT. Intracoronary eptifiblite given as double dose. Rx: repeated added injection clexane 60 mg sc. Planned for staged PTCA stent lad after 48 hrs. Other day IV dopamine was given 25 ml/hr. NTG was stopped. Pt was stable – no angina. Dopamine was tapered and stopped. Vitals were checked reguraly. Staged PTCA to lad was done iv 1 ½ NS 30 ml/hr started. Added tab. Trika (Al prazolam) 0.5mg p/o. The patient had bed sores So added- T. betaloc 25 mg p/o, Inj. Monecef 1g, Inj. Nikoran 4mg (Nicorandil) iv. Psychological support was given to patient. Good prognosis was seen. No chest pain/ dyspnea. Patient was stable. Vitals were normal. Procedural and post procedural hospital stay was good, the patient is asymptomatic and been discharged in a stable condition. Discharge medications were given and asked for investigations and check up regularly.

Medication chart:

Tab Ecospirin (Aspirin) 75mg OD	Tab Axel (Aceclofenac) 200mg BD
Tab Storvas (Atorvastatin) 40mg OD	Inj Clexane (Enoxaparin) 60mg sc BD
Inj Lasix (Furosemide) 20mg iv BD	Inj Pantocid (Pantaprazole) 40mg iv BD
Tab Restyl (alprazolam) 0.25mg HS	Syp Cremaffin plus (Liquid paraffin) 15ml HS
Tab Taxim (cefixime) 200mg BD	Syp Mucaine gel (AlOH3)10ml TID
Tab Befolac (Multivitamin) 25mg BD	Tab Trika (Alprazolam) 0.5mg

Tab Monocef (Ceftriaxone) 1g

Inj Fentanyl   50ml IV

Inj NTG (Nitroglycerine) 25mg

Tab Clonotril (Clonazepam) 0.25mg p/o

Inj Nikoran (Nicorandil) 4mg IV

Inj Heparin

Inj Dopamine   200mg

Discharge Medication

Tab Ecospirin (Aspirin) 75mg OD

Tab Atoravas (Atorvastatin) 40mg OD

Tab Metocard xl (Metoprolol) 50mg OD

Tab Pantodal (Pantaprazole) 40mg OD

Syp Mucaine gel Aluminium hydroxide (AlOH$_3$) 10 ml TID - 5 Days

Tab Axel (Aceclofenac) 200mg BD

Tab Losar (Losartan)   25mg OD

Tab Clonotril (Clonazepam)0.25mg OD 2 weeks

Syp Cremaffin plus (Liquid paraffin) 15 ml HS/SOS

Tab Taxim O (cefixime) 200mg BD - 3 Days

Assignment

1. **What pharmacotherapeutic options are available for treating this patient? Discuss the agents in each class with doses routes?**

Initial management include

-   Intravenous access, supplemental oxygen if oxygen saturation is less than 90%
-   Immediate administration of non enteric coated aspirin
-   Nitroglycerine for active chest pain, either sublingually or iv injection 25 mg

Classes of Drugs

1. Aspirin sose 162-325mg maintenance dose 75-81mg chewable aspirin is preferred as it promotes rapid absorption into blood stream to achieve faster therapeutic levels.
2. Reduction of cardiac pain: Nitrates- are potent vasodilators reduces venous blood return to heart ie reduces ventricular preload. Reduction in work load of the heart, leads to less oxygen demand and reduction in ischemic pain. Nitrate dose -0.4mg sublingually
3. Anticoagulants important adjuvant therapy for reperfusion therapy - Drugs like heparin, Low Molecular Weight Heparin (LMWH) are available options
4. Anti platelet drugs apart from aspirin other drugs are P2Y$_{12}$ receptor inhibitors ex. Clopidogrel, ticlopidine, prasugrel

    Loading doses of clopidogrel 600mg, ticagrelor 180mg, prasugrel 60mg are given

    Daily doses- 75mg clopidogrel, 90mg ticagrelor, 10mg prasugrel.

    Maintenance doses are continued for 1 year or minimum of 14 days

    Others like iv glycoprotein IIb/IIIa receptor antagonist

5. Beta-blockers: Works by reduction of oxygen consumption of the myocardium by decreasing heart rate, BP and myocardial contractility
   - These are given orally with in 24 hours; initiated with low doses
   - e.g. Metoprolol, Carvediol, Bisoprolol
6. Calcium channel blockers - For recurrent myocardial ischemia if beta blockers are contraindicated
- Unfractionated heparin - Initial loading doses of 60 IU/kg with an initial infusion of 12 IU/kg/hr continued for 48 hours
- Fondaparinoux-Selective factor X inhibitor once daily SC inj of 2.5mg
7. Statins- Atorvastatin 40mg -80mg; Rosuvastatin 20 mg are recommended

Nicorandil - Has nitrate action dose of 10 mg can be given

2. What are the goals of pharmacotherapy for Ischemic Heart Disease (IHD)?

The goals of pharmacotherapy for patients with IHD are-
- Prevent premature cardiovascular death of other complications
- Maintain and restore a quality life while eliminating avoidable adverse effects of tests and treatment.
- Reduce the symptom and pain
- Slowing of the progression of atherosclerosis by controlling risk factors
- Widening or bypassing narrowed arteries
- Decreasing myocardial oxygen demand and for increasing oxygen supply.

3. What are the modifiable risk factors for IHD?

Risk factors-
- Smoking/ Diabetes/ High BP/ Obesity/ Lack of physical activity.

This patient showed high BP, high blood glucose levels and stress.

4. When the patient returns to the clinic in 2wks for follow up visit, how will you evaluate the response to his new antianginal regimen for efficacy and adverse effects?

Follow up evaluation-
- Improved symptoms of angina, improved cardiac performance and longer duration exercise capacity is subjective evidence that therapy is working.
- There are several instruments (ex- Seattle angina questionnaire, specific activity scale) and Canadian classification system to assess the symptoms and reproducibility.
- Objective assessment is obtained through increased exercise duration by Exercise Tolerance Test (ETT) and absence of ischemic changes in ECG.
- Echocardiography and cardio imaging may also be used.

The Seattle Angina Questionnaire-7

1. The following is a list of activities that people often do during the week. Although for some people with several medical problems it is difficult to determine what it is that limits them, please go over the activities listed below and indicate how much limitation you have had **due to chest pain, chest tightness or angina** <u>over the past 4 weeks</u>.

Place an X in one box on each line.

Activity	Extremely limited	Quite a bit limited	Moderately Limited	Slightly limited	Not at all limited	Limited for other reasons or did not do the activity
a. Walking indoors on level ground	☐	☐	☐	☐	☐	☐
b. Gardening, vacuuming or carrying groceries	☐	☐	☐	☐	☐	☐
c. Lifting or moving heavy objects (e.g. furniture, children)	☐	☐	☐	☐	☐	☐

2. Over the <u>past 4 weeks</u>, on average, how many times have you had **chest pain, chest tightness or angina?**

I have had **chest pain, chest tightness or angina**...

4 or more times per day	1-3 times per day	3 or more times per week but not every day	1-2 times per week	Less than once a week	None over the past 4 weeks
☐	☐	☐	☐	☐	☐

3. Over the <u>past 4 weeks</u>, on average, how many times have you had to take nitroglycerin (nitroglycerin tablets or spray) for your **chest pain, chest tightness or angina?**

I have taken nitroglycerin...

4 or more times per day	1-3 times per day	3 or more times per week but not every day	1-2 times per week	Less than once a week	None over the past 4 weeks
☐	☐	☐	☐	☐	☐

4. Over the <u>past 4 weeks</u>, how much has your **chest pain, chest tightness or angina** limited your enjoyment of life?

It has **extremely** limited my enjoyment of life	It has limited my enjoyment of life **quite a bit**	It has **moderately** limited my enjoyment of life	It has **slightly** limited my enjoyment of life	It has **not** limited my enjoyment of life at all
☐	☐	☐	☐	☐

5. If you had to spend the rest of your life with your **chest pain, chest tightness or angina** the way it is right now, how would you feel about this?

Not satisfied at all	Mostly dissatisfied	Somewhat satisfied	Mostly satisfied	Completely satisfied
☐	☐	☐	☐	☐

Chan et al.

Fig. 4.1 Evaluation Questionaire for Antianginal regimen efficacy.

Source: Paul S chanet al., Development and Validation of a Short Version of the Seattle Angina Questionnaire, Circulation: Cardiovascular Quality and Outcomes. 2014;7:640–647.

5. What is the recommended duration of dual antiplatelet therapy with aspirin and clopidogrel in percutaneous coronary intervention with drug eluting stents?

Dual anti-platelet therapy including aspirin and a $P2Y_{12}$ receptor inhibitor has been consistently shown to reduce recurrent major adverse cardio vascular events in patients with Acute Coronary Syndrome (ACS) or undergoing Percutaneous Coronary Intervention (PCI) for stable Coronary Artery Diease (CAD).

Among patients with stable CAD undergoing PCI with drug eluting stents, shorter duration of Dual Antiplatelet Therapy (DAPT) 3-6 months showed Good Results. Non inferior to 12-24 months duration with respect to Major Adverse Cardiovascular Events (MACE), but reduced the rate of major bleeding.

Prolonged Dual Antiplatelet Therapy (DAPT) durations (18-48 months) reduced the incidence of MI and stent thrombosis but at a cost of major bleedings.

12months duration of Dual Antiplatelet Therapy (DAPT) is currently recommended.

6. **What information will you communicate to the patient about his antianginal regimen to help him experience few adverse effects and good benefits?**
   - Take anti-anginal drugs as prescribed and follow your doctor's advice to prevent your heart disease and angina from getting worse.
   - Adhere to your drug therapy for other diseases that can increase your risk to angina such as diabetes high BP and high cholesterol.
   - Do not take vitamin or fish oil supplement to treat stable angina.
   - If you feel light headed after taking Nitroglycerin (GTN) sit down or find something to hold on.
   - Place yourself and take rest breaks as angina is often brought on by exertion.
   - Eat a balanced and healthy diet.
   - Eat lots of fiber with whole grains and variety of fruits and vegetables.
   - Avoid foods high in saturated fats, Cut down on the amount of salt in food as it can raise BP. Adopt a healthy life style as its is the most effective way of reducing your risk of angina. Limit alcohol consumption.
   - Stop smoking and exposure to second hand smoke.
   - Maintain a healthy weight/Exercise regularly.
   - Avoid stress, engage in healthy activities to reduce tension and stress.

7. **Describe the role of Low Molecule Weight heparins and fondaparinux in the management of ACS?**
   - Low Mollecule Weight Heparin and fondaparinux are anticoagulants used in the management of ACS LMWH –Bind to antithrombin and inhibit both factor Xa and IIa. They preferentially inhibit factor Xa over IIa. The benfit was apparent after 48hrs of treatment but has significant increased risk of bleeding.
   - Fondaparinux-Indirect acting specific inhibitor of factor Xa. It does not cause heparin induced thrombocytopenia unlike LMWH.

8. **What are the precautions to be taken with the use of sildenafil, Vardenafil in IHD patient?**
   - Sildenafil is contraindicated in patient using long or short acting nitrates due to possibility of developing potentially fatal severe hypotension.
   - Patients not using long acting nitrates but requiring nitrates sublingual for treatment of episodes of angina should be informed about the hazard of using these drugs.

- Any use of nitrate is contraindicated in the 24hrs following the use of Sildenafil.
- High risk Cardiovascular patients including patient with HTN, Diabetes, Obesity should be informed about the potential severe risk of Sildenafil and Nitrate interaction.
- Patients using vasodilation of diuretics simultaneously should be monitored for a hypotensive response to sildenafil.
- Physicians and Health Personnel Emergency departments should be instructed to routinely ask patients about the use of these drugs (Sildenafil & Nitrates Combination).
- An initial dose of 25mg should be recommended in all situations.

References

1. [Guideline] Ibanez B, James S, Agewall S, et al, for the ESC Scientific Document Group . 2017 ESC guidelines for the management of acute myocardial infarction in patients presenting with ST-segment elevation: The Task Force for the management of acute myocardial infarction in patients presenting with ST-segment elevation of the European Society of Cardiology (ESC). *Eur Heart J*. 2018 Jan 7. 39 (2):119-77.
2. Krumholz HM, Anderson JL, Brooks NH, et al. ACC/AHA clinical performance measures for adults with ST-elevation and non-ST-elevation myocardial infarction: A report of the American College of Cardiology/ American Heart Association Task Force on Performance Measures (Writing Committee to Develop Performance Measures on ST-Elevation and Non-ST-Elevation Myocardial Infarction). J Am Coll Cardiol 2006;47:236–265.
3. Levine GL, Berger PB, Cohen DJ, et al. Newer pharmacotherapy in patients undergoing percutaneous coronary interventions: A guide for pharmacists and other health care professionals. Pharmacotherapy 2006;26:1537–1556.
4. Spinler SA. Acute coronary syndromes. In: Shumock GT, Brundage DM, Chapman MM, et al., eds. Pharmacotherapy Self-Assessment Program, Book 1: Cardiovascular I, Cardiovascular II, 5th ed. Kansas City: American College of Clinical Pharmacy, 2004:1–40.
5. Awtry EH, Loscalzo J. Aspirin. Circulation 2000;101:1206–1218.
6. O'Gara PT, Kushner FG, Ascheim DD, et al. 2013 ACCF/AHA guideline for the management of ST-elevation myocardial infarction: A report of the American College of Cardiology Foundation/American Heart Association Task Force on Practice Guidelines. J Am Coll Cardiol 2013;**61**:e78–e140.
7. Jneid H, Anderson JL, Wright RS, et al . 2012 ACCF/AHA focused update of the guideline for the management of unstable angina/non-ST segment myocardial infarction (updating the 2007 guideline and replacing the 2011 focused update): A report of the American College of Cardiology Foundation/American Heart Association Task Force on Practice Guidelines J Am Coll Cardiol. 2012;**60**:645–681.
8. Cabello JB, Burls A, Emparanza JI, Bayliss S, Quinn T. Oxygen therapy for acute myocardial infarction. *Cochrane Database Syst Rev*. 2013 Aug 21. 8:CD007160.

CHAPTER - 5

Congestive Heart Failure

Introduction to Congestive Heart Failure (CHF)

Congestive Heart Failure (CHF) is a condition in which the cardiac output is inadequate to body demands and there is poor cardiac contractility and relaxation, resulting in symptoms of low cardiac out and congestion. It is a common heart disease that carries significant morbidity and mortality. CHF increases risk of death by 3 times and 60% of the patients die within 5 years of the diagnosis. Therefore it requires careful management by drugs and nondrug modalities.

Acute v/s Chronic Failure: Patients with acute failure present with breathlesness, pulmonary congestion and elevation of ventricular filling pressures. The objective of treatment is to provide immediate relief from dyspnoea and inotropic support to failing heart. In chronic heart failure symptoms of peripheral pooling of blood (oedema, hepatomegaly) and fatigue can be improved by long term use of drugs that provide functional and structural support to the failing heart and improve quality of life.

Systolic v/s Diastolic Failure: Systolic failure is a common abnormality characterized by low left ventricular ejection fraction Left Ventricular Ejection Fraction (LVEF <40%, Normal 65±8%). It is due to a large but poorly contracting heart and the predominant symptoms are fatigue and low effort tolerance. In contrast to this, the diastolic failure is characterized by near normal sized heart and LVEF but there is stiffness of ventricles, which relax poorly. This is seen as a result of persistent hypertension, aortic stenosis, chronic myocardial ischemia and cardiomyopathy. It is seen in about 40%-60% of patients with CHF. The objective of therapy is to regress hypertrophic changes so that LV relaxation improves [1].

Other terms used are high v/s low output failure; forward v/s backward failure and right v/s left heart failure. The right-sided failure is characterized by pedal oedema, distended neck veins, congestive hepatomegaly and dyspnoea. The left heart failure manifests as orthopnoea, paroxysms of nocturnal dyspnoea and pulmonary oedema. In many cases of CHF there is involvement of both the ventricles.

Epidemiology and etiology: Life time to risk of developing heart failure is 20% for Americans >40years of age Heart failure increases with age.

(a) Coronary artery disease: Arteries supply blood to heart causes decreased blood flow to heart muscle. Arteries become narrow and blocked. Heart becomes starved for oxygen and nutrients

(b) Heart attack: Coronary artery is suddenly blocked. Stopping of flow of blood to heart muscle. Arteries become narrow and blocked.

(c) Cardiomyopathy: Damage of heart muscle due to usage of more number of antibiotics or other drugs and alcoholism. Arteries become narrow and blocked. Heart becomes starved for oxygen and nutrients

(d) Conditions that over work the heart: Diabetes mellitus, hypertension and kidney diseases, Obesity, allergic reactions may also contribute Congestive Heart Failure (CHF).

Pathophysiology of Heart Failure [2]

In order to understand the role of pharmcotherapeutic agents in CHF, it is important to understand the haemodynamic and structural compensatory changes which occur in CHF. Normally cardiac output (4-6 lit/min) and stroke output (70 ml per beat) are determined by factors such as myocardial contractility, ventricular filling pressure, heart rate and peripheral vascular resistance. Diseases of heart muscle and adrenergic activity determine myocardial contractility. Two terms are commonly used:

Preload: It is Left ventricular end diastolic Pressure (LVEDP) and is determined by *venous return* and size of ventricular cavity (myocardial fiber length).

Afterload: It is the tension developed by ventricles during ejection and is determined by *peripheral vascular resistance*, ventricular wall thickness and compliance (or distensibility).

The key factor is poor myocardial contractility. This initiates a series of short and long-term compensatory neurohumoral responses in order to maintain cardiac output. However, these compensatory responses cannot sustain adequate cardiac output for a long period and thus a vicious cycle is maintained which further deteriorate cardiac performance.

Structural Changes in Chronic CHF

Hypertrophy and remodeling: Remodeling includes slow structural changes, which occur in stressed myocardium and vascular tissues. These changes are due to growth of connective tissue, apoptosis, loss of normal myocytes and vascular intimal thickening with increased wall: lumen ratio. Normal cells are replaced by fibrous tissue, which cannot contract. A-II, aldosterone, TGF and IGF play role in inducing remodeling changes. Remodeling leads to concentric hypertrophy in diseases such as hypertensive heart failure (pressure overload) and eccentric hypertrophy in cases of aortic or mitral regurgitation with CHF (volume overload).

Cardiac enlargement: Compensatory hypertrophy and dilatation of heart to normalize cardiac output, puts stress on myocardium because it has to generate extra wall tension.

$$\text{Laplace law indicates that Wall tension} = \frac{\text{Intraventricular Pressure} \times \text{Ventricular Radius}}{\text{Wall Thickness}}$$

That means a dilated heart (radius more) with normal wall thickness has to generate greater wall tension and the afterload on hypertrophied heart is less.

Contractile dysfunction: There is abnormality of contraction and relaxation, which is caused by
   (a) Reduced Ca^{++} sequestration in sarcoplasmic reticulum and greater $Na^{+}Ca^{++}$ exchange leading to accumulation of Ca^{++} inside cells. Sarcoplasmic calcium channel dysfunction is found in CHF.
   (b) Production of poorly contractile proteins by altered gene transcription, which is further contributed by activation of metalloproteinases. These result in a marked derangement of alignment of sarcomeres with matrix.
   (c) Disturbed Ca^{++} delivery to the contractile proteins

Adrenergic receptor dysfunction: β_{1-} receptors are down regulated in heart failure. Therefore, reduced Cyclic Adenosine Monophosphate (cAMP) production and subnormal Ca^{++} release and sequestration with each cardiac cycle leads to poor contractions.

Clinical Manifestation and Features

Symptoms

Dyspnea, particularly on exertion, Orthopnea, Paroxysmal nocturnal dyspnea, Exercise intolerance, Tachypnea, Cough, Fatigue, Nocturia, Hemoptysis, Abdominal pain, Anorexia, Nausea, Bloating, Poor appetite, Early satiety, Ascites, Mental status changes

Signs

Pulmonary rales, Pulmonary edema, Cool extremities, Pleural effusion, Cheyne-Stokes respiration, Tachycardia, Narrow pulse pressure, Cardiomegaly Peripheral edema, Jugular venous distension, Hepatojugular reflux, Hepatomegaly

Diagnosis with Algorithm

1. If the patient is suspected with heart failure because of history, symptoms and signs.
   - Tests to be conducted are 12-lead ECG, and/or natriuretic peptides Brain Natriuretic Peptide (BNP) N-terminal Pro-B type Natriuretic Peptide (NT pro BNP).
   - Other tests include chest X-ray, Blood tests: electrolytes, creatitnine, Full Blood Count (FBC) Liver Function Tests (LFTs), glucose, lipids, urinalysis, peak flow or spirometry.
2. If the results all are normal, heart failure unlikely, consider alternative diagnosis.
   - But if one or more abnormal results are seen, imaging by echocardiography to be done.
   - If no abnormality detected, heart failure unlikely, but if diagnostic doubt persists consider diastolic dysfunction and consider referral for specialist assessment.
3. If abnormal results are seen, assess heart failure severity, etiology, precipitating and exacerbating factors and type of cardiac dysfunction. Corelatable cause to be identified and consider referral.

Tests

Electrocardiogram: Electrocardiogram records hearts rhythm such as rapid heart beat irregular rhythm could suggest that the walls of the heart chamber are thicker than normal

Echocardiogram: An echocardiogram uses sound waves to record the hearts structure and motion. The test can determine if you already have poor blood flow, muscle damage or a heart muscle that doesn't contract normally

MRI: MRI takes pictures of heart with both still and moving pictures this allows your doctor to see if there's damage to your heart

Stress test: Stress tests show how well heart performs under different levels of stress. Making heart work harder makes it easier for your doctor to diagnose problems

Blood Tests: Blood tests can check for abnormal blood cells and infections. They can also check the level of BNP a hormone that rises with heart failure. Hyponatremia, serum sodium <130 mEq/L, is associated with reduced survival and may indicate worsening volume overload and/or disease progression

Cardiac catheterization: Cardiac catheterization can show blockage of the coronary arteries. Insertion of small tube into blood vessels and thread it from upper thigh, arm or wrist.

Management

Goals of Therapy

The therapeutic goals for chronic HF are

1. To improve quality of life,
2. Relieve or reduce symptoms, prevent or minimize hospitalizations,
3. Slow disease progression, and
4. Prolong survival.

General Approach to Treatment of Diastolic Heart Failure

(a) Symptom-Targeted Treatment:
- Decrease pulmonary venous pressure:
  Reduce left ventricular volume- Diuretics, salt restriction
  Maintain atrial contraction- Cardioversion of atrial fibrillation
  Reduce heart rate -β-Blockers, diltiazem, verapamil
- Use positive inotropic agents with caution

(b) Disease-Targeted Treatment:
- Prevent/treat myocardial ischemia- β-Blockers, diltiazem, verapamil, nitrates
- Prevent/regress ventricular hypertrophy Antihypertensive therapy

(c) Mechanism-Targeted Treatment

- Modify myocardial and extramyocardial mechanisms- Possibly ACE inhibitors or ARBs, diuretics, spironolactone
- Modify intracellular and extracellular mechanisms Possibly ACE inhibitors or ARBs, spironolactone

Pharmacological Therapy

1. **Angiotensin-converting enzymes inhibitors (ACE):** Angiotensin-II (A-II) formation is increased in CHF. Tissues can generate angiotensin-II by ACE and non ACE pathways. Angiotensim-II (A-II) has multiple deleterious effects on cardiovascular system. It is responsible for hypertrophy, remodeling and rise in peripheral vascular resistance (PVR). Renin-angiotensin system is activated early in the course of CHF and plays critical role in haemodynamic and structural changes in chronic CHF. ACE-Is are indicated in patients with systolic dysfunction (EF<40%) and are considered to be the first drug of choice for the treatment of mild to severe heart failure New York Heart Association (NYHA class I-IV). There is reduction in systemic vascular resistance (preload), heart size, and ventricular end diastolic pressure. Cardiac output increases gradually. Diuresis occurs with reduction in oedema and body weight. Heart rate is reduced and exercise capacity is increased.

   In asymptomatic patients, ACE-Is delay occurrence of frank CHF and hospitalization. They can be given with β-blockers, diuretics and digoxin. ACE inhibitors (ACE-Is) are effective in diastolic dysfunction when used along with other agents. These beneficial effects are attributed to the reductions in levels of A-II, aldosterone and sympathetic over-activity.

   Beneficial effects of ACE-Is: ACE-Is are indicated in all grades of severity of heart failure with EF<40% and left ventricular dysfunction after myocardial infarction. They are indicated even in asymptomatic patients with low ejection fraction because these agents reduce occurrence of clinical heart failure. In addition ACE-Is have protective effects in coexistent conditions like diabetic mellitus (nephropathy and retinopathy). There are several benefits with these drugs:

   1. Reversal of A-II induced cardiac structural and functional changes.
   2. Reduction in preload and afterload with subsequent reduction in cardiac work.
   3. Reduction in adrenergic overactivity and aldosterone secretion
   4. Reduced myocardial fibrosis
   5. Improvement in well-being and quality of life.

Adverse effects of ACE-Is: Hypotension may occur if diuretics are already given. Dry cough occurs in about 10-20% cases and is due to bradykinin-induced secretion of prostaglandins. Maculopapular skin rash, angioedema, neutropenia and dysguesia occur more frequently with captopril.

Table 5.1 ACE-Is Dosage regimen.

Drug	Starting dose	Target dose
Captopril	6.25-12.5 mg TID	25-50mg TID
Enalapril	1.25-2.5 mg BID	10mg BID
Ramipril	1.25-2.5mg BID	5mg BID
Lisinopril	2.5-5mg OD	20-35mg OD

Beta-Blocker

These drugs have proved to be beneficial in many ways and are now a part of standard drug treatment of CHF, along with ACE-Is and diuretics.

1. Reduction in cardiac contractions reduces wall stress, increase diastolic time for adequate cardiac filling and reduce tachycardia.
2. Reduce cardiac excitation due to sympathetic overactivity thus prptect myocardium.
3. Reverse defects in β-receptor signaling (c'AMP, β-ARK), ultimately improves c'AMP production which enhances cardiac contractions.
4. Carvedilol reduces β_3 overactivity (β_3 receptors have negative inotropic effects) and has antioxidant property also.
5. Antiarrhythmic actions of β-blockers prevent arrhythmia-induced sudden death.
6. Anti apoptotic and anti-remodeling actions are important for reversal of structural changes in CHF.
7. Overactive renin-angiotensin system is normalized.
8. Reduced β_1 receptor gene expression. Reversal of downregulation of β_1 receptors on chronic administration.

β-blockers reduce all cause mortality by 35-40%, reduce hospitalizations, worsening of CHF and prevent sudden death. There is increased exercise capacity and Cardiac Output (CO) rises gradually along with a fall in heart rate. Full benefits occur slowly over a period of 2-4 weeks. Initial doses of β-blockers are very small and dose increments are done gradually once in 2-4 weeks

Table 5.2 Beta Blockers dosage regimen.

Drug	Starting dose	Target dose
Carvedilol	3.125 mg BID	25 mg OD
Bisoprol	1.25mg OD	10mg OD
Metoprolol CR/XL	1.25-25mg OD	200mg OD

Aldosterone Antagonist

Aldosterone levels are markedLy raised (10-20 times normal) in heart failure. It is responsible for some of haemodynamic (volume overload, sodium retention & oedema) and structural changes.

Aldosterone antagonists (spironolactone and eplerenone) can reverse the structural and functional changes induced by aldosterone excess in CHF. Spironolactone is a mild K^+ conserving diuretic, which is given with thiazides or loop acting diuretics to antagonize their hypokalemic effects. It has shown a significant additional improvement as reduction in hospitalization, mortality by 30% and prevention of progression of heart failure when added in low doses (25 mg/day) with ACE-Is, diuretics, digoxin and β-blockers in resistant cases of CHF. This beneficial effect is not due to reduction in edema alone but mainly due to reduction in myocardial fibrosis and remodeling.

Eplerenone: It is another K+sparing diuretic is also found to be as effective in improving left ventricular function given after myocardial infarction in a dose of 25-50 mg/day. The advantage with eplerenone is that it does not have endocrine adverse effects (gynecomastia, impotence, menstrual disturbance) of spironolactone. Spironolactone and eplerenone are life saving agents in patients with advanced heart failure.

K+and renal function must be routinely assessed to minimize the risk of life threatening hyperkalaemia

Drug	Starting dose	Target dose
Spiranolactone	12.5 mg OD	50 mg OD
Eplerenone	25 mg OD	50 mg OD

Angiotensin Receptor Blockers (ARBs) in CHF

These agents competitively block the Angiotensin 1 (AT_1) receptors, which are responsible for mediation of actions of angiotensin-II. Candesartan induced block is surmountable while with others there is insurmountable block of Angiotensin (AT_1) receptors. ARBs are found to be as effective as ACE-Is and are indicated when the latter are not tolerated because of dry cough, angioedema or drug rashes. AT_2 receptors are not blocked by ARBs so that these receptors continue to exert cardioproective and antiproliferative effects. ARBs are slow acting thus full effects occur in 3-4 weeks.

Drug	Starting dose	Target dose
Candesartan	4 mg OD	32 mg OD
Valsartan	40 mg BID	160 mg BID

Role of Diuretics in CHF

These drugs are time-tested drugs for CHF and increase urine output, reducing oedema and breathlessness in heart failure. There is reduction in blood volume (preload) also.

Thiazides: Thiazides are effective in mild to moderate CHF. Hydrochlorothiazide (HCTZ) is commonly used agent. The diuretic dose of HCTZ is higher than antihypertensive doses. Clopamide, chlorthalidone and metolazone are other agents. Thiazides are not effective when GFR is low. Metolazone acts even when GFR is low. A small dose of K+retaining diuretic is also added to reduce hypokalemic effect. If thiazides fail or there is severe CHF then loop diuretics are needed. Thiazides show synergism with frusemide and combination is used in diuretic resistant oedema.

Loop diuretics: Frusemide, bumetanide, torasemide and ethacrynic acid are potent diuretics, which inhibit $Na^+ K^+ 2Cl^-$ symporter in the ascending limb of loop of Henle. As such these agents are effective even when Glomerular Filtration Rate (GFR) is low. Frusemine is started in low dose of 20-40 mg/day and dose increased to achieve desired volume reduction. Frusemide and bumetanide are short acting that means if these are given as a single morning dose then action wears off by afternoon and there is post dose retention of Na^+ from all segments of nephron. This Na^+ retention causes loss of diuretic efficacy and can be avoided by giving frusemide twice a day. Hypokalemia can be prevented by combining loop diuretics with spironolactone, amiloride or triamterene. Frusemide is the diuretic of choice in acute left ventricular failure/pulmonary oedema. It rapidLy reduces dyspnoea and pulmonary congestion by its venodilatory action that is observed earlier to diuretic effect. It is given as 20-40 mg i.v. and may also be given by continuous infusion at a rate of 10 mg/hr. This method reduces risk of ototoxicity and there is sustained natriuretic action.

Loop diuretics-enhance the synthesis of prostataglandins cause renal and venous dilation

Drug	Oral	Intra venal	Infusion
Furosemide	20-40 mg	40 mg	10-40g/hr
Torsemide	10-20 mg	20 mg	5-20 mg/hr
Bumetanide	1-5 mg	1mg	0.5-2 mg /hr
Ethacrynic acid	50-400 mg	0.5-1 mg	-

Thiazide Diuretics and Metolazone

Benzothiazide diuretic: Inhibit $Na^+ Cl^-$ transporter at distal portion of ascending limb and first part of the distal tubule.

Drug	Dose/PO
Metolazone	2.5-20mg
Chlorlidone	25-200mg
Hydrochlorothiazide	12.5-100mg
Chlorothiazide	500-1000mg

Limitations of diuretics: Diuretics increase renin and angiotensin-II secretion because of reduction in blood volume. Chronic use causes electrolyte disturbances (hypokalemia), raise LDL and uric acid levels and worsen diabetes mellitus. There is no reduction in mortality on long-term use. Diuretic resistance may occur.

Inotropic Drugs

Digoxin

Digoxin has positive inotropic effects; its benefits in Heart Failure (HF) are related to its neurohormonal effects. Digoxin attenuates the excessive sympathetic nervous system activation present in HF patients, by reducing central sympathetic outflow and improving impaired baroreceptor function.

It also increases parasympathetic activity in HF patients and decreases heart rate, thus enhancing diastolic filling. Digoxin does not improve survival in patients with HF but does provide symptomatic benefits.

- In patients with HF and supraventricular tachyarrhythmias such as atrial fibrillation, digoxin should be considered early in therapy to help control ventricular response rate.
- For patients in normal sinus rhythm, effects on symptom reduction and quality-of-life improvement are evident in patients with mild to severe HF. Therefore, it should be used together with standard HF therapies (ACE inhibitors, β-blockers, and diuretics) in patients with symptomatic HF to reduce hospitalizations.
- Doses should be adjusted to achieve plasma digoxin concentration of 0.5to 1 ng/mL.

Dobutamine: It is a derivative of dopamine and has β_1-agonistic action. It increases cardiac contractility but heart rate does not rise much in usual doses. It is therefore a cardiotonic agent. It reduces sympathetic activity in CHF. It must be given intravenously in a dose of 2.5 μg/kg/minute and can be increased upto 20 μg/kg/minute. It may stimulate vascular β_2 receptors and thus causes hypotension.

It is indicated in the treatment of acute heart failure with systolic dysfunction and pump failure in acute myocardial infarction.

It is also used in β-blocker poisoning and, as a short-term inotropic drug in severe acute decompensation in chronic heart failure and during cardiac surgery.

Adverse effects are cardiac rhythm disturbances, hypotension, nausea and vomiting.

Dopamine: It is used in shock to raise blood pressure and to improve renal perfusion by acting on renal vascular dopaminergic receptors in low doses causing renal vasodilation. A higher dose stimulates heart by β_1 agonist action and in still higher doses α-adrenergic action causes peripheral vasoconstriction and raises PVR. In refractory heart failure with hypotension it is used in a dose of 0.5-1.0 μg/kg/minute and dose increased upto 5-10 μg/kg/minute. It is contraindicated in ventricular extrasystoles and VT.

Milrinone: It is a bipyridine and is more selective inhibitor of PDE-III than amrinone. It is about 10 times more potent and can be used orally. Its half-life is short (1 hour). It does not cause thrombocytopenia so is a preferred inotrope.

In acute heart failure i.v. milrinone is given as a freshly prepared solution in a dose of 50 µg/kg in 10 minutes, initially and then as an infusion at a rate of 0.25-1.00 µg/kg/minute for 1-2 days. It can be given concurrently with ACE Inhibitors (ACE-Is), dobutamine or dopamine.

Vasodilators

Nitroprusside

- **Sodium nitroprusside** is a mixed arterial-venous vasodilator that acts directly on vascular smooth muscle to increase cardiac index and decrease venous pressure.
  Hypotension is an important dose-limiting adverse effect of nitroprusside and other vasodilators.
  Nitroprusside is effective in the short-term management of severe HF in a variety of settings (e.g., acute MI, valvular regurgitation, after coronary bypass surgery, decompensated HF). Nitroprusside has a rapid onset and a duration of action of less than 10 minutes, used as continuous IV infusions.
  It should be initiated at a low dose (0.1 to 0.2 mcg/kg/min) to avoid excessive hypotension, and then increased by small increments (0.1 to 0.2 mcg/kg/min).

Nitroglycerin

- The major hemodynamic effects of IV **nitroglycerin** are decreased preload and Pulmonary Artery Occulusion Pressure (PAOP) because of functional venodilation and mild arterial vasodilation. It is used primarily as a preload reducer for patients with pulmonary congestion.

Nesiritide: A family of endogenous neurohormones such as atrial natriuretic peptide (ANP), brain natriuretic peptide (BNP) and C-type peptide are secreted by atrial and ventricular myocytes. BNP is secreted in response to stretch and its circulating levels parallel with severity of heart failure. Circulating BNP opposes actions of angiotensin-II and noradrenaline. Recombinant form of human-BNP has diuretic, natriuretic and vasodilatory actions. Vasorelaxation is mediated by activation of guanylate cyclase and production of NO. Nitric Oxide has a short half-life of 18 minutes and has to be given i.v.. It is administrered in a dose of 25 µg/kg initially and then as an infusion of 0.01-0.03 µg/kg/minute.

It reduces right and left ventricular End Diastolic Volume (EDVs) and pulmonary capillary pressure. There is fall in Peripheral Vascular Resistance (PVR), rise in cardiac output and diuresis in acute heart failure.

Treatments Recommended in All Symptomatic Patients (New York Heart Association Class II-IV) with Heart Failure with Reduced Ejection Fraction (HFrEF)

- ➤ An ACE Inhibitor is recommended, in addition to a beta-blocker, for symptomatic patients with hfref to reduce the risk of HF hospitalization and death
- ➤ A beta-blocker is recommended, in addition an ACE-I, for patients with stable, symptomatic HFrEF to reduce the risk of HF hospitalization and death

➢ A Mineralocorticoid receptor antagonist (MRA)is recommended for patients with HFrEF, who remain symptomatic despite treatment with an ACE-I and a beta-blocker, to reduce the risk of HF hospitalization and death

Other Pharmacological Treatments Recommended in Selected Patients with Symptomatic (NYHA Class II-IV) Heart Failure with Reduced Ejection Fraction

➢ Diuretics are recommended in order to improve symptoms and exercise capacity in patients with signs and/or symptoms of congestion. Diuretics should be considered to reduce the risk of HF hospitalization in patients with signs and/or symptoms of congestion.

➢ Angiotensin receptor neprilysin inhibitor Sacubitril/Valsartan is recommended as a replacement for an ACE Inhibitors (ACE-I) to further reduce the risk of Heart Failure (HF) hospitalization and death in ambulatory patients with HFrEF who remain symptomatic despite optimal treatment with an ACE-I, a beta-blocker and an Magnetic Resonance Angiography (MRA)

➢ HCN channel Blocker inhibitor Ivabradine should be considered to reduce the risk of Heart Failure (HF) hospitalization or cardiovascular death in symptomatic patients with LVEF ≤35%, in sinus rhythm and a resting heart rate ≥70 bpm despite treatment with an evidence-based dose of betablocker (or maximum tolerated dose below that), ACE-I (or ARB), and an MRA (or ARB)

➢ Angiotensin Receptor Blocker (ARB): An ARB is recommended to reduce the risk of (HF) hospitalization and cardiovascular death in symptomatic patients unable to tolerate an ACE-I (patients should also receive a beta-blocker and an MRA). An ARB may be considered to reduce the risk of (HF) hospitalization and death in patients who are symptomatic despite treatment with a beta-blocker who are unable to tolerate an MRA.

➢ Hydralazine and isosorbide dinitrate: Hydralazine and isosorbide dinitrate may be considered in symptomatic patients with HFrEF who can tolerate neither an ACE-I nor an ARB (or they are contra-indicated) to reduce the risk of death.

➢ Digoxin: Digoxin may be considered in symptomatic patients in sinus rhythm despite treatment with an ACE-I (or ARB), a beta-blocker and an MRA, to reduce the risk of hospitalization (both all-cause and (HF) hospitalizations)

➢ N-3 PUFA: An n-3 PUFAe preparation may be considered in symptomatic HF patients to reduce the risk of cardiovascular hospitalization and cardiovascular death.

Treatments (or Combinations of Treatments) That May Cause Harm in Patients with Symptomatic (NYHA Class II–IV) Heart Failure with Reduced Ejection Fraction

➢ Thiazolidinediones (glitazones) are not recommended in patients with HF, as they increase the risk of HF worsening and HF hospitalization.

➢ NSAIDs or COX-2 inhibitors are not recommended in patients with HF, as they increase the risk of HF worsening and HF hospitalization.

➢ Diltiazem or verapamil are not recommended in patients with HFrEF, as they increase the risk of HF worsening and HF hospitalization

> The addition of an ARB (or renin inhibitor) to the combination of an ACE-I and an MRA is not recommended in patients with HF, because of the increased risk of renal dysfunction and hyperkalaemia.

Treatment of Heart Failure with Preserved Ejection Fraction

Recommendations for treatment of patients with heart failure with preserved ejection fraction and heart failure with mid-range ejection fraction

> It is recommended to screen patients with (HFpEF) or (HFmrEF) for both cardiovascular and noncardiovascular comorbidities, which, if present, should be treated, provided safe and effective interventions exist to improve symptoms, well-being and/or prognosis.

> Diuretics are recommended in congested patients with (HFpEF) or (HFmrEF) in order to alleviate symptoms and signs.

Recommendations for initial management of a rapid ventricular rate in patients with heart failure and atrial fibrillation in the acute or chronic setting

> Urgent electrical cardioversion is recommended if Atrial Fibranation (AF) is thought to be contributing to the patient's haemodynamic compromise in order to improve the patient clinical condition.

> For patients in NYHA Class IV, in addition to treatment for AHF, an intravenous bolus of amiodarone or, in digoxin-naïve patients, an intravenous bolus of digoxin should be considered to reduce the ventricular rate.

> For patients in NYHA Class I–III, a beta-blocker, usually given orally, is safe and therefore is recommended ventricular rate, provided the patient is euvolaemic.

> For patients in NYHA Class I–III, digoxin, should be considered when ventricular rate remains highd despite beta-blockers or when beta-blockers are not tolerated or contra-indicated.

> AV node catheter ablation may be considered to control heart rate and relieve symptoms in patients unresponsive or intolerant to intensive pharmacological rate and rhythm control therapy, accepting that these patients will become pacemaker dependent.

> Treatment with dronedarone to improve ventricular rate control is not recommended due to safety concerns.

References

1. Seth SD &Seth S. Drug therapy of heart failure. In Seth SD, Text book of Pharmacology, 2nd Ed, New Delhi, Elsevier, 1999, pp 305-317.

2. Masse BM, Granger CB. Cardiac failure. In Tierney, McPhee SJ Papadkis MA, Editors, Current Medical diagnosis and treatment, 44th Ed, New Delhi, Lange 2005, pp 374-386.

CHAPTER - 6

Hypertension

Introduction to Hypertension

Hypertension also known as high blood pressure, in which there is Persistently elevated arterial blood pressure, which can lead to increase in risk of heart disease, stroke and death.

During systole, the left ventricle contracts, ejecting blood systemically into the arteries, causing a sharp rise in arterial BP. This is the systolic BP (SBP). The left ventricle then relaxes during diastole, and arterial BP decreases to a trough value as blood returns to the right atria and ventricle of the heart from the venous system. This is the diastolic BP (DBP). When recording BP (e.g., 120/76 mmHg), the numerator refers to SBP and the denominator refers to DBP. BP has a predictable diurnal rhythm, with fluctuations throughout the day. Values are lowest during the nighttime, sharply rise starting in the early morning, and peak in the late morning to early afternoon. Mean arterial pressure (MAP) is sometimes used to represent BP. MAP collectively reflects both SBP and DBP, with one-third of the pressure from SBP and two-thirds from DBP. It is calculated using the following equation

$$MAP = ([SBP] \cdot [1/3]) + ([DBP] \cdot [2/3])$$

An increase in cardiac output (CO) normally results in a compensatory decrease in total peripheral resistance (TPR); likewise, an increase in TPR results in a decrease in CO. These events regulate MAP, as is represented in the following equation

$$MAP = CO \cdot TPR$$

Hypervolemia due to renal artery stenosis, renal disease, hyperaldosteronism, aortic coarction, pregnancy); stress; pheochromocytoma lead to increased cardiac output.

Stress (sympathetic activation); atherosclerosis; renal artery disease; thyroid dysfunction; diabetes; cerebral ischemia lead to incresed systemic vascular resisitance.

	SYSTOLIC	DIASTOLIC
Normal blood pressure	less than 120 mmHg	less than 80 mmHg
Elevated	between 120 to 129 mmHg	less than 80 mmHg
Stage-1 HTN	between 130 to 139 mmHg	between 80 and 89 mmHg
Stage-2 HTN	at least 140 mmHg	at least 90 mmHg
HTN crisis	over 180 mmHg	over 120 mmHg

Epidemology

Overall prevalence of hypertension in India is 29.8%. Men are prone to high BP compared to women before the age of 45 years. But between 45 and 54 years it is slightly higher in women. After 55 years of age, still higher percentage than men. BP increases with age and it is very commonly seen in the elderly population.

Types

1. **Essential hypertension:** Higher blood pressure without any identifiable cause is called Primary Hypertension (90-95%).
2. **Secondary Hypertension:** If hypertension is caused by specific identifiable cause it is called Secondary Hypertension. Accounts for 5-10% of total cases.
3. **Pseudohypertension:** In this condition the blood vessels become stiff and thick because of calcification and resist compression from the bladder of the inflatable BP cuff. But it is very rare.
4. **White–coat hypertension:** The patients who have consistently elevated BP values when measured

in a clinical environment in the presence of health care professional. But when measured elsewhere or with 24-hour ambulatory monitoring, BP is not elevated. At minimum, patients with white-coat hypertension should be treated with lifestyle modifications.

Hypertensive Crisis: If BP is markedLy elevated i.e. BP >180/110 mm Hg it is called hypertensice crisis. It is classified as a) Hypertensive emergency, where there is acute or progressive target organ damage or b) Hypertensive urgency where there is no acute or progressive target organ damage. Hypertensive emergencies require hospitalisation for lowering of BP by using IV medictions. Hypertensive urgencies do not require hospitalisation and BP can be reduced within 24 hrs by using medications.

Etiology

Primary Hypertension (90-95%)

- **Genetic:** May be due to mutations or genetic abnormalities inherited from the parents
- **Environment:** Unhealthy lifestyle like lack of physical activity and poor diet can lead to weight problems. Overweight can cause increase in the blood pressure.

Secondary Hypertension (5-10%)

- **Chronic kidney disease:** Any pathologic processes (e.g., diabetic nephropathy, glomerulonephritis) can damage nephrons in the kidney. When this occurs, the kidney cannot excrete normal amounts of sodium which leads to sodium and water retention, increased blood volume, and increased cardiac output by the Frank-Starling mechanism. Renal disease may also result in increased release of renin leading to a renin-dependent form of hypertension.

- **Hyperaldosteronism:** Increased secretion of aldosterone generally results from adrenal adenoma or adrenal hyperplasia. Increased circulating aldosterone causes renal retention of sodium and water, so blood volume and arterial pressure increase.
- **Hyperglucocorticoidism (Cushing's Syndrome):** In this disease, excess of cortisol hormone is released in the body. Cortisol main function is to maintain blood sugar level, water balance and salt balance so that blood pressure can be maintained. so excess salt retention and increase in blood pressure.
- Growth hormone excess: Acromegaly
- **Pheochromocytoma:** Catecholamine secreting tumors in the adrenal medulla can lead to very high levels of circulating catecholamines (both epinephrine and norepinephrine). This leads to alpha-adrenoceptor mediated systemic vasoconstriction and beta-adrenoceptor mediated cardiac stimulation, both of which contribute to significant elevations in arterial pressure.
- Pre-eclampsia: This is a condition that sometimes develops during the third trimester of pregnancy that causes hypertension due to increased <u>blood volume</u> and tachycardia.
- **Renal artery stenosis (Renovascular disease):** Renal artery disease can cause of narrowing of the vessel lumen (stenosis). The reduced lumen diameter increases the pressure drop along the length of the diseased artery, which reduces the pressure at the afferent arteriole in the kidney. Reduced arteriolar pressure and reduced renal perfusion stimulate renin release by the kidney. This increases circulating angiotensin II (AII) and aldosterone. These hormones increase blood volume by enhancing renal reabsorption of sodium and water. Increased AII causes systemic vasoconstriction and enhances sympathetic activity. Chronic elevation of AII promotes cardiac and vascular hypertrophy. The net effect of these renal mechanisms is an increase in blood volume that augments cardiac output by the Frank-Starling mechanism. Therefore, hypertension caused by renal artery stenosis results from both an increase in systemic vascular resistance and an increase in cardiac output.
- **Hyper- or hypothyroidism:** Excessive thyroid hormone induces systemic vasoconstriction, an increase in blood volume, and increased cardiac activity, all of which can lead to hypertension. It is less clear why some patients with hypothyroidism develop hypertension, but it may be related to decreased tissue metabolism reducing the release of vasodilator metabolites, thereby producing vasoconstriction and increased systemic vascular resistance.
- **Obstructive sleep apnoea:** There is sympathetic activation and hormonal changes due to repeated hypoxia, stress associated from loss of sleep.
- **Coarction of the aorta:** There is reduced systemic blood flow, esp. renal blood flow. So leads to release of renin and activation of Renin-Angiotensin-Aldosterone System (RAAS) pathway. Inturn elevation of blood volume and arterial pressure.

Prescription Drugs
- Adrenal steroids (e.g., Prednisone, Fludrocortisone, triamcinolone)
- Calcineurin inhibitors (Cyclosporine and Tacrolimus)

- Amphetamines/anorexiants (e.g., Phendimetrazine
- Decongestants (Phenylpropanolamine and Analogs)
- Erythropoiesis stimulating agents (Erythropoietin and Darbepoietin)
- Nonsteroidal antiinflammatory drugs, cyclooxygenase-2 inhibitors
- Others: venlafaxine, bromocriptine, bupropion, buspirone, carbamazepine, clozapine, desulfrane, ketamine, metoclopramide

Street Drugs and other Natural Products

- Cocaine and cocaine withdrawal
- Ephedra alkaloids (e.g., Ma-huang), "herbal ecstasy,"
- Phenylpropanolamine analogs-methylphenidate, phencyclidine, ketamine, ergotamine and other ergot-containing herbal products

Risk Factors

- Age (>55 years for men and > 65 years for women): Age increases the arteries to stiffen and narrow due to plaque buildup.
- Family history: High BP is seen commonly in families.
- Being obese: The more the weight of the person, the more blood supply is needed to supply oxygen and nutrients to the tissues. As the amount of blood flow increases through the blood vessels the pressure also increases.
- Physical inactivity: If physical inactive, there is increased heart rate. There is increased workload on the heart to pump the blood.
- Using tobacco: Smoking or chewing tobacco increases BP, and the chemicals in tobacco damage the lining of artery walls. So there is narrrowing of arteries and causes increased risk of heart disease.
- Alcohol: Heavy drinking usually causes damage to heart and affects the Blood pressure.
- Dyslipidemia (elevated low-density lipoprotein-cholesterol, total cholesterol, and/or triglycerides; low highdensity lipoprotein-cholesterol): High levels of lipids increase the likelyhood of plaques or blood clots forming in the arteries.
- Hypokalemia: Potassium balances the amount of sodium in cells. Less amount of potassium due to dehydration, or from diet, sodium builds up in the cells.
- **Stress:** High levels of stress can lead to a temporary increase in blood pressure. Stress-related habits such as eating more, using tobacco or drinking alcohol can lead to further increases in blood pressure.

Pathophysiology for Hypertension [1]

Arterial Blood Pressure

Arterial BP is hemodynamically generated by the interplay between blood flow and the resistance to blood flow. It is mathematically defined as the product of cardiac output and total peripheral resistance according to the following equation:

$$BP = \text{Cardiac Output (CO)} \times \text{Total Peripheral Resistance (TPR)}$$

Cardiac output is the major determinant of SBP, whereas total peripheral resistance largely determines DBP. In turn, cardiac output is a function of stroke volume, heart rate, and venous capacitance.

Blood pressure is the mathematical product of cardiac output and peripheral resistance. Elevated blood pressure can result from increased cardiac output and/or increased total peripheral resistance.

Increased Cardiac Output

Increased cardiac preload:
- Increased fluid volume from excess sodium intake or renal sodium retention (from reduced   number of nephrons or decreased glomerular filtration)

Venous constriction:
- Excess stimulation of the RAAS
- Sympathetic nervous system overactivity

Increased peripheral resistance

Functional vascular constriction:

- Excess stimulation of the RAAS
- Sympathetic nervous system overactivity
- Genetic alterations of cell membranes
- Endothelial-derived factors

Structural vascular hypertrophy:

- Excess stimulation of the RAAS
- Sympathetic nervous system overactivity
- Genetic alterations of cell membranes
- Endothelial-derived factors
- Hyperinsulinemia resulting from obesity or the metabolic syndrome

Neurogenic Control

The baroreceptor reflex system is the major negative-feedback mechanism that controls sympathetic activity. Baroreceptors are nerve endings lying in the walls of large arteries, especially in the carotid arteries and aortic arch. Changes in arterial pressure rapidLy activate baroreceptors that then transmit impulses to the brainstem through the ninth cranial nerve and vagus nerves. In this reflex system, a decrease in arterial BP stimulates baroreceptors, causing reflex vasoconstriction and increased heart rate and force of cardiac contraction. These baroreceptor reflex mechanisms may be blunted (less responsive to changes in BP) in the elderly and those with diabetes.

Renin-angiotensin Aldosterone System (RAAS)

The RAAS regulates sodium, potassium, and fluid balance. Juxtaglomerular cells function as a baroreceptor-sensing device. Decreased renal artery pressure and kidney blood flow are sensed by these cells and stimulate secretion of renin. decrease in sodium and chloride delivered to the distal tubule stimulates renin release. Catecholamines increase renin release probably by directly stimulating sympathetic nerves on the afferent arterioles that in turn activate the juxtaglomerular cells. Decreased serum potassium and/or intracellular calcium are detected by the juxtaglomerular cells resulting in renin secretion.

Renin catalyzes the conversion of angiotensinogen to angiotensin I in the blood. Angiotensin I is then converted to angiotensin II by angiotensin-converting enzyme (ACE). After binding to specific receptors (classified as either AT1 or AT2 subtypes), angiotensin II exerts biologic effects in several tissues. The AT1 receptor is located in brain, kidney, myocardium, peripheral vasculature, and the adrenal glands. These receptors mediate most responses that are critical to CV and kidney function. The AT2 receptor is located in adrenal medullary tissue, uterus, and brain. Stimulation of the AT2 receptor does not influence BP regulation.

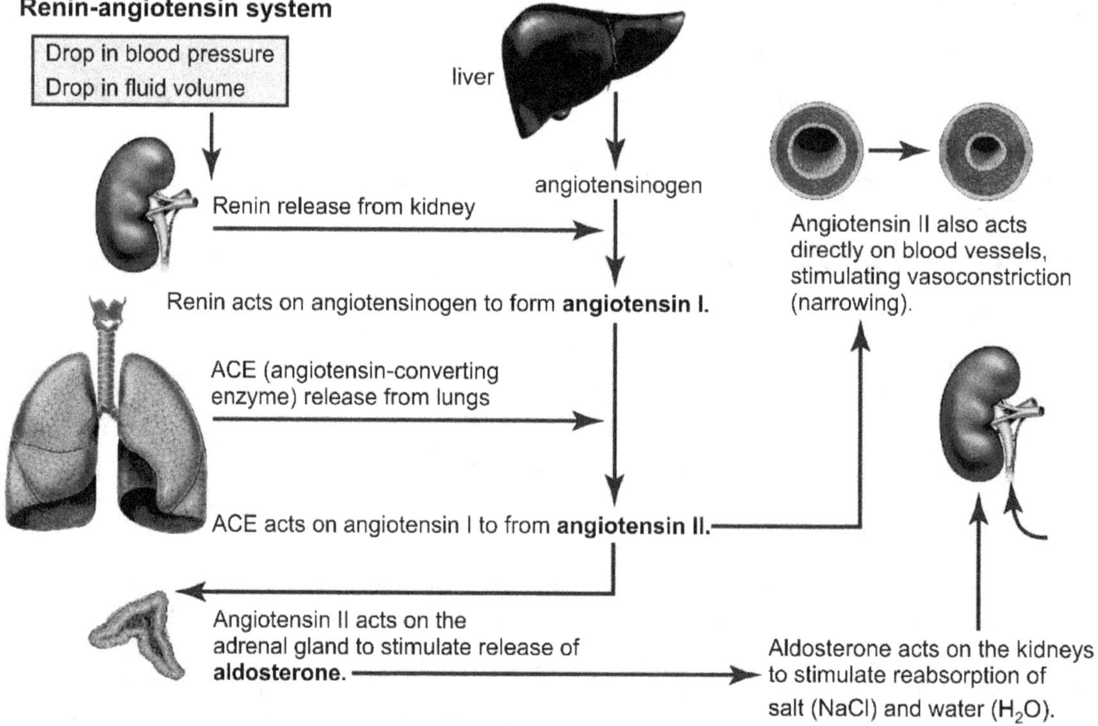

Fig. 6.1 Regulation of blood pressure.

Source: By Renin-angiotensin-aldosterone system. Britannica, The Editors of Encyclopaedia. "renin-angiotensin system". Encyclopedia Britannica, 11 Feb. 2023.

Circulating angiotensin II can elevate BP through pressor and volume effects. Pressor effects include direct vasoconstriction, stimulation of catecholamine release from the adrenal medulla, and centrally mediated increases in sympathetic nervous system activity.

Angiotensin II also stimulates aldosterone synthesis from the adrenal cortex. This leads to sodium and water reabsorption that increases plasma volume, total peripheral resistance, and ultimately BP.

Atrial Natriuretic Peptide

Atrial natriuretic peptide (ANP) is released from atrial granules. It produces natriuresis, diuresis and a modest decrease in blood pressure, while decreasing plasma renin and aldosterone. Natriuretic peptides also alter synaptic transmission from the osmoreceptors. ANP is released as a result of the stimulation of atrial stretch receptors. ANP concentrations are increased by raised filling pressures and in patients with arterial hypertension and left ventricular hypertrophy as the wall of the left ventricle participates in the secretion of ANP.

Eicosanoids

Arachidonic acid metabolites alter blood pressure through direct effects on vascular smooth muscle tone and interactions with other vasoregulatory systems: autonomic nervous system, renin–angiotensin–aldosterone system, and other humoral pathways. In hypertensive patients, vascular endothelial cell dysfunction could lead to reduction in endothelium-derived relaxing factors such as nitric oxide, prostacyclin, and endothelium-derived hyperpolarizing factor, or increased production of contracting factors such as endothelin-1 and thromboxane A2.

Kallikrein-kinin Systems

Tissue kallikreins act on kininogen to form vasoactive peptides. The most important is the vasodilator bradykinin. Kinins play a role in the regulation of renal blood flow and water and sodium excretion. ACE inhibitors decrease the breakdown of bradykinin into inactive peptides.

Endothelial Mechanisms

Nitric oxide is produced in the endothelium, relaxes the vascular epithelium, and is a very potent vasodilator. The nitric oxide system is an important regulator of arterial BP. Patients with hypertension may have an intrinsic deficiency in nitric oxide, resulting in inadequate vasodilation.

Peripheral Autoregulatory Components

Local autoregulatory processes maintain adequate tissue oxygenation. When tissue oxygen demand is normal to low, the local arteriolar bed remains relatively vasoconstricted. However, increases in metabolic demand trigger arteriolar vasodilation that lowers peripheral vascular resistance and increases blood flow and oxygen delivery through autoregulation. Intrinsic defects in these renal adaptive mechanisms could lead to plasma volume expansion and increased blood flow to peripheral tissues, even when BP is normal.

Adrenal Steroids

Mineralo- and glucocorticoids increase blood pressure. This effect is mediated by sodium and water retention (mineralocorticoids) or increased vascular reactivity (glucocorticoids). In addition, glucocorticoids and mineralocorticoids increase vascular tone by upregulating the receptors of pressor hormones such as angiotensin II.

Renomedullary Vasodepression

Renomedullary interstitial cells, located mainly in the renal papilla, secrete an inactive substance medullipin I. This lipid is transformed in the liver into medullipin II. This substance exerts a prolonged hypotensive effect, possibly by direct vasodilatation, inhibition of sympathetic drive in response to hypotension, and a diuretic action. It is hypothesized that the activity of the renomedullary system is controlled by renal medullary blood flow.

Sodium and Water Excretion

Sodium and water retention are associated with an increase in blood pressure. It is postulated that sodium, via the sodium–calcium exchange mechanism, causes an increase in intracellular calcium in vascular smooth muscle resulting in increased vascular tone.

The primary cause of sodium and water retention may be an abnormal relationship between pressure and sodium excretion resulting from reduced renal blood flow, reduced nephron mass, and increased angiotensin or mineralocorticoids. Altered calcium homeostasis also may play an important role in the pathogenesis of hypertension. A lack of dietary calcium hypothetically can disturb the balance between intracellular and extracellular calcium, resulting in an increased intracellular calcium concentration. This imbalance can alter vascular smooth muscle function by increasing peripheral vascular resistance.

Clinical Manifestation and Features

Symptoms

- Most patients are asymptomatic.

Signs

- Previous BP values in the prehypertension or hypertension category.

Diagnosis with Algorithm[2]

- Elevated BP may be only sign of primary HTN
- Signs of end organ damage occurs in eye, brain, heart and kidneys
- Fundoscopic examination:
    - Reveals arteriolar narrowing (or) focal artery narrowing (or) constriction
    - Papilledema indicates hypertensive emergency

- Cardiopulmonary examination:
  - Reveals abnormal heart beat and Left Ventricular (LV) hypertrophy
- Peripheral examination of vessels:
- Reveals abdominal (or) aortic Bruits

Laboratory Tests

- BUN/Serum creatinine test
- Fasting blood glucose
- Albumin to creatine ratio
- Glomerular Filtration Rate (GFR)
- Serum electrolytes

Laboratory Tests for Secondary HTN

- Plasma norepinephrine and urinary meta epinephrine levels in pheochromocytoma
- Plasma and urinary aldosterone concentration in primary aldosteronism
- Plasma renin activity
- Captopril stimulation test

Diagnostic Algorithm for Hypertension

- ➤ If a person identifies elevated BP reading –office, home or pharmacy.
- ➤ If it is the first visit, history, physical examination and diagnostic tests to be performed. If BP ≥ 180/110 it is confirmed as hypertension.
- ➤ And if automated office BP ≥ 135/85 and office BP measurement is ≥ 140/90, the person has to be tested for "out of office assessment". By ambulatory BP measurement (ABPM) and home BP measurement (HBPM) methods.
- ➤ Now in the 2nd visit within 1 month to the clinic daytime ABPM or HBPM ≥ 135/85, it is confirmed as hypertension. If the BP is not ≥ 135/85, it is decided as person does not have hypertension.

Evaluation Pattern for Hypertension in Childhood (Secondary Hypertension)

- ➤ Check accuracy of blood pressure measurements, rule out diet and drug-related causes.
- ➤ History, physical examination and laboratory tesing to be done
- ➤ No clinical clues, but secondary hypertension, remains a concern
  - (a) Child/adolescent: perform urinalysis/urine culture/renal ultrasonsography and followed by echocardiography.
  - (b) Young adult: MRI with gadolinium contrast media or CT renal artery and echocardiography.

(c) MiddLe aged adult: Rennin and aldosterone levels, polysomnography, 24-hour urinary cortisol.

(d) Older adult: MRI with gadolinium contrast media or CT renal artery, TSH analysis, urinalysis, 24-hour urinary cortisol.

Diagnostic Algorithm for Hypertensive emergency

If the patient is suspected with possible hypertensive emergency-Evaluate specific condition causing/associated with hypertension:

- Pregnancy
- Aortic dissection
- Acute pulmonary edema
- Type-I myocardial infacrtion
- Cerebrovascular accident
- Sclerodera renal crisis
- Sympathomimetic intoxication
- Pheocromocytoma
- Hypertension due to uncontrolled pain/anxiety

If any of the above conditions are met, he is a candidate of secondary hypertension. Evaluate and treat using specific strategies.

If he is not having any of the above conditions described, meets the criteria for hypertensive emergency. Check for any target organ damage like acute kidney injury, type 1 myocardial infacrtion, hypertensive encephalopathy or pulmonary edema. He is a candidiate for primary hypertensive emergency and immediate BP control required using IV antihypertensives-nicardipine infusion.

Management

Non Pharmacological

Includes life style modifications such as

- Weight loss in case of over weight
- Dietary sodium restriction ideally 1.5g-3.8g/day
- Regular physical activity
- Moderate alcohol consumption
- Smoking cessation
- Changes in the diet plan

Lifestyle modification alone is appropriate therapy for patients with prehypertension. Patients diagnosed with stage 1 or 2 hypertension should be placed on lifestyle modifications and drug therapy concurrently.

Pharmacological Therapy

Most patients with stage 1 hypertension should be treated initially with a thiazide diuretic, angiotensin-converting enzyme (ACE) inhibitor, angiotensin II receptor blocker (ARB), or calcium channel blocker (CCB). Combination therapy is recommended for patients with stage 2 disease, with one of the agents being a thiazide-type diuretic unless contraindications exist.

Classes of drugs used in the treatment of hypertension are listed below.

1. Diuretics
   - thiazide diuretics (Hydrochlorothiazide)
   - loop diuretics (Furosemide)
   - potassium-sparing diuretics (Spironolactone)
2. Vasodilators
   - alpha-adrenoceptor antagonists (alpha-blockers) [Prazosin]
   - angiotensin converting enzyme inhibitors (ACE inhibitors) [Enalapril]
   - angiotensin receptor blockers (ARBs) [Losartan]
   - calcium-channel blockers (Nifedipine)
   - direct acting arterial dilators (Hydralazine)
   - ganglionic blockers
   - nitrodilators
   - potassium-channel openers
3. Cardioinhibitory drugs
   - beta-blockers (Propranolol)
   - calcium-channel blockers (Verapamil)
4. Centrally acting sympatholytics (Clonidine)
   1. **Diuretics**
      (i) **Thiazides and Related Agents:** Primary Mechanisms of Action: Thiazide diuretics reduce the reabsorption of sodium and chloride in the early part of the distal convoluted tubule of the kidney by inhibiting Na^+Cl^- symport at the luminal membrane. This results in the delivery of increased amounts of sodium to the distal tubule, where some of it is exchanged for potassium. The net result is increased excretion of sodium, potassium and water. Circulating volume is diminished, reducing preload on the heart and, thus, cardiac output and blood pressure. With long-term therapy, autoregulation by the body's own compensatory mechanisms results in vasodilatation, reduction of peripheral vascular resistance and return of the cardiac output to normal. Thiazides also have some direct vasodilatory properties. They've efficacy of up to 10-15 mm Hg when administered alone and perhaps more when used in combination with other agents. Pharmacokinetics - Thiazides are rapidLy absorbed orally and pro duce a prolonged diuresis. They tend to produce a maximal response at relatively low

doses, such as 12.5mg hydro-chlorothiazide or 1.25mg Bendroflumethiazide. Further increases in dose simply increase side effects with little further effect on blood pressure.

On the whole, standard doses of thiazides lower blood pressure as much as other first-line antihypertensives. In some patient groups, such as blacks and the elderly, the thiazides are particularly efficacious. However, they tend to be less effective in younger, white patients. Thiazides are used in patients with mild to moderate hypertension and normal cardiac/renal function.

Side effects: Hypokalaemia Acute gout, Impotence Thiazides can increase serum LDL-cholesterol and triglyceride levels. Rarer side effects include nausea, headache, rashes, photosensitivity and blood dyscrasias.

(ii) **Loop Diuretics (High ceiling diuretics):** Loop diuretics act by inhibiting Na^+-K^+-$2Cl^-$ transporter in the thick ascending limb of the loop of Henle and inhibit the reabsorption of chloride, sodium and potassium. They produce a brisk but short-lived diuresis and are thus unsuitable as first-line agents for hypertension, as they do not provide 24-hour control. However, they do have a role in patients with impaired renal function in whom thiazides are ineffective, and in patients with hypertension resistant to multiple drug therapy, who are often fluid overloaded. They may be synergistic with agents such as the ACE inhibitors.

Furosemide

Side Effects: dehydration, most metabolic effects are same as in case of thiazides (i.e., hypokalemia, impaired diabetes control, increased LDL/HDL)

(iii) **Potassium-Sparing Diuretics:** Potassium-Sparing Diuretics are often used: 1) in combination with other diuretics (i.e., thiazides) to prevent or correct hypokalemia; 2) to avoid potassium depletion in patients taking digitalis.

Spironolactone: Spironolactone antagonizes effect of aldosterone, with a particular role in primary hyperaldosteronism or Conn's syndrome.

Side Effects: Hyperkalemia, gynecomastia

Triamterene: Weak antihypertensive activity of its own.

Side Effects: Hyperkalemia, gastrointestinal disturbances

Thiazide diuretics are available as fixed-dose combinations with potassium-sparing or other antihypertensive drugs. Thiazide diuretics Often used in combination with antihypertensive agents that impair vascular responsiveness (i.e., vasodilators) since blood pressure can become very sensitive to blood volume in the presence of these agents. Potassium supplements can be prescribed to compensate for hypokalemia. The thiazides are not useful in patients with renal insufficiency (glomerular filtration rate < 40 ml/min).

Vasodilators

(i) **Alpha-blockers**

Alpha 1 Blockers Usual Dosage range

Prazosin 1-10 mg BID

Terazosin 1-20 mg daily

Doxazosin 1-16 mg daily

The α_1 adrenoceptor blockers produce vasodilatation by blocking the action of noradrenaline at post-synaptic α_1 receptors in both arteries and veins. This results in a fall in peripheral resistance, without a compensatory rise in cardiac output. The prototype α_1-blocker — prazosin — is short acting and tends to produce precipitous falls in blood pressure. Doxazosin combines the advantage of a more gentle reduction in blood pressure with the longer duration of action, permitting once daily dosing.

Side effects: Dizziness (10% of patients), headaches (8% of patients), weakness (7% patients); decrease LDL/HDL. α_1-blockers are, on the whole, well tolerated. In women-urinary incontinence. In men-they may improve the symptoms of benign prostatic hypertrophy.

(ii) **ACE inhibitors:** ACE Inhibitors Usual Dosage Range

Quinapril 5-40 mg daily

Ramipril 1.25-10 mg daily

Captopril 12.5-50 mg daily

Perindopril 2-8 mg daily

Benazepril 5-40 mg daily

Cilazapril 1-10 mg daily

Enalapril 5-40 mg daily -converted to metabolite enalaprilat

Lisinopril 5-40 mg daily - lysine derivative of enalaprilat

Fosinopril 10-40 mg daily

Angiotensin converting enzyme (ACE) inhibitors work by blocking the renin-angiotensin system, inhibiting the conversion of the inactive angiotensin I to the powerful vasoconstrictor and stimulator of aldosterone release, angiotensin II. This results in decreased peripheral vascular resistance and reduction in the levels of the sodium-retaining hormone — aldosterone.

ACE inhibitors may improve endothelial function and reduce central adrenergic tone. They also have beneficial effects on renal haemodynamics, reducing intraglomerular hypertension, resulting in improvements in proteinuric renal disease. ACE inhibitors are effective as single agents in hypertension. This class of drugs is one of the first choice drugs in all grades of essential as well as renovascular hypertension (except in bilateral renal artery stenosis). There is generally little to choose between the large number of ACE inhibitors available. Agents, such as fosinopril, have the advantage of hepatic as well as renal excretion and are less likely to accumulate in patients with renal failure. Perindopril, ramipril and trandolapril are agents with long half-lives, which provide good 24 -hour antihypertensive coverage.

There is useful synergism between the ACE inhibitors and diuretics and between ACE inhibitors and calcium channel blockers. The ACE inhibitors are particularly useful in diabetic hypertensives, in which they may be renoprotective, as they slow the progression of diabetic nephropathy. Furthermore, these agents have shown some benefits in improving diabetic retinopathy and even diabetic neuropathy.

Side effects: Dry cough caused by the inhibition of bradykinin breakdown, **angioedema, deterioration in renal function can occur in patients with bilateral renal artery stenosis.**

Hyperkalaemia because they reduce aldosterone and, thus, potassium excretion. Rarer side effects include rash, taste disturbance, blood dyscrasias, fever and vasculitis.

Contraindicated in second and third trimesters of pregnancy due to fetopathic potential.

(iii) **Angiotensin II antagonists:** Losartan 25-100 mg daily

Irbesartan

Candesartan

Valsartan

Telmisartan

This class of drugs is also called ARB (Angiotensin II Receptor Blockers). Like the ACE inhibitors, these drugs act on the renin-angiotensin system, blocking the action of angiotensin II at its peripheral receptors. Although binding of ARBs to angiotensin receptors is competitive, the inhibition by ARBs of biological responses to angiotensin II often is insurmountable. Candesartan exerts the maximum blockade to angiotensin II.

Possible advantages of ARBs could be:

ARBs do not inhibit the breakdown of bradykinin, therefore they do not cause cough. They have similar physiological effects to ACE inhibitors and produce similar falls in blood pressure. There is synergism of antihypertensive effect with thiazide diuretics. There is also evidence that they may regress LVH and improve proteinuria.

Possible disadvantages of ARBs could be:

ARBs stimulate renin release and this result in increased circulating levels of angiotensin II, which may act on some angiotensin receptors.

Side effects: Hyperkalaemia, renal impairment and hypotension. Well tolerated. angioedema. Like ACE inhibitors, ARBs also have teratogenic potential.

(iv) **Calcium Channel Blockers (CCBs):** Nifedipine - relatively selective vasodilator and less cardiac depression than verapamil or diltiazem

Diltiazem - intermediate action on heart and blood vessels

Verapamil – greatest effect on heart. Decreases heart rate effectively.

Primary Mechanisms of Action: inhibit Ca^{++} influx into vascular smooth muscle; relax peripheral arteriole smooth muscle and thereby decrease total peripheral resistance; interfere with both angiotensin II and $alpha_2$-mediated vasocontriction, and perhaps $alpha_1$-mediated vasoconstriction.

Calcium channel blockers may be divided into two classes — the dihydropyridines and the non-dihydropyridines. The dihydropyridines, such as nifedipine and amlodipine, act predominantly by causing peripheral vasodilatation. The non-dihydropyridines, such as verapamil and diltiazem, also slow the heart rate and atrio-ventricular node conduction. All calcium channel blockers are efficacious at reducing blood pressure as single agents. The older drugs, such as nifedipine, have short half-lives and may cause rapid vasodilatation, a reflex tachycardia and catecholamine surges. This may increase adverse effects and aggravate myocardial ischaemia. Longer-acting agents, such as amlodipine or slow-release preparations of nifedipine, partially overcome these problems.

Ca^{++} channel blockers are useful in hypertensive patients with a wide variety of concomitant illnesses including ischemic heart disease, chronic pulmonary disease, diabetes mellitus and variant angina.

Side effects: Ankle oedema. headache, flushing and palpitation,

Verapamil reduces intestinal motility and, thus, can cause significant constipation, heart block,

Diltiazem can similarly cause gastrointestinal and conduction problems,

(v) **Direct acting arterial dilators (Direct Vasodilators):** Usual Dosage Range

Hydralazine 25-100 mg BID

Minoxidil 2.5-40 mg daily

These agents act directly to relax vascular smooth muscle, thereby reducing peripheral vascular resistance. Side effect is a lupus-like syndrome.

Cardioinhibitory Drugs

Beta-blockers

Beta-blockers act by blocking the action of noradrenaline at β adrenoceptors throughout the circulatory system and elsewhere. Their major effect is to slow the heart rate and reduce its force of contraction. Beta-blockers also cause some reduction in renin release and central sympathetic tone.

Atenolol, betaxolol, bisoprolol, and **metoprolol** are cardioselective at low doses and bind more avidLy to $\beta1$-receptors than to $\beta2$-receptors. As a result, they are less likely to provoke bronchospasm and vasoconstriction and may be safer than nonselective β-blockers in patients with asthma, chronic obstructive pulmonary disease, diabetes, and Peripheral Artery Disease (PAD).

Acebutolol, carteolol, penbutolol, and **pindolol** possess intrinsic sympathomimetic activity (ISA) or partial β-receptor agonist activity these drugs may have advantages in patients with heart failure or sinus bradycardia.

Beta-blockers are useful as first-line antihypertensive agents, although they tend to be less effective in the elderly and in black hypertensives. For the treatment of hypertension it is best to choose a beta-blocker with high cardioselectivity and low lipid solubility to reduce side effects. A long half-life also allows once daily dosing.

Side effects:
- They slow the rate of conduction at the atrio-ventricular node and are thus contraindicated in patients with second- and third-degree heart block.
- Sinus bradycardia, bronchospasm Lipid-soluble agents can cause central nervous system side effects of insomnia, nightmares and fatigue.
- Exercise capacity may be reduced by beta-blockers and patients may experience tiredness and fatigue.
- β-blockers can worsen glucose intolerance and hyperlipidaemia.

Central and Peripheral Sympatholytics

Usual Dosage Range

Reserpine 0.0625-0.25 mg daily

Methyldopa 125 mg - 1 g daily

Clonidine 0.05-0.3 mg BID.

These drugs stimulate central α_2 adrenoceptors, resulting in a decrease in central sympathetic tone. This leads to a fall in both cardiac output and peripheral vascular resistance. Examples of such drugs include methyldopa and clonidine. The drugs cause sedation, dry mouth and fluid retention. Methyldopa can also cause autoimmune hepatic derangement and haemolytic anaemia.

Adrenergic Neurone Blockers

Such agents are now rarely used. Reserpine and guanethidine inhibit the release of noradrenaline from peripheral nerves. This reduces sympathetic tone, peripheral vascular resistance and cardiac output. They cause postural hypotension and central nervous system depression.

Compelling Indications

1. **Left Ventricular Dysfunction (Systolic Heart Failure)**
   - ACE inhibitor with diuretic therapy is recommended as the first-line regimen of choice.
   - β-Blocker therapy is appropriate to further modify disease in LV dysfunction and is a component of this first-line regimen (standard therapy) for these patients
   - ARBs are acceptable as alternative therapy for patients who cannot tolerate ACE inhibitors
   - An aldosterone antagonist may be considered in addition to a diuretic, ACE inhibitor or ARB, and β-blocker.
2. **Postmyocardial Infarction**
   - β-Blocker (without ISA) and ACE inhibitor therapy is recommended. β-Blockers decrease cardiac adrenergic stimulation and reduce the risk of a subsequent MI or sudden cardiac death. ACE inhibitors improve cardiac function and reduce CV events after MI. ARBs are alternatives to ACE inhibitors in postmyocardial patients with LV dysfunction.
3. **Coronary Artery Disease**
   - β- Blockers (without ISA) are first-line therapy in chronic stable angina and have the ability to reduce BP, improve myocardial consumption, and decrease demand.
   - Long-acting CCBs are either alternatives (the nondihydropyridines verapamil and diltiazem) or add-on therapy (dihydropyridines) to β-blockers in chronic stable angina.

4. **Diabetes Mellitus**
   - The BP goal in diabetes is less than 130/80 mm Hg.
   - All patients with diabetes and hypertension should be treated with either an ACE inhibitor or an ARB. Both classes provide nephroprotection and reduced CV risk.
   - A thiazide-type diuretic is recommended as the second agent to lower BP and provide additional CV risk reduction.
   - Clacium Channel Blockers (CCBs) are useful add-on agents for BP control in hypertensive patients with diabetes.
5. **Chronic Kidney Disease**
   - Renin-Angiotensin-Aldosteron System (RAAS) blockers are more effective at reducing albuminuria than other antihypertensive agents, and are recommended as part of the treatment strategy in hypertensive patients in the presence of microalbuminuria or proteinuria. A combination of a RAS blocker with a CCB or a diuretic is recommended as initial therapy.
   - Either an ACE inhibitor or ARB is recommended as first-line therapy to control BP and preserve kidney function in chronic kidney disease
6. **Acute stroke and cerebrovascular disease**
   - In patients with acute intracerebral haemorrhage: Immediate BP lowering is not recommended for patients with SBP>220 mmHg, careful acute BP lowering with i.v. therapy to <180mm Hg should be considered.
   - In patients with acute ischaemic stroke who are eligible for i.v. thrombolysis, BP should be carefully lowered and maintained at <185mm Hg for at least the first 24 h after thrombolysis.
   - The recommended antihypertensive drug treatment strategy for stroke prevention is a RAAS blocker plus a CCB or a thiazide like diuretic
7. **Atrial fibrillation**
   - A beta-blocker or non-dihydropyridine CCB should be considered as part of the treatment of hypertension if rate control is needed
   - Stroke prevention with oral anticoagulation is recommended in patients with Atrial Fibrillation (AF) and hypertension

Special Populations

1. **Older People:** Elderly patients may present with either isolated systolic hypertension or an elevation in both SBP and DBP. Diuretics and ACE inhibitors provide significant benefits and can be used safely in the elderly.
2. **Children and Adolescents:** Secondary hypertension is much more common in children than in adults. Kidney disease (e.g., pyelonephritis, glomerulonephritis) is the most common cause of secondary hypertension in children. ACE inhibitors, ARBs, β-blockers, CCBs, and thiazide-type diuretics are all acceptable drug therapy choices.

3. **Pregnant Women:** Preeclampsia, defined as BP ≥140/90 mm Hg that appears after 20 weeks' gestation accompanied by new-onset proteinuria (≥300 mg/24 hours), can lead to life-threatening complications for both the mother and fetus.

   Management consists of restricting activity, bedrest, and close monitoring. Salt restriction or other measures that contract blood volume should be avoided.

   Antihypertensives are used prior to induction of labor if the DBP is >105–110 mm Hg, with a target DBP of 95–105 mm Hg.

   Methydopa, CCBs, IV hydralazine is most commonly used; IV labetalol is also effective. ACE inhibitors, ARBs, or direct renin inhibitors are not recommended during pregnancy In severe hypertension, drug treatment with i.v. labetalol, oral methyldopa, or nifedipine is recommended. The recommended treatment for hypertensive crisis is i.v. labetalol or nicardipine and magnesium. In pre-eclampsia associated with pulmonary oedema, nitroglycerin given as an i.v. infusion is recommended.

4. **Peripheral Arterial Disease**
   - ACE inhibitors may be ideal in patients with symptomatic lower-extremity Peripheral Artery Disease (PAD); CCBs may also be beneficial

Hypertensive Urgencies and Emergencies

Hypertensive urgencies are ideally managed by adjusting maintenance therapy by adding a new antihypertensive and/or increasing the dose of a present medication.

- Acute administration of a short-acting oral drug (captopril, clonidine, or labetalol) followed by careful observation for several hours to ensure a gradual BP reduction is an option.
- Oral captopril doses of 25 to 50 mg may be given at 1- to 2-hour intervals. The onset of action is 15 to 30 minutes.
- Labetalol can be given in a dose of 200 to 400 mg, followed by additional doses every 2 to 3 hours.

Hypertensive emergencies require immediate BP reduction to limit new or progressing target-organ damage.

- The goal is not to lower BP to normal; instead, the initial target is a reduction in mean arterial pressure of up to 25% within minutes to hours.
- If BP is then stable, it can be reduced toward 160/100– 110 mm Hg within the next 2 to 6 hours.
- Nitroprusside is the agent of choice for minute-to-minute control in most cases. It is usually given as a continuous IV infusion at a rate of 0.25 to 10 mcg/kg/min. Its onset of hypotensive action is immediate and disappears within 1 to 2 minutes of discontinuation. When the infusion must be continued longer than 72 hours, serum thiocyanate levels should be measured,

2018 Europeon Society of Cardiology/Europeon Society of Heart (ESC/ESH) Guidelines for the Management of Arterial Hypertension

Initiation of hypertension treatment according to office BP

- Prompt initiation of BP-lowering drug treatment is recommended in patients with grade 2 or 3 hypertension at any level of Cardio Vascular (CV) risk, simultaneous with the initiation of lifestyle changes.
- In patients with grade 1 hypertension: Lifestyle interventions are recommended to determine if this will normalize BP. In patients with grade 1 hypertension at low–moderate-risk and without evidence of Hypertension Mediated Organ Damage (HMOD), BP-lowering drug treatment is recommended if the patient remains hypertensive after a period of lifestyle intervention. In patients with grade 1 hypertension and at high risk or with evidence of HMOD, prompt initiation of drug treatment is recommended simultaneously with lifestyle interventions.
- BP-lowering drug treatment and lifestyle intervention are recommended for older patients (>65 years but not >80 years) when SBP is in the grade 1 range (140–159 mmHg), provided that treatment is well tolerated.
- In patients with high–normal BP (130–139/85–89 mmHg): Lifestyle changes are recommended. Drug treatment may be considered when their Cardiovascular Risk (CV) is very high due to established Cardiovascular Disease (CVD), especially CAD.

Lifestyle Modifications to Prevent and Treat Hypertension

- Weight management: Lose weight if overweight or obese, ideally attaining a $BMI < 25 Kg/m^2$.
- Adopt DASH-type dietary patterns: Consume a diet that is rich in fruits and vegetables (8–10 servings/day), rich in low-fat dairy products (2–3 servings/ day), but has reduced amounts of saturated fat and cholesterol.
- Reduced sodium intake: Reduce daily dietary sodium intake as much as possible; ideally to no more than 65 mmol/day (equal to 1.5 g/day sodium, or 3.8 g/day sodium chloride)
- Increased dietary potassium intake: Increase daily dietary potassium intake to 120 mmol/day (4.7 g/day), which is also the amount provided in a DASH-type diet.
- Moderation of alcohol consumption: For patients who drink alcohol, limit consumption to no more than two drinks/day in men and no more than one drink/day in women and lighter-weight persons. Do not recommend alcohol consumption in patients that do not drink alcohol.
- Regular physical activity: Regular moderate-intensity aerobic physical activity; at least 30 min of continuous or intermittent 5 days/wk, but preferably daily.

Common Combination Antihypertensive Agents

➢ ACEI with thiazide diuretic: Benazepril/HCTZ

Captopril/HCTZ

Enalapril/HCTZ

Lisinopril/HCTZ

Moexipril/HCTZ

Quinapril/HCTZ

ARB with thiazide diuretic: Olmesartan medoxomil/HCTZ

Telmisartan/HCTZ

Valsartan/HCTZ

ACEI with CCB: Amlodipine besylate/Benazepril hydrochloride

Enalapril/Felodipine

CCB with ARB: Amlodipine/Valsartan

Amlodipine/Olmesartan medoxomil

The Drug Treatment Algorithm for Hypertension

1. The initiation of treatment in most patients with two drugs, to improve the speed, efficiency, and predictability of BP control.
2. Preferred two-drug combinations are a RAAS blocker with a CCB or a diuretic. A beta-blocker in combination with a diuretic or any drug from the other major classes is an alternative when there is a specific indication for a beta-blocker, e.g. angina, post-myocardial infarction, heart failure, or heart rate control.
3. Use monotherapy for low-risk patients with stage 1 hypertension whose SBP is <150mm Hg. very high-risk patients with high–normal BP, or frail older patients.
4. The use of a three-drug comprising a Renin-Angiotensin-Aldostere System (RAAS) blocker, a Calcium Channel Blocker (CCB), and a diuretic if BP is not controlled by a two-drug combination.
5. The addition of spironolactone for the treatment of resistant hypertension, unless contraindicated.

Treatment of Resistant Hypertension

➢ It is defined as : Optimal doses (or best-tolerated doses) of an appropriate therapeutic strategy, which should include a diuretic (typically an ACE inhibitor or an ARB with a CCB and a thiazide/thiazide-type diuretic), fails to lower. SBP and DBP values to <140mm Hg and <90mmHg respectively and inadequte control of BP has been confirmed by Ambulatory BP Measurement/Clinical (ABPM) or Home BP Measurement (HBPM).
➢ Management: Reinforcement of lifestyle measures, especially sodium restriction.
- Addition of low-dose spironolactonec to existing treatment;

- Or the addition of further diuretic therapy if intolerant to spironolactone, with either eplerenone, amiloride, a higherdose thiazide/thiazide-like diuretic, or a loop diuretic;
- Or the addition of bisoprolol or doxazosin.

Management of White Coat and Masked Hypertension

Management of white-coat hypertension: In patients with white-coat hypertension: • Drug treatment may be considered in people with evidence of Hypertension Mediated Organ Damage (HMOD) or in whom CV risk is high or very high. Routine drug treatment is not indicated.

Management of masked hypertension: Antihypertensive drug treatment should be considered in masked hypertension to normalize the out-of-office BP, based on the prognostic importance of out-of-office BP elevation

Case Study of Meningoencephalitis/Hypertension/Stroke

Summary

A patient named xyz was admitted into the Intensive Unit (ICU) chief complaints of fever since 1day, altered sensorium since bpm, episode of seizure like activity, fever with chills a/w myalgias patient took OTC drugs. Patient past medical history: bronchial asthma. Appetite: poor, Build: normal. Diagnostic tests are performed and the abnormal results are shown below: ESR: 25mm/hr, WBC: leucocytosis, RBC: 173 mg/dL, Neck rigidity: aPTT: 35 sec, MRI: s/o diffuse decrease in calibre flow of left vasospasm. Lumbar puncture and CSI analysis: showed increased protein and 5 cells was suggestive of a viral etiology.

Cerebral   RBC: 4.1 million/L

Diagnosis: Based on the investigations and symptoms the condition was confirmed as CVA with hemiparesis associated with viral encephalitis

Daily progress: Patient is under medication, vitals checked and recorded, irrelevant talk occasionally. He is under physiotherapy session, Checked for any adverse drug reactions. Monitor aPT levels and other abnormalities induced by Heparin (INR must be assessed). The body movements, neck rigidity are assessed.

Drug interactions between:

1. Quetiapine and ondansetron - Prolonged QTc interval
2. Ceftriaxone and enoxaparin - Anti coagulation
3. Methyl prednisolone and Quetiapine - Decreased Quetiapine levels by affecting CYP enzymes

Discharge medications:

Tab Levipil (Levtiracetam)- 500 mg BD
Tab Lacosamide (Lacosamide) - 100mg TID
Tab Qutipin (Quetiapine) - 50 mg OD Bed time

Tab Zelfresh (Zolpidem) - 10mg OD H/S

Cap Surbex gold (Supplment) OD after breakfast *2weeks

Tab Rantodac (Ranitidine) 40mg OD before breakfast *1 week

HTN with Stroke

1. Treatment options available for HTN treatment in stroke?

For patients with a systolic blood pressure above 220mmHg (or) a diastolic blood pressure greater than 120 mm Hg.

1. Labetalol 100mg(doubled or repeated every 10mins) IV for 1-2 mins
2. Nicardipine IV(15mg/h) 5mg/h
3. Nitroprusside: 0.5 mg/kg/min IV infusion

HTN control for candidate without Fibrinolysis:

1. Nicardipine 5mg/h titrate- 2.5 mg/h every 5-15mins Maximum 15 mg/hr

   HTN treatment is indicated only if active MI, or hypertensive encephalopathy is present.

Table 6.1 Treatment options for patients with Hypertension and stroke.

Hypertensive Emergency Treatment *Diseases-specific Recommendations*			
Conditions	**Preferred Agent**	**Goal**	**Risks**
Acute ischemic stroke	Nicardipine, labetalol	Treat when > 220/120 except w/thrombolytics > 185/110	Excessive BP decrease may worsen ischemia
Intracranial Hemorrahge	Nicardipine, labetalol, esmolol	Treat to target MAP 130	Precipitous BP fall may increase mortality
Sub arachnoid Hemorrhage	Nicardipine, labetalol, esmolol	SBP < 160	Keep SBP > 120 to maintain Cerebral Perfusion Pressure (CPP)
Hypertensive Encephalopathy	Nicardipine, labetalol, esmolo	Decrease Mean Arterial Pressure MAP 15-20%	Aggressive BP fall may produce ischemia

2. What is appropriate antiplatelet therapy?

Acute Antiplatelet Therapy

(i)   All patients with acute ischemic stroke or transient ischemic attack not already on an antiplatelet agent should be treated with at least 160 mg of acetylsalicylic acid immediately as a one-time loading dose after brain imaging has excluded intracranial hemorrhage.

(ii)   For patients with dysphagia, acetylsalicylic acid (80 mg daily) or clopidogrel (75 mg daily) may be administered by enteral tube or acetylsalicylic acid by rectal suppository (325 mg daily). Note acetylsalicylic acid should only be administered orally once dysphagia screening has been performed and indicates absence of potential dysphagia.

(iii)   Antiplatelet therapy should be started as soon as possible after brain imaging has excluded hemorrhage, within 24 hours of symptom onset (ideally within 12 hours).

(iv) For patients receiving intravenous thrombolysis therapy, avoid antiplatelet therapy within the first 24 hours; antiplatelet therapy could then be initiated after brain imaging has excluded secondary hemorrhage.

(v) For transient ischemic attack or minor ischemic stroke patients who are being discharged from the emergency department, antiplatelet therapy should be started prior to discharge.

Antiplatelet Therapy for Secondary Stroke Prevention

(i) For patients with ischemic stroke or transient ischemic attack, antiplatelet therapy is recommended for long-term secondary stroke prevention to reduce the risk of recurrent stroke and other vascular events unless there is an indication for anticoagulant therapy.

(ii) Antiplatelet therapy should be started as soon as possible after brain imaging has excluded hemorrhage, within 24 hours of symptom onset (ideally within 12 hours).

(iii) For long-term secondary stroke prevention, either acetylsalicylic acid (80 mg – 325 mg daily), or clopidogrel (75 mg daily), or combined acetylsalicylic acid and extended-release dipyridamole (25mg/200 mg BID), are all appropriate treatment options and selection depends on patient factors or clinical circumstances.

3. What are Risk factors for stroke

Nonmodifiable

- Age, Race, Sex, H/O migraine, Heredity
- Modifiable
- HTN, DM, Cardiac diseases
- Transient ischemic attacks (TIA)
- Carotid stenosis, obesity

4. What are Goals of therapy:

- ➢ To preserve tissue in the ischemic penumbra, where perfusion is decreased but sufficient to stave off infarction.
- ➢ To establish revascularization.
- ➢ To limit duration of ischemia or usage of neuroprotective agents.

5. Write the Non pharmacological measures:

Diet:

- ➢ 3 servings of whole grains a day and 2 servings of berries, 6 servings of green leafy vegetables a week.
- ➢ Fish, poultry, beans and nuts can also be given.
- ➢ Restrict intake of redmeats, fastfoods, cheese, desserts and butter.

Lifestyle modifications:

- ➢ Stop smoke and alcohol consumption.
- ➢ Exercise regularly

6. What are the Complications of stroke

1. Pneumonia, urinary tract infections/venous thrombosis/immobility related complication
2. Contractures/ Orthopaedic problems/Pressure sores/Pressure palsies
3. Malnutrition

References

1. Massie BM. The Safety of Calcium Channel Blockers. Clin Cardiol. 1998 Dec;21(12 Suppl 2):II12-7.

2. Lever AF, Brennan PJ. MRC Trial of Treatment in Elderly Hypertensives. Clin Exp Hypertens. 1993 Nov;15(6):941-52.

3. Wang Y, Pan Y, Zhao X, et al.; CHANCE Investigators. Clopidogrel with aspirin in acute minor stroke or transient ischemic attack (CHANCE) trial: one-year outcomes. *Circulation*. 2015;132(1):40–46.

CHAPTER - 7

Stroke

Introduction to Stroke

Definition: The sudden death of brain cells due to lack of oxygen, caused by blockage of blood flow or rupture of an artery to the brain. Sudden loss of speech, weakness, or paralysis of one side of the body can be **symptoms**. Also known as cerebrovascular accident.

Stroke can be either ischemic or hemorrhagic (88% and 12%, respectively, of all strokes in the 2003 American Heart Association report).

Hemorrhagic strokes include subarachnoid hemorrhage, intracerebral hemorrhage, and subdural hematomas.

- **Subarachnoid hemorrhage** occurs when blood enters the subarachnoid space (where cerebrospinal fluid is housed) owing to trauma, rupture of an intracranial aneurysm, or rupture of an arteriovenous malformation (AVM).
- By contrast, intracerebral hemorrhage occurs when a blood vessel ruptures within the brain parenchyma itself, resulting in the formation of a hematoma. These types of hemorrhages are associated with uncontrolled high blood pressure and antithrombotic or thrombolytic therapy.
- Subdural hematomas are due to collections of blood below the dura, and are caused by trauma.
- Hemorrhagic stroke is significantly more lethal than ischemic stroke, two to six times higher.
- **Ischemic strokes** are due either to local thrombus formation or to embolic phenomenon, resulting in occlusion of a cerebral artery.
- **Atherosclerosis,** particularly of the cerebral vasculature, is a causative factor for ischemic stroke, 30% are cryptogenic. Emboli can arise either from intra- or extracranial arteries (including the aortic arch) or, as is the case in 20% of all ischemic strokes, the heart. Cardiogenic embolism can occur if the patient has concomitant atrial fibrillation, valvular heart disease, or any other condition of the heart that may lead to clot formation.

Classification of Stroke

1. Ischemic stroke:
   - Cardiogenic embolic stroke
   - Cryptogenic stroke
   - Large artery thrombosis
   - Small penetrating artery thrombosis
2. Primary hemorrhagic stroke
   - Subarachnoid haemorrhage
   - Intracranial hemorrhage

Risk Factors

(A) Single Risk Factors:
   - Nonmodifiable risk factors 1or risk markers
   - Age, Gender, Race, Ethnicity, Heredity.

(B) Potentially modifiable

   - **Hypertension**—single most important risk factor for ischemic stroke, Cardiac disease, Atrial fibrillation—most important and treatable cardiac cause of stroke, Mitral stenosis, Mitral annular calcification, Left atrial enlargement, Structural abnormalities such as atrial-septal aneurysm, Myocardial disease 1% to 6% of myocardial infarction patients develop a stroke,
   - **Transient ischemic attacks**—major independent risk factor,
   - Diabetes—independent risk factor,
   - Hypercholesterolemia—positive risk factor for extracranial atherosclerosis
   - Cigarette smoking,
   - Alcohol and Illicit drug use—cocaine, heroin, amphetamines, LSD, PCP and others linked with stroke,
   - **Lifestyle factors**—associated with stroke risk, Obesity, Physical inactivity, Diet Acute triggers—emotional stress,
   - Oral contraceptives—positive only with estrogen content >50 µg,
   - Migraine—risk not clear,
   - Hemostatic and inflammatory factors—fibrinogen linked to increased risk; elevated hematocrit and sickle cell disease are positive risk factors,
   - Homocysteine—hyperhomocysteinemia may be related to increased stroke risk, Asymptomatic carotid stenosis, Subclinical disease—aortic arch atheromas.

(C) Multiple Risk Factors—Stroke Is Increased by the Presence of Multiple Risk Factors Framingham profile: Elevated systolic blood pressure, Elevated serum cholesterol, Glucose intolerance, Cigarette smoking, Left ventricular hypertrophy.

Pathophysiology

(A) **Ischemic stroke [1, 2]:** In carotid atherosclerosis, progressive accumulation of lipids and inflammatory cells in the intima of the affected arteries, combined with hypertrophy of arterial smooth muscle cells, results in plaque formation. Eventually, sheer stress may result in plaque rupture, collagen exposure, platelet aggregation, and clot formation. The clot may remain in the vessel, causing local occlusion, or travel distally as an embolism, eventually lodging downstream in a cerebral vessel. In the case of cardiogenic embolism, stasis of blood in the atria or ventricles of the heart leads to the formation of local clots that can become dislodged and travel directly through the aorta to the cerebral circulation. The final result of both thrombus formation and embolism is an arterial occlusion, decreasing cerebral blood flow and causing ischemia distal to the occlusion.

  - Normal cerebral blood flow averages 50 mL/100 g per minute, and this is maintained over a wide range of blood pressures (mean arterial pressures of 50 to 150 mm Hg) by a process called cerebral autoregulation.
  - Cerebral blood vessels dilate and constrict in response to changes in blood pressure, but this process can be impaired by atherosclerosis and acute injury, such as stroke. When local cerebral blood flow decreases below 20 mL/100 g per minute, ischemia ensues, and when further reductions below 12 mL/100 g per minute persist, irreversible damage to the brain occurs, and this is called infarction.
  - Tissue that is ischemic but maintains membrane integrity is referred to as the ischemic penumbra because it usually surrounds the infarct core. This penumbra is potentially salvageable through therapeutic intervention.

(B) **Hemorrhagic stroke:** The presence of blood in the brain parenchyma causes damage to the surrounding tissue through the mechanical effect it produces (mass effect) and the neurotoxicity of the blood components and their degradation products. Compression of the tissue surrounding the hematoma also may lead to secondary ischemia. Approximately 30% of intracerebral hemorrhages continue to enlarge over the first 24 hours, and clot volume is the most important predictor of outcome, regardLess of location. Much of the early mortality of hemorrhagic stroke (up to 50% at 30 days) is due to the abrupt increase in intracranial pressure that can lead to herniation and death.

  Blood vessel ruptures and bleeds so increase in intracranial pressure. This results in cytotoxicity and sudden focal internal brain trauma from hematoma mass effect.

  - There is RBC lysis-cytotoxic Hb release, fenton type free radical generation-oxidative damage to proteins, nucleic acids, carbohydrates, lipids leading to necrosis.
  - Increased lactate, so astrocyte death, release of inflammatory markers like Tumor Necrosis Factor (TNF) alpha, Interferon (IFN γ). So there will be increased intracranial pressure.
  - Decreased ATP- astrocytes release Calcium causing excititoxicity. Because of excessive influx of calcium it causes oxidative damage.

Clinical Manifestation and Features

General: The patient may not be able to reliably report the history owing to cognitive or language deficits. A reliable history may have to come from a family member or another witness.

Symptoms: The patient may complain of weakness on one side of the body, inability to speak, loss of vision, vertigo, or falling. Ischemic stroke is not usually painful, but patients may complain of headache, and with hemorrhagic stroke, it can be very severe.

Signs: patients usually have multiple signs of neurologic dysfunction, and the specific deficits are determined by the area of the brain involved. Hemi- or monoparesis occurs commonly, as does a hemisensory deficit. Patients with vertigo and double vision are likely to have posterior circulation involvement. Aphasia is seen commonly in patients with anterior circulation strokes. Patients also may suffer from dysarthria, visual field defects, and altered levels of consciousness.

Diagnosis with Algorithm

1. Identify signs and symptoms of possible stroke, activate emergency response.
2. Crirtical EMS asessements and actions:
   - support Airway, Breathing, Circulation (ABC,s), give oxygen if needed
   - Perform prehospital stroke assessment
   - Establish time of symptom onset
   - Triage to stroke center
   - Alert hospital consider direct transfer to CT scan
   - Check glucose if possible
3. Immediate general assessment and stabilization:
   - Assess ABCs, vital signs
   - Provide oxygen if hypoxemic
   - Obtain IV access and perform laboratory assessments
   - Check glucose, treat if needed
   - Perform neurogenic screening assessment
   - Activate stroke team
   - Order emergency CT scan or MRI of brain
   - Obtain 12-lead ECG
4. Immediate neurologic assessment by stroke team
   - Review patient history
   - Establish time of symptom onset or last known normal Naional Institutes of Health.
   - Perform neurologic examonation NIH stoke scale or canadian neurological scale
5. Does CT scan show hemorrhage- if yes consult neurologist or surgeon. Begin stroke or hemorrhage pathway, and shift to intensive care unit.
6. If CT scan does not show any hemorrhage, possible acute ischemic stroke. Consider fibrinolytic therapy. If pateint remain candidate for fibrinolytic therapy, review risk

benefits with patient and family and give (Recombinant Tissue Plasminogen Activator (rtPA), no anticoagulants or antiplatelet treatments for 24 hours, begin post rtPA stroke pathway, emergency admission to stroke unit. If patient is not a candidate for fibrinolytic therapy, administer aspirin and shift to intensive care unit.

Laboratory Tests

Tests for hypercoagulable states [3, 4, 5]

- Protein C, protein S, and antithrombin III are best measured in the "steady state," not in the acute stage.
- Antiphospholipid antibodies as measured by anticardiolipin antibodies, $\beta2$-glycoprotein I, and lupus anticoagulant screen are of higher yield than protein C, protein S, and antithrombin III but should be reserved for patients who are young (may take 24 hours (and rarely longer) to reveal the area of infarction.

MRI of the head will reveal areas of ischemia with higher resolution and earlier than the CT scan. Diffusion-weighted imaging (DWI) will reveal an evolving infarct within minutes.

Carotid Doppler (CD) studies will determine whether the patient has a high degree of stenosis in the carotid arteries supplying blood to the brain (extracranial disease).

The electrocardiogram (ECG) will determine whether the patient has atrial fibrillation, a potent etiologic factor for stroke.

A transthoracic echocardiogram (TTE) will determine whether valve abnormalities or wall motion abnormalities are sources of emboli to the brain. A "bubble test" can be done to look for an intraatrial shunt indicating an atrial septal defect or a patent foramen ovale.

A transesophageal echocardiogram (TEE) is a more sensitive test for thrombus in the left atrium. It is effective at examining the aortic arch for atheroma, a potential source of emboli.

Transcranial Doppler (TCD) will determine whether the patient is likely to have intracranial arterial sclerosis (e.g., middLe cerebral artery stenosis).

Management

Goals of Treatment:

1. To reduce the ongoing neurologic injury and decrease mortality and long-term disability,
2. Prevent complications secondary to immobility and neurologic dysfunction, and
3. Prevent stroke recurrence.
4. Primary prevention of stroke is reviewed elsewhere reperfusion therapy. Patients with elevated blood pressure should remain untreated unless their blood pressure exceeds 220/120 mm Hg or they have evidence of aortic dissection, acute myocardial infarction (AMI), pulmonary edema, or hypertensive encephalopathy. If blood pressure is treated, short-acting parenteral agents, such as labetalol, nicordipine, and nitroprusside, are favored.

Non Pharmacological Therapy

Ischemic Stroke

Surgical interventions in the acute ischemic stroke patient are limited.

Craniectomy-to release some of the rising pressure

- ➢ In cases of significant swelling associated with a cerebellar infarction, surgical decompression can be lifesaving.
- ➢ In secondary prevention, carotid endarterectomy of an ulcerated and/or stenotic carotid artery to reduce stroke incidence and recurrence
- ➢ In ischemic stroke patients with 70% to 99% stenosis of an ipsilateral internal carotid artery, recurrent stroke risk can be reduced by up to 48% compared with medical therapy alone when combined with aspirin 325 mg daily.

Hemorrhagic Stroke [6]

In patients with subarachnoid hemorrhage owing to a ruptured intracranial aneurysm or an AVM, surgical intervention to either clip or ablate the offending vascular abnormality substantially reduces mortality owing to rebleeding.

- Insertion of an extraventricular drain (EVD) and subsequent monitoring of intracranial pressure are done commonly and are the least invasive of the procedures done in these patients.
- Surgical decompression of a hematoma is done when it is a last option in a life-threatening situation.

Pharmacological Therapy

A. Ischemic Stroke: according to 'The Stroke Council of the American Stroke Association guidelines'
- Grade A recommendation are intravenous tissue plasminogen activator (tPA) within 3 hours of onset and aspirin within 48 hours of onset.
- Early reperfusion with intravenous tPA reduces the ultimate disability due to ischemic stroke.
- The essentials of the treatment protocol can be summarized as
  1. Stroke team activation,
  2. Onset of symptoms within 3 hours,
  3. CT scan to rule out hemorrhage,
  4. Meet inclusion and exclusion criteria
  5. Administer tPA 0.9 mg/ kg over 1 hour, with 10% given as initial bolus over 1 minute,
  6. Avoid antithrombotic (anticoagulant or antiplatelet) therapy for 24 hours, and

7. Monitor the patient closely for response and hemorrhage.

- Early aspirin therapy also has been shown to reduce long-term death and disability but should never be given within 24 hours of the administration of tPA because it can increase the risk of bleeding in such patients.
- All three currently used agents, aspirin, clopidogrel, and extended-release dipyridamole plus aspirin (ERDP + ASA), are considered first-line antiplatelet agents by the ACCP. In patients with atrial fibrillation and a presumed cardiac source of embolism, warfarin is the antithrombotic agent of first choice.

I. Acute Treatment [7, 8, 9]:

(a) tPA 0.9 mg/kg IV (maximum 90 kg) over 1 hour in selected patients within 3 hours of onset.

(b) ASA 160–325 mg daily started within 48 hours of onset tPA (various doses) intraarterially up to 6 hours after onset in selected patients

II. Secondary Prevention

(a) **Noncardioembolic** Aspirin 50–325 mg daily, Ticlopidine 250 mg twice daily, Clopidogrel 75 mg daily, Asprin 25 mg + extended-release dipyridamole 200 mg twice daily.

(b) **Cardioembolic** (esp. atrial fibrillation) Warfarin (INR = 2.5)6 All ACE inhibitor + diuretic or ARB blood pressure lowering, Statin.

(c) **Warfarin:** Warfarin is the most effective treatment for the prevention of stroke in patients with atrial fibrillation and a presumed cardiac source of embolism.

(d) **Blood Pressure Lowering:** Elevated blood pressure is very common in ischemic stroke patients, and treatment of hypertension in these patients is associated with a decreased risk of stroke recurrence.

- Blood pressure lowering in the acute stroke period (first 7 days) may result in decreased cerebral blood flow and worsened symptoms; therefore, recommendations are limited to patients out of the acute stroke period.

(e) **Statins:** The statins reduce the risk of stroke by approximately 30% in patients with coronary artery disease and elevated plasma lipids.

(f) **Heparin for Prophylaxis of Deep Vein Thrombosis (DVT):** The use of low-molecular-weight heparins or low-dose subcutaneous unfractionated heparin (5000 units twice daily) can be recommended for the prevention of DVT in hospitalized patients with decreased mobility owing to their stroke and used in all but the most minor strokes.

(g) **Clopidogrel:** Clopidogrel has a unique platelet antiaggregatory effect in that it is an inhibitor of the adenosine diphosphate (ADP) pathway of platelet aggregation and inhibits known stimuli to platelet aggregation.

(h) **Ticlopidine:** Ticlopidine, another thienopyridine, inhibits activation of the ADP receptor on the platelet, as does clopidogrel. Side effects include suppression of bone marrow, rash and diarrhea, and elevation of serum cholesterol levels.

(i) **Angiotensin II Receptor Antagonists (ARBs):** Angiotensin II receptor antagonists (ARBs) also have been shown to reduce the risk of stroke.

ASPIRIN PLUS CLOPIDOGREL: In the MATCH study, clopidogrel in combination with aspirin 75 mg daily was no better than clopidogrel alone in secondary stroke prevention.

Alteplase Prescribing Guidelines [10]

Dosage: 0.9 mg /kg IV, max 90mg; 10% given as bolus, 90% given over 60min.

Contraindications:

➢ Hypersensitivity to alteplase/ evidence of Intracranial Hemorrhage (IH) on pretreatment evaluation

➢ Suspicion of Subarachroid Hemorrhage (SH) on pretreatment evaluation

➢ Recent intracranial or intraspinal surgery, serious head trauma, or previous stroke within 3 months

➢ History if Intracranial Hemorrhage (IH) uncontrolled hypertension at time of treatment

➢ Seizure at onset of stoke/active internal bleeding

➢ Intracranial neoplasm, aneurysm

➢ Platelet count $<100,000/mm^3$

Direct Oral Anticoagulants for Secondary Stroke Prevention [11]

The drugs are summarized in Table 7.1.

(B) **Hemorrhagic stroke [12]:** There are currently no proven pharmacologic strategies for treating intracerebral hemorrhage (ICH). Medical guidelines for the management of blood pressure, raised intracranial pressure, and other medical complications of ICH are those required for the management of any acutely ill patient in a neurointensive care unit.

- Subarachnoid hemorrhage (SAH) owing to aneurysm rupture is associated with a high incidence of delayed cerebral ischemia (DCI) in the 2 weeks following the bleeding episode. Vasospasm of the cerebral vasculature is thought to be responsible for DCI and occurs between 4 and 21 days after the bleed, peaking at days 5 through .

- The calcium channel blocker nimodipine is recommended to reduce the incidence and severity of neurologic deficits owing to DCI.

- Nimodipine at a dose of 60 mg every 4 hours should be initiated on diagnosis and continued for 21 days in all SAH patients. Administration of nimodipine therapy is complicated by a fairly high incidence of hypotension.

- This can be managed by reducing the dosing interval to 30 mg every 2 hours (same daily dose), reducing the total daily dose (30 mg every 4 hours), and maintaining intravascular volume and pressor therapy.

Table 7.1 Summary of currently available direct oral anticoagulants.

d FDA oval	Target	FDA-approved indications	Available Strengths	Half-life[b]	Dosing Frequency	Renal Dosing Adjustments	Drug Interactions
n Oct	Thrombin	NVAF, treatment Secondary prevention of DVT and PE VTE prevention after hip replacement	75 mg 100 mg 150 mg	12-17 hr	Twice Daily	Contraindicated if CrCl < 30 mL/min	PPI, antacids dronedarone, P-gp inhibitors
an July	Factor Xa	NVAF, treatment and secondary prevention of DVT and PE, VTE prevention after hip and knee replacement	10 mg 15 mg 20 mg	9hr	Once Daily[c]	Avoid use if CrCl < 30 mL/min	CYP3A4 inhibitors, P-gp inhibitors
Dec	Factor Xa	NVAF, treatment and secondary prevention of DVT and PE, VTE Prevention after hip and knee replacement	25 mg 5 mg	12 hr	Twice Daily	Limited data for serum creatnine > 25 mg/dL and CrCl < 25 mL/min	CYP3A4 inhibitors P-gp inhibitors
Jan	Factor Xa	NVAF, treatment of DVT and PE	15 mg 30 mg 60 mg	10-14 hr	Once Daily	CrCl < 15-50mL/min: 30 mg once daily CrCl < 15 mL/min: not recommended	CyP3A4 inhibitors P-gp inhibitors
n June	Factor Xa	Prevention of DCT and PE in hospitalized, medically-ill patients	40 mg 80 mg	20 hr	Once Daily[c]	Not reported	Not reported

nded strength varies on indication, [b]Assuming normal renal function, [c]May require higher, more frequency dosing at initiation based on reviations: CrCl, creatinine clearance calculated by the Cockcroft-Gault formula; CYP, cytochrome, P450; DVT, deep vein thrombosis; NVAF: trial fibrillation; PCC; protjrombin complex concentrate, PE, pulmonary embolism, P-gp, P-Glycoprotein; PPI, proton pump inhibitors; VTE: venos thromboembolism

Barr. D., EPPS DJ. Direct oval anticoagulants: A review in common medication errors. J Throm b Thromblysis 2018 Oct 8. DOI: 10.1007/S11239-018-1752-9.

Case of Recurrent Ischaemic Stroke with Dysphagia

Summary

A Male patient of age 65yrs was admitted in the hospital with the chief complaints of c/o Decrease intake of food, generalised weakness, decreased responsiveness, vomitings since days, throat pain+ 2days, difficulty in talking from 1 week. On examination-hypotension (BP 90/60mm/hg). Past History: Recurrent ischaemic stroke, Type 2 DM; HTN; Hypothyroidisim; Dyslipididemia. Past Medication History: Novorapid 10u BD; Telma 40 mg; Thyronorm 75mg; Tonact 40mg. On Examination: Conscious, coherent, cooperative, oriented, PR:95/60mm hg; BP:90/60mm hg, Temperature: 99 °f, CVS:S1 S2+ No murmurs, peripheral pulses palpable, RS:B/L Airway Entry+,Wheezes present, GIS:P/A-Soft, No Organomegaly, Bowel sounds heard, CNS:Left upper limb weakness+(present)

Course in Hospital

- TLC and Sr. creatinine-increase, Patient was started on IV Antibiotics, IV Proton Pump Inhibitors (PPI'S) RT feeds Supportive care, Dysphagia+, Urine culture: E.COLI and sensitive to magnex forte, Hematemesis, GIT:Hiatus hernia and esophagitis, PPI'S, Regular physiotherapy

  DIAGNOSIS: Recurrent ischaemic stroke with dysphagia; T2 DM; HTN; Hypothyroidisim, Severe GERD; UTI

TREATMENT CHART

- Inj.Magnex Forte -1.5gm-multivitamin
- Inj.PAN (Pantaprazole)-40mg
- T.Deplatt A (Aspirin+clopidogrel)-150mg
- Tonact (Atorvastatain) -40mg
- T. Eltroxin (Thyroxine) -50mcg
- Pulmoclear (acebrophylline 100mg+Acetylcysteine 600mg) 1tab
- Nephroadd (Taurine 500mg+acetylcysteine 150mg) -1tab
- Inj.Zosyn (piperacillin+tazobactum)-4.5 mg
- Inj. Zofer (Ondansteron)-4 mg
- Neb with Duolin (Levosalbutamol+ ipratropium) -2.5mg/500mg
- Syp.Sucralset Plus (Sucralfate+oxetacaine)-10 ml
- Inj.Pan (Pantaprazole) -8mg/hr
- Inj.Novorapid (Insulin) -6U
- Inj.Novomix (Insulin) -6U
- Inj.Lesuride (levosulpiride)25mg
- T.Galvus Met (Metformin+ vildagliptin)   -50/1000mg
- T.Reneguard (Cefixime+K.Clavulanate)-200mg
- T.Niftas(Nitrofurantoin) -500mg

- T.Sompraz D (Domperidone 30mg + esomeprazole 40mg)
- T.Forcan(Fluconazole) -150 mg
- Zytee (Choline salicylate) mouth paint - for local application
- Neb with Formonide -0.5 mg
- Limcee (Vitamin C) -500mg
- Syp.Broncorex -5ml (Expectorant-Guafenesin, Terbutaline, Bromhexime)
- T.Pantodac (pantaprazole) -40 mg-

Investigations

DAY	INVESTIGATION
D1	Difficulty in talking :1 week, Throat pain:2days
D2	Physiotherapy, no feeding, Ultra sound abdomen, Dysphagia+
D3	Cough while swalloving
D5	Patient is stable, RT feeding+, Verbal Communication+
D7	GRBS:140MG/DL, HBAIC:7.7, Dysphagia decrease Urine Output good (creatinine-1.5)
D8	Throat irritation, cough+, Mild relief of dysphagia edema-present-
D9	Dysphagia decreased, oral feeds, no other fresh issues.
D10	GRBS: 193mg/dL, urine culture: E.coli($7*10^5$ CFU/ml), senstive to the magnex forte
D11	Physiotherapy mobilisation silicon catheters
D12	Patient is stable vitals stable no fresh issues
D13	Cognitive language aspect, speech, mild dysarrthymia, conscious, coherent urine output good (creatinine 1.2)
D20	Vomiting-1 episode GRBS:54mg/dL
D23	Severe GERD, Wheezing
D24	Endoscopy-Hiatus hernia GRBS-22 (General Random Blood Sugar)

Discharge Medication

1. T.Clopilet (Clopidogrel) -75mg
2. T.Tonact (Atorvastatain) -40mg
3. T.Eltroxin (Thyroxine) -50mcg
4. T.Pulmoclear (acebrophylline 100mg+Acetylcysteine 600mg)
5. T.Nephroadd (Taurine 500mg+acetylcysteine 150mg)
6. Syp.Sucralset plus (Sucralfate 500mg+ oxetacaine 10mg) -10ml
7. Neb with Duolin (Levosalbutamol+ ipratropium)
8. T.Niftas (Nitrofurantoin) -50mg
9. Neb with formonide –0.5mg (Formeterol + Budesonide)
10. Zytee (Choline salicylate) mouth paint for local application
11. T.Forcan (Fluconazole) - 150mg

12. T.Claribid (Clarithromycin)
13. T.Sampraz D (Domperidone 30mg + esomeprazole 40mg)
14. Inj.Novorapid SC 10 units (BBF)- Insulin
15. T.Galvusmet-50/500mg (Metformin+ vildagliptin)
16. GRBS-check TID

Assignment

1. Specific pharmacotherapeutic treatment to reduce risk of stroke for this patient?

Table 7.2 Comparion of Antithrombotic Agents for the Prevention of Recurrent Ischemic Stroke.

Agent	Effectiveness	Tolerability
Aspirin	Aspirin, 50 to 325 mg daily, is recommended for initial therapy to prevent recurrent ischemic stroke.	GI upset (17.6%)
Clopidogrel	Clopidogrel monotherapy, 75 mg daily, is recommended for secondary prevention of stroke and can also be used in patients who are allergic to aspirin	GI upsent (15%), diarrhea (4.5%), Rash (6%)
Aspirin plus clopidogrel	The CHANCE (Clopidogrel in High-Risk Patients with Acute Nondisabling Cerebrovascular Events) trial demonstrated that starting aspirin plus clopidogrel within 24 hours of a minor ischemic stroke or TIA and continuing it for up to 21 days may prevent recurrent stroke	GI upset, diarrhea, rash
Aspirin/ dipyridamole	Aspirin/dipyridamole, 25 mg/200 mg twice daily, is indicated for initial therapy after TIA or ischemic stroke for recurrent stroke prevention	Headache (26%), GI upset

Source: Dickerson LM, Carek PJ, Quattlebaum RG. Prevention of recurrent ischemic stroke. Am Fam Physician. 2007;76(3):386.

2. Prevention of TIA?

- Stop smoking; Limit cholesterol and fat diet; Eat plenty of fruits and vegetables and whole grains
- Limit sodium intake; Exercise regularly; Limit alcohol intake
- Maintain healthy weight; Control diabetes; Dont use illicit drugs

3. Initial and long term goals in treating the patient?

- Initially start with antiplatlet therapy include asprin, clopidogrel, ticlodipine, aspirin-dypridamole or tissue plasminogen activator is preferred

Long Term Treatment

- Antiplatlet therapy;
- Anticoagulation: for patients with atrial fibrillation
- Antihypertensives;

- Statin therapy;
- Diabetic care
- Life style modifications;
- Stroke education

4. Non Pharmacolagical Interventions available to prevent another TIA?

- Reducing vascular risk factors is often a complex process
- This cardiac rehabilitation programs designed for people with heart disease. Tends to be multi-faceted, involving combination of exercise, dietary advice, lifestyle counseling with patient education and aerobic training
- Exercise based Cardiac rehabilitation (CR), with or with out patient education and lifestyle counseling has been shown to induce favorable effects on total cholesterol, triglyceride, systolic blood pressure

5. Role of Aspirin in TIA in Preventing Ischaemic Stroke?

- The primary role of aspirin is for secondary prevention rather than for treatment for acute minor stroke or TIA. Any dose of aspirin reduce the risk of any stroke by 23% among patient with prior stroke or TIA. Immediate treatment with aspirin can substantially reduce the risk and severity of early recurrent stroke. MOA: Inhibition of PGI synthesis action to prevent formation of platelet aggregating substance Thromboxane A2

6. What is the recommended dose of aspirin?

1. Mostly recommended are 80mg/160mg/325mg/day
2. Appropriate dose is lowest dose that is effective in preventing both MI and stroke
3. In men:160mg/d – lowered risk of MI

In women: 50mg,75mg and 100mg – did not significantly decrease risk of MI The appropriate dose in women, must exceed 100mg/d so appropriate dose in men and women must be atleast 160mg/d

7. Patient Councelling Measures?

- Educating patients about risk of recurrence and discussing ways they can reduce their risk is essential
- Patient are often concerned about antiplatelet agents
- Due to potential for bleeding and may discontinue these agents
- Chronic headache is common side effect of dipyridamole, causing patients to discontinue this potentially life saving medication
- It is also common for patients to experience GI upset with aspirin therapy and pharmacists can recommended patients take their aspirin with food or suggest their physician about changing to clopidogrel which is reasonable alternative
- Monitoring patient's blood pressure, offering smoking cessation counseling as well as counseling on weight loss and exercise would prove beneficial in reducing risk of stroke and improving patients over all health

8. What subjective and objective data of patient history are consistent with recurrent ischaemic stroke?

Subjective Data

- Chief complaints of decreased intake of food, generalized weakness, decrease responsiveness, vomiting (2 days), throat pain (2 days) and difficulty in talking

The patient history of patient is recurrent ischemic stroke, type2 DM, HTN, Hypothyrodisim and dyslipidemia

Objective Data

- Consicious, coherent, cooperative, oriented
- BP:90/60mm hg
- RS:B/L Airway entry, wheezes present
- CVS: S_1S_2, sounds normal, no murmurs, peripheral pulses palpable
- CNS:Left upper limb weakness
- TLC and Sr.Creatinine – Increases
- Dysphagia

References

1. Dirnagl U, Iadecola C, Moskowitz MA. Pathobiology of ischemic stroke: An integrated view. Trends Neurosci 1999; 22:391–397.
2. Update. Stroke 2007; 38:2001–2023.
3. Juvela S, Kase CS. Advances in intracerebral hemorrhage management. Stroke 2006; 37:301–304.
4. Feuerstein GZ, Wang X. New opportunities for stroke prevention and therapeutics: A hope from anti-inflammatory drugs? In: Feuerstein GZ, ed. Inflammation and Stroke. Basel: Birkhauser-Verlag, 2001:3– 10.
5. Broderick J, Connelly S, Feldman E, et al. Guidelines for the management of spontaneous intracerebral hemorrhage in adults: 2007
6. Chinese Acute Stroke Trial (CAST) Collaborative Group. CAST: A randomized, placebo-controlled trial of early aspirin use in 20,000 patients with acute ischemic stroke. Lancet 1997; 349:1641–1649.
7. Adams HP Jr, del Zoppo G, Alberts MJ, et al. Guidelines for the early managment of adults with ischemic stroke: A guideline from the American Heart Association. Stroke 2007;38:1655–1711.
8. Khaja AM, Grotta JC. Established treatments for acute ischemic stroke. Lancet 2007;369:319–330.
9. Miller J, Diringer M. Management of aneurysmal subarachnoid hemorrhage. Neurol Clin 1995;13:451–478.

10. The National Institute of Neurological Disorders and Stroke rt-PA Stroke Study Group. Tissue plasminogen activator for acute ischemic stroke. N Engl J Med 1995;333:1581–1587.

11. Mayer SA, Brun NC, Begtrup K, et al. Recombinant activated factor VII for acute intracerebral hemorrhage. N Engl J Med 2005;352:777–785.

12. Badjatia N, Rosand J. Intracerebral hemorrhage. Neurologist 2005; 11(6):311–324.

13. Barr D, Epps QJ. Direct oral anticoagulants: a review of common medication errors. *J Thromb Thrombolysis* 2018 Oct 8. doi: 10.1007/s11239-018-1752-9.

CHAPTER - 8

Venous Thromboembolism

Introduction to Venous Thromboembolism (VTE)

Venous thromboembolism results from clot formation in the venous circulation. It is manifested as Deep Vein Thrombosis (DVT) and Pulmonary Embolism (PE). A DVT is a thrombus composed of cellular material (RBC, WBC, platelets) bound together with fibrin strands. A PE is a thrombus that arises from systemic circulation and lodges in the pulmonary artery or one of its branches causing partial or complete obstruction of pulmonary blood flow.

Epidemiology

VTE is a spectrum: simple superficial thrombophlebitis to fatal PE. VTE incidence among whites of European origin exceeds 1 per 1000; the incidence among persons of African and Asian origin may be higher and lower, respectively. VTE incidence over recent time remains unchanged. Survival after VTE is worse than expected, especially for pulmonary embolism where one-quarter of patients present as sudden death. Of those patients who survive, 30% develop VTE recurrence and venous stasis syndrome within 10 and 20 years, respectively.

Estimated incidence: 100/100000. 1/3 cases are PE. Increase dramatically with age.

Etiology and Risk Factors [1, 2]

Three primary factors influence the formation of pathological clots and are described as Virchow's triad:

1. **Stasis:** Mainly caused by heart failure; any major surgery with general anesthesia for greater than 30 minutes; paralysis due to stroke or spinal cord injury; prolonged immobility; polycthemia vera and obseity
2. **Endothelial injury:** Mainly caused by either trauma (esp. fractures of pelvis, hip, or leg); local irritation (by chemotherapy, past DVT, Phlebitis); any major orthopedic surgery (e.g. knee and hip replacement); indwelling venous catheters
3. **Hypercoagulability:** Inherited or acquired. Antithrombin (AT) 3 deficiency, protein C or protein S deficiency; antiphospholipid antibodies; plasminogen activator inhibitor excess;

pregnancy; factor V laiden; malignancy; estrogen therapy; homocysteinemia

4. **Others:** Immobility, surgery with in last three months, stroke, history of VTE, CHF, HTN, varicose veins, superficial vein thrombosis, heavy smoking, pregnancy, obesity, age greater than 60.

5. **Heriintrinsic and extrinsic pathwditary:** Factor 5 leiden, pro thrombin deficiency.

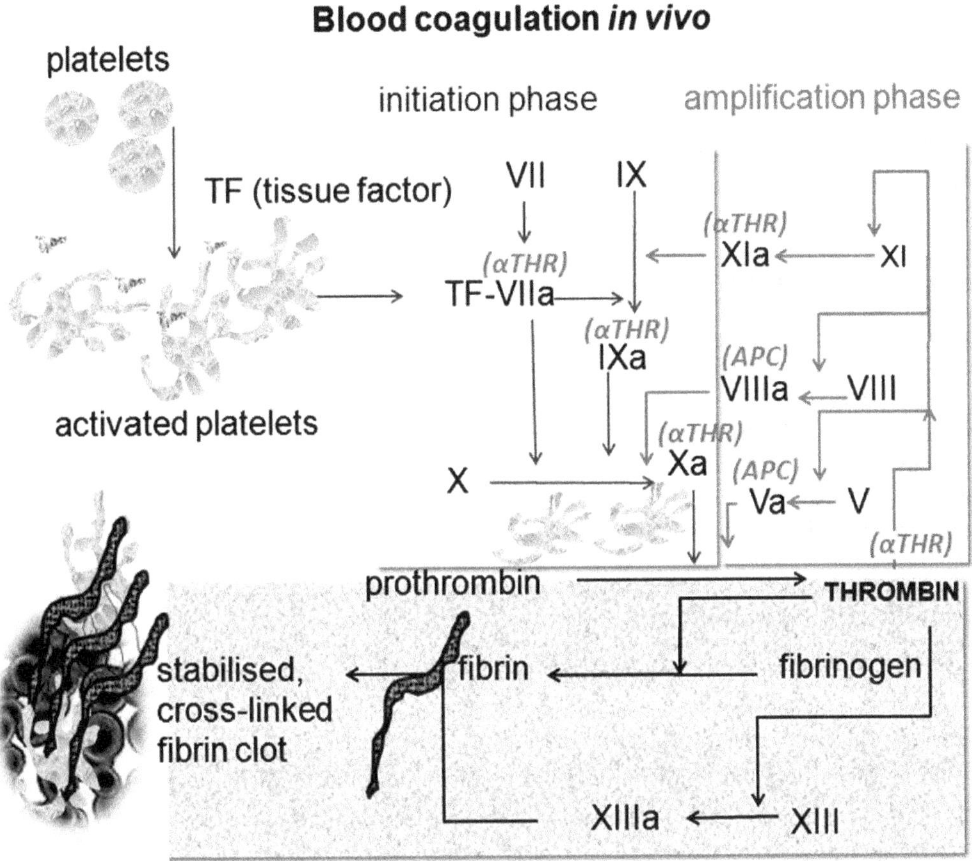

Fig. 8.1 Intrinsic and extrinsic pathways of blood coagulation.

Clotting cascade: The coagulation cascade has been divided into three distinct parts: the intrinsic, extrinsic, and common pathways. This artificial division is somewhat misleading, as there are numerous interactions between the three pathways. The extrinsic pathway, sometimes referred to as the tissue factor pathway, appears to be the principal mechanism that triggers the coagulation cascade. Tissue factor, released from the subendothelium, forms a complex with factor VIIa. The factor VIIa–tissue factor complex activates factor X in the common pathway and factor IX in the intrinsic pathway. The intrinsic pathway plays a key role in the propagation of clot formation. The activation and inhibition of factor X in the common pathway is a key step in the regulation of clot formation. With its cofactor, factor Va, factor Xa converts prothrombin

(II) to thrombin (IIa), which then cleaves fibrinogen to form fibrin monomers. Finally, as the fibrin monomers reach a critical concentration, they begin to precipitate and polymerize to form fibrin strands. Factor XIIIa covalently bonds these strands to one another.

Normally, a number of tempering mechanisms control coagulation. Without effective self regulation, the coagulation cascade would proceed unabated until all the clotting factors and platelets were consumed. The intact endothelium adjacent to the damaged tissue actively secretes several anti-thrombotic substances. As its name implies, thrombomodulin modulates thrombin activity by converting protein C to its active form. When joined with its cofactor protein S, protein C enzymatically inactivates factors Va and VIIIa. Activated protein C also stimulates the release of tissue plasminogen activator. Antithrombin is a circulating protein that inhibits thrombin and factor Xa. Heparan sulfate, a heparin-like compound secreted by endothelial cells, exponentially accelerates antithrombin activity. By a similar mechanism, heparin cofactor II also inhibits thrombin. Tissue factor pathway inhibitor plays an important role by regulating the initiation of the coagulation cascade. When these self-regulatory mechanisms are intact, the formation of the fibrin clot is limited to the zone of tissue injury. However, disruptions in the system, so-called hypercoagulable states, often result in thrombosis.

The fibrinolytic protein plasmin degrades the fibrin mesh into soluble end products collectively known as fibrin split products or fibrin degradation products. The fibrinolytic system is also under the control of a series of stimulatory and inhibitory substances. Tissue plasminogen activator and urokinase plasminogen activator convert plasminogen to plasmin. Plasminogen activator inhibitor-1 inhibits the plasminogen activators, and α2-antiplasmin inhibits plasmin activity. Aberrations in the fibrinolytic system have also been linked to hypercoagulability.

Inhibitors of Clotting Mechanisms

- Antithrombin: Inhibits factors IIa, IXa, and Xa
- Protein S: Cofactor for activation of protein C
- Protein C: Inactivates factors Va and VIIIa
- Tissue factor pathway inhibitor: Inhibits activity of factor VIIa
- Plasminogen: Converted to plasmin via tissue plasminogen activator
- Plasmin: Lyses fibrin into fibrin degradation products

Pathological Thrombi

Pathological thrombi are sometimes classified according to location and composition. Arterial thrombi are composed primarily of platelets, although they also contain fibrin and occasional leukocytes. Arterial thrombi generally occur in areas of rapid blood flow (i.e., arteries) and are typically initiated by spontaneous or mechanical rupture of atherosclerotic plaques. Venous thrombi are found primarily in the venous circulation and are composed almost entirely of fibrin and erythrocytes. Venous thrombi have a small platelet head and generally form in response to either venous stasis or vascular injury after surgery or trauma. The areas of stasis prevent dilution of activated coagulation factors by normal blood flow

Pathophysiology of DVT [3]

Deep venous thrombosis usually arises in the lower extremities. Most DVTs form in the calf veins, particularly in the soleus sinusoids and cusps of the valves.

- Venous valves are avascular, which, in conjunction with reduced flow of oxygenated blood in veins, predisposes the endothelium to be hypoxemic. The endothelium around valves responds by expressing adhesion molecules that attract leukocytes. These cells transfer tissue factor to the endothelium, which can complex with activated factor VII to begin the coagulation cascade via the extrinsic pathway. The main component of these venous thrombi is fibrin (as product of coagulation cascade) and red blood cells, which get trapped in the clot. *Platelets* also contribute, but to a lesser extent.
- The skeletal muscle pump helps prevent DVT by moving blood past the valves (i.e. reducing venous stasis), which washes away activated clotting factors that can otherwise propagate the initial thrombus.
- If a clot forms and does not resolve, it will extend proximally into the popliteal and femoral veins ("proximal veins"). 25% of calf DVTs will extend proximally within 7 days. While calf DVTs are usually asymptomatic and do not give rise to significant PEs, proximal DVTs are more likely symptomatic and can embolize to form dangerous PEs.

Resolution and Consequences

The initial thrombus can lead to complete resolution, clot extension/embolization, or organization.

- Complete resolution: Fibrinolysis is a dynamic process where *plasminogen* is converted into plasmin, an enzyme that degrades fibrin into soluble peptides. Fibrinolysis starts within hours, and it can lead to complete or partial resolution of the thrombus. Partial resolution may lead to any one of these 3 consequences.
- Clot extension and embolization: Proximal flow of the venous blood sweeps the thrombus in the same direction, extending it into the proximal veins.
- Organization: Thrombi that do not resolve begin to *retract* within days. At the same time, inflammatory cells infiltrate the thrombi and cause remodeling. The residual clot is incorporated into the vessel wall and a layer of endothelial cells forms on top (re-endothelialization). This process, called organization, allows some blood flow to resume, but it destroys valves along the length of the clot and causes scarring of the veins. The hemodynamic changes to the vein causes post-thrombotic syndrome.
  - ➤ Post-thrombotic syndrome is a consequence of DVTs, and the clinical features include *pain, leg edema,* and other *signs of venous insufficiency.* It occurs in approximately 1/3 of DVT cases. The cause is a combination of *venous obstruction* by residual clots or venous scarring and *venous reflux* due to valve destruction. Prevention of this sequela includes *adequate anticoagulation* to prevent VTE recurrence and *compression stockings* to improve venous return.

Pathophysiology of PE [4, 5]

Patients with risk factors (Virchow's triad) develop DVT, which ascends up the inferior venacava to the right heart and lodges in the pulmonary vasculature.

V-Q mismatch: Large emboli get stuck in the central vessels, which more likely leads to hemodynamic consequences. Small emboli clear the large vessels and lodges in the peripheral vessels, leading to irritation of the pleural. The primary defect is V-Q mismatch because parts of lung are not perfused and as a result of vascular compromise and inflammation, some parts are not ventilated. Arterial hypoxemia follows and leads to more CO_2 than necessary leading to hypocapnia.

Hemodynamic consequences: Mechanical occlusion of the vessels and response vasoconstriction causes pulmonary resistance and sunsequent right heart overload. If the occlusion is significant, forward flow to the left heart is reduced, causing heart failure and shock.

Clinical Manifestation and Features

Signs and Symptoms of DVT

1. Symptom: asymmetric leg/calf swelling
   Sign: pitting edema on affect side
   Mechanism: swelling and pitting edema are caused by venous obstruction. Calf circumference is measured 10cm below the tibial tuberosity.
2. Symptom: Pain, erythema
   Sign: Localized tenderness along deep venous system.
   Mechanism: Pain, erythema and tenderness are caused by vascular inflammation. Recruitment of inflammatory cellsto thrombus and venous stasis causes phlebitis.
3. Sign: homan's sign
   Mechanism: the sign is elicited by passive dorsiflexion of the ankle.
   Positive signs include increased resistance to dorsiflexion or knee flexion both in response to irritation of the posterior calf muscles.
4. Symptom: dilated superficial veins (non varicose)
   Sign: palpable cord
   Mechanism: dilated superficial veins are caused by obstruction of deep venous system. Palpable cords refer to palpable superficial veins which is sign of superficial phlebitis.

Clinical Features of PE

1. Symptom: dyspnea
   Sign: tachypnea
   Mechanism: hyperventilation to compensate for increased deadspace and in response to chemical mediators from platelets.

2. Symptom: palpitations

   Sign: tachycardia

   Mechanism: it is a sympathetic response to decreased cardiac output.

3. Symptom: pleuriticchest pain

   Sign: pleural friction rib,; pleural effusion.

   Mechanism: inflammation in the pleural region is responsible for pleuritic chest pain.

4. Symptom: hemoptysis and cough

   Mechanism: damage to pulmonary vasculature, which leads to bleeding into the airways.

   Cough is nonproductive and may be triggered by irritation of the pleura.

5. Symptom: syncope

   Sign: hypertension, cyanosis

   Mechanism: decreased left ventricular filling causing forward heart failure.

6. Sign: parasternal heave, loud P2, increased Jugular venous pressure (JVP)

   Mechanism: increased pulomonary pressure causes right ventricular overload and right ventricular dilatation.

Diagnosis with Algorithm

Step wise approach for diagnosis of Pulmonary embolism [6]:

1. If there is clinical suspicion for pulmonary embolism, perform clinical probability assessment.

2. If the patient is hemodynamically stable and has low clinical probability, perform D-dimer assay. If it is normal, then pulmonary embolism excluded. But if it is elevated, multidetector Computed Tomography (CT) should be performed. If the result is negative, it is confirmed as PE excluded. But if it is positive, then it is confirmed as Pulmonary Embolism (PE).

   If the patient is with intermediate/ high clinical probability, perform multidetector CT scan to confirm if the patient is positive for PE.

3. If the patent is hemodynamically unstable but not critically ill, perform multidetector CT scan to confirm if he is positive for PE.

4. If the patient is hemodynamically unstable, critically ill and with high clinical probability, perform transthoracic or transesophageal echocardiography to assess the ventricular dysfunction and confirm it as positive for PE.

Step wise approach for diagnosis of DVT [7]

- If there is clinical suspicion for DVT, determine pretest probability.
- If the probability is low, perform d-dimer assay to confirm it as DVT. Ultrasonography also can be done to confirm DVT in the patient.
- But if the probability is intermediate or high, perform compression ultrasonography to

confirm as DVT. If the ultrasonography result is negative, additionally perform d-dimer assay. If the result is negative DVT is excluded. But if it is positive, repeat the compression ultrasonography in one week and confirm if the test is positive.

Laboratory Tests

1. **Compression ultrasound** (CUS) and computed tomography pulmonary angiography (CTPA) are used most often for initial evaluation of suspected VTE.
2. Venography, pulomonary angiography are the most accurate and reliable diagnostic methods but are expensive, invasive and difficult to perform and evaluate.
3. TheV/Q (Ventilation-perfusion) scans for PE
4. Sr conc of D-dimer if >500ng/dL – VTE
5. **WELL's risk score [8]:**

Variable	Points
1. Previous deep vain thrombosis or PE	1.5
2. Recent surgery or immobilsation	1.5
3. Cancer	1
4. Haemoptysis	1.5
5. Heart rate > 100 beats/min	1.5
6. Clinical signs of deep vein thrombosis	3
7. Alternative diagnosis less likely than PE	3

Clinical probability: Low   0-1   Intermediate 2-6   High > 7.

6. Bleeding and coagulation profile: may show prolongation of PT and APTT.

7. Troponin: high in moderate to large PE.

8. ABG (arterial blood gases): May show hypoxemia, hypocapnia, respiratory alkalosis or respiratory failure.

9. Echocardiography: may show right ventricular enlargement, right atrial enlargement or tricuspid regurgitation. Regurgitant Volume (RV) Right Ventricular Outflow Tract (RVOT) thrombus may be rarely be seen.

Clinical Assessment Models for DVT and PE (Clinical features with score)

1. Pretest Probability of DVT
    - (a) Tenderness along entire deep vein system 1.0
    - (b) Swelling of the entire leg 1.0
    - (c) Greater than 3-cm difference in calf circumference 1.0
    - (d) Pitting edema 1.0
    - (e) Collateral superficial veins 1.0
    - (f) Risk factors present:

Active cancer 1.0

Prolonged immobility or paralysis 1.0

Recent surgery or major medical illness 1.0

Alternative diagnosis likely (ruptured Baker's cyst, rheumatoid arthritis, superficial thrombophlebitis, or infective cellulitis) −2.0

Score $\geq$3 = high probability; 1–2 = moderate probability; $\leq$0 = low probability

1. Pretest Probability of PE
   (a) Clinical features of deep vein thrombosis 3.0
   (b) Recent prolonged immobility or surgery 1.5 Active cancer 1.0
   (c) History of deep vein thrombosis or pulmonary embolism 1.5
   (d) Hemoptysis 1.0
   (e) Resting heart rate > 100 beats per minute 1.5
   (f) No alternative explanation for acute shortness of breath or chest pain 3.0

Score $\geq$6 = high probability; 2–6 = moderate probability; $\leq$1.5 = low probability

Management: The goals of treatment for VTE are

(i) Anticoagulation to prevent further clot generation and
(ii) Thrombolysis if the thrombus is large enough to cause hemodynamic compromise.

Treatment with Algorithm

Treatment clinical Algorithm for DVT

The patient should be tested for Pretest probability for deep vein thrombosis.

1. If probability is low:
   (i) Is he D-dimer positive-perform emergency bedside ultrasoiund for DVT. If the test is negative repeat in 5-7 days. But if he is pested positive, anticoagulant therapy to be initiated.
   (ii) Is he D-Dimer negative- DVT is excluded.
2. If probability is Modearte to high: Perform emergency bedside ultrasound for DVT.
   (i) Is he positive- anticoagulant therapy to be initiated.
   (ii) Is he negative-obtain D-Dimer. If he is tested negative for D-Dimer then DVT is excluded in the patient. Id D-Dimer is positive – repeat ultrasound in 5-7 days or obtain confirmatory study.

Pharmacological Treatment Options

1. **Unfractionated Heparin**: Extracted from porcine gut mucosa or beef lung. 80 units/kg IV bolus than continuous infusion of 18units/kg/h
2. **Low molecular weight heparins (LMWH):** Enoxaparin-1 mg/kg SC twice daily OR 1.5mg/kg SC once daily
   Tinzaparin

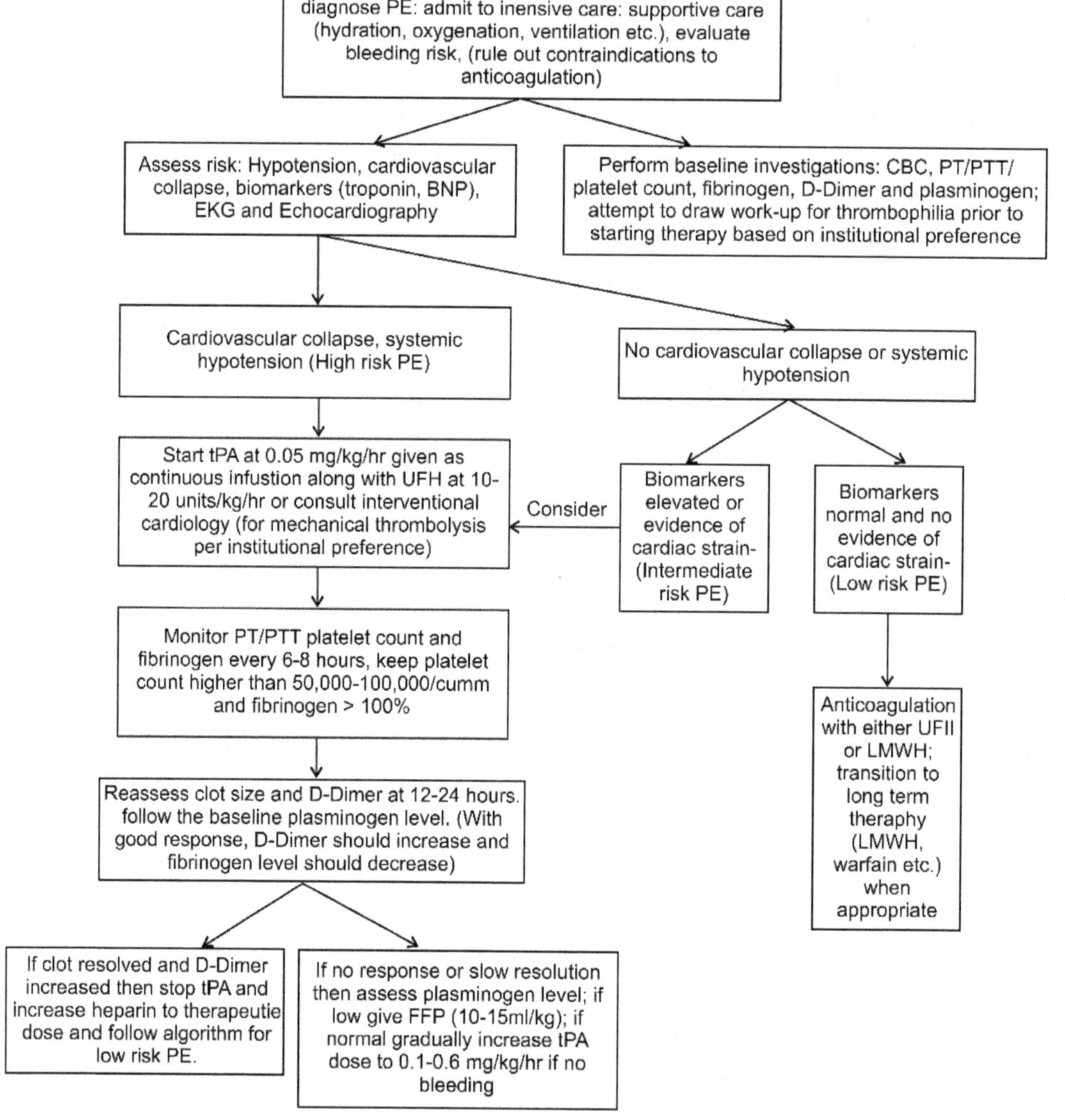

Fig. 8.2 Treatment algorithm for Pulmonary embolism.

Source: Ahmar Zaidi et al., Pulmonary embolism in children, Frontiers in Pediatrics. 2017; 5: 10-20.

3. **Anti-factor Xa Inhibitors**: Foundaparinox: <50kg-5 mg SC once daily; 50-100 kg: 7,5 mg SC once daily; 100kg: 10mg SC once daily
   Indaparinox
4. **Direct thrombin inhibitors**: Argatroban, Bivalirudin, Lepirudin
5. **Vitamin K antagonists**: Warfarin: patient specific dosing based on INR
   Rivaroxaban: 15mg twice daliy for 21 days then 20mg daily
   Dabigatran: 150mg twice daily after parateral anticoagulation
6. **Thrombolytics:** Alteplase: 100mg IV infusion over 2 h

Pharmacolgical Treatment

1. **Unfractionated heparin (UFH):** UFH is a heterogeneous mixture of sulfated glycosaminoglycans of variable lengths and pharmacologic properties. Each heparin molecule is composed of repetitive units of D-glycosamine and uronic acid. The molecular weights of these molecules range from 5000 to 30,000 Daltons, with a mean of 15,000 Daltons. It binds to antithrombin, provoking a conformational change. The UFH-antithrombin complex is 100 to 1000 times more potent as an anticoagulant compared with antithrombin alone. UFH prevents the growth and propagation of a formed thrombus and allows the patient's own thrombolytic system to degrade the clot. Factors IIa and Xa are the most sensitive to inhibition by the UFH-antithrombin complex.

   Weight-Based Dosing for UFH Administered by Continuous Intravenous Infusion
   For Deep Vein Thrombosis (DVT) Pulmonary Embolism (PE) Initial Loading Dose is 80–100 units/kg and Maximum = 10,000 units
   Initial Infusion Rate 17–20 units/kg/h Maximum = 2300 units/h
   aPTT (s): maintenance infusion rate
   1. If < 37: 80 units/kg bolus; then increase infusion by 4 units/kg/h
   2. 37-47: 40 units/kg bolus; then increase infusion by 2 units/kg/h
   3. 48-71: No change
   4. 72–93: Decrease infusion by 2 units/kg/h
   5. >93: Hold infusion for 1 h; then decrease by 3 units/kg/h

   Risk Factors for Major Bleeding While Taking Anticoagulation Therapy
   Anticoagulation intensity (e.g., INR > 4.0), Unstable anticoagulation response, Age > 65 years, Concurrent antiplatelet 2drug or NSAID use, History of gastrointestinal bleeding, Recent surgery or trauma, Heavy alcohol use, Renal failure, Cerebrovascular disease, Malignancy

   Contraindications to Anticoagulation Therapy
   a) Active bleeding b) Hemophilia or other hemorrhagic tendencies c) Severe liver disease with elevated baseline Prothrombin Time (PT) d) Severe thrombocytopenia (platelet count < 20,000/mm^3) e) Malignant hypertension f) Inability to meticulously supervise and monitor treatment.
   ADRS: Bleeding in GIT, urinary tract and soft tissues, severe headache, joint pain, chestpain etc.

Monitering parameters: Activated Partial Thromboplastin Clotting Time (Aptt) must be checked, 2. Thrombocytopenia :<15,000/mm^3

2 types: 1) heparin associated thrombocytopenia (HAT): it is a benign, transient and mild phenomenon that usually occurs with in the first 5days of treatment. 2) Heparin induced thrombocytopenia (HIT): it is a serious problem that required immediate intervention. Platelet count goes as low as 20,000/mm^3 with in 5 days of Heparin use.

Long-term UFH has been reported to cause alopecia, priapism, and suppressed aldosterone synthesis with subsequent hyperkalemia. The use of UFH for longer than 1 month has been associated with significant bone loss and may lead to osteoporosis.

Management of Bleeding and Excessive Anticoagulation

When major bleeding occurs, UFH should be discontinued immediately, and the underlying source of bleeding should be identified and treated. Intravenous protamine sulfate, 1 mg/100 units of UFH up to a maximum of 50 mg can be administered to reverse the anticoagulant effects of UFH.

2. **Low molecular weight heparin (LMWH):** Produced by either chemical or enzymatic depolymerization. LMWHs are fragments of UFH. They are heterogeneous mixtures of sulfated glycosaminoglycans with approximately one-third the molecular weight of UFH. Functions similar to UFH, but due to the smaller average heparin chain length, accelerates the bridging of Antithrombin Activity (AT) with Xa only, and not thrombin and LMWHs have greater anti-factor Xa activity only. Compared to UFH, the LMWHs have more predictable anti-coagulation response.

Indications and Doses for the Low-Molecular Weight Heparins (LMWHs): Enoxaparin

(a) Hip replacement surgery (prophylaxis) 30 mg SC q 12 h initiated 12–24 h after surgery OR 40 mg SC q 24 h initiated 12 h prior to surgerya. Extended prophylaxis may be given for up to 3 weeks

(b) Knee replacement surgery (prophylaxis) 30 mg SC q 12 h initiated 12–24 h prior to surgery

(c) Abdominal surgery (prophylaxis) 40 mg SC q 24 h initiated2h prior to surgery

(d) Acute medical illness (prophylaxis) 40 mg SC q 24 h

(e) Trauma (prophylaxis) 30 mg SC q 12 h starting 12–36 hours after injury

(f) DVT treatment (with or without PE) 1 mg/kg SC q 12 h

(g) Unstable angina or non-Q-wave Ml 1 mg/kg SC q 12 h

Adverse effects: Bleeding is common, thrombocytopenia can occur, osteoporosis lower compared to UFH.

3. **Fondaparinux:** Fondaparinux, also known as pentasaccharide, is a synthetic molecule consisting of the five critical saccharide units that bind specifically but reversibly to antithrombin. A pentasaccharide sequence that directly binds to AT (at an allosteric site) and induces a conformational change allowing it to bind and inhibit factor Xa only. It prevents thrombus generation and clot formation.

Fondaparinux is approved by the FDA for the prevention of VTE following orthopedic surgery (e.g., hip fracture, hip replacement, and knee replacement) and for the treatment of Deep Vein Thrombosis (DVT) and Pulmonary Embolism (PE). Dosing: 2.5 mg injected subcutaneously once daily starting 6 to 8 hours following surgery. Adverse effects: Bleeding.

4. **Direct thrombin inhibitors (e.g. Dabigatran):** Directly block thrombin function by blocking the active site. Dabigatran is equivalent to warfarin in both prevention of recurrent clots and bleeding risk in patients with acute VTE, but it does not require monitoring due to its predictable therapeutic effect (RE-COVER trial).

   1. lepirudin : 0.4mg/kg slow IV bolus titrated to 0.15mg/kg per hour continuous IV

   2. Argatroban : 2microgram/kg/min until App is 1.3-3times control.

5. **Direct Xa inhibitors (e.g. Rivaroxaban):** Directly inhibit the function of Xa by blocking the active site. Unlike warfarin and dabigatran, rivaroxaban does not require overlapping with heparins. Rivaroxaban is equivalent to warfarin in short- and long-term prevention of PE in symptomatic patients, but it does not require monitoring or overlapping, and has significantly lower bleeding risk compared to warfarin

6. **Aspirin:** Although this antiplatelet agent is classically used to prevent **arterial thrombosis**, new evidence suggests that it can also be used for recurrent Venous Thromboembolism (VTE) prevention. Daily aspirin (100mg/day used in trials) can reduce VTE recurrence by approximately 1/3. Aspirin, although not as effective as other anticoagulants, may be used if the patient is intolerant of anticoagulants.

7. **Vitamin K antagonists (e.g. Warfarin)**: Warfarin inhibits the vitamin K dependent synthesis of calcium dependent clotting factors (II, VII, IX and X). Furthermore, warfarin also inhibits Protein S (PS) and Protein C (PC) (part of the endogenous anticoagulation pathway). The inhibition of Protein C and Protein S occurs faster than the other clotting factors, making warfarin acutely a procoagulant. Therefore, warfarin must be given concomitantly with acute anticoagulants at first (a process known as "overlapping") to (i) prevent acute procoagulant effect and (ii) allow time for inhibition of vitamin K dependent factors. Once the patient's international normalized ratio (INR) is therapeutic (2-3), acute anticoagulants can be discontinued.

   Warfarin has been the mainstay of chronic VTE therapy for over 50 years, but there are several issues with its use: (i) increased bleeding risk, (ii) teratogenicity in pregnancy, (iii) interaction with many foods and drugs, and (iii) close monitoring required because anticoagulation effect is not reliably predictable by dosage. New antithrombotic medications have been developed that are potentially safer than warfarin. Dose: 2 or 2.5mg. ADRs: Purple toe syndrome and skin necrosis.

Risk Classification and Consensus Guidelines for VTE Prevention

1. **Risk low:** Minor surgery, age < 40 years, and no clinical risk factors- ambutation is preferred.

2. **Moderate:** Major or minor surgery, age 40–60 years, and no clinical risk factors

   Major surgery, age < 40 years, and no clinical risk factors

   Minor surgery, with clinical risk factor(s)

   Acutely ill (e.g., MI, ischemic stroke, CHF exacerbation), and no clinical risk factors

   Prevention strategies: UFH 5000 units SC q12h

   Dalteparin 2500 units SC q24h

   Enoxaparin 40 mg SC q24h

   Tinzaparin 3500 units SC q24h

   Graduated compression stockings.

3. **High risk:** Major surgery, age > 60 years, and no clinical risk factors

   Major surgery, age 40–60 years, with clinical risk factors

   Prevention strategies: UFH 5000 units SC q8h

   Dalteparin 5000 units SC q24h

   Enoxaparin 40 mg SC q24h

   Tinzaparin 3500 units SC q24h

4. **Highest:** Major lower extremity orthopedic surgery

   Hip fracture

   Multiple trauma

   Major surgery, age > 40 years, and prior history of VTE

   Major surgery, age > 40 years, and malignancy

   Major surgery, age > 40 years, and hypercoagulable state

   Spinal cord injury or stroke with limb paralysis

   Prevention strategies: Adjusted dose UFH SC q8h (aPTT > 36 s)

   Dalteparin 5000 units SC q24h

   Desirudin 15 mg SC q12h

   Enoxaparin 30 mg SC q12h

   Fondaparinux 2.5 mg SC q24h

   Tinzaparin 75 units/kg SC q24h

   Warfarin (INR = 2.0–3.0)

   IPC with UFH 5000 units SC q8h

General Approach to The Treatment of VTE

Anticoagulation therapy remains the mainstay of treatment for VTE. DVT and PE are manifestations of the same disease process and are treated similarly.

1. Acute anticoagulation

Table 8.1 Recommended Anticoagulants for the Acute Management of DVT.

Drug	Dosage
Heparin	80 IU/kg IV (max 10,000 U) for the bolus dose followed by a continuous infusion of 18 IU/kg/h. The aim oif therapy is to achieve an aPTT of 1.5–2 × baseline
Dalteparin sodium	200 U/kg/day SC divided qd-bid. Max: 18,000 U/dose. Continue for <5 days and overlap witg warfarin until INR 2-3
Enoxaparin sodium	1 mg/kg SC q12h. Alt: 1.5 mg/kg SC qd. Continue for > 5 days and overlap with warfarin until INR 2-3
Rivaroxaban	20 mg po qd. Start: 15 mg po bid × 21 days; give 15 abd 20 mg tabs with food. Consider D/C >24 h before surgery or invasive procedure.
Dabigatran	For patients with CrCl > 30 mL/min: 150-mg orally, twice daily after 5-10 days of parenteral anticoagulation.
Fondaparinux	5 mg (body weight < 50 kg), 7.5 mg (50-100 kg), or 10 mg (>100 kg) SC once daily

Alt: alternative: aPTT: activated partial thromboplastin time; CrCl: creatinine clearance; D/C: discontinue: DVT: deep venoses thrombosis; INR: international normalized ratio

Source: Guy att GH, AKIEA, Crowther M, et al. Executive Summary: Antithrombotic therapy and prevention of thrombosis, 9th ed. American College of Chest Physicans. Evidence based clinical practice guidelines chest 2012; 14/(2 Suppl), 75-47S.

2. Duration of acute treatment

- Treatment with UFH, LMWH, or fondaparinux should be overlapped with warfarin for at least 5 days and can be stopped when the INR is >2.0. Most patients should have warfarin started at the same time as UFH, LMWH, or fondaparinux.
- Patients with cancer should be treated with a LMWH for at 1A least 6 months.
- A longer period of heparin therapy (approximately 10 days) is recommended for massive PE or severe iliofemoral thrombosis

3. Long-term anticoagulation

- Oral anticoagulation therapy (target INR 2.5; range 2.0–3.0) should be continued for at least 3 months. If oral anticoagulation therapy is contraindicated (e.g., pregnancy), a treatment dose of LMWH or adjusted-dose UFH should be used.
- Patients with an idiopathic VTE, an inherited disorder of hypercoagulability, or antiphospholipid antibodies should be treated for at least 6 to 12 months and considered for indefinite therapy.
- Patients with two or more episodes of documented DVT should be treated indefinitely

Thrombolysis for the treatment of VTE: Breaks down the thrombus [11, 12, 13]

Thrombolytic therapy should be reserved for patients who present with shock, hypotension, right ventricular strain, or massive DVT with limb gangrene. Diagnosis must be confirmed objectively before initiating thrombolytic therapy. Thrombolytic therapy is most effective when administered as soon as possible after PE diagnosis, but benefit may extend up to 14 days after symptom onset. **Tissue plasminogen activator (tPA):** activates plasminogen (Pg) to plasmin (Pn), which cleaves the thrombus, generating soluble D-dimer products.

- **Alteplase:** for PE: 0.9mg/kg/hr over 24hrs with 10% of the total dose administered as an initial IV dose over 1 min **DVT:** 0.9mg/kg/hr over 24hrs
- **Reteplase:** for PE: 10 units IV bolus followed 30mins later by second 10units IV bolus
- **Streptokinase:** 250,000 units bolus infusion over 30min followed by **100000 units/h for 24hts IV infusion**
- **Tenecteplase: 30-50 mg IV bolus over 5 sec as a single dose**

UFH and LWMH Use during Pregnancy

(A)   Acute treatment:

- LMWH - Enoxaparin 1 mg/kg SC q12h or 1.5 mg/kg q24h or Dalteparin 100 units/kg SC q12h or 200 units/kg q24h or Tinzaparin 175 units/kg SC q24h or
- UFH- Initiate using weight-based intravenous therapy, and adjust dose to achieve therapeutic aPTT for at least 5 days. Transition to SC adjusted-dose UFH administered q8–12h with midinterval a PTT in the therapeutic range.

(B)   Long-term treatment:

- LMWH - Maintain initial LMWH dose regimen throughout pregnancy or Alter LMWH dose in proportion to any weight change (usually gain) or Obtain monthly anti-Xa level measurements 4 to 6 hours after morning dose and adjust LMWH dose to achieve an anti-Xa level of 0.5 to 1.2 units/mL if twice-daily dosing or 1.0 to 2.0 units/mL if once-daily dosing or
- UFH: Obtain monthly aPTT at the midpoint of the dosing interval and adjust UFH dose as indicated.

(C)   Issues at time of delivery:

- Elective induction of labor- Discontinue UFH or LMWH 24 hours prior to induction. Initiate therapeutic doses of UFH by IV infusion and discontinue 4 to 6 hours prior to expected time of delivery if risk of recurrent VTE is deemed high.
- Spontaneous labor- For LMWH, if there is a reasonable expectation that significant anticoagulant effect will be present at time of delivery, (1) epidural should be avoided, and (2) reversal with protamine sulfate may be considered. For UFH, monitor the aPTT and reverse with protamine sulfate if aPTT is prolonged near the time of delivery.
- Postpartum - Commence UFH or LMWH as soon as safely possible (usually 12 hours following delivery). Concurrently initiate warfarin therapy and discontinue UFH or LMWH when the INR is 2.0 or greater. Continue anticoagulants for at least 4 weeks following delivery. Warfarin can be used safely by women who are breast-feeding.

Recommendations for the regimen and the duration of anticoagulation after pulmonary embolism in patients with active cancer

- For patients with PE and cancer, weight-adjusted subcutaneous LMWH should be considered for the first 6 months over Vitamin K Antagonists (VKAs).
- A Edoxaban should be considered as an alternative to weight-adjusted subcutaneous LMWH in patients without gastrointestinal cancer.
- Rivaroxaban should be considered as an alternative to weight-adjusted subcutaneous LMWH in patients without gastrointestinal cancer.
- For patients with PE and cancer, extended anticoagulation (beyond the first 6 months) should be considered for an indefinite period or until the cancer is cured.

References

1. Eric wong, Sultan chowdary. 2011 Apr;105(4):586-96.
2. Tapson VF Acute pulmonary embolism. N Engl J Med. 2008 Mar 6;358(10):1037-52.
3. Line BR. Pathophysiology and diagnosis of deep venous thrombosis. Semin Nucl Med. 2001 Apr;31(2):90-101.
4. Charlebois D[1]. Early recognition of pulmonary embolism: the key to lowering mortality. J Cardiovasc Nurs. 2005 Jul-Aug;20(4):254-9.
5. Kostadima E[1], Zakynthinos E. Pulmonary embolism: pathophysiology, diagnosis, treatment. Hellenic J Cardiol. 2007 Mar-Apr;48(2):94-107.
6. Algorithm for the diagnosis of pulmonary embolism. (CT = computed tomography.) *Adapted from Agnelli G, Becattini C. Acute pulmonary embolism. N Engl J Med. 2010; 363(3):267.*
7. Algorithm for the diagnosis of deep venous thrombosis (DVT). *Adapted with permission from Institute for Clinical Systems Improvement. Copyright 2012. Health care guideline: venous thromboembolism diagnosisantreatment.*
   http://www.icsi.org/venousthromboembolism/venousthromboembolism_4.html.
8. Kline JA, Mitchell AM, Kabrhel C, Richman PB, Courtney DM. Clinical criteria to prevent unnecessary diagnostic testing in emergency department patients with suspected pulmonary embolism. J Thromb Haemost 2004;2:1247-55.
9. Guyatt GH, Akl EA, Crowther M, et al. Executive summary: Antithrombotic therapy and prevention of thrombosis, 9th ed: American College of Chest Physicians Evidence-Based Clinical Practice Guidelines. *Chest.* 2012; 141(2 suppl) :7S-47S.
10. Kearon et al., Antithrombotic therapy for VTE disease: Antithrombotic Therapy and Prevention of Thrombosis, 9th ed: American College of Chest Physicians Evidence-Based Clinical Practice Guidelines. Chest. 2012 Feb;141(2 Suppl):e419S-e496S. doi: 10.1378/chest.11-2301.

11. Kearon C, Alk EA, Ornelas J, et al. Antithrombotic therapy for VTE disease. CHEST Guideline and Expert Panel Report. *Chest* 2016;149(2):315-352.
12. Kearon C, Alk EA, Comerota AJ, et al. Antithrombotic therapy for VTE disease: antithrombotic therapy and prevention of thrombosis. 9th ed: American College of Chest Physicians Evidence-Based Clinical Practice Guidelines. *Chest.* 2012;142(6):1698-1704.
13. PaloVA.Thromboembolism. *Medscape.Reference.* http://emedicine.medscape.com/article/1267714-overview#aw2aab6b2b6. Accessed March 15, 2014.

CHAPTER - 9

Asthma

Introduction to Asthma

Asthma is a chronic inflammatory disorder of airways causing airflow obstruction and recurrent episodes of wheezing, breathlessness, chest tightness and coughing.

Asthma is characterised by inflammation and spasms of the airways (tubes that carry air in and out of the lungs) which makes them very sensitive and react strongly to allergic things and difficulty in air passage.

When asthma symptoms become worse than usual is called asthma attack.

In severe asthma attack, the airways can close so that the vital organs do not get enough oxygen and may lead to death.

Severe asthma is term used when patients have trouble with frequent asthma symptoms or flare ups even when taking highest levels of recommended treatment, so have to be treated for other conditions that can make asthma worse.

Types of Asthma

> **Allergic Asthma:** The people with allergic asthma have their airways extra sensitive to certain allergens making immune system over reactive and airway tightened and flooded with thick mucus. Allergens include windblown pollen from trees grasses, spares and fragments, animal dander, dust, mites etc.
> **Exercise Induced Asthma:** Triggered by exercise or physical exertion, patient's airway narrowing peaks 5 to 20 min after exercise begins, making it difficult to catch your breath.
> **Cough Variants Asthma**: Severe coughing is main symptoms. Other causes post nasal drip, chronic rhinitis, sinusitis or GERD or heart burn.
> **Occupation Asthma**: Results from workplace triggers (jobs associated as animal breeders, farmers, hairdressers, nurses, painters, woodworkers.) Has difficulty in breathing and asthma symptoms just on days of the jobs.

- ➤ **Night Time (Nocturnal) Asthma**: Chances of having symptoms are much higher during sleep because asthma is powerfully induced by sleep work cycle (cardiac rhythms). Trouble breathing, cough, wheezing are dangerous symptoms particularly at night time. Sometimes heart burn can cause asthma at night.
- ➤ **Aspirin induced asthma**: Taking aspirin or other NSAIDs triggers an asthma attack. More common in adults than children. Signs include asthma, ongoing sinus infection, nasal polyp, sensitive to NSAIDs, runny or stuffy nose, watery eyes,
- ➤ **Adult Onset Asthma**: Usually, asthma symptoms can appear at any time in life. Some people develop asthma at age 50-60 or even later. Hormonal fluctuations in women, exposure to viral infections or workplace materials causes this.

Epidemiology: Prevalence rate for reported cases of **asthma** was 4 to 9 times higher than the rate observed for diagnosed cases for **India** and its sub-geographies. The **prevalence** rate varied from 54.9 per 1000 population for reported cases and 9.1 for diagnosed cases for **India.** About 6% of children and 2% of adults have asthma.

Etiology

Causes of Asthma Include

- ➤ **Genetics and Heriditary Factors**: More likely to develop if family members had asthma or have been allergic or certain immunological reactions. Develop in obese people.
- ➤ **Allergies:** Most common cause of asthma attacks by airborne particles, dust and pollen. Sometimes certain food or additives causes airway (bronchi) lining swollen, muscle spasms.
- ➤ **Other Coexisting Conditions:** Viral flu can develop asthma symptoms, sinusitis, nasal polyp, GERD.
- ➤ **Pollution:** Home, work place chemicals, tobacco smoke, exhaust fumes, chemical gases, induce ASTHMA.
- ➤ **Sports and Exercise:** Particularly in cold weather can set an asthma attack.
- ➤ **Drugs /Medications:** Aspirin and other NSAIDs may trigger asthma, also beta blockers, eye drops for glaucoma may cause bronchoconstriction and thus asthma. Occupational hazards, working with plastic resins, wood dust, grains, metals, insecticides can induce.

Risk Factors

- ➤ **Family history:** Person with asthma affected parent are 3 to 6 times more likely to develop asthma than non asthma parent.
- ➤ **Viral respiratory infections:** Some children having viral respiratory infections have risk of asthma.
- ➤ **Allergies:** Having allergic condition like atopic dermatitis, allergic rhinitis is risk factor to develop asthma.
- ➤ **Occupational exposure** to dust, chemical fumes, moulds in workplace cause asthma developed first time

➢ **Smoking:** Cigarette smoking irritates Airways. Smokers are at high risk of asthma development.

➢ **Air pollution** exposure to main component of smog (Ozone) raises risk in people of urban areas

➢ **Obesity -** Children and adult who are obese or overweight are at greater risk of asthma.

Pathophysiology

Allergens inhaled in allergic patents leads to early phase allergic reactions and late phase allergic reactions.

Early Phase Allergic Reactions: After exposure to an asthma precipitating factor (aeroallergen), there is rapid activation of IgE bearing cells. Mast cells, macrophages of airways release proinflammatory mediators (histamine, eicosonoids). These mediators cause contraction of airway smooth muscle mucous, secretion, vasodilation, exudation of Plasma in Airways. This leads to thickened, engorged, edematous airway wall and narrowing lumen, reduced mucous clearance. (Acute Inflammation)

Late Phase Allergic Reactions: Occurs 6 to 9 hrs after allergen provocation, there is activation of eosinophils, T lymphocytes, Basophils, neutrophils, macrophages. The mediators released form them cause air flow obstruction like bronchospasms, oedema, bronchial hyper responsiveness (BHR), airway inflammation hyper secretion.

Airway Inflammatory Reactions:
➢ **T lymphocytes activation causes**: Cytokine release from TH2 cells, mediate allergic inflammation by releasing interleukins- IL-4, IL-5, IL-13. Where as IL-2 and interferon gamma from TH1 cell are responsible for cellular defense mechanism. Imbalance between TH1 and TH2 leads to Allergic Asthmatic inflammation.

➢ **Mast cell degranulation: Mast cells release** mediators like histamine, eosinophils, neutrophils, chemotactic factors, prostaglandins, platelet activating factor (PAF), Leukotrienes LT-C4, D4 and E4. Histamine induces smooth muscle constriction, bronchospasms, mucosal edema, and mucosal secretion.

➢ **Alveolar macrophages:** Release mediators like PAF, LT-B4, C4, D4, neutrophilic and eosinophilic chemotactic factors. Leukotrienes cause bronchospasms, mucus secretions, microvascular permeability, and airway edema.

➢ **Bronchial epithelial cells:** Release eicosonoids, peptidases, matrix proteins, cytokine, NO causing inflammation and release epithelial cell shedding in lumen of airway causing lightened airway response, altered permeability of airway mucosa finally leading to impaired mucociliary transport, bronchial gland increase in size, goblet cell increase in number and size.

➢ **AIRWAY innervated by para sympathetic, sympathetic, non adrenergic inhibitory nerves**: Normal resting tone of airway smooth muscle maintained by vagal afferent activity and bronchoconstriction maintained by vagal stimulation in small bronchi. Innervation of beta 2 adrenergic receptor, produce bronchodilation. Non cholinergic, non adrenergic nervous system in trachea, bronchi amplify inflammation by release of Nitric Oxide (NO).

Clinical Presentation[1]

Chronic Asthma

Symptoms: Dyspnea, chest tightness, coughing (night particularly), wheezing, whistling sounds. May occur when exposed to Allergens during exercise or spontaneously.

Signs: Expiratory wheezing, auscultation, dry cough, atopy (eczema, rhinitis)

Symptoms can be chronic daily, intermittent or with interval of days months, weeks or years.

Mild intermittent symptoms require no medication or beta 2 agonists severity determined by lung function, night awakening etc.

Classification of Asthma Severity by Clinical Features before Treatment

Step 1: Intermittent

Symptoms less than once a week/Brief exacerbations/Nocturnal symptoms not than twice a month/ FEV1 or PEF $\geq$ 80% predicted/ PEF or FEV1 variability < 20%

Step 2: Mild persistent

Symptoms more than once a week but less than once a day/exacerbations may affect activity and sleep/ nocturnal symptoms more than twice a month/ FEV1 or PEF $\geq$ 80% predicted/ PEF or FEV1 variability < 20-30%

Step 3: Moderate persistent

Symptoms daily/ Exacerbations may affect activity and sleep/ nocturnal symptoms more than once a week/ FEV1 or PEF 60-80% predicted/ PEF or FEV1 variability > 30%

Step 4: Severe persistent

Symptoms daily/frequent exacerbations/frequent nocturnal asthma symptoms/ limitation of physical activities/ FEV1 or PEF $\leq$ 60% predicted/ PEF or FEV1 variability >30%.

Acute Severe Asthma [2]

Uncontrolled asthma can progress to acute state in which inflammation, airway edema, mucus accumulation, severe bronchospasms result in profound airway narrowing which is poorly responsive to bronchodilator therapy.

Symptoms: Severe Dyspnea, Shortness of breadth (SOB), chest burning/tightness, speak few words with each breath, unresponse to usual measures (short acting inhaled beta 2 agonists)

Signs: Expiratory /inspiratory wheezing on auscultation, dry cough, tachypnea, tachycardia, pallor, cyanosis, hyperinflated chest with inter coastal and supra clavicular retraction. Breath sounds diminished with severe obstructions.

Diagnosis with Algorithm

- If the patient is with dyspnoea and suspected of Asthma based on history and physical examination. Spirometry assessment has to be done.
- If FEV1/FVC < lower limit of normal: a bronchodilator response on pulmonary function testing is done.
- If increase in FEV1 ≤ 200mL or <12 % from baseline is observed. Then alternative diagnosis or categorised as severe Asthma.
- If increase in FEV1 > 200 mL or > 12% from baseline, it is diagnosed as Asthma.

Chronic Asthma

- Primarily by history of recurrent coughing wheezing shortness of chest tightness and spirometry.
- Spirometry demonstrated obstruction:
- FEV1/FVC GREATER THAN 80% with reversibility after inhaled beta 2 agonists administration. (atleast 12% improved FEV1)
- If baseline spirometer normal then, challenge testing with exercise, histamine done to elicit Brondial Hyperresponsiveness (BHR).
- Patient history of elevated symptoms during specific allergen seasons, exercise, family history of allergy/asthma

Acute Severe Asthma

- PEF and FEV1 greater than 40% which after inhaled beta 2 agonists FEV1 improved at 30 min.
- Arterial blood gases reveals metabolic acidosis, decreased PO_2
- History of previous asthma and exacerbations.
- Hydration status checked, if presence of cyanosis, pneumonia, pneumothorax, upper airway obstruction.
- CBP appropriate is present if fever and purulent sputum present in the patient.

Factors contributing to asthma severity

1. Viral infections: Involved in 20 – 40 % of acute episodes. The most common cause of exacerbations in both children and adults is the common rhinovirus.
2. Environmental and Occupational Factors
3. Psychological Factors: Bronchoconstriction from psychological factors appears to be mediated primarily through excess parasympathetic input.
4. Sinusitis and Rhinitis: 40% to 50% of asthmatics have abnormal sinus radiographs.
5. Gastroesophageal Reflux: Nocturnal asthma may be associated with nighttime reflux
6. Menstruation-Related Asthma: Seen in 30% to 40% of women

Management

Goals of Treatment

Chronic Asthma

- **Reduce impairment:** (a) Prevent chronic and troublesome symptoms (e.g., coughing or breathlessness in the night, in the early morning, or after exertion), (b) maintain (near) "normal" pulmonary function, (c) maintain normal activity levels (including exercise, other physical activities, and attendance at work or school), (d) require infrequent use of short-acting inhaled $\beta2$-agonist ([SABAs], ≤ 2 days a week for quick relief of symptoms).
- Reduce risk and prevent recurrent exerbations, decrease need for emergency department, reduce loss of lung function, lung growth prevent adverse effects of therapy.

Acute Asthma

- Correct the hypoxia
- Rapidly reverse within min. Airway obstruction.
- Reduce reoccurrence of airflow obstruction.

Non Pharmacological Therapy

- Patient education given to better medication adherence, self management skills, use of health care services.
- Avoid exposure to allergic triggers, decrease Brondial hyperresponsiveness (BHR)
- Avoid smoking
- Patient with acute severe asthma should receive O_2 to maintain PO_2 greater than 90%
- Dehydration should be corrected.
- Urine specific gravity may help guide therapy in children.

Pharmacological Therapy [3, 4]

Pharmacological treatment of chronic asthma in adults aged 17 and over according to NICE guidelines

- Offer a short-acting beta$_2$ agonist (SABA) as reliever therapy to adults (aged 17 years and over) with newly diagnosed asthma
- For adults (aged 17 years and over) with asthma who have infrequent, short-lived wheeze and normal lung function, consider treatment with SABA reliever therapy alone
- Offer a low dose of an ICS (inhaled corticosteroid) as the first-line maintenance therapy to adults (aged 17 years and over) with:
  - symptoms at presentation that clearly indicate the need for maintenance therapy (for example, asthma-related symptoms 3 times a week or more, or causing waking at night) **or**
  - asthma that is uncontrolled with a SABA alone

- If asthma is uncontrolled in adults (aged 17 years and over) on a low dose of ICS as maintenance therapy, offer a leukotriene receptor antagonist Leukotriene Receptor Antagonist (LTRA) in addition to the ICS and review the response to treatment in 4 to 8 weeks
- If asthma is uncontrolled in adults (aged 17 years and over) on a low dose of ICS and an LTRA as maintenance therapy, offer a long-acting beta$_2$ agonist (LABA) in combination with the ICS, and review LTRA treatment as follows:
  - o   discuss with the person whether or not to continue LTRA treatment
  - o   take into account the degree of response to LTRA treatment
- If asthma is uncontrolled in adults (aged 17 years and over) on a low dose of ICS and a LABA, with or without an LTRA, as maintenance therapy, offer to change the person's ICS and LABA maintenance therapy to a Maintenance and Reliever Therapy (MART) regimen with a low maintenance ICS dose
- If asthma is uncontrolled in adults (aged 17 years and over) on a MART regimen with a low maintenance ICS dose, with or without an LTRA, consider increasing the ICS to a moderate maintenance dose (either continuing on a MART regimen or changing to a fixed-dose of an ICS and a LABA, with a SABA as a reliever therapy)

  If asthma is uncontrolled in adults (aged 17 years and over) on a moderate maintenance ICS dose with a LABA (either as MART or a fixed-dose regimen), with or without an LTRA, consider:
  - o   increasing the ICS to a high maintenance dose (this should only be offered as part of a fixed-dose regimen, with a SABA used as a reliever therapy) **or**
  - o   a trial of an additional drug (for example, a long-acting muscarinic receptor antagonist or theophylline) **or**
  - o   seeking advice from a healthcare professional with expertise in asthma

Pharmacological treatment of newly diagnosed asthma in children aged 5-16 years according to NICE guidelines

- Newly diagnosed asthma in children and young people (aged 5-16 years), for symptoms that indicate need for maintenance therapy. At presentation offer pediatric Short acting B$_2$ agonist SABA. Next if uncontrolled - low dose ICS is preffered. Alternative is cromolyn, LTRA or theophylline.
- If asthma is uncontrolled in 4-8 weeks-consider pediatric low dose ICS + either (Leukotriene receptor antagonist) LTRA, LABA, or theophylline.
- If asthma is uncontrolled in 4-8 weeks, consider pediatric moderate dose ICS + LABA ; alternative is medium dose ICS+ either LTRA or theophylline
- If asthma is uncontrolled in 4-8 weeks. Consider high dose ICS + LABA.
- If asthma is not controlled in 4-8 weeks, consider high dose ICS + LABA + oral systemic corticosteroid. Alternative: high dose ICS+ LTRA or theophylline + oral systemic corticosteroid.

Pharmacological treatment of chronic asthma in children under 5 years of age

- Offer a SABA as reliever therapy to children under 5 with suspected asthma. This should be used for symptom relief alongside all maintenance therapy

Management of Acute Asthma

Baseline assessment: Must not delay institution of treatment.

(i) Nebuliser with salbutamol 5mg dailypreferably with O2 driven nebuliser or 20 puffs salbutamol MD with large volume soacer.

(ii) Oral prednisolone 0.5mg/kgstat or hydrocortisone 100-200mg IV immediately if severe or unable to swallw. Monitor peak flow.

   (a) **If no improvement is seen**: Nebulise with salbuatamol every 20 minutes or continuously. Add ipratropium bromide0.5mg. IV lines give fluids. Oxygen therapy. Measure arterial blood gases. Antibiotics inly if infection is present.

      If still there is no improvement: Continuous nebulisation with salbutamol and ipratropium bromide. Magenesium sulphate 1-2 g IV. Hydrocortisone IV 100-200mg 6-hourly. Oxygen, IV fluids and calories to be given. Continuous review for complications.

      If still no improvement: Continuous nebulisation with salbutamol and ipratropium bromide. IV Aminophylline-loading dose 5mg/kg over 30 minutes. Maintenance infusion of 0.5mg/kg/h. Continue Hydrocortisone IV 100-200mg 6-hourly. Magenesium sulphate 1-2 g IV in 12 hours. Oxygen, IV fluids and calories to be given. Continuous review for complications. Consider salbuatamol IV infusion.

      Transfer to high care/ICU with ventilation facility.

   (b) **If improvement is seen:** Improvement in symptoms and signs; pulse <120resp rate. O$_2$ saturation > 90% on room air. Able to converse in full sentences. Prepare discharge plan. Prednisolone 20-40mg/day for 7-14 days. Commence controller medications.

(Source: Global Initiative for Asthma. i) GINA Report: Global strategy for asthma management and prevention (2011 Update). http://www.ginasthma.com. ii) Shim CS, Williams MH. Evaluation of the severity of asthma: Patients versus physicians. Am J Med 1980;68(1):11-13).

- Consider an 8-week trial of a paediatric low dose of an ICS in children under 5 years with:
  - symptoms at presentation that clearly indicate the need for maintenance therapy (for example, asthma-related symptoms 3 times a week or more, or causing waking at night) or
  - suspected asthma that is uncontrolled with a SABA alone
- After 8 weeks, stop ICS treatment and continue to monitor the child's symptoms:
  - if symptoms did not resolve during the trial period, review whether an alternative diagnosis is likely
  - if symptoms resolved then reoccurred within 4 weeks of stopping ICS treatment, restart the ICS at a paediatric low dose as first-line maintenance therapy

- o   if symptoms resolved but reoccurred beyond 4 weeks after stopping ICS treatment, repeat the 8-week trial of a paediatric moderate dose of ICS
- If suspected asthma is uncontrolled in children under 5 on a paediatric moderate dose of ICS as maintenance therapy add either an LTRA (Montelukast) or LABA in addition to the ICS
- If suspected asthma is uncontrolled in children under 5 then high dose of ICS + either LABA or montelikast
- If uncontrolled; high dose ICS+ either LABA or montelikast; consider oral corticosteroids.

Beta 2 Agonists

Albuterol is inhaled short acting beta 2 agonists for bronchospasms and acute severe asthma and Exercise Induced Bronchoconstriction (EIB) treatment.

Formeterol, Salmeterol are long acting beta 2 agonists for log term patients.

In acute severe asthma continuous nebulisation of Albuterol is given for patients having unsatisfactory response after three doses (every 20 minutes) of aerosolized Beta 2 agonist and patient initially with PEF/FEV1 values less than 30%.

In nocturnal asthma long acting inhaled Beta 2 agonist preferred over oral sustained release Beta 2 agonist.

Corticosteroids [5, 6]

Inhaled corticosteroids are preferred long term control therapy for persistent asthma because of potency and consistence effectiveness. They are only therapy shown to reduce risk of dying from asthma.

Toxicity is minimal with low to moderate dose but risk of systemic effects increased with high doses.

Maximum improvement in FEV1 and PEF rates may require 3 to 6 weeks.

Adverse Effects of Chronic Systemic Glucocorticoid Administration

Hypothalamic–pitutitary-adrenal suppression, Hypertension, Skin striae, Growth retardation, Impaired wound healing, Skeletal muscle myopathy, Inhibition of leukocyte and monocyte function, Osteoporosis/fractures, Aseptic necrosis of bone, Subcutaneous tissue atrophy, Pancreatitis, Glaucoma, Pseudotumor cerebri, Posterior subcapsular cataracts, Psychiatric disturbances, Moon facies, Sodium and water retention, Central redistribution of fat.

Methyl Xanthines

Theophylline (5mg//kg) and theobromine (10 mg/kg) appears to produce bronchodilation through non selective phosphodiesterase inhibition by methyl xanthene ineffectiveness as aerosol and must be taken systematically (orally or IV).

Anticholinergicss

Ipratropium bromide is a nonselective muscarinic receptor blocker, and blockade of inhibitory muscarinic receptors theoretically could result in an increased release of acetylcholine and overcome the block on the smooth muscle receptors. Ipratropium Bromide and Tiotropium Bromide produced bronchodilation only in cholinergic mediated bronchoconstriction.

Inhaled Ipratropium Bromide is only indicated as adjunctive therapy in severe acute asthma.

Mast Cell Stabilizers

Cromolyn sodium has effects resulting from stabilization of mast cell membrane.

It inhibits the response to allergen challengeas well as EIB but does not cause bronchodilation.

Effective by inhalation

Cromolyn initially taken four times daily after symptoms stabilization reduced to three times daily.

Leukotriene Modifiers

Zafirlukast (Aceolate) and Montelukast (singulair) are Oral Leukotriene receptor antagonists that are oral Leukotriene receptor antagonists that reduce the proinflammatory (increased micro vascular and permeability and airway edema) and bronchoconstriction effects of LD4.

Montelukast Adult dose 10 mg once daily (evening after food)

Children dose 6 - 14 yrs 5 mg chewable tablets (daily eve)

Zileuton (Zyflo) – 5 lipo oxygenase inhibitor

600 mg 4 times daily. Extended release 600 mg tablets twice daily within 1 hr.

Omalizumab[7]

Omalizumab (Xolair) is an anti IgE Ab for treatment of allergic asthma.

Dosage - determined by baseline total serum IgE (International units/mL) and body weight (kg)

Dose- 150 to 375 mg subcutaneously at either 2 or 4 week interval.

Table 9.1 Therapy with Imuunomodulators.

Biologic	Mechanism of action	Indication	Dose	Evidence
Omalizumab	Monoclonal antibody against IgE	Poor control on ICS or LABA, positive perennial aeroallergen testing, total serum IgE level > 30 IU/μL	Subcutaneously once every 2-4 week a based on IgE level and weight	Reduced all exacerbations by 25% and severe exacerbations by 50%
Mepolizumab	Monoclonal antibody against IL-5	Poor control on ICS or LABA, > 2 exacerbations per year, eosinophilia > 150 cells/μL	100 mg subcutaneously once every 4 weeks.	>50% reduction in overall exacerbation rate and a > 60% reduction in hospitalisation/emergency department visits
Reslizumab	Monoclonal antibody against IL-5	Poor control on ICS or LABA, multiple exacerbations peripheral eosinophilia > >400 cells/μl	Intravenous infusion once every weeks, based on weight	>50% improvement in quality of life and an FEV_1, improvement by 90-160 mL
Benralizumab	Monoclonal antibody against Il-5 receptor	Poor control on ICS or LABA, >2 exacerbations per year, eosinophilia > 300 cells/μL.	Subcutaneous 30 mg once every 4 weeks (first three doses) the once every 8 weeks.	>50% reduction in exacerbations and a lung function improvement of 24%
Dupilumab	Monoclonal antibody against Il-4 receptor alpha subunit	Eosinophilia > 300 cells/μL, FeNO > 25 ppb	Not approved in the USA or Eurepoe for asthma (200-300 mg once every 2 weeks, subcutaneously)	Improved severe exacerbation rates by >47% and an improved FEV_1 by 320 mL
Tezepelumab	Monoclonal antibody against thymic stromal lymphopoietin	Poor control on ICS/LABA, >2exacerbations per year	Phase III testing (70 mg versus 210 mg once every 4 weeks or 280 mg once every 2 weeks)	Exacerbation lowered by >60% and FEV_1 improved by >100 mL in all groups

Management of Asthma Exacerbations:
Emergency Department and Hospital-Based Care.

(National Institutes of Health. Expert Panel Report 3. Guidelines for the Diagnosis and Management of Asthma. NIH Publication No. 08-4051.0; 2007)

Initial Assessment Brief history, physical examination (auscultation, use of accessory muscles, heart rate, respiratory rate), PEF or FEV1, oxygen saturation, and other tests as indicated.

- FEV1 or PEF 40% (Mild-to-Moderate) Oxygen to achieve SaO2 90%; Inhaled SABA by nebulizer or MDI with valved holding chamber, up to 3 doses in first hour; Oral systemic corticosteroids if no immediate response or if patient recently took oral systemic corticosteroids.
- FEV1 or PEF < 40% cases (severe): Oxygen to achieve SaO2 90%; High-dose inhaled SABA plus ipratropium by nebulizer or Metered Dose in haler (MDI) plus valved holding chamber, every 20 minutes or continuously for 1 hour; Oral systemic corticosteroids.
- Impending or Actual Respiratory Arrest: Intubation and mechanical ventilation with 100% oxygen; Nebulized SABA and ipratropium; Intravenous corticosteroids; Consider adjunct therapies. Admit the patient to hospital intensive care.

After initial treatment, assessment is repeated and the patient is now confirmed as

1. Moderate Exacerbation FEV1 or PEF 40–69% predicted/personal best Physical exam: moderate symptoms Inhaled SABA every 60 minutes; followed by Oral systemic corticosteroid; Continue treatment 1–3 hours, provided there is improvement; make admit decision in < 4 hrs.
2. Severe Exacerbation FEV1 or PEF < 40% predicted. Physical exam: severe symptoms at rest, accessory muscle use, chest retraction History: high-risk patient No improvement after initial treatment; Oxygen Nebulized SABA + ipratropium, hourly or continuous; followed by Oral systemic corticosteroids; Consider adjunct therapies.

After the respective treatments,

- Good Response FEV1 or PEF 70% Response sustained 60 minutes after last treatment No distress; Physical exam: normal. The patient is discharged home. Continue treatment with inhaled SABA. Continue course of oral systemic corticosteroid and Consider initiation of an ICS. Patient education – Review medications, including inhaler technique. – Review/initiate action plan. – Recommend close medical followup.
- Incomplete Response FEV1 or Peak Expiratory Flow (PEF) 40–69% Mild-to-moderate symptoms are observed. Hospitalisation is required. He should be admitted to hospital ward. Oxygen; Inhaled SABA Systemic (oral or intravenous) corticosteroid; Consider adjunct therapies; Monitor vital signs, FEV1 or PEF, (Oxygen Saturation of Arterial Bllod) SaO$_2$. If it is improved, he can be discharged.

- Poor Response FEV1 or PEF <40%. PCO_2 > 42mmHg Physical exam: symptoms severe, drowsiness, confusion. The patient should be admitted to hopital intensive care unit for further treatment. Inhaled SABA hourly or continuously; Intravenous corticosteroid; Consider adjunct therapies Possible; intubation and mechanical ventilation. If the condition is improved, he can be discharged home.

Table 9.2 Dosages of drugs for Asthma Exacerbations.

Medications:	Dosages	
	Adult dose	**Child dose**
Inhaled short acting Beta 2 Agonists		
Albuterol Nebuliser Solution (5mg/ml,0.63 mg/3ml, 1.25mg/3ml)	2.5-5mg every 20 min for 3 doses then, 2.5-10mg every 1-4hrs as needed.	0.15 mg/kg every 20 min for 3 doses, then. 0.15-0.3mg/kg up to 10 mg every 1-4 hrs or 0.5/mg/kg/hr continuously
Albuterol MDI(90mcg/puff)	4-8 puffs every 30 min upto 4 hrs,then every 1-4hr as needed	4-8puffs every 20 min for 3 doses, then1-4 hr as needed
Levalbuterol Nebuliser Solution (0.31 mg/3ml,0.63 mg/3ml,2.5 mg/1ml,1.25 mg/3ml)	Given 1 half mg dose of Albuterol above	Given 1 half the mg dose of Albuterol above
Levalbuterol MDI(45 mcg/puff)	4-8 puffs every 30 min upto 4 hrs, then every 1-4hr as needed	4-8puffs every 20 min for 3 doses, then1-4 hr as needed
Pirbuterol(200 mcg/puff)	4-8 puffs every 30 min upto 4 hrs, then every 1-4hr as needed	4-8puffs every 20 min for 3 doses, then1-4 hr as needed
Systemic Beta 2 Agonists		
Epinephrine (1mg/ml)	0.3-0.5mg every 20 min for 3 doses subcutaneous	0.01mg/kg upto 0.5mg every 20 min 3 doses subcutaneous
Terbutaline (1mg/ml)	0.25mg every 20 min 3 doses, subcutaneous	0.01mg/kg upto 0.5mg every 20 min 3 doses subcutaneous
Anticholinergics		
Ipratropium Bromide Nebuliser Solution (0.25 mg/ml)	500 mcg every 20 min for 3 doses then 2-4 hrs	250mcg every 20 min for 3 doses, then 250mcg every 2-4 hr
Ipratropium BromideMDI (18mcg/puff)	8 puffs every 20 min as needed for upto 3 hr	4-8 puffs every 20 min as needed upto 3 hr
Systemic Corticosteroids		
Prednisone, Prednisolone, Methyl Prednisolone	40-80 mg/day in 1 or 2 divided doses till PEF reach 70% of personal best	1-2 mg/kg in 2 divided doses(max. 60 mg/day) until PEF reach 70% of normal predicted

Life-Threatening Asthma

Treatment of life-threatening episode should be immediate and no time should be spent on detailed clinical history.

- Oxygen inhalation 4 L/min to maintain SpO2–>90%.
- Inj. Terbutaline 10 mcg/kg subcutaneously or IV (maximum 40 mcg/day).
- Inhaled Salbutamol/Terbutaline preferably by nebulizer (as discussed above).
- Ipratropium Bromide 250 mcg by nebulizer with Salbutamol.
- Inj. Hydrocortisone 10 mg/kg IV. Inj. Aminophylline 5 mg/kg bolus slowly followed by 0.8-1.2 mg/kg/hour slow infusion (If patient has received theophylline preparation in last 72 hours; reduce bolus dose to 2.5 mg/kg).
- Inj. Magnesium sulphate 40 mg/kg in 50 ml 5% dextrose as slow infusion over 30 minutes can be considered.
- If no response do arterial blood gas analysis, X-raychest and serum electrolytes. Intubate the patient if no or poor respiratory effort, increased carbon dioxide with respiratory acidosis. Transfer to intensive care unit as early as possible.
- If above therapy fails. Transfer should be arranged so that oxygen and inhalation therapy can be continued on the way

References

1. NHLBI, National Asthma Education and Prevention Program, Expert Panel Report 2. Guidelines for the Diagnosis and Management of Asthma. NIH Publication No. 97–4051. Bethesda, MD: U.S. Department of Health and Human Services, 1997.

2. National Institutes of Health, National Heart, Lung, and Blood Institute. National Asthma Education and Prevention Program. Full Report of the Expert Panel: Guidelines for the diagnosis and management of asthma (EPR-3) 2007. 2007, *http://www.nhlbi.nih.gov/guidelines/asthma*.

3. National Institutes of Health, National Heart, Lung, and Blood Institute. Global Initiative for Asthma (GINA). Global Strategy for Asthma Management and Prevention Revised (2002). NHLBI/WHO Workshop Report. NIH publication No. 02–3659. Bethesda, MD: U.S. Department of Health and Human Services, 2002.

4. https://www.guidelines.co.uk/respiratory/nice-asthma-guideline-chronic-asthma-management/453885.article

5. Busse WW, Lemanske RF Jr. Asthma. N Engl J Med 2001;344:350–362.

6. Rowe BH, Edmonds ML, Spooner CH, Diner B, Camargo CA Jr. Corticosteroid therapy for acute asthma. Respir Med 2004;98:275–284.

7. Humbert M et al. Benefits of omalizumab as add-on therapy in patients with severe persistent asthma who are inadequately controlled despite best available therapy (GINA 2002 step 4 treatment): INNOVATE. Allergy. 2005;60(3):309-16

CHAPTER - 10

Chronic Obstructive Pulmonary Disease

Introduction to COPD

Chronic obstructive pulmonary disease (COPD) is a lung disease characterized by chronic obstruction of lung airflow that interferes with normal breathing and is not fully reversible. The airflow limitation is usually both progressive and associated with an abnormal inflammatory response of the lungs to noxious particles or gases. Emphysema and chronic bronchitis are the two most common conditions that contribute to COPD.

Chronic bronchitis is inflammation of the lining of the bronchial tubes, which carry air to and from the air sacs (alveoli) of the lungs. It's characterized by daily cough and mucus (sputum) production.

Emphysema is a condition in which the alveoli at the end of the smallest air passages (bronchioles) of the lungs are destroyed as a result of damaging exposure to cigarette smoke and other irritating gases and particulate matter.

Epidemiology

- The Global Burden of Disease Study reports a prevalence of 251 million cases of COPD globally in 2016.
- Globally, it is estimated that 3.17 million deaths were caused by the disease in 2015 (that is, 5% of all deaths globally in that year).
- More than 90% of COPD deaths occur in low and middleincome countries.
- The primary cause of COPD is exposure to tobacco smoke (either active smoking or secondhand smoke).
- Other risk factors include exposure to indoor and outdoor air pollution and occupational dusts and fumes.
- Exposure to indoor air pollution can affect the unborn child and represent a risk factor for developing COPD later in life.
- Some cases of COPD are due to long-term asthma.

Etiology

- Emphysema (destruction of alveoli/lungs over time), bronchitis (inflammation of the lining of the bronchial tubes), genetic disorder
- Only about 20 to 30 percent of chronic smokers may develop clinically apparent COPD, although many smokers with long smoking histories may develop reduced lung function. Causes of airway obstruction include:
- **Emphysema.** This lung disease causes destruction of the fragile walls and elastic fibres of the alveoli. Small airways collapse when exhaled, impairing airflow out of the lungs.
- **Chronic bronchitis.** The bronchial tubes become inflamed and narrowed and lungs produce more mucus, which can further block the narrowed tubes producing more chronic cough.
- Cigarette smoke
- Other irritants can cause COPD, including cigar smoke, second-hand smoke, pipe smoke, air pollution and workplace exposure to dust, smoke or fumes.
- Alpha-1-antitrypsin deficiency: In 1 % of people with COPD, the disease results from a genetic disorder that causes low levels of a protein called alpha-1-antitrypsin. Alpha-1-antitrypsin (AAt) is made in the liver and secreted into the bloodstream to help protect the lungs. Alpha-1-antitrypsin deficiency can affect the liver as well as the lungs. Damage to the lung can occur in infants and children, not only adults with long smoking histories.

Risk Factors

- **Exposure to tobacco smoke.** The most significant risk factor for COPD is long-term cigarette smoking. Inhalation of noxious agents, such as cigarette smoke, leads to the activation of resident immune and parenchymal cells, which in turn, recruit additional inflammatory cells from the systemic compartment into the resident tissue and airway causing obstruction to airways.
- **People with asthma who smoke.** The combination of asthma, a chronic inflammatory airway disease, and smoking increases the risk of COPD even more.
- **Occupational exposure to dusts and chemicals.** Long-term exposure to chemical fumes, vapours and dusts in the workplace can irritate and inflame the lungs.
- **Exposure to fumes from burning fuel.** People exposed to fumes from burning fuel for cooking and heating in poorly ventilated homes are at higher risk of developing COPD.
- **Age.** COPD develops slowly over years, so most people are at least 40 years old when symptoms begin.
- **Genetics.** The uncommon genetic disorder alpha-1-antitrypsin deficiency is the cause of some cases of COPD. Other genetic factors likely make certain smokers more susceptible to the disease.

Etiology of Airflow Limitation in COPD

1. **Reversible:** Presence of mucus and inflammatory cells and mediators in bronchial secretions

   Bronchial smooth muscle contraction in peripheral and central airways

   Dynamic hyperinflation during exercise

2. **Irreversible:** Fibrosis and narrowing of airways

   Reduced elastic recoil with loss of alveolar surface area

   Destruction of alveolar support with reduced patency of small airways

Pathophysiology: Chronic bronchitis is defined clinically as the presence of a chronic productive cough for 3 months during each of 2 consecutive years. Emphysema is defined pathologically as an abnormal, permanent enlargement of the air spaces distal to the terminal bronchioles, accompanied by destruction of their walls and without obvious fibrosis.

Emphysema

The inflammatory response, mediated by neutrophils, macrophages and CD8+ T-cells, release inflammatory mediators and enzymes that damage the lung parenchyma. Proteases like elastase and matrix metalloproteinases (MMPs) released by these inflammatory cells break down the connective tissue of the alveolar walls and the septae. **A loss of elastic recoil** leads to **diminished expiratory flow rates, air trapping and airway collapsing.**

Parenchymal destruction: Recurrent damage to the alveoli eventually leads to septal destruction along with the capillary bed also.

Matched V/Q defect: Since both the terminal bronchioles and alveoli along with the capillary bed have been destroyed, a matched defect exists between the ventilation and perfusion; areas of low ventilation also have poor perfusion.

Mild hypoxia: Despite the "matched" V/Q defect, overtime hyperventilation develops and cardiac output (CO) drops which leads to areas of poor blood flow in relatively well oxygenated areas. Due to this poor CO, the rest of the body suffers from tissue hypoxia.

Cachexia: At the pulmonary level, the low CO leads to pulmonary cachexia; which induces weight loss and muscle wasting. This gives these patients the characteristic **"pink-puffer"** appearance.

Chronic Bronchitis

Mucous gland enlargement, goblet cell hyperplasia and mucociliary dysfunction occur in larger airways, causing excessive mucus production and build-up reducing the airway lumen. Although these pathological changes in the large airways, it appears that the major site of increased airway resistance is the small airways ($\leq$ 2mm). Fibrosis and smooth **muscle hypertrophy** may occur along with **excess mucus production** and **cellular infiltration** in the peripheral airways.

Small airway inflammation: Mechanisms discussed above lead to inflammation in the smaller bronchioles and mucus secretions further narrow the airway lumen. Despite this, the parenchyma is relatively less damaged.

V/Q mismatch: The physiologic response leads to a drop in ventilation and compensation with the rise in CO. Increased perfusion in the areas of poor ventilation takes place eventually causing hypoxia and secondary polycythemia.

Severe hypoxia and hypercarbia: Chronic Ventilation and Perfusion Ratio) V/Q mismatch leads to decreased oxygenation/deoxygenation of the blood resulting in hypoxemia and increased CO2 retention (respiratory acidosis ensues).

Pulmonary hypertension and cor pulmonale: Chronic hypercapnia and respiratory acidosis lead to arterial vasoconstriction in the lungs. With the retrograde pressure build-up, the right ventricular pressures continue to rise and eventually causing RV failure. Otherwise, known as **cor pulmonale.**

Pathophysiology of Exacerbation

A working definition of a COPD exacerbation is a sustained worsening of the patient's condition from the stable state and beyond normal day-to-day variations that is acute in onset and necessitates a change in regular medication. The primary physiologic change is often a worsening of arterial blood gas results owing to poor gas exchange and increased muscle fatigue. In a patient experiencing a severe exacerbation, profound hypoxemia and hypercapnia can be accompanied by respiratory acidosis and respiratory failure.

Clinical Manifestations and Features [1]

Signs and Symptoms

For chronic bronchitis, the main symptom is a daily cough and mucus (sputum) production at least three months a year for two consecutive years.

Other signs and symptoms of COPD may include:
- Shortness of breath, especially during physical activities
- Wheezing
- Chest tightness
- Having to clear your throat first thing in the morning, due to excess mucus in your lungs
- A chronic cough that may produce mucus (sputum) that may be clear, white, yellow or greenish
- Blueness of the lips or fingernail beds (cyanosis)
- Frequent respiratory infections
- Lack of energy
- Unintended weight loss (in later stages)
- Swelling in ankles, feet or legs

Diagnosis with Algorithm

1. Any known risk factors: a) current or former smoker; b) personal or familier risk factors or occupational exposure c) passive exposure to tobacco smoke d) biomass smoke e) environmental or occupational exposure
2. **Has the patient had any of these symptoms?** Cough, sputum, shortness of breath; emergency visit for dyspnoea of probable respiratory origin.
3. Perform post bronchodilator spirometry
4. If $FEV1/FVC$ (Post)< 0.70 possible COPD.
5. Differential diagnosis to be performed: asthma, A1-antitrypsin deficiency, CVS diseases, anemia, bronchoectasis
6. If they are ruled out, then it is confirmed as COPD
7. Lung (pulmonary) function tests. Pulmonary function tests measure the amount of air inhaled and exhaled.

Three types of pulmonary function tests are used in the diagnosis of COPD:

1. Spirometry
2. Diffusion studies
3. Body plethysmography

Spirometry is the most common lung function test. During this test, the person has to blow air into a large tube connected to a small machine called a spirometer. This machine measures how much air lungs can hold and how fast the air can be blown out of the lungs.

Other lung function tests include measurement of lung volumes, diffusing capacity and pulse oximetry.

Gold Spirometry Criteria for COPD Severity

1. **Mild COPD:** $FEV1/FVC < 0.7$ $FEV1 \geq 80\%$ predicted

    At this stage, the patient is probably unaware that lung function is starting to decline.
2. **Moderate COPD:** $FEV1/FVC < 0.7$ $FEV1$-50%

    Symptoms during this stage progress, with shortness of breathe developing upon exertion.
3. **Severe COPD:** $FEV1/FVC < 0.7$ $FEV1$-30%

    Shortness of breath becomes worse at this stage and COPD exacerbations are common.
4. **Very severe COPD:** $FEV1/FVC < 0.7$ $FEV1< 30\%$ predicted

    Quality of life at this stage is gravely impaired. COPD exacerbation can be life-threatening.

Along with spirometry, two other pulmonary function tests are important in the diagnosis of lung disease:

1. Diffusion studies—This PFT tells how much oxygen moves into the bloodstream.

2. Body plethysmography—A test which determines how much air is present in lungs when a deep breath is taken and how much air is left in the lungs after exhaled.

- Chest X-ray
- CT scan.
- Arterial blood gas analysis-Patients with severe COPD can have a low arterial oxygen tension (PaO2 45to 60 mm Hg) and an elevated arterial carbon dioxide tension (PaCO2 50 to 60 mm Hg). Hypoxemia results from hypoventilation (V) of lung tissue relative to perfusion (Q) of the area. The low V: Q ratio progresses over several years, resulting in a consistent decline in the PaO_2.
- Laboratory tests- alpha-1-antitrypsin (AAt) deficiency, which may be the cause of some cases of COPD. This test is done if there is family history of COPD.

Procedures for Reversibility Testing

1. **Preparation**
   - Tests should be performed when patients are clinically stable and free from respiratory infection.
   - Patients should not have taken inhaled short-acting bronchodilators in the previous 6 hours, long-acting β-agonists in the previous 12 hours, or sustained-release theophylline in the previous 24 hours.

2. **Spirometry**
   - FEV1 should be measured before bronchodilator is given.
   - Bronchodilators can be given by either metered-dose inhaler or nebulization.
   - Usual doses are 400 mcg of β-agonist, 80 mcg of anticholinergic, or the two combined.
   - FEV1 should be measured again 30–45 minutes after bronchodilator is given.

3. **Results**
   - An increase in FEV1 that is both greater than 200 mL and 12% above the prebronchodilator FEV1 is considered significant.

Clinical Presentation of COPD Exacerbation

Symptoms: Increased sputum volume, Acutely worsening dyspnea, Chest tightness, Presence of purulent sputum, Increased need for bronchodilators, Malaise, fatigue, Decreased exercise tolerance

Physical Examination: Fever, Wheezing, decreased breath sounds

Diagnostic Tests: Sputum sample for Gram stain and culture, Chest radiograph to evaluate for new infiltrates

Staging Acute Exacerbations of COPD

1. Mild (type 1)-One cardinal symptom plus at least one of the following: URTI within 5 days, fever without other explanation, increased wheezing, increased cough, increase in respiratory or heart rate >20% above baseline
2. Moderate (type 2) - Two cardinal symptoms
3. Severe (type 3) - Three cardinal symptoms

Cardinal symptoms include worsening of dyspnea, increase in sputum volume, and increase in sputum purulence

Management

Goals of COPD Management

Prevent disease progression

Relieve symptoms

Improve exercise tolerance

Improve overall health status

Prevent and treat exacerbations

Prevent and treat complications

Reduce morbidity and mortality

Nonpharmacologic Therapy

1. Smoking cessation is the most effective strategy to reduce the risk of developing COPD and the only intervention proven to affect the long term decline in FEV1 and slow the progression of COPD.
   Five-Step Strategy for Smoking-Cessation Program (5 A's)
   Ask: Use systematic approach to identify all tobacco users.
   Advice: Urge all tobacco users to quit.
   Assess: Determine willingness to make a cessation attempt.
   Assist: Provide support for the patient to quit smoking.
   Arrange: Schedule follow-up and monitor for continued abstinence.
   First-Line Pharmacotherapies for Smoking Cessation
   1. Bupropion SR 150 mg orally daily for 3 days, then twice daily 12 weeks, up to 6 months Side Effects (SE): Insomnia, dry mouth
   2. Nicotine gum 2–4 mg dose, up to 24 pieces daily upto 12 weeks SE: Sore mouth, dyspepsis
   3. Nicotine inhaler 6–16 cartridges daily Up to 6 months SE: Sore mouth and throat
   4. Nicotine nasal spray 8–40 doses daily upto 3 to 6 months SE: Nasal irritation
   5. Nicotine patches, 7–21 mg every 24 hours Up to 8 weeks SE: Skin reaction, insomnia

2. **Pulmonary rehabilitation** programs include exercise training along with smoking cessation, breathing exercises, optimal medical treatment, psychosocial support, and health education.

3. **Annual vaccination** with the inactivated intramuscular influenza vaccine is recommended. Annual vaccination with the inactivated intramuscular influenza vaccine is recommended.

4. **Long-term oxygen therapy:** The use of supplemental oxygen therapy increases survival in COPD patients with chronic hypoxemia. Before patients are considered for long-term oxygen therapy, they should be stabilized in the outpatient setting, and pharmacotherapy should be optimized. Once this is accomplished, long-term oxygen therapy should be instituted if either of two conditions exists:

   1. A resting PaO2 of less than 55 mm Hg
   2. Evidence of right-sided heart failure, polycythemia, or impaired neuropsychiatric function with a PaO2 of less than 60 mm Hg

   The most practical means of administering long-term oxygen is with the nasal cannula, at 1 to 2 L/min which provides 24% to 28% oxygen. The goal is to raise the PaO2 above 60 mm Hg. Patient education about flow rates and avoidance of flames (i.e., smoking) is of the utmost importance. There are three different ways to deliver oxygen, including (1) in liquid reservoirs, (2) compressed into a cylinder, and (3) via an oxygen concentrator

5. **Adjunctive Therapies:** Psychoeducational care and nutritional support. Psychoeducational care (such as relaxation) has been associated with improvement in the functioning and well-being of adults with COPD.

Pharmacologic Therapy

1. **Sympathomimetics:** β2-Selective sympathomimetics cause relaxation of bronchial smooth muscle and bronchodilation by stimulating the enzyme adenyl cyclase to increase the formation of cyclic adenosine monophosphate and produces functional antagonism to bronchoconstriction. They may also improve mucociliary clearance.

   Albuterol, levalbuterol, bitolterol, pirbuterol, and terbutaline are the preferred short-acting agents because they have greater β2 selectivity and longer duration of action.

   Formoterol and salmeterol are long-acting inhaled β2-agonists that are dosed every 12 hours.

   There are short acting (SABA) and long acting (LABA) beta-agonists.

   Resting sinus tachycardia, and has the potential to precipitate cardiac rthym disturbances in susceptible patients. Exacerbated somatic tremor is troublesome in some older patients treated with higher doses.

2. **Anticholinergics:** When given by inhalation, anticholinergic agents produce bronchodilation by competitively inhibiting cholinergic receptors in bronchial smooth muscle. This activity blocks acetylcholine, with the net effect being a reduction in cyclic guanosine monophosphate, which normally acts to constrict bronchial smooth muscle.

   Ipratropium bromide has a slower onset of action than short-acting β2-agonists. The recommended dose via MDI is two puffs four times a day with upward titration often to 24 puffs/day [2].

Tiotropium bromide is a long-acting agent that protects against cholinergic bronchoconstriction for more than 24 hours. One capsule once daily [3].

Adverse effects: Inhaled drugs are poorly absorbed so less systemic effects. Dryness of mouth.

3. **Methylxanthines [4, 5]:** Theophylline and aminophylline may produce bronchodilation by inhibition of phosphodiesterase (thereby increasing cyclic adenosine monophosphate levels), inhibition of calcium ion influx into smooth muscle, prostaglandin antagonism, stimulation of endogenous catecholamines, adenosine receptor antagonism, and inhibition of release of mediators from mast cells and leukocytes.

   200 mg twice daily and titrated upward every 3 to 5 days to the target dose;

   Adverse effects: The most common side effects of theophylline include dyspepsia, nausea, vomiting, diarrhea, headache, dizziness, and tachycardia.

   Combination bronchodilator therapy: Combination increases the degree of bronchodilation with a lower risk of side effects compared to increasing the dose of a single bronchodilator. Combination of SABAs and short acting anticholinergics are superior compared to either medication alone in improving FEV1 and symptoms. Formeterol and tiotropium has bigger impact on FEV1 than either component alone.

   Combination of LABA and LAMA also are efficacious.

4. **Corticosteroids [6]:** The antiinflammatory mechanisms whereby corticosteroids exert their beneficial effect in COPD include reduction in capillary permeability to decrease mucus, inhibition of release of proteolytic enzymes from leukocytes, and inhibition of prostaglandins.

   Appropriate situations to consider corticosteroids in COPD include (1) short term systemic use for acute exacerbations; and (2) inhalation therapy for chronic stable COPD.

   Inhaled corticosteroids: ICS in combination with LABA in patients with moderate to severe COPD and exacerbations is more effective than either component alone in improving lung function, health staus and exacerbations.

   Side effects of inhaled corticosteroids are relatively mild and include hoarseness, sore throat, oral candidiasis, and skin bruising.

5. **Phosphodiesterase inhibitors:** Roflumilast reduces moderate and severe exacerbations. Adverse effects include nausea, reduced appetite, weight loss, abdominal pain, diarrhea, headache.

6. **Antibiotics:** Use of macrolide antibiotics may reduce exacerbations. Azithromycin 250 mg/day or 500 mg TID per week.

7. **α1-Antitrypsin Replacement Therapy:** In patients with inherited AAT deficiency–associated emphysema, treatment focuses on reduction of risk factors such as smoking, symptomatic treatment with bronchodilators, and augmentation therapy with replacement AAT

Algorithm for Management of COPD [7]

If diagnoisis of COPD is confirmed,

➤ Fundamentals of COPD care are advised: i) offer treatemnt and support to stop bleeding ii) offer pneumococcal and influnza vaccinations iii) offer pulmonary rehabilitationif indicated iv) optimize treatment for co-morbidities.

➤ Inhaled therapies is to be initiated only if: i) all the above interventions have been offered ii) people have been trianed to use inhalers.

➤ Offer SABA or SAMA to use as needed.

If the patient is limited by symptoms or no asthmatic features – Offer LABA+ LAMA.

(a) Assess if the person has day to day symptoms that adversely impact quality of life. Then 3 month trial of LABA+LAMA+ICS is initiated. If no improvement then revert to LABA+LAMA.

(b) Assess if the patient has 1 severe or 2 moserate exacerbations within a year. Consider LABA+LAMA+ICS

If the patient has exacerbations despite treatment and has asthmatic features or features suggesting steroid responsiveness; consider LABA+ICS

➤ Assess if the person has day to day symptoms that adversely impact quality of life, or has 1 severe or 2 moserate exacerbations within a year: offer LABA+ LAMA+ ICS

Management of Stable COPD [8]

(a) **Bronchodilators:** *Short-acting (4-6 hours for ß2 adrenergics and 6-8 hours for anticholinergics):* Inhaled ß2 adrenergics (salbutamol 100-200 mcg e.g. ventolin, terbutaline 400-500 mcg), Inhaled anticholinergics (ipratropium 20-40 mcg), Oral ß2 adrenergics (salbutamol 2 or 4 mg e.g. ventolin, terbutaline 2.5 or 5 mg); Combination of salbutamol/ipratropium (100/20 mcg)

- *Long-acting (12 hours for ß2 adrenergics and 24 hours for anticholinergics:* Inhaled ß2 adrenergics (Salmeterol 25-50 mcg, Formoterol 4.5-12 mcg), Inhaled anticholinergics (Tiotropium 18 mcg e.g. tiova)

Other medications:

1. Short acting beta adrenergics: Fenoterol, Levalbuterol
2. Short acting anticholinergics: Oxitropium
3. Long acting beta adrenergics (once daily): Indacaterol, Oladaterol, Vilanterol
4. Long acting anticholinergics: Aclidinium, Glycopyrronium, Umeclidinium

(b) **Inhaled corticosteroids:**

- Beclomethasone 50-400 mcg
- Budesonide 100, 200, 400 mcg
- Fluticasone 50-500 mcg

Foracort is a combination of formoterol (fixed 6 mcg) and budesonide (100, 200 or 400 mcg)

(c) Oral methylxanthines:
- Aminophylline 200-600 mg pill
- Theophylline 100-600 mg pill
- Doxofylline 400 mg (PO BD)

(d) Systemic steroids: Prednisolone 5-60 mg (pill), Methylprednisolone 4, 8, 16 mg (pill)
- Long term use of systemic steroids is not recommended

(e) Phosphodiesterase-4 inhibitor (new class): Roflumilast 500 mcg (duration 24 hours)

More recent studies have shown that regular use of macrolide antibiotics may reduce exacerbation rate.

(f) Symptomatic measures:
- Hot drinks or steam inhalation to liquefy sputum
- Mucolytics: bromhexine, N-acetylcysteine, carbocysteine, ambroxol, erdosteine

Treatment of Acute Exacerbation of COPD (AECOPD) if Present

Classification of AECOPD:

(a) No respiratory failure: Respiratory rate: 20-30 breaths per minute; no use of accessory respiratory muscles; no changes in mental status; hypoxemia improved with supplemental oxygen given via Venturi mask 28-35% inspired oxygen (FiO2); no increase in PaCO2.

(b) Acute respiratory failure – non-life-threatening: Respiratory rate: > 30 breaths per minute; using accessory respiratory muscles; no change in mental status; hypoxemia improved with supplemental oxygen via Venturi mask 25-30% FiO2; hypercarbia i.e., PaCO2 increased compared with baseline or elevated 50-60 mmHg.

(c) Acute respiratory failure – life-threatening: Respiratory rate: > 30 breaths per minute; using accessory respiratory muscles; acute changes in mental status; hypoxemia not improved with supplemental oxygen via Venturi mask or requiring FiO2 > 40%; hypercarbia i.e., PaCO2 increased compared with baseline or elevated > 60 mmHg or the presence of acidosis (pH < 7.25).

(a) Oxygen:
- Aim: Oxygen saturation of 88-92%

(b) Bronchodilators
- Nebulized Short Acting Beta-Adrenergics/SABAs (Salbutamol 2.5 mg i.e. 0.5 ml) and Anticholinergics (Ipratropium 0.5 mg i.e. 2.5 ml) every 20 minutes for initial 1-2 hours
  - o SABAs: fast onset of action but short-lived
  - o Anticholinergics: delayed onset of action but prolonged effect

(c) Antibiotics: Indicated if 2 out of 3 symptoms of exacerbation- Increased dyspnea Increased sputum production Increased sputum purulence

(d) Corticosteroids: For patients with advanced lung disease or less severe lung disease with severe exacerbation:
- Oral Prednisolone: start at 0.5-1 mg/kg/day and taper slowly OR
- IV Methylprednisolone: 40-125 mg every 8-12 hours OR
- IV Hydrocortisone: 100 mg every 6-8 hours

They shorten the recovery time and improve lung function (FEV1) and hypoxemia. Limit the duration of therapy to: 5-7 days

(e) Methylxanthines: are not recommended due to side effect profiles

(f) Diuretics: in patients with gross right ventricular failure (cor-pulmonale)

Recommended Antimicrobial Therapy in Acute Exacerbations of COPD

1. Uncomplicated exacerbations < 4 exacerbations per year No comorbid illness FEV1 > 50% of predicted: Macrolide (Azithromycin, Clarithromycin) or Second- or third-generation cephalosporin or Doxycycline
2. Complicated exacerbations Age ≥ 65 > 4 exacerbations per year FEV1 < 50% but > 35% of predicted: Amoxicillin/clavulanate, Fluoroquinolone with enhanced pneumococcal activity (Levofloxacin, Gatifloxacin, Moxifloxacin
3. Complicated exacerbations with risk of P. Aeruginosa: Fluoroquinolone with enhanced pneumococcal and P. aeruginosa activity (levofloxacin, gatifloxacin, moxifloxacin). IV therapy if required: Third- or fourth-generation cephalosporin.

Case Study of COPD

A 71 years old male patient was admitted in the general ward with the chief complaints of general weakness, shortness of breath (SOB), vomiting's. past history: COPD, HTN. Past medication history: Acebropyhlline, rabiwox dsr, telma h, combihale ff 250. Social history:- smoker. His objective data shows: Temperature : 98.6 ° f, BP : 114/58mm hg, pulse rate : 119 Beats per minute (bpm), SPO_2 : 95% on room air, CVS : S_1 S_2 heard, peripheral pulses palpable, RS : b/l airway entry + , GIT : Per abdomen (p/a) – soft, no organomegaly, bowel sounds heard. CNS: Glassglow Coma Scale (CGS) 15/15, pupils: b/l Normal Size/Normal Reaction (ns/nr). Ocular movements intact, b/l plantar flexor normal.

Lab reports:

chest x-ray: Opacification is seen in the left mid & lower lung zones – possibly consolidation.

2 d echo: Good lv systolic function, grade i lv diastolic dysfunction.

USG abdomen: Hepatomegaly with fatty infiltration

Mild splenomegaly

Left kidney is not visualized? Ectopic/ agenesis/ atropic

CBP:

	D1	D2	D3	D4	D5
Hb (g/dl)	15.5	14.7	14.0	15.8	16.1 (normal)

PCV	46	44	44.6	46.4	47.7
WBC (cells/cumm)	8,600	6,100	4,600	5,100	4,640
Platelets	57,000	1.2	1.5	72,000	58,000 (decreased)
Serum creatinine (mg/dL)	1.3	1.5	1.2 (normal)		
Urea (mg/dL)		42	-	45 (normal)	
Sodium (mmols/lit)	130.7	133.5	131.4		
Potassium	4.7	4.76	5.14		
Chlorides	97.0	101.1	96.9		
Total bilirubin	0.5mg				
Direct	0.1mg/dL			Globulin : 3.5 gm/dL	
Indirect	0.4 mg/dL			AG ratio : 1.0	
ABT	41 IU/L				
ALT	39 IU/L				
ALP	48 IU/L				
Proteins	7.2 gm/dL				
Albumin	3.7 gm/dL				

Diagnosis

Viral fever with thrombocytopenia, COPD – Acute Exacerbation, AKI, HTN

Treatment

STAT drug orders-

Injection Hydrocortisone IV 100 mg OD

Injection PCM (paracetamol) IV 1gm OD

Injection Magnex Forte IV 1.5gm

Injection PAN (Pantaprazole) IV 40mg OD

Injection Zofer (Ondansetron) IV 8 mg

Nebulizer: Duolin (Levosalbutamol + ipratropium) + budecort (Budesonide)

Progress chart:

D1: Viral pyrexia

Bronchospasm

Motion not passed

D2 : SOB(decreased) No c/o fever, motion not passed

Syrup Duphalac 25 ml PO stat

D3: Stop budecort neb

Add formonide neb

Table 10.1 Treatment initiated in the patient.

Drug Name	Generic Name	Route	Frequency	Dose	Indication
Inj Magnex Forte	Cefperazone + salbactum	IV	BD	1.5gm	Antibiotic: treat respiratory tract infection
Injclarithromycin	Clarithromycin	IV	BD	500mg	Antibiotic
Inj PCM	Paracetamol	IV	TID	1gm	Treat fever
Inj Zofer	Ondansetron	IV	TID	4mg	Antiemetic
Inj Solumedrol	Methyl prednisolone	IV	TID	40mg	Anti-inflammatory
Inj Mgso$_4$	Magnesium sulphate	IV	TID	1gm	Bronchodilatory effect in COPD condition
Inj Deriphylline	Theophylline	IV	TID	1amp	Acute bronchopasm
Neb duolin	Salbutamol sulpahte+ ipratopium bromide	P/N	TID	200mcg	COPD (bronchodilator)
Neb budecort	Budesonide	P/N	BD	200mcg	Treatment of airway obstruction
Neb formonide	Formoterol+ Budesonide	P/N	BD	200mcg	Treatment of airway obstruction

Discharge Advice

TIOVA (tiotropium bromide) 9mcg inhaler 2 puffs OD- BRONCHODILATOR

SEROFLO (salmeterol+ fluticasone propionate) 250 mcg inhaler 2 puffs BD

Duolin (Salbutamol sulpahte+ ipratopium bromide) inhaler 2 puffs TID with space

Tablet Zostum -O (cefditoren pivoxil) 200 mg OD 5 days

Tablet omnacortil (prednisolone) 20 mg OD 5 days

Tablet PAN pantaprazole 40 mg OD bbf

Tablet Unicontin-E (theophylline) 400 mg OD (night) – bronchodilator

Tablet DOLO 650 mg (if necessary)

Continue old HTN medication

Assignment

1. **What are the Signs & Symptoms of the Patient?**

   General weakness, SOB.

2. **What are the Laboratory tests for diagnosis?**

   FEV1/FVC < 70% > FEV1 <50% > PaCo2 44mmHg

PaO2 < 55mmHg/ Chest X-ray: opacification is seen in the left mid and lower lung zones – possibly consolidation.

3. Goals of Therapy for COPD:
- Relieve symptoms/ Reduce symptoms / Improve exercise tolerance
- Improve health status / Reduce risk/ Prevent disease progression
- Prevent and treat exacerbations / Reduce mortality

4. Non-Pharmacological Therapy for COPD:
- Smoking cessation
- Pulmonary rehabilitation – improve exercise tolerance and exercertional dyspnea
- Long term oxygen therapy (18 or more hours of O2 everday) Improves exercise performance and survival short term oxygen therapy: improve dyspnea and exercise tolerance and do not improve survival.
- Treatment of acute exacerbations of COPD: Non-invasive, positive pressure, ventilation (NIV) has been effective.
- Lung transplantation: If PaCo2 > 55 mmHg

5. What are the Pharmacotherapeutic Regimens available for the patient? [9, 10]
(a) SABA's - albuterol, levalbuterol
(b) LABA's - salmeterol, formeterol
(c) Short actinf anti-cholinergics- ipratropium bromide
(d) LAMA's - acridinium, glycopyrolate. Tiotropium
(e) LABA+ICS- Salmeterol + Fluticasone/Formeterol + Budosenide

Table 10.2 Pharmacologic Treatment for Inpatient COPD exacerbations.

	Medication	Dose and Frequency
Bronchodilator	Albuterol	2.5 mg/3 mL NS nebulized or MDI 1 puff every hour × 2-3 doses, then every 2-4 hours
	Ipratropium	500 mcg nebulized or inhaled every 6-8 hours or MDI 1 puff every hour × 2-3 doses
Glucocorticoids[a]	Methylprednisolone	60-125 mg IV daily for no more than 5-7 days OR 40 mg IV daily × 1 day, then prednisone 40 mg PO daily × 4 days (total 5 days)
	Prednisone	40 mg PO daily × 5 days
Antibiotics (nonpseudomonal coverage)	Ceftriaxone Moxifloxacin	1-2 g IV daily × 5-7 days 400 mg IV or PO daily × 5-7 days
Antibiotics (pseudomonal coverage)	Cefepime Ceftazidime Piperacillin-tazobactam Levofloxacin	1-2 g IV q 8-12 hours × 5-7 days 1-2 g IV q 8 hours × 5-7 days 4.5 g IV q6 hours × 5-7 days 750 mg IV or PO daily × 5-7 days

Source: [a]Might be less efficacious in acute COPD exacerbations in patientswith lower levels of blood eosinophils. COPD: chronic obstructive pulmonary disease; MDI: metered-dose inhaler

6. When is Oxygen Therapy prescribed for the patients?

Oxygen therapy is prescribed for people who cannot get enough oxygen on their own. This is often because of lung conditions that prevent the lungs from absorbing oxygen Symptoms of low oxygen in the patients are – SOB, wheezing.

- Nocturnal continuous and day time intermittent Bi PAP oxygen therapy is prescribed for this patient
- Oxygen therapy improves the quality and the length of life for people with COPD
- Bi PAP- Bi level positive airway pressure

7. Is Alpha 1 – Antitrypsin Therapy indicated for the patient?

- This therapy is medically necessary for adults with emphysema due to congenital deficiency of alpha 1- antitrypsin
- This therapy is not needed in this patient because there is no evidence for deficiency of alpha 1 antitrypsin emphysema
- If the lung disease is very severe, then the alpha 1 trypsin therapy may be initiated

8. What are the Clinical Parameters to Assess COPD Regimen?

SOB; Bronchospasm

9. What are the lab tests to assess the efficacy of the regimen?

- For patients on home oxygen: arterial blood gases are checked yearly or with any change in condition
- FEV1- measured both pre and post bronchodilators, checked regularly during treatment period. Mostly FEV1 (spirometry) and arterial blood gases test are done to assess the efficacy of the therapy. Other test may include lung volumes and chest X ray

10. Discuss the patient counselling measures.

- To improve adherence to COPD therapy
- Device education and selection: correct use of inhaler and nebulizer devices is crucial for the efficacy of inhaled medication.
- Inhalers should be selected properly as per the patient need.
- Technique of inhalation is important in the COPD patients similar devices for inhaled medications should be used.
- The patients will adhere to COPD therapy if their inhalers are simple to use and manage.
- Information about dosing frequency should be provided to the patient.
- Information about drug therapy and possible adverse effects should be provided

11. What is the Drug therapy related problems

- Drug- drug interactions:
  - Clarithromycin + Ondansetron:
- Both increase QTc interval (irregular heart beat)
  - Pantoprazole + Theophylline
- Pantoprazole increases toxicity of theophylline
- Prolonged use of proton pump inhibitors cause hypochlorhydria.

A Case Study of COPD Exacerbation

Summary

Male patient of 71 years old came to hospital with the following complaints i.e generalized weakness, shortness of breath, platelet count 57 thousand and no history of Vomiting and loose stools and has past medical history of hypertension, COPD and also history of dengue NS + and on medication with combihale FB 250, RabiwokDSR, Acebrophyllin, Telma H and he is also having habit of smoking. He has gone under following test: Complete blood picture : WBC count is decreased – 3640cells/cu.mm, Platelet count : 57,000 cells/cumm -decreased, Serum creatinine : 1.5mg/dL- increased, ECG: Sinus Tachycardia , Chest x ray: opacification is seen, USG Abdomen: Hepatomegaly with fatty infiltration.

Diagnosis: With the undergone test the patient was diagnosed with viral fever with thrombocytopenia, COPD – Acute Exacerbation and AKI

Treatment Plan:

His treatment plan includes:

Magnex forte   Clarithromycin   Inj. PAN (Pantaprazole)

Inj. Zofer (Ondansetron)   Inj. Solu-Medrol (Methylprednisolone) Inj. PCM (Paracetamol)

Inj. MgSO$_4$ Inj. Deriphylline (Etophylline + Theophylline)

Inj. Hydrocortisone   Inj. Clexane (Enoxaparin)

With the day to day investigation on the 1st day of admission the patient urine output is poor. Viral pyrexia and C/O SOB and decreased platelets count and inflammation so he is on treatment with Inj. Solu-Medrol which prevents inflammation and on nebulization with decrease SOB and also Inj. Paracetamol.

On 2nd day investigation patient is advised with low potassium diet and has complaints of SOB and fever.

On 3rd day investigation his platelet count is increased 72K and patient is conscious coherent and no fresh complaints as of now and advised with low potassium diet.

On 4th day patient is conscious and coherent and fresh complaints

On 5th day patient was discharged with the following medications.

Nocturnal continuous and day time intermittent BiPAP & Oxygen therapy

TIOVA (Tiotropium) 9 mcg – 2 puffs OD

Seroflo (Salmeterol + Fluticasone) 250 mcg 2 Puffs BD with water

Duolin inhaler (Salbutamol sulpahte + ipratopium bromide)2 puffs TID

Tab. Zostum O (Cefoperazone + Sulbactam) 200 mg BID 3 days

Tab. Omnacortil (Prednosolone) 20mg OD and stop after 5 days

Tab. PAN 40 mg Pantaprazole OD before food

Tab. Unicontin E (Theophylline) 400mg OD H/S

Tab. Dolo 650mg (Paracetamol) SOS

Continue old HTN medication

Pharmacist intervention

As Clarithromycin interacts with the Budesonide and increases its absorption into the blood stream. Side effects as swelling high B.P. are observed the dose of Clarithromycin should be tapered.

Patient counselling measures:

Stop smoking

Regular exercise should be done

Medication should be taken properly

Take more fluids

Take low potassium diet

Assignment

1. **Create a list of this patients drug related problems?**
   - Ondansetron using together with lactulose may cause an irregular heart rhythm and may be serious and life threatening
   - Clarithromycin when taken together with methyl prednisolone can increase the blood levels of methyl prednisolone and effects such as swelling and weight gain.
   - Clarithromycin when taken together with budesonide may increase the absorption of budesonide into the blood stream and side effects as swelling and high blood pressure
   - Methyl prednisolone and magnesium sulphate together may cause laxative effects
   - Theophylline and formetrol can increase the cardiovascular side effects such as heart palpitations
   - The major risk of having COPD to the patient is smoking

2. **What signs and symptoms and lab data provide evidence that this patient is having stable COPD status?**
   Signs and symptoms of this patient include: Weakness SOB wheezing sound
   Lab data
   Chest X ray; Opacification is seen in the left mid and lower lung zone possibly consolidation
   Opacification is the process of becoming cloudy or opaque
   Pulmonary opacification represents the results of a decrease in the ratio of gas of soft tissues
   Pulmonary consolidation means lung tissue that has filled with liquid instead of air the condition is marked by induration
   With the above chest x ray examination the patient was diagnosed with COPD

3. **What are the desired goals for the treatment of COPD?**

   The desired goals of medication use is to prevent symptoms reduce the frequency and severity of exacerbation and improve both health status and exercise tolerance

   It improve the quality of life

   It prevents the recurrence of Exacerbation

4. **What Non Pharmacological theripies would be useful to improve his copd status?**

   Non pharmacological therapy

   Quit smoking;   Regular exercise in the morning;   Avoid fumes and odour

   Eat healthy food;   Minimize milk to limit mucous production;

   Cut cruciferous vegetable's to reduce bloating;   Avoid fried foods

   Avoid alcohol;   Oxygen therapy

5. **Should home oxygen therapy is considered at this time?**

   The patient should be given oxygen therapy as he was suffering with acute exacerbation. It is given when there is not enough oxygen in blood we need to supplement oxygen. There are several devices to deliver oxygen to lungs including light weight portable units that one can take to run. Oxygen therapy can improve quality of life and is the only COPD therapy proven to extend life.

6. **Is this patient a candidate for Alpha 1 Anti trypsin therapy?**

   He is not the candidate for a 1 antitrypsin therapy because he is not having alpha one antitrypsin deficiency it occurs in less than 2% of all COPD cases

7. **What clinical parameters will you monitor?**

   Clinical parameters to be monitored are -As he is having acute Exacerbation we should monitor whether the Exacerbation is prevented or not. Weather the symptoms are relieved or not

   WBC and platelet count has to be evaluated.

8. **What lab tests should be performed?**

   The lab test to be performed is WBC count platelet count chest x ray and Physical examination

9. **What information should be provided to the Patient to enhance adherence and ensure successful therapy and minimize adverse effects?**

   Patient should stop smoking

   Regular exercise to prevent Exacerbation

   Follow medical instructions and regarding nebulisation properly

   Patient should not over use or under use forgetfulness and alteration of schedules and doses

Inhaled corticosteroid medication should include side effects like bruising oral infection and hoarseness so these medications are useful for people with frequent Exacerbation of COPD.

Oral steroids short course only should be given for acute Exacerbation more than 5 days usage may cause serious side effects such as weight gain diabetes.

References

1. Celli BR. The importance of spirometry in COPD and asthma. Chest 2000;117:15S–19S.

2. Dolovich MB, Ahrens RC, Hess DR, et al. Device selection and outcomes of aerosol therapy: Evidence-based guidelines. Chest 2005;127:335–271.

3. Barnes PJ. The pharmacological properties of tiotropium. Chest 2000;117:63S–66S.

4. Van Noord JA, de Munck DRAJ, Bantje TA, et al. Long-term treatment of chronic obstructive pulmonary disease with salmeterol and the additive effect of ipratropium. Eur Respir J 2000;15:880–885.

5. Barnes PJ. Theophylline in chronic obstructive pulmonary disease: New horizons. Proc Am Thorac Soc 2005;2:334–339.

6. https://www.guidelines.co.uk/respiratory/nice-copd-guideline/454912.article. © NICE 2019. Chronic obstructive pulmonary disease in over 16s: diagnosis and management. Available from: www.nice.org.uk/guidance/NG115

7. Callahan CM, Dittus RS, Katz BP. Oral corticosteroid therapy for patients with stable chronic obstructive pulmonary disease: A metaanalysis. Ann Intern Med 1991;114:216–223.

8. Robert burkes., An Update on the Global Initiative for Chronic Obstructive Lung Disease 2017 Guidelines With a Focus on Classification and Management of Stable COPD. June 2018. Respiratory care 63(6):749-758.

9. https://www.who.int/news-room/fact-sheets/detail/chronic-obstructive-pulmonary-disease-(copd)

10. Micromedex Solutions. Truven Health Analytics, Inc. Ann Arbor, MI. www.micromedexsolutions.com.

CHAPTER - 11

Pulmonary Function Tests

Introduction to Pulmonary Function Test

Pulmonary function test is a complete evaluation of the respiratory system including patient history, physical examination, and tests of pulmonary function. The primary purpose of pulmonary function testing is to identify the severity of pulmonary impairment.

There are two types of disorders that cause problems with air moving in and out of the lungs.

Obstructive: This is when air has trouble flowing out of the lungs due to airway resistance. This causes a decreased flow of air.

Restrictive: This is when the lung tissue or chest muscle can not expand enough. This creates problem with air flow, mostly due to lower lung volumes.

Pulmonary Function Tests

Spirometry: It measures the amount of air you breathe in and out. For this test the patient will sit in front of a machine and be fitted with a mouth piece. It's important that the mouthpiece fits snugly so that all the air he breathes goes into the machine. He will also wear a nose clip to keep you from breathing air out through your nose. The respiratory technologist will explain how to breathe for the test.

The measurements taken by spirometry device are used to generate pheumotochograph that can help to assess lung conditions such as asthma. Pulmonary fibrosis, cystic fibrosis, COPD.

FVC: Forced vital capacity

The determination of the vital capacity from a maximally forced expiratory effort.

Normal value: 80 to 120%

Mild: 70 to 79%

Moderate: 50 to 69%

Severe: Less than 50%

FEV t: forced expiratory volume time

The volume of air exhaled under forced condition in the first 't' seconds.

FEV 1: Volume maximum of air that has been exhaled at the end of the first second of forced expiration.

Normal value: 75 to 85%

FEV x: Forced expiratory flow related to some portion of the FVC curve, modifiers refer to amount of Fvc already exhaled.

FEF max: The maximum instantaneous flow achieved during a FVC maneuverer.

PEF: Peak expiratory flow

The highest forced expiratory flow measured with a peak flow meter.

MVV: Maximal voluntary ventilation.

Volume of air expired in a specified period during repetitive maximal effort.

Lung Volumes

TV: Tidal volume

The volume of air moved into or out of the lungs during quiet breathing.

Normal volume: 6 to 8 ml/ kg.

RV: Residual volume.

The volume of air remaining in the lungs after a maximal exhalation.

Normal value: 20 to 25 ml / kg.

ERV: Expiratory reserve volume.

The maximal volume of air that can be exhaled from the end expiratory position.

Normal volume: 700 to 1000 ml / kg.

IRV: Inspiratory reserve volume

The maximal volume that can be inhaled from the end Inspiratory level.

Normal value: 1900-3300 ml/kg.

Lung Capacity

TLC: Total lung capacity.

The volume in the lungs at maximal inflation,

$$TLC = RV + ERV + TV + IRV$$

$$TLC = RV + VC$$

Normal value: 4-6 litres.

VC: Vital capacity

The volume of air exhaled after the deepest inhalation

Normal value: 60-70ml/kg.

Formula: TLC -RV.

$$VC = TV + IRV + ERV$$

IC: Inspiratory capacity

The sum of T V + IRV.

$$IC = IRV + TV$$

Normal Value: 2400 to 3800 ml

EC: Expiratory capacity.

The sum of Tidal volume + expiratory reserve volume.

$$EC = TV + ERV$$

FRC: Functional residual capacity.

The volume in the lungs at the end expiratory position.

$$FRV = ERV = RV$$

Normal volume: 30 to 35 ml / kg.

Diffusing Capacity

Measurement of the single breathe diffusing capacity for carbon monoxide is a fast and safe tool in the evaluation of both restrictive and obstructive lung disease.

Oxygen Desaturation during Exercise

The six-minute walk test is a good index of physical function and therapeutic response in patient's with chronic lung disease, such as COPD or idiopathic pulmonary fibrosis.

Arterial Blood Gases

This is a helpful measurement in pulmonary function testing in selected patients. The primary role of measuring arterial blood gas in individuals that are healthy and stable is to confirm hypoventilation. When it is suspected on the basis of medical history, such as respiratory muscle weakness or advanced copd.

Arterial blood gas also provide a more detailed assessment of the severity of hypoxia in patient's who have low normal oxyhemoglobin saturation.

Other Techniques

Helium Dilution

The helium dilution technique for measuring lung volumes uses a closed rebreathing circuit. This technique is based on the assumption that a known volume and concentration of helium in air begin in the closed spirometer, that the patient has no helium in their lungs, and that an equilibration of helium can occur between the spirometer and the lungs.

Formula:

$$V_2 = V_1 \times \left(\frac{C_1 - C_2}{C_2} \right)$$

V_1 = volume of spirometer
V_2 = FRC
C_1 = concentration of helium in the spirometer before equilibrium
C_2 = concentration of helium in the spirometer after equilibrium.

Nitrogen Washout

Nitrogen Washout (or Fowler's method): It is test for measuring anatomic dead space in the lung during respiratory cycle.

The nitrogen washout technique uses a non breathing open circuit. The technique is based on the assumption that the nitrogen concentration in the lungs is 78% and in equilibrium with the atmosphere, that the patient inhales 100% oxygen and that the oxygen replaces all of the nitrogen in the lungs.

Plethysmography

The plethysmography technique applies boyle' s law and uses measurements of volume and pressure changes to determine lung volume, assuming temperature is constant.

VQ Scan

A pulmonary ventilation or perfusion VQ scan is a series of two lung scans. The scans are either performed together or one after the other, but are often referred to as one procedure.

A Ventilation-perfusion (VQ) scan is a nuclear medicine scan that uses radioactive material to examine air flow (ventilatin) and blood flow (perfusion) in the lungs.

Both scan involves the use of a low risk radioactive substance that can be traced by a special type of scanner. The substance will show up in the scanned image and can tell information about how well the lungs are working. The substance will gather at areas of abnormal blood or airflow which may indicate a blockage in the lung.

Values of Pulmonary Function Test in Case of

Obstructive and Restrictive Disorders

FEV 1/ FVC: In case of obstructive disorder FEV 1/FVC is decreased
In case of restrictive disorder FEV 1/FVC is normal or increased.

FEV1: In case of obstructive disorder FEV 1 is decreased.
In case of restrictive disorders FEV1 is decreased, normal, increased.

FVC: In case of obstructive disorder FVC is decreased or normal
In case of restrictive disorders FVC is decreased.

TLC: In case of obstructive disorder TLC is normal or increased
In case of restrictive disorders TLC is decreased.

Residual Volume (RV): In case of obstructive disorder RV is normal or increased
In case of restrictive disorders RV is decreased.

CHAPTER - 12

Diabetes Mellitus

Introduction to Diabetes Mellitus

Diabetes Mellitus (DM) is a group of metabolic disorders characterized by hyperglycemia and abnormalities in carbohydrate, fat, and protein metabolism. It results from defects in insulin secretion, insulin sensitivity, or both.

Epidemiology [1]: Globally, the prevalence of diabetes for all ages is estimated to be 2.8% in 2000 and projected to increase to 4.4% by 2030. The Centers for Disease Control and Prevention predicts the national incidence of diabetes will rise by 37.5% by the year 2025. The incidence of type 2 diabetes is now epidemic, with alarming increases in prevalence in both adults and children. The dramatic increase in type 2 diabetes is related to obesity and decreased physical activity levels. Additional factors include genetic predisposition, increased insulin resistance, and progressive β-cell failure. Approximately 5% to 10% of the diagnosed diabetic population has type 1 diabetes. In type 2 diabetes mellitus the prevalence of self-reported diagnosed diabetes is 1.7% among persons 20 to 39 years of age and 15.8% among persons over 65 years of age.

Table 12.1 Types of Diabetes.

Type 1 diabetes [Insulin Dependent]	Type 2 diabetes [Non-Insulin Dependent]
• It occurs when the pancreas does not produce enough insulin properly to control blood sugar levels.	• It occurs due to the high glucose levels in the context of insulin resistance.

Gestational Diabetes Mellitus (GDM): In which there is glucose intolerance that has its onset during pregnancy. GDM affects about 7% of all pregnancies and is defined as "any carbohydrate intolerance with onset or first recognition during pregnancy.

Table 12.2 Distinguishing features of 2 major types of diabetes mellitus.

	Insulin-dependent type 1[IDDM]	Non-insulin dependent type 2[NIDDM]
Age of onset	Usually, but not always, during childhood or puberty.	Frequently over 35.
Type of onset	Abrupt	Usually gradual
Prevalence	0.5%	5-6%

Contd...

	Insulin-dependent type 1[IDDM]	Non-insulin dependent type 2[NIDDM]
Incidence	<10-15%	>75%
Family history of diabetes	Infrequently positive	Commonly positive
Primary cause	Pancreatic beta cell deficiency	End-organ[insulin receptors] unresponsiveness to insulin action
Etiology	Unknown; possible factors include:- inheritance: associated with specific HLA tissue types, but only 40-50% concordance in twins.Viral Infections: mumps, influenza.	Unknown; possible factors include:- inheritance: 95-100% concordance in twins but not associated with specific HLA tissue types.
Diet	Mandatory in all patients.	If diet is utilized fully, hypoglycaemic drug therapy may not be needed.
Symptoms	Polydipsia, polyphagia and polyuria.	Maybe unknown.
Insulin	Necessary for all patients	Necessary for 20-30% of patients.
Oral agents	Rarely efficacious	Efficacious

Type I Diabetes Mellitus

Etiology and risk factors [2, 3, 4]:

1. **Genetic risk factors:**

   - Predisposition to destruction of beta cells – increased cytokine mediated beta cell death

   - Defective immunoregulatory mechanisms- decreased binding to antigenic epitopes resulting in ineffective tolerance induction

   - Altered insulin expression levels-by modulating thymic expression of insulin and affecting recognition by cytotoxic T-lymphocytes.

2. **Epigenetic risk factors:** Histone post-translational modifications/ DNA methylation/ non-coding RNAs-so there is decreased production of insulin.

   Predisposing factors and biomarkers-

   - Altered methylation levels of INS gene promoter

   - Type 1 Diabetes (T1D) specific in the T1D affected co-twins and in the islet autoantibody positive individuals many years before clinical diagnosis.

   - Altered methylation and acetylation profiles of histones upstream from Human Leukocyte antigen Class II-Histocompatibility-D related beta chain 1 (HLA-DRB1) and Human Leukocyten Antigen DQHLA- DQB1 and Cytotoxic-T-lymphocyte-associated antigen-4 (CTLA4) genes in monocytes of T1D patients.

3. **Exogenous risk factors:** Virusus/dietary factors/ intestinal microbiota/ antibiotic use. Predisposing factors:

   - Enteroviruses trigger beta cell autoimmnity

   - Altered bacteriodetes/fiemicutes ratio; low mucin, low microbial diversity affect innate immunity

- Early exposure to complex dietary proteins and short duration of breastfeeding are risk factors for Beta cell autoimmunity.

All these risk factors activate the autoimmune response against beta cell of pancreas. There is development of autoantibodies, and subsequent Type 1 diabetes

Pathogenesis: Type 1 Diabetes Mellitus is a syndrome characterized by hyperglycemia and insulin deficiency resulting from the loss of beta cells in pancreatic islets. Type 1 diabetes is less hereditary than type 2 but 7-13% of patients also have a first degree relative with type 1 diabetes.

What is evident are four main features: (1) a long preclinical period marked by the presence of immune markers when β-cell destruction is thought to occur; (2) hyperglycemia when 80% to 90% of β cells are destroyed; (3) transient remission (the so-called, "honeymoon" phase); and (4) established disease with associated risks for complications and death.

The destruction of insulin-producing beta cells in the pancreas starts with the formation of autoantigens. These autoantigens are ingested by antigen-presenting cells which activate T helper 1 (Th1) and T helper 2 (Th2) lmphocytes. Activated Th1 lymphocytes secrete interluekin-2 (IL-2) and interferon. IL-2 activates autoantigen-specific T cytotoxic lymphocytes which destroy islet cells through the secretion of toxic perforins and granzymes. Interferon activates macrophages and stimulates the release of inflammatory cytokines (including IL-1 and tumor necrosis factor [TNF]) which further destroy beta cells. Activated Th2 lymphocytes produce IL-4 which stimulates B lymphocytes to proliferate and produce islet cell autoantibodies (ICAs) and anti-glutamic acid decarboxylase (antiGAD65) antibodies. AntiGAD65 is an enzyme that helps control the release of insulin from beta cells and can be used to determine the cause of diabetes. Insulin autoantibodies [IAAs]) and zinc transporter 8 (Znt8) protein are also associated with type 1 diabetes mellitus. Without insulin or amylin the body cannot promote glucose disappearance or limit glucose appearance from the bloodstream, respectively, resulting in hyperglycemia.

Clinical Manifestation and Features

Type 1 diabetics may present with abrupt onset of diabetic ketoacidosis, polyuria, polyphagia, polydipsia, or rapid weight loss with marked hyperglycemia.

System	Symptom/Physical Exam
Central	Polydipsia, Polyphagia, Lethargy, Fatigue, **Acute Confusion**
Systemic	Weight Loss
Respiratory	**Kussmaul Breathing, Hyperventilation**
EENT	Blurred Vision, **Smell Acetone**
Cardiovascular	Tachycardia
Gastrointestinal	**Nausea, Vomiting, Abdominal Pain**
Gastrourinary	Polyuria, Glycosuria, Nocturia, Ketonuria
Musculoskeletal	**Muscle Wasting**

Long Term Consequences of Hyperglyceamia:

- Diabetes often develop kidney failure (Nephropathy), lesions of the eye (Retinopathy) and atrophy of the peripheral nerves (Neuropathy).
- Diabetic patients have a high frequency of gangrene. Gangrene results from a combination of factors including atherosclerosis, decreased pain sensation due to neuropathy and trauma.

Type II Diabetes Mellitus

Etiology and risk factors

1. **Modifiable risk factors:** Overweight: Being obese can cause insulin resistance. Sedentary lifestyle, previously identified glucose intolerance,
2. **Metabolic syndrome:** Persons with insulin resisitance have a group of conditions including high blood sugar, high blood pressure, high cholesterol and triglycerides. Intrauterine environment, smoking
   Non-modifiable risk factors: ethnicity, family history of type-2 DM, age, gender, history of gestational diabetes, polycystic ovarian syndrome, inflammation

Pathogenesis of type II DM:

1. **Type 2 DM (90% of cases) is characterized by multiple defects:**
   - ✓ *Impaired insulin secretion* is a hallmark finding; β-cell mass and function are both reduced, and β-cell failure is progressive.
   - ✓ Normally, the gut incretin hormones glucagon-like peptide-1 (GLP-1) and glucose-dependent insulinotropic peptide (GIP) are released and stimulate insulin secretion when nutrients enter the stomach and intestines. Patients with type 2 DM have a *reduced incretin effect* due to decreased concentrations of or resistance to the effects of these incretin hormones.
   - ✓ *Insulin resistance* is manifested by excessive hepatic glucose production, decreased skeletal muscle uptake of glucose, and increased lipolysis and free fatty acid production. The association of insulin resistance with a clustering of cardiovascular risk factors including hyperinsulinemia, hypertension, abdominal obesity, dyslipidemia, and coagulation abnormalities has been referred to by a variety of names including "the insulin resistance syndrome," "the metabolic syndrome.
   - ✓ *Excess glucagon secretion* occurs because type 2 DM patients fail to suppress glucagon in response to meals because of GLP-1 resistance/deficiency and insulin resistance/deficiency, which directly suppress glucagon.
   - ✓ *Sodium-glucose cotransporter-2 (SGLT-2) upregulation in the kidney* increases reabsorption of glucose by proximal renal tubular cells, which may worsen hyperglycemia.
2. **Unhealthy life style** i,e, over-eating, obesity, inactivity cause the intraperitoneal cavity accumulation of visceral fat, which is an endocrine organ that secretes- inflammatory mediators/ adipokines/ free fatty acids. FFAs inhibit function of GLUT-2 on beta cells

and decrease glucose import. The above secreted substances are also responsible for the development of insulin resistance (Liver, muscle, adipose tissue become less responsive to insulin and thus less able to use glucose as a fuel source). In this situation-Initially beta cells of the pancreas work overtime to increase insulin secretion and blood glucose is kept normal. Over many years, as insulin resistance worsens, beta cells "tire out", decrease insulin secretion (relative insulin deficiency). Now hyperglycemia ensues. Hyperglycemia is directly toxic to beta cells. Since cells can't use glucose body perceives a state of 'starvation', thus mobilizing triglycerides into FFAs, to be used as fuel by the cells. Again excessively produced FFAs further inhibit glucose import, and beta cells do not recognise high blood glucose and there is decreased insulin secretion.

3. Over many more years, beta cells deteriorate until they finally stop producing insulin (Absolute insulin defect). This leads to finally Type II diabetes Mellitus.

4. **Genetic susceptibility:** Polygenetic or monogenetic factors can predispose insulin resistance.

5. **Aging:** Beta cell mass dceclines with aging, so those predisposd to insulin resisitance may develop type II diabetes.

6. **Medication:** Corticosteroids, anti-psychotics, highly active retrovirals, oral contraceptives also predispose to insulin resistance.

7. **Uncommon causes of diabetes** (less than 5% of cases) include gestational diabetes mellitus (GDM), maturity onset diabetes of youth (MODY), endocrine disorders (eg, acromegaly, Cushing syndrome), pancreatic exocrine dysfunction, infections, and medications (eg, glucocorticoids, thiazides, niacin).

8. **Microvascular complications** include retinopathy, neuropathy, and nephropathy. Macrovascular complications include coronary heart disease, stroke, and peripheral vascular disease.

Diagnosis of Diabetes with Algorithm [5, 6]: Type 1 diabetes is usually easy to diagnose because they present with all of the classic symptoms of diabetes and high amount of glucose in blood and urine. Type 2 diabetes is more of challenge because they often do not present with the classic symptoms.

Screening and diagnosis algorithm for type 2 diabetes

1. Screen every 3 years in individuals $\geq$ 40 yrs of age or in individuals at high risk using a risk calculator

2. Screen earlier and/or more frequently (every 6-12 months) in people with additional risk factors for diabetes or for those at very high risk using a risk calculator

   (a) FPG < 5.6mmol/L and/or HbA_1C <5.5%: considered as "normal" and can be rescreened as recomended.

   (b) If FPG is 5.6 -6.0 mmol/L and/or HbA_1C 5.5 – 5.9%: the patient is considered as "at risk".

   (c) If FPG is 6.1 -6.9mmol/L and/or HbA_1C is 6.0 -6.4%-the patient is in "Prediabetic" stage and should be rescreened more often.

   (d) If FPG $\geq$ 7.0 mmol/L and/or HbA_1C is $\geq$ 6.5%- he is considered as "Diabetic"

The Expert Committee of the **American Diabetic Association** has established the diagnostic criteria for diabetes for nonpregnant individuals of any age. For these individuals, a diagnosis of diabetes can be made when one of the following is present.

Criteria for the Diagnosis of Diabetes Mellitus

1. Classic signs and symptoms of diabetes (polyuria, polydipsia, ketonuria, and unexplained weight loss) combined with a random plasma glucose ≥200 mg/dL (11.1 mmol/L).
2. A FPG≥126 mg/dL (7.0 mmol/L). Fasting means no caloric intake for at least 8 hours.
3. After a standard oral glucose challenge (75 g glucose for an adult or 1.75 g/kg for a child), the venous plasma glucose concentration is ≥200 mg/dL (11.0 mmol/L) at 2 hours and >200 mg/dL (11.0 mmol/L) at least one other time during the test (0.5, 1, 1.5 hours); this is the OGTT.

The diagnosis must be confirmed on a subsequent day by any one of these conditions in the absence of unequivocal hyperglycemia with acute metabolic complications.

The categories of FPG values are as follows:

1. A normal FPG is <100mg/dL
2. An FPG of 100 to 125 mg/dL (5.6–6.9 mmol/L) is Impaired Fasting Glucose.
3. An FPG ≥126 mg/dL (7.0 mmol/L) indicates a provisional diagnosis of diabetes that must be confirmed, as described.

The corresponding categories when the OGTT is used for diagnosis are as follows:

1. A 2-hour postload glucose (2-hPG) <140mg/dL (7.8 mmol/L) indicates normal glucose tolerance.
2. A 2-hPG 140-199 mg/dL (7.8-11.1 mmol/L) indicates Impaired Glucose Tolerance.
3. A 2-hPG ≥200 mg/dL (11.1 mmol/L) indicates a provisional diagnosis of diabetes, which must be confirmed by a second test.

Diagnosis of Gestational Diabetes Mellitus with a 100-g or 75-g Glucose Load

100-g Glucose load

Fasting: ≥95 mg/dL (5.3 mmol/L)
1 hour ≥180 mg/dL (10.0 mmol/L)
2 hours ≥155 mg/dL (8.6 mmol/L)
3 hours ≥140 mg/dL (7.8 mmol/L)

75-g Glucose load

Fasting ≥95 mg/dL (5.3 mmol/L)
1 hour ≥180 mg/dL (10.0 mmol/L)
2 hours ≥155 mg/dL (8.6 mmol/L)

Women is considered gestationally diabetic if plasma glucose ≥140 mg/dL (7.8 mmol/L) at 2 hr post prandial.

Oral Glucose Tolerance Test: The OGTT measures a person's ability to handle a glucose load over a period of time. Following on overnight fast, a morning fasting blood sugar is drawn and a 75g glucose load is ingested by the patient; blood samples are then drawn at 30-min intervals for 2 hr and at 3hr. Urine samples are often taken at the same time and tested for the glucose.

Fasting Plasma Glucose: No food or drink for 8 to 12hrs prior to test. Blood is drawn and tested for the levels of glucose in blood. Normal value: - <100mg/dl. This test is used in non-pregnant patients only

Two Hour Post Prandial Blood Glucose: It is used as the screening test. A blood glucose level is drawn after 2hr following a 100gm glucose load. In non-diabetics blood glucose levels return to normal in less than 2 hr

Glycosylated Hemoglobin A_1C test [HbA_1C]: It is the test that measures the amount of glycated Hb in the blood. It is a substance in red blood cells that is formed when blood sugar is attached to Haemoglobin. If >6.5% then DM

Urinalysis: Glycosuria, Ketone bodies

Management

The goals of therapy in DM are:

- To Ameliorate symptoms of hyperglycemia,
- Reduce the onset and progression of microvascular and macrovascular complications,
- Reduce mortality, and improve quality of life.

Glycemic Goals of Therapy by American Diabetes Association

1. Hemoglobin A1C <7%
2. Preprandial plasma glucose 90–130 mg/dL
3. Postprandial plasma glucose <180mg/dL

Non Pharmacological Therapy

- Aerobic exercise can improve insulin resistance and glycemic control
- Avoid fat diets and prolonged fasting
- Avoid quick-acting(simple)sugars
- Decrease consumption of animal (saturated)fats
- Increase amount of fiber in the diet
- Control calories
- Avoid smoking
- Take vitamin-mineral supplements

Management of Diabetes Mellitus

I. Classification of Oral Hypoglycaemic Drugs

1. Insulin seretagogues:
   (a) Sulfonylureas: tolbutamide, chlorpropamide, glipizide, glimepiride, glyburide
   (b) Meglitinides: repaglinide, D-phenylalanine derivatives: nateglinide
2. Biguanides: metformin
3. Thiazolidinediones: pioglitazone, rosiglitazone
4. Alpha – glucosidase inhibitors: acarbose, miglitol

1. **Sulphonyl Ureas:** Sulphonyl urea stimulates insulin secretion by the pancreas and potentially increase the number of insulin receptors. Therefore a minimum of pancreatic function is a prerequisite to sulphonylureas therapy.

Table 12.3 Dosage and Pharmacokinetics of Sulphonyl Ureas.

Drug	Recommended dose (gm.)	Dosing
Tolbutamide	500 mg	0.5-1.5g daily in divided oses. Dose to be given with or immedialtely after meals. Maximum 2 g/day
Glipizide	5 mg	Initially 2.5-5mg daily, take shortly befrore breakfast or lunch, upto 15mg may be given as a single dose. Max 20mg/day.
Glimepiride	1mg, 2mg. 3mg, 4mg	Once daily with first main meal.
Gliclazide (immediate release)	40mg 80mg 160mg	Initially 40-80mg daily; increased, if necessary upto 160mg once daily; with breakfast. Max 320mg/day.
Gliclazide (modified release)	30mg 60mg	Initially 30mg daily with breakfast. Adjust dose every 4 weeks. Max. 120mg/day.

Source: Joint Formulary Committee (2022) British National Formulary. Available at: www.medicinescomplete.com

Mechanism of Action: They cause hypoglycemia by stimulating insulin release from pancreatic beta cells by binding to the ATP sensitive K^+ channel and inhibiting it. Reduced K^+ conductance lead to membrane depolarization which allows Ca^{2+} to enter the cell and then insulin is released. They also decrease the hepatic clearance of insulin whereby increasing insulin level in the body. They also stimulate the secretion of somatostatin and suppress glucagon. They also have extra pancreatic actions.

Absorption, Fate and Excretion: All sulfonylureas are well absorbed from the gastrointestinal tract. Food and hyperglycemia may retard their absorption. They are largely bound to plasma protein (90-99%). They are metabolized mainly in liver; some metabolites are active and then excreted in urine. Hence they should be used cautiously in patients in hepatic and renal dysfunction

Efficacy: When given in equipotent doses, all sulfonylureas are equally effective at lowering blood glucose. Sulfonylureas showed a reduction of microvascular complications in type 2 DM patients.

Adverse effects: Hypoglycemia is common. Hyponatremia (serum sodium < 129mEq/L is seen with tolbutamide. Weight gain. Less common - skin rash, hemolytic anemia, gastrointestinal upset, and cholestasis. Disulfiram-type reactions and flushing

2. **Short Acting Insulin Secretagogues (Meglitinides or Glinides):** These are benzoic acid derivatives and unrelated to sulfonylureas. Repaglinide is the drug of this class. But like

sulfonylureas, repaglinide increases insulin secretion by inhibiting ATP dependent K^+ channels in pancreatic cells. It is rapidly absorbed from the intestines and has a fast onset of action. Peak effect comes within 1 hr and duration of action is 5-8 hr. Because of this it is mainly used to control post prandial rise in blood glucose concentration. It is metabolized by hepatic CYP3A4 and renal tissue. Therefore needs caution in patients with hepatic and renal insufficiency.

Ex: Repaglinide – Normal dose - 2 to 4 mg with meals

Elderly dose - 0.5 to 1 mg with meals

Nateglinide – Normal dose – 60 to 120 mg with meals

Elderly dose – 120 mg with meals

D-Phenylalanine Derivatives

Nateglinide is a D-phenylalanine derivative and is effective orally. Like sulfonylureas and repaglinide, nateglinide stimulates insulin secretion by inhibiting ATP sensitive K^+ channels in pancreatic cells. Nateglinide is primarily metabolized in liver by CYP 2C9, 3A4 system and therefore dose adjustment is needed in patients with hepatic insufficiency. No dosage adjustment is needed in renal failure.

Therapeutically nateglinide is primarily used for controlling postprandial hyperglycemia in patients of type 2 diabetes mellitus and it produce even fewer episodes of hypoglycemia than other secretagogues as its ability to release insulin is markedly decreased in presence of normoglycemia.

Efficacy: In monotherapy, both significantly reduce postprandial glucose excursions and reduce HbA1c levels. Repaglinide, dosed 4 mg three times a day, when compared to glyburide in diet-treated drug-naïve patients reduced HbA1c levels. Nateglinide, dosed 120 mg three times a day in a similar population reduced HbA1c values by 0.8%.

Adverse effects: Hypoglycemia is main side effect. Weight gain with repaglinide is more compared to nateglinide.

3. **Biguanides:**

Mechanism of Action: Metformin is an antihyperglycemic agent and does not cause hypoglycemia as it does not lead to release of insulin. It also has no significant effect on other counter regulatory hormones like glucagon and cortisol or somatostatin. It primarily causes decrease in hepatic glucose production ($\downarrow$ gluconeogenesis) and increasing insulin action in muscle and fat. These actions are mediate by activation of cellular kinase, AMP-activated protein kinase. It may also decrease uptake of glucose from small intestines.

Absorption, Fate and Excretion: Drug is primarily absorbed from small intestines. It does not bind to plasma proteins and excreted unchanged in urine.

Efficacy: Metformin consistently reduces HbA1c levels by 1.5% to 2.0%, fasting plasma glucose levels by 60 to 80 mg/dL, and retains the ability to reduce fasting plasma glucose levels when they are extremely high (>300 mg/dL). Metformin also has positive effects on several components of the insulin resistance syndrome. Metformin decreases plasma triglycerides and LDL-C by approximately 8% to 15%, as well increasing HDL-C very modestly (2%).

Acute side effects that can occur with metformin include diarrhea, abdominal pain, nausea, metallic taste, and anorexia. Intestinal absorption of B12 and folate is decreased with chronic metformin therapy.

Ex. Metformin – immediate release -500 mg BID with meals with max dose 2000mg/day.

Extended release- 500mg with evening meal, titrated to 2000mg/day

4. **Thiazolidinediones [Glitazones]:** Thiazolidinediones are selective agonist for nuclear peroxisomal proliferator activated receptor-γ (PPAR- γ). These drugs binds to PPAR- γ, which activates genes that regulate carbohydrate and fat metabolism. They increase the uptake of glucose into muscle and fat by increasing the expression of specific transporters.

   Efficacy: Pioglitazone and rosiglitazone, given for about 6 months, reduce HbA1c values ~1.5% and reduce FPG levels by approximately 60 to 70 mg/dL at maximal doses. Glycemic-lowering onset is slow, and maximal glycemic-lowering effects may not be seen until 3 to 4 months of therapy. Thiazolidinediones improve endothelial function, raise HDL levels, slightly lower blood pressure.

   Adverse effects: weight gain, retention of sodium and water, edema.

   Ex: Pioglitazone – decreases plasma triglycerides

   Normal dose -15 -45 mg – OD

   Elderly dose -15 mg

   Rosiglitazone –decrease plasma triglycerides

   Normal dose -2-8 mg – OD

   Elderly dose -2 mg-   BD

5. **Alpha- Glucosidase Inhibitors:** These delay breakdown of sucrose and prolongs carbohydrate absorption in intestine (small intestine). net effect from this action is to reduce the postprandial blood glucose rise.

   Efficacy: Postprandial glucose concentrations are reduced (40 to 50 mg/dL), while fasting glucose levels are relatively unchanged (~10% reduction). Efficacy on glycemic control is modest. α-Glucosidase inhibitors modestly reduce HbA1c levels.

   Adverse effects: GI side effcts- flatulence, bloating, abdominal discomfort, diarrhoea.

   Ex: Acarbose – Normal dose – 25 to 100 mg – OD/TID

            Elderly/adult dose – 25 mg – OD/TID

            Miglitol – Normal dose – 25 to 100 mg- 1 to 3 times/day

            Elderly dose – 25 mg – OD to TID

6. **Dipeptidyl Peptidase –IV Inhibitors:** These reduce in appropriately elevated post prandial glucagon and improves β-cell response to hyperglycaemia. The drugs are well tolerated.

   Ex: Sitagliptin – Normal dose -100mg OD

            Elderly dose -25 to 100 mg daily

            Saxagliptin – Normal dose – 5mg OD

            Elderly dose – 2.5mg to 5mg

7. **Insulin [7]: Mechanism of Action of Insulin** After reaching the target cell insulin binds to its receptor. Insulin receptor is a transmembrane glycoprotein composed of two alpha

subunits and two beta subunits linked by disulphide bonds forming a beta-alpha-alpha-beta tetramer. After insulin binds to the receptor, insulin-receptor complex is internalized and undergoes autophosphorylation. This leads to activation of tyrosine kinase activity, which in turn leads to activation of various MAP kinases and phosphoinositol phosphate 3 kinase (PI3 kinase). It stimulates glucose transport across cell membrane by ATP dependant translocation of glucose transporter GLUT4 to the plasma membrane.

Glucose enters with GLUT4 protein and is taken up by skeletal muscle, liver and adipose tissues.

Insulin Preparations

All insulins available are manufactured using recombinant DNA technology and are highly purified.

1. Regular insulin – given SC
   - Pharmacokinetics forms- hexamer- dimers- monomers- absorbed
   - Slow on set of action and given 30 mins before meal
   - It's concentration is U-500
   - Available as vials(20ml) ,insulin pen (3ml)
2. Rapid acting insulins
   - Dissociates rapidly into monomers, shows rapid onset of action and peak effect with a shorter duration of action than regular insulin
   - Sub cutaneously dose with in 10 mins of meal
   - Better efficacy in lowering post prandial blood glucose than regular insulin in type 1 DM, minimizes delayed post meal hypoglycaemia
     - Ex: Humalog (insulin lispro) – Insulin pen (3ml), vials, pen, carbidge
              Novolog (insulin apart) – Insulin pen (3ml) 10- ml vials, 3-ml pen carbidge
              Apidra (insulin glulisine) – Insulin pen (3ml) 10 ml vials, 3ml carbidge
3. Intermediate acting
   - Variable in absorption and pharmacokinetics
   - Labile glucose response,nocturnal hypoglycaemia, fasting hyperglycaemia
     - Ex: Neutral protamine Hagedorn (NPH)
              Humulin N – 3ml and 10ml vial, Insulin pen 3ml
              Novolin N – 10 ml vial
4. Long -Acting
   - Peak less insulin
   - Result is less nocturnal hypoglycaemia than NPH insulin when given at bed time
     - Ex: Insulin Glargine
              Insulin Degludec
              Insulin detemir (Levemir)– low doses -< 0.3 U/kg -BD
5. Inhaled Insulin
   - Dry powder of regular insulin is inhaled and absorbed through pulmonary tissue
   - Rapid absorption and reaches max blood concentration in 12 to 15 mins

> Common adverse effects:- cough, URTI
> Contraindicated in patients with asthma and COPD

Dose: 4-U carbidge before each meal

6. Premixed Inhibitors

Ex: Humalog mix- 75/25 -75% neutral protamine lispro+ 25% lispro
50/50- 50% neutral protamine lispro + 50%lispro
Novolog mix -70/30 – 70% aspart protamine suspension + 30% aspart

Common Adverse Effects of Insulin

> Hypoglycaemia – treatment – Glucose – 10 to 15 mg – P/O

Dextrose – IV   unconscious patients

Glycagon -1g

Weight gain

> Allergies, lipo hypertrophy – uncommon effects

> Site of infections and injection using should be changed regularly.
> Lipo atrophy – uncommon effect

Patient Who Should Use Human Insulin

- Patient with insulin resistance [using more than 100-200 units /day]
- Patient with insulin allergy
- Patient with lipoatrophy
- All newly diagnosed type 1 patient
- Pregnant diabetics – antibodies are passed to foetus

Table 12.4 Different types of Insulin Preperations.

Product	Manufacturing	Purity	Species	Strength

• Rapid acting:
(Onset - 0.5- 4Hrs,
  Duration-5-6 hrs)
  ➤ Humulin BR
	Lilly	0	Recombinant-DNA human	U100

➤ Humulin Regular	Lilly	0	Recombinant-DNA human	U100
➤ Novolin R (Regular)	Squibb/Nova	<1	Semisynthetic Human	U100
• Intermediate Acting: (onset 1-4 hr, duration 16-18 hr) ➤ Humulin L	Lilly	0	Recombinant-DNA human	U100
➤ Humulin NPH	Lilly	0	Recombinant-DNA human	U100
• Long Acting: (onset 4-6 hr , duration 36hr) ➤ Iletin II PZI	Lilly	<1	beef or pork	U100
➤ Ultralene	Squibb/	<20	beef	U100
➤ Iletin I PZI	NovoLilly	<1	beef or pork	U40,U100

Pharmacotherapy of Type 1 Diabetes Mellitus

Nonpharmacological

Principles of dietary therapy
- Carbohydrate 45-65% of total calories; Protein—10-35% of total Kcal/day (10% for those with nephropathy); 20-35% from fat: saturated fat<7% of total Kcal/day polyunsaturated fat 10% of Kcal/day. Intake of trans-fats should be minimized.
- Low carbohydrate diets (<130g/day) not recommended in the treatment of overweight/obesity. Routine supplementation with antioxidants (vitamins E, C and carotene) not advised.
- Use of caloric sweetners including sucrose is safe when consumed within the intake levels recommended by FDA. Fibre 20-35 g/day and sodium 3000 mg/day. Cholesterol 300 mg/day.

Pharmacological

Insulin therapy

1. Therapy should be started with insulin (human) in a dose of 0.5 units/kg/day to 1.0 unit/kg/day.
2. Combination of regular + lente/semilente insulin should be used (now available as Premix preparation as well).
3. One-third of the total insulin requirement is given as regular and two-thirds as lente/semilente.
4. One-third of the total dose is used before dinner and two-thirds before breakfast.
5. Insulin is given SC 30-45 min before meals.
6. Medial aspect of thigh and abdominal wall are generally used for injection. Rotate injection site frequently. There is no need to use spirit swab, if the skin is clean.
7. Dose, type and timing of insulin is adjusted according to pre-prandial blood sugar levels (80-150 mg%). Level of blood glucose estimated depends on dose of plain insulin taken 3-4 hours before or intermediate/long-acting insulin taken 8-12 hours before the test.
8. Increment of dose should not be more than 10% of existing dose and dose readjustment should not be made earlier than 3 days.
9. Use of insulin analogs in select cases when it is justified on clinical grounds, preferably under guidance of a specialist. Patients must be properly trained for administration of SC injections.
10. Meals must be ensured after injection.
11. Explain features of hypoglycaemia to the patient.
12. Diabetes self-management and adjustment of Insulin dose based on self-monitoring of glucose and carbohydrate count.

Pharmacotherapy of Type 2 Diabetes Mellitus

Nonpharmacological

Diet: Basic principles of the diet are same as in DM Type 1. Most of the patients in DM type 2 are, however, obese and should be put on dietary restrictions for weight reduction as above.

Exercise: Regular physical exercise for 1/2 to 1 hour (for sedentary workers): at least 150 min/week of moderate-intensity aerobic physical activity (50-70% of maximum heart rate) and/or at least 90 min/week of vigorous aerobic exercise (>70% of maximum heart rate). At least for 3 days/week.

Pharmacological

Level of hyperglycaemia influences the initial choice of oral hypoglycaemic agents. Treatment may be started with any of the following drugs and dose individualized and dose can be increased every 2-3 weeks as determined by blood glucose response:

Tab. Metformin 500 mg once or twice a day in obese patients and increase the dose to 1000 mg 2 times a day with meals.

or

Tab. Glimepiride 1-8 mg/day once daily to be taken at the same time every day with breakfast or Tab. Glipizide 2.5-40 mg/day before breakfast or Tab. Glipizide ER 5-10 mg/day with breakfast or Tab. Gliclazide MR 30 mg-120 mg/day as single dose at breakfast time. (Caution: MR and ER tablets should be swallowed whole and not broken, chewed or crushed, as this would damage the modified release action)

or

Tab. Glyburide (Glibenclamide) 1.25-20 mg/day administered with breakfast or with the first main meal. Or

Tab Pioglitazone initially 15-30 mg, up to 45 mg usually once daily without regard to meals.

Combination therapy. If monotherapy fails with oral hypoglycaemics at maximaltolerated doses as does not achieve or maintain A1C target over 3-6 months, add a second oral agent or GLP-1 receptor agonist or insulin. Following combination can be given, if inadequate glycaemic control with single oral hypoglycaemic agent:

Sulphonylurea + metformin

Sulphonylurea + pioglitazone

Sulphonylurea + alpha glucosidase inhibitor (Acarbose)

Insulin + metformin

Insulin may be required in patients with primary (markedly symptomatic and/ or elevated blood glucose levels or A1C) or secondary failure to oral agents; often as single dose of intermediate acting insulin 0.3-0.4 units/kg/day either before breakfast or at bedtime in combination with Tab. Metformin. Insulin is also required in situations like pregnancy, surgery, infection, etc.

Consider insulin as initial therapy in patients with:

1. Fasting plasma glucose >250-300 mg/dl since more rapid glycaemic control will reduce glucose toxicity to islet cells, improve insulin secretion and possibly make oral hypoglycaemic agents more effective.
2. Lean patients or those with severe weight loss.
3. Underlying renal or hepatic disease, or acutely ill or hospitalized patients

Glycaemic goals Glycaemic control is fundamental to the management of diabetes and glycaemic goals

Summary of recommendations on glycaemic goals for adults with diabetes

Glycaemic control

A1C	< 7.0%
Preprandial capillary plasma glucose	90-130 mg/dl (5.0-7.2 mmol/L)
Peak postprandial capillary plasma glucose	<180mg/dL (10mmol/L)
Blood pressure	< 130/80 mmHg
Lipids	
LDL	<100 mg/dl (2.6mmol/L)
Triglycerides	<150mg/dL (<1.7mmol/L)
HDL	>40mg/dL(>1.0mmol/L)

Prevention and Management of Diabetes Complications [8, 9, 10]

Cardiovascular disease (CVD)

1. **Hypertension/blood pressure control:** Patients with diabetes should be treated to a systolic blood pressure <140mg/Hg and diastolic blood pressure <90mg/Hg
2. **Dyslipidaemia/lipid management:** In individuals without overt CVD
   - The primary goal is an LDLC< 89 mg/dL (2.6 mmol/l).
   - For those over the age of 40 years, statin therapy to achieve an LDL reduction of 30-40% regardless of baseline LDL levels is recommended.
   - For those under the age of 40 years but at increased risk due to other cardiovascular risk factors who do not achieve lipid goals with lifestyle modifications alone, the addition of pharmacological therapy is appropriate.
   - In individuals with overt CVD- All patients should be treated with a statin to achieve an LDL reduction of 30-40%.
   - Lower triglycerides to 40 mg/dL (1.0 mmol/L). In women, an HDL goal 10 mg/dL higher (>50 mg/dL) should be considered.
   - Statin therapy is contraindicated in pregnancy.

3. **Antiplatelet agents** - Use aspirin therapy (75-162 mg/day) as a secondary prevention strategy in those with diabetes with a history of CVD. Use aspirin therapy (75-162 mg/day) as a primary prevention strategy in those with: Type 1 and 2 diabetes at increased cardiovascular risk, including those who are¬ >40 years of age or who have additional risk factors (family history of CVD, hypertension, smoking, dyslipidaemia, or albuminuria).

4. **Smoking cessation**

5. **Coronary heart disease (CHD) screening and treatment** - In patients >55 years of age, with or without hypertension but with another cardiovascular risk factor (history of CVD, dyslipidaemia, microalbuminuria, or smoking), an ACE inhibitor (if not contraindicated) should be considered to reduce the risk of cardiovascular events.

   In patients with a prior myocardial infarction or in patients undergoing major surgery, β-blockers, in addition, should be considered to reduce mortality.

   In asymptomatic patients, consider a risk factor evaluation to stratify patients by 10 year risk and treat risk factors accordingly.

6. **Nephropathy screening and treatment**
   Screening
   - Perform an annual test for the presence of microalbuminuria in type 1 diabetic patients with diabetes duration of $\geq$ 5 years and in all type 2 diabetic patients, starting at diagnosis and during pregnancy.
   - Serum creatinine should be measured at least annually for the estimation of glomerular filtration rate (GFR) in all adults with diabetes regardless of the degree of urine albumin excretion. The serum creatinine alone should not be used as a measure of kidney function but instead used to estimate GFR and stage the level of chronic kidney disease (CKD).
   - For individuals with diabetic kidney disease dietary protein should be maintained at recommended daily allowance of 0.8 g/kg body weight per day. Reducing the amount is not recommended because it does not alter glycemic measures, cardiovascular risk measures or the rate at which GFR declines.

7. **Retinopathy screening and treatment**
   Screening – Adults and adolescents with type 1 and 2 diabetes should have an initial dilated and comprehensive eye examination by an ophthalmologist or optometrist within 1-2 years after the onset of diabetes.
   Treatment
   - Laser therapy can reduce the risk of vision loss in patients with high-risk characteristics (HRCs).
   - Promptly refer patients with any level of macular oedema, severe non-proliferative diabetic retinopathy (NPDR) or any PDR to an ophthalmologist.

8. **Neuropathy screening and treatment**
   Recommendations
   - All patients should be screened for distal symmetric polyneuropathy (DPN) at diagnosis¬ and at least 1-2 times a year thereafter, using simple clinical tests.

- Once the diagnosis of DPN is established, special foot care is appropriate for insensate feet to decrease the risk of amputation.
- Simple inspection of insensate feet should be performed at 3- to 6-month intervals. An abnormality should trigger referral for special footwear, preventive specialist, or podiatric care.
- Screening for autonomic neuropathy should be instituted at diagnosis of type 2 diabetes and 5 years after the diagnosis of type-1 diabetes.

Diagnosis of neuropathy

Screened annually for Diabetic Periopheral Neuropathy (DPN) using tests such as pin-prick sensation, temperature and vibration perception (using a 128-Hz tuning fork), and 10 g monofilament pressure sensation at the distal plantar aspect of both great toes and ankle reflexes. Loss of 10 g monofilament perception and reduced vibration perception predict foot ulcers.

Diabetic autonomic neuropathy

1. Tricyclic drugs	Amitryptilline	10-75mg at bedtime
	Imipramine	25-75 mg at bedtime
2. Anti-convulsants	Gabapentin	300-1200mg 3 times daily
	Carbamazepine	200-400mg 3 times daily
	Pregabalin	100mg 3 times daily
3. SNRIs	Duloxetine	60-120mg daily

Diabetic Ketoacidosis [11]

Ketoacidosis is acute complication of diabetes, usually occurs in type 1 but can occur in type 2 and characterized by hyperglycaemia, hyperketonaemia and acidosis.

Clinical Features Nausea, vomiting, abdominal pain, Dehydration and altered sensorium.

Treatment

1. Confirm the diagnosis (increased plasma glucose, positive serum ketones, metabolic acidosis). Admit to hospital; intensive care setting necessary for frequent monitoring or if pH < 7 or unconscious.
2. Asess serum electrolytes(K^+, Na^+, Mg^{++},Cl^-, bicarbonate, phosphates), acid base status (pH,HCO_3^-, pCO_2, β hydroxybutyrate), Renal function(creatinine, urine output)
3. Replace fluids 2-3 L of 0.9% saline over first 1-3 hrs (10-20 ml/kg/hr) then 0.45% saline at 150-250 ml/hr when plasma glucose reaches 250 mg/dl.
4. Administer short acting insulin: IV (0.1 U/kg) then 0.1U/kg/hr by continous IV infusion; increase 2-3 fold if no response by 2-4 hrs. If the initial serum K^+ < 3.3 mEq/L .Do not administer insulin until K^+ is corrected.

5. Asess patient: what precipitated the episode (non-compliance, infection, trauma, pregnancy, infarction, cocaine)? Initiate appropriate workup for precipitating event (cultures, chest X ray, ECG).

6. Measure capillary glucose every 1-2 hrs; measure electrolytes (especially K^+, bicarbonate, $PO4^-$) and anion gap every 4 hrs for first 24 hrs.

7. Monitor blood pressure, pulse, respiration, mental status, fluid intake & output every 1-4 hrs.

8. Replace K^+ =10 mEq/hr when plasma K^+ < 3.5 mEq/L or if bicarbonate is given. If initial serum K^+ is > 5.2 mmol/L do not supplement K^+ until K^+ is corrected.

9. Continue above until patient is stable, glucose goal is 150-250 mg/dL and acidosis is resolved. Insulin infusion may be decreased to 0.05-0.1 U/kg/hr.

10. Administer long acting insulin as soon as patient is eating. Allow for a 2-4 hr overlap in insulin infusion and subcutaneous insulin injection.

Case Study of Diabetic Foot

Summary

An 86 year old male patient was admitted, with chief complaints of swelling of left limb 4 days associated with pain and fever and chills, he has a history of HTN and DM and is on Tab. Aten. (OD) and Tab. Glucored forte (OD), vitals are stable with normal temperature, BP of 130/70 and pulse rate 82. His CBP reports an increase in WBC count that is 12,100 cells/cu mm, increase in neutrophils (76%), decrease in lymphocytes (18%) and an increase in platelet count that is 5.2 lakh/cu mm. Blood sugar reports showed increased fasting blood sugar (115mg/dL), increase post lunch blood sugar (212mg/dL) and increase in RBS (154mg/dL). His ECG showed sinus rhythm.

Diagnosis: By above subjective and objective data patient was diagnosed with " DIABETIC FOOT on his Left leg."

Therapy includes:

Drugs	Drug name	Route	Dose	Frequency
T. ATEN	Atenolol	PO	125mg	OD
T. PAN	Pantaprazole	PO	40mg	OD
T. ULTRACET	Paracetamol+tramadol	PO	1 tab	BD
T.ECOSPORIN	Aspirin+atorcastatin	PO	1 tab	OD
T.SEPTRAN DS	Sulfamethoxaole+trimethoprim	PO	1 tab	BD
T.NORFLOX	Norfloxacin+lactobacillus	PO	20mg	BD
INJ. HMI	Insulin	IV	14U + 16U	BD

On day 1 -the patient was admitted with c/o diabetic foot(left), on day 2- Complete Blood Picture (CBP) was done, on day 4- below knee amputation of wound necrosis was done. Patient is on fluids. On day5- patient is stable with c/c, on day 7- patient is on fluid flow. Surgical drain is present.

Discharge Medications:

Tab. Aten (OD)-atenolol

Tab. Liquiprine - paracetamol

Tab. Septran DS (BD)- Sulfamethoxaole+trimethoprim Septran

Patient education: Patient Education

- Regular medical exams.
- Monitor blood sugar daily.
- Eat a balanced diet rich in fruits.
- Avoid walking bare foot.
- Never use heating pad, hot water bottle on feet.
- Protect feet from heat and cold.
- Don't sit with legs crossed or in one position for a longer time.

Assignment

1. **What signs and symptoms lab values indicate the presence of infection?**

   Fever, chills and sweat, sore throat, SOB, Malaise, muscle weakness, sharp pain or burning sensation in legs, temperature changes, discolouration, increased WBC, increased ESR and increase in CRP. (C-Reactive Protein)

2. **What risk factors for infection does this patient have?**

   Diabetes mellitus, swelling of limbs, fever with chills, increased WBC and increased neutrophil count.

3. **What organisms are most likely involved in an infection?**

   Diabetic foot commonly experience infection with gram positive bacteria such as Staphylococcus aureus, Enterococcus and gram negative bacteria like Pseudomonas aeruginosa, Klebsiella, Escherichia coli, Proteus species etc and anaerobes. These organisms show multidrug resistance. Imipenem was the most effective drug against gram negative and vancomycin was most effective against gram positive.

4. **What are the therapeutic goals for this patient?**
   - Maintaining tight glycemic control and performing proper foot care are critical to decrease the incidence of foot infection.
   - Improving the condition of patient.
   - Decreasing the complaints like swelling, pain and fever.
   - Decreasing sugar levels.
   - Decreasing the complications like amputations, loss of sensation etc
   - Maintain blood pressure.

5. What feasible pharmacotherapeutic alterations are available for empiric treatment of diabetic foot infection?

- Patient with mild infection can be treated in outpatient sittings with oral antibiotics that cover skin flora including Staphylococcus aureus and Streptococcus.
- Eg: cefalexin, Amoxicillin-clavulanate, clindamycin for 7-14 days.
- For methicillin resistant Staphylococcus aureus strains drugs such as clindamycin, linezolid, minocycline, co-trimoxazole can be given for 7-14 days.

Table 12.5 Empirical antibiotic regimen for a diabetic foot infection.

Type of infection	Likely pathogens(s)	Class of antibiotic(s)
Acute, antibiotic-naïve; low-risk MRSA	Aerobic Gram-positive ciccu	Penicillins; first-generation cephalosporins
Healthcare-associated; high local rates of MRSA	MRSA	Co-trimoxazole; doxycycline; clindamycin; glycopeptide; linezolid; daptomycin
Chronic, previous antibiotic treatment	Gram-negative bacilli, Gram-positive cocci and anaerobes	b-Lactam, b-lactamase inhibitor; second- or third-generation cephalosporin; group 1 carbapenem, fluoroquinolone
Necrotic, gangrenous ischaemic limb; foul odour	Gram-nagative bacilli, Gram-positive cocci and obligate anaerobes	Clindamycin (+fluoroquinolone), metronidazole (+fluoroquinolone), b-lactam, b-lactamase inhibitor, carbapenem
Hydrotherapy; green-blue-coloured drainage	Pseudomonas aeruginosa	Anti-pseudomonal fluroquinolone, penicillin or cephalosporin

- Gram negative aerobes and anaerobes are present drugs like clindamycin+ levo/morifloxacin or co-trimoxazole+ amoxicillin clavulanate for 7-14 days can be used.
- Patients with moderate to severe infections must be hospitalized for parenteral antibiotic therapy.
- Empiric choices that cover streptococci, MRSA, aerobic gram negative bacteria, anaerobes are ampicillin, sulbactam, piperacillin, tazobactam, meropenem, carbapenem for 2-4 weeks.
- Amoxiciilinclavulanate for streptococcus and gram positive aerobes for 2-4 weeks.
- Vancomycin, linezolid, daptomycin for MRSA for 2-4 weeks.
- Alternatively for gram negative aerobes and anaerobes ceftriaxone, cefepime, levofloxacin, morifloxacin or aztreonam +metronidazole for 4-6 weeks.

6. **Optimal therapeutic plan to take care of the diabetic foot with hypertension?**
   - Proper foot care using light paraffin oil.
   - Take Atenolol 125mg PO, OD for hypertension.
   - Glucored forte 1mg for diabetes.
   - If ulcer is infected, T. Septran –DS, PO 1 Tab BD.
   - T.Tramadol 1tab for pain.
   - T.Quiprime for irregular rhythms.
   - Follow up after one week.

7. **Describe how would you educate the diabetic patient about proper foot care to prevent further skin infection?**
   - Take care of the infection properly/ Clean it everyday with saline.
   - Avoid walking barefoot/ Never use heating pad or hot water bottle on feet.
   - Protect feet from heat and cold/ Do not sit with legs crossed or stand in one position for long time.
   - Wear orthocare footwear/ Keep feet moisturized with paraffin oil.
   - Take medication regularly/Keep feet dry and clean. / Maintain your blood sugar.

References

1. Wild S et al. Global prevalence of diabetes: Estimates for the year 2000 and projections for 2030. Diabetes Care 2004;27:1047.
2. Karmen Stankov, Damir Benc and Dragan Draskovic. Genetic and Epigenetic Factors in Etiology of Diabetes Mellitus Type 1. Pediatrics December 2013, 132 (6) 1112-1122.
3. Mapes, S. & Faulds, E. *Dysfunction of endocrine pancreas: Diabetes mellitus* [PDF document]. Retrieved from https://carmen.osu.edu.
4. McCance, K.L. & Huether, S.E. (2014). *Pathophysiology: The biological basis for disease in adults and children* (7th ed.). St. Louis, MO: Mosby.
5. American Diabetes Association. Diagnosis and classification of diabetes mellitus. Diabetes Care 2008;31(Suppl 1):S55.
6. American Diabetes Association. The Expert Committee on the Diagnosis and Classification of Diabetes Mellitus: follow-up report on the diagnosis of diabetes. Diabetes Care 2003;26:3160.
7. Glycemic control algorithm from the AACE/ACE.[4] AACE/ACE = American Association of Clinical Endocrinologists/American College of <u>Endocrinology</u>; Garber AJ, brahamson MJ, Barzilay JI, et al. AACE/ACE comprehensive type 2 diabetes management algorithm. 2017. *Endocr Pract.* 2017;23:207-238.
8. Pravin kumar V.I er al., Current Trends in Pharmacological Treatment of Type II Diabetes Mellitus. International Journal of Pharma Research & Review, Jan 2018;7(1): 1-15
9. Executive Summary: Standards of Medical Care in Diabetes—2012. Diabetes Care 2012; 35 2001; (Suppl. 1).
10. American Diabetes Association: Clinical Practice Recommendations update 2016.
11. Diabetes Mellitus. In: Harrison's Principles of Internal Medicine. Fauci, Braunwald, Kasper et al (eds), 19th Edition, McGraw Hill Company Inc., New York, 2012; pp. 2419.

CHAPTER - 13

Thyroid Disorders

Introduction to Thyroid disorders

Thyroid gland is one of the largest and highly vascularised. Endocrine gland present in the body. It is made up of functional units called follicles or acinus.Thyroid gland is controlled and maintained by pituitary gland and hypothalamus. Thyroid gland produces 3 hormones Thyroxine (T4), Triiodothyronine (T3), Calcitonin. These hormones are nonsteroidal and chemically regarded as amino acids containing iodinated diphenyl ethers. T4 is the major form of thyroid hormone found in circulation.

Thyroid Hormone Biosynthesis

1. **Iodine Trapping:** Thyroid follicular cells trap the plasma iodide between the thyroid follicular cells and plasma. This is taken up by the Na/I- symporter. This process is stimulated by thyroid stimulatinghormone and inhibited by certain inorganic ions like thiocyanates, perchlorates etc

2. **Oxidation and Iodintion:** Iodide trapped by follicular cells is oxidised to hypoiodate under the influence of H2O2 and thyroid peroxidase hypoiodate binds to tyrosine residues of thyroglobulin molecule and forms monoiodotyrosine and diiodotyrosine

3. **Coupling:** One DIT molecule is coupled with MIT molecule to form T3 or two DIT molecules are coupled with each other to form T4. It is an oxidative process catalysed by thyroid peroxidase and is stimulated by TSH

4. **Secretion:** T3 and T4 bound to thyroglobulin are taken up from the colloidal material in to the follicular cells lysosomal proteases act on the intracellular TG and release T3, T4, MIT and DIT directly in to the circulation DIT and MIT are deiodinated and iodine thus removed re-enter the cycle

5. **Peripheral Conversion of T4 TO T3:** T3 is principle hormone and physiologically more active but is formed in lesser amounts than T4 hence the T4 gets converted in to T3 in the peripheral tissues especially liver and kidney. This process in inhibited by drugs such as propranolol, glucocorticoids and propylthiouracil.

Disorders

Hyperthyroidism: It occurs when the thyroid makes too much T3, T4 or both

Causes:

- Graves diseases
- Thyroiditis
- Excess iodine
- Tumours of the ovaries
- Tumours of thyroid or pituitary gland
- Large amount of tetraiodothyronine through diet

Symptoms: Due to hyperthyroidism metabolic rate increases this can lead to

- Rapid heart rate/Elevated blood pressure/Hand tremors/Sweating
- Low tolerance for heat/Weight loss/Irregular menstrual cycle
- Swelling of thyroid gland/ Hair loss/Increases appetite/Nervousness
- Anxiety/ Palpitations/ Tachycardia/Lagging of upper lid

Pathophysiology: (Hyperthyroidism) Thyrotoxicosis results when tissues are exposed to excessive levels of serum T4, T3 and low levels of TSH in serum.

Types of Hyperthyroidism [1]

1. **Graves Disesase (Exophthalmic goiter):** It is an autoimmune syndrome that may include hyperthyroidism, diffuse thyroid enlargement. It results in the production of autoantibodies called thyroid stimulating antibodies. These Abs mimic the actions of TSH and continuously stimulate the thyroid gland to enlarge its size.

   B & T lymphocyte mediate autoimmunity and attack TSH receptor. There is continuous stimulation of thyrotropin receptor by circulating autoantibodies. Because of this- a) increase in Na-I symporter, increasing iodine uptake and intracellular iodine b) increase in thyrogloulin synthesis c) upregulation of Nosine Monophosphate Protein Kinase C (cAde) cAMP amd PKc pathway, increasing TH synthesis, secretion and cell proliferation. Consequently there is increase in iodination of thyroglobulin and thyroid gland hyperplasia. This results in Grave's disease.

2. **Toxic Adenoma:** It is a benign tumor of thyroid gland. An autonomous thyroid nodule is a discrete thyroid mass whose function is independent of pituitary gland. TSH receptor mutation occurs. These depend on mass of nodule. Hyperthyroidism usually occurs with large nodules.

3. **Multinodular Goiter:** It is the second most common cause of hyperthyroidism after grave's disease. In this thyroid gland becomes autonomous i.e. independent of control of anterior pituitary. Follicles with a very high degree of autonomous function coexist with normal or even non-functioning follicles. Thyrotoxicosis is a multinodular goiter which occurs when the follicles with high degree or autonomy generate enough thyroid hormone to exceed needs of patient [autonomous follicles generate more thyroid hormones than required]. Disease is characterized by multinodular enlargement of thyroid gland.

4. **Subacute Thyroiditis:** Thyroiditis may be caused by viral invasion of thyroid parenchyma. Thyroiditis symptoms can be relieved by using beta-blockers. Prednisolone must be used to supress the inflammatory process.

5. **Pituitary Adenomas:** These are tumors of pituitary gland, which may be benign, invasive 35% or carcinomas 0.1-0.2%. there is an excessive release of TSH from pituitary adenoma cells that causes persistant stimulation of thyroid gland to increase the release of thyroid hormones. Along with typical symptoms of hyperthyroidism, there are symptoms due to excessive release of growth hormones (acromegaly) and glucoocrticoids (Cushing's syndrome).

6. **Thyroid storm:** It is not a separate type of throtoxicosis. It is a life threatening medical emergency characterized by severe thyrotoxicosis, high fever, tachycardia, tachypnoea and diarrhea resulting in dehydration, mental agitation, delitium and coma.

7. **Drug Incuced:** Amiodarone may induce thyrotoxicosis. Amiodarone interferes with I 5'-deiodianase leading to reduced conversion of T4-T3, and iodine released from the drug owing to deiodination contributes to excess iodine.

Diagnosis with Algorithm [2, 3]

➢ When the Signs and/or symptoms of hyperthyroidism are identified in the patient, TSH level has to be estimated.

➢ If there is Low TSH level, elevated or normal free T4 and total T3 levels, radioactive iodine uptake has to be obtained, and scan of the thyroid gland has to be done.

- If low uptake is identified- then it can be confirmed as thyroiditis/ ectopic thyroid homone/exogenous thyroid hormone.
- If high uptake is identified-
- It can be confirmed as graves' disease OR toxic multinodular goitre OR Toxic adenoma

➢ If elevated TSH level, elevated free T4 and total T3 levels- A TSH –secreting pituitary adenoma can be suspected.

Physical Examination: Weight loss, rapid pulse, elevated blood pressure, protruded eyes, and enlarged thyroid gland.

Free T3, T4: This test measures the amount of thyroid hormone in the body.

TSH Level: TSH is a pituitary gland hormone that stimulates the thyroid gland to produce hormones. When thyroid hormone levels are normal or high TSH should be lower. Abnormally low TSH means first sign of hyperthyroidism.

Cholesterol Test: Low cholesterol can be a sign of elevated metabolic rate in which our body is burning through cholesterol quickly

Tyhroid Scan: This allows to see the thyroid over activity and to know single area or entire gland is causing the over activity.

Ultrasound: Can measure the size of thyroid gland.

CT OR MRI: This can show if a pituitary tumor is present that is causing hyper thyroidism

Management

Nonpharmacologic Therapy

- Surgical removal of the thyroid gland should be considered in patients with a large gland (>80 g), severe ophthalmopathy, or a lack of remission on antithyroid drug treatment.
- If thyroidectomy is planned, **propylthiouracil** (PTU) or **methimazole** (MMI) is usually given until the patient is biochemically euthyroid (usually 6 to 8 weeks), followed by the addition of **iodides** (500 mg/day) for 10 to 14 days before surgery to decrease the vascularity of the gland. **Levothyroxine** may be added to maintain the euthyroid state while the thionamides are continued.

Pharmacological Treatement

Thionamides [4]

Examples		Initial Dose
Propyl thiouracil	:	900-1200/day orally in 4 or 6 divided doses
Methimazole	:	90-120mg/day orally in 4 or 6 divided doses
Mechanism of Action	:	These drugs block hormone synthesis by inhibiting the peroxidase enzyme.
Adverse Effect	:	Agranulocyctosis, GI intolerance, hepatotoxicity, rashes, fever; etc.

Propyl thiouracil considered as 1st line therapy except in case of 1st trimester.

Iodides

KI [saturated solution] 38 mg iodide per drop   3-10 drops in water / juice.

Lugols solution 6.3 mg of iodide per drop 5-10 drops

Mechanism of Action: Block thyroid hormone release; inhibit thyroid hormone biosynthesis by interfering with intrathyroidal iodide. And decreases size and vascularity of gland.

Adverse Effects: Salivary gland swelling, iodism, burning mouth, sore teeth, diarrhoea, hyper sensitive reactions.

Radioactive Iodine (RAI)

Sodium iodide-131 is an oral liquid that concentrates in the thyroid and initially disrupts hormone synthesis by incorporating into thyroid hormones and thyroglobulin. Over a period of weeks, follicles that have taken up RAI and surrounding follicles develop evidence of cellular necrosis and fibrosis of the interstitial tissue. Mainly used for graves disease. Goal of therapy is to destroy overactive cells at a single dose of 4000-8000 rad results in a euthyroid state in 60% of patients.

Adrenergic Blockers: They are used as adjunctive therapy with anti-thyroid drugs, Radioactive (RAI), or iodides when treating Graves' disease or toxic nodules; in preparation for surgery; or in thyroid storm.

Propranolol: 20-40 mg intial per oral 4 times

Nodolol

Mechanism of Action: These drugs block conversion of T4-T3.

Adverse Effects: Nausea, Vomiting, anxiety, insomnia, bradycrdia.

Table 13.1 Benefits and Risks of Graves Disease Treatment Options.

Treatment options	Benefits	Risks
Antithyroid medication (methimazole [Tapazole] or propylthiouracil	No exposure to radiation or to surgical risks No permanent hypothyroidism Prophylthiouracil is safe for the fetus in the first trimester of pregnancy	Agranulocytosis, hepatotoxicity (especially with propylthiouracil), rash Methimazole can cause aplasia cutis and other birth defects in the first trimester of pregnancy
Radioactive iodine ablation	No exposure to potential adverse effects of an antithyroid medication or to surgical risks Treatment of choice in the United States	Aggravation of Graves orbitopathy, especially in smokers Permanent hypothyroidism (oocurs in most patients) Radiation exposure Failure to cure hyperthyroidism if the radioactive iodine dose is insufficient Risk of Graves disease recurrence even after successful treatment Contraindicated in pregnancy
Thyroidectomy	No exposure to adverse effects of an antithyroid medication or to radiation Little chance of Graves disease recurrence	Risk of general anesthesia Risk of damaging recurrent laryngeal nerve leadig to hoarse voice (if famage is unilaternal) or of respiratory distress (if damage is bilateral) Risk of inadvertent damage or removal of parathyroid glands leading to permanent hypoparathyroidism

Information from:

Abraham P. Avenell A, Park CM, Watson WA, Bevan JS. A systematic review of drug therapy for Grave's hyperthyroidism. Eur J Endocrinol. 2005, 153(4): 489-498.

Bartalena L. Diagnosis and management of Graves disease: a global overview. Nat Rev Endocrinol 2013;9(12):724-734

Cappelli C, Pirola J, De Martino E, et al. The role of imaging I Grave's disease: a cost-effectiveness analysis. Eur J Radiol. 2008;65(1)99-103.

Nakamura H, Noh JY, Itoh K, Fukata S, Miyauchi A, Hamada N. Comparison of methimazole and propylthiouracil in patients with hypoerthroidism caused by Grave's disease. J Clin Endocrinol Metab. 2007;92(6);2157-2162.

Treatment of Thyroid Storm

The following therapeutic measures should be instituted promptly:
1. Suppression of thyroid hormone formation and secretion;
2. Antiadrenergic therapy;
3. Administration of corticosteroids; and
4. Treatment of associated complications or coexisting factors that may have precipitated the storm

Drug Dosages Used in the Management of Thyroid Storm
1. Propylthiouracil: 900–1200 mg/day orally in four or six divided doses
2. Methimazole 90–120 mg/day orally in four or six divided doses
3. Sodium iodide Up to 2 g/day IV in single or divided doses
4. Lugol's solution 5–10 drops three times a day in water or juice
5. Saturated solution of potassium iodide 1–2 drops three times a day in water or juice
6. Propranolol 40–80 mg every 6 h
7. Dexamethasone 5–20 mg/day orally or IV in divided doses
8. Prednisone 25–100 mg/day orally in divided doses
9. Methylprednisolone 20–80 mg/day IV in divided doses
10. Hydrocortisone 100–400 mg/day IV in divided doses

Hypothyroidism

This is the most common thyroid disorder where the thyroid gland produces inadequate quantity of thyroid hormone and there is a significant reduction in the levels of T3 and T4 in the serum, along with a rise in serum TSH levels.

Epidemiology

More common in women. 4.3%-8.5% have overt hypothyroidism.

Causes: Primary hypothyroidism (95%of cases)
- Idiopathic hypothyroidism,
- Hashimoto's thyroiditis,
- surgical removal of gland
- Iatrogenic Hypothyroidism
- Iodine deficiency
- drug therapy(lithium)
- Cretinism (congenital hypothyroidism)

Secondary hypothyroidism (5% of cases)
- Deficiency of Thyroid Stimulating Hormone (TSH) due to Pituitary dysfunction
- Deficiency of Thyroid Releasing Hormone (TRH) due to hypothalamic dysfunction

Risk factors:

- Woman older than age 60, having an autoimmune disease, family history of thyroid disease, have been treated with radioactive iodine or antithyroid medications, received radiation to neck or upper chest, pregnancy

Pathophysiology

Secretion of thyroid hormones are regulated by the hypothalamic pituitary thyroid axis. In primary hypothyroidism, the following changes occur- Destruction of the thyroid gland leads to decreased secretion of thyroid hormones T3 and T4. In response, TSH secretion increases. Effects of hypothyroidism-

1. Generalized decrease in the basal metabolic rate, so decreased oxygen and substrate consumption leading to:
   CNS: apathy, slowed cognition
   Skin and appendages: skin dryness, alopecia
   Lipd profile: increased LDL, triglycerides
   Cold intolerance
2. Decreased sympathetic activity leads to decreased sweating, cold skin, constipation, bradycardia.
3. Decreased transcription of sarcolemnal genes, so decreased cardiac output and myopathy.
4. Myxedema: Due to accumulation of glycosaminoglycans and hyluronic acid within the reticular layer of the dermis, complex protein mucoplysaccharides bind water leading to nonpitting edema.

Types of Hypothyroidism [5]

1. **Chronic autoimmune thyroiditis (Hashomoto's disease):** There is a specific defect in functioning of suppressor T cells, which leads to over-activity of immune system and some of these cells attack thyroid gland. Once these T lymphocytes interact with thyroid membrane antigen, B lymphocytes are stimulated to produce thyroid antibodies Antimicrosomal antibodies are present in virtually all patients with Hashimoto's thyroiditis and appear to be directed against the enzyme thyroid peroxidase, thyroglobulin, and other thyroid cell membrane antigens. These antibodies are capable of fixing complement and inducing cytotoxic changes in thyroid cells. Patients have either enlargement of thyroid gland (goiter), hypothyroidism or shrinking of thyroid gland (Atrophy).
2. **Iatrogenic hypothyroidism:** there is destruction of thyroid gland due to surgery or exposure to radiations for hyperthyroidism. It may occur within 3 months to 1 yr after radioactive therapy for grave's disease.
3. **Iodine deficiency goiter:** due to deficiency of iodine there is reduced synthesis of thyroid hormones and in order to restore the levels thyroid hormones, there is excessive release of TSH from anterior pituitary. In turn, TSH stimulates thyroid gland and it increases in size.

4. **Congenital hypothyroidism:** cretinism is a congenital hypothyroidism due to maternal hypothyroidism. May be due to iodine defeiency or enzymatic defects or exposure to goitrogens.

5. **Myxedema coma:** it is a life threatening state of extreme hypothyroidism and is characterized by very low body temperature, confusion, slow heart rate and reduced breathing effort.

6. Due to the drugs which are used in treatment of hyperthyroidism Eg: thioamides (when taken in larger dose) produces Iodine deficiency

7. **Pituitary Disease**: Pituitary insufficiency may be caused by destruction of thyrotrophs by functioning or nonfunctioning pituitary tumors, surgical therapy, external pituitary radiation, postpartum pituitary necrosis. In all these situations, TSH deficiency most often occurs in association with other pituitary hormone deficiencies. In most hypothyroid patients with pituitary disease, serum TSH concentrations are low or normal.

Clinical Manifestations and Features

- Adult manifestations of hypothyroidism include dry skin, cold intolerance, weight gain, constipation, weakness, lethargy, fatigue, muscle cramps, myalgia, stiffness, and loss of ambition or energy.
- In children, thyroid hormone deficiency may manifest as growth retardation.
- Physical signs include coarse skin and hair, cold or dry skin, periorbital puffiness, bradycardia, and slowed or hoarse speech.
- Objective weakness (with proximal muscles being affected more than distal muscles) and slow relaxation of deep tendon reflexes are common.
- Reversible neurologic syndromes such as carpal tunnel syndrome, polyneuropathy, and cerebellar dysfunction may also occur.

Diagnosis with Algorithm:

Observe the signs and symptoms of hypothyroidism, serum TSH levels should be measured.

(a) If TSH >5.5mIU per L, then serum free T4 should be measured.

If Free T_4 is below normal range. It is confirmed as primary hypothyroidism.

If free T_4 is within normal range, it is confirmed as subclinical hypothyroidism. Treatment should be initiated with Levothyroxine if TSH > 10 mIU per L.

If T_4 is above normal range, it is considered as not primary hypothyroidism and endocrinologist consultation should be preferred.

(b) If TSH is in normal range, patient is euthyroid.

(c) If TSH is < 0.35 mIU per L, it is considered as hyperthyroid state.

Normal Levels

TSH: 0.55-4.7 mIU/mL   T3: 60-181ng/dL   T4: 7.3-15ug/dL

Blood test: That measures the level of TSH, T3, T4. A high level of TSH and low level of T3, T4 means underactive thyroid gland. Antithyroid peroxidise antibodies and antithyroglobulin antibodies are elevated.

Treatment [6, 7]

Algorithm for the treatment of primary hypothyroidism

1. If the patient is diagnosed with primary hypothyroidism
   - (a) Child or adolescent patient-treatment based on patients weight
   - (b) If adult patient and < 50 yrs follow the guidelines below.
   - (c) If patient age > 50 to 60 yrs- start levothyroxine 25 to 50mcg daily. Increase the dosage by 25 mcg every 3 to 4 weeks until TSH is within normal range.
   - (d) If the patient is suspected with ischemic heart disese- start levothyroxine 25 to 50 mcg daily. Increase the dosage by 25 mcg every 3 to 4 weeks until TSH is within normal range.
   - (e) If patient is pregnant and on previously stable dosage of levothyroxine: increase levothyroxine to 9 doses weekly.
   - (f) If patient is presented with stupor and other mental status changes and hypothermia: it can be inferred as myxedema coma. Patient has to be admitted in intensive care unit and referred by endocrinologist.

Thyroid Preparations Used in the Treatment of Hypothyroidism

1. Thyroid USP made with Desiccated beef or pork thyroid gland. 1 grain (60mcg of T4)
2. Thyroglobulin made with partially purified pork thyroglobulin- 1 grain
3. Levothyroxine- synthetic T4- 50-60 mcg: drug of choice for thyroid replacement and suppressive therapy because it is chemically stable, relatively inexpensive, and free of antigenicity, and has uniform potency.
4. Liothyronine- synthetic T3 – 15 – 37.5 mcg: Liothyronine (T3) is chemically pure with known potency and has a shorter half-life of 1.5 days.
5. Liotrix: Liotrix is a combination of synthetic T4 and T3 in a 4:1 ratio that attempts to mimic natural hormonal secretion. It is chemically stable and pure and has a predictable potency. The major limitations to this product are high cost and lack of therapeutic rationale, because about 35% of T4 is peripherally converted T3.

Adverse effects: Serious untoward effects are unusual if dosing is appropriate and the patient is carefully monitored during initial treatment. Excessive doses of thyroid hormone may lead to heart failure, angina pectoris, and myocardial infarction; rarely, the latter may be caused by coronary artery spasm. Allergic or idiosyncratic reactions can occur with the natural animal-derived products such as desiccated thyroid and thyroglobulin, but these are extremely rare with the synthetic products used today

Levothyroxine Dosing Guidelines for Hypothyroidism in Adults

1. **Non pregnant patients:** 1.6 mcg per kg per day initial dosage.
2. **Older patients with known or suspected cardiac disease:** 50-100mcg/kg/day starting dosage; increase by 25 mcg every 3-4 weeks until full replacement dosage reached.
3. **Pregnant patients:** increase to nine doses weekly at earliest knowledge of pregnancy
4. **Pregnant with subclinical hypothyroidism:** If TSH < 10mIU/per L- 50 mcg daily; increase by 25mcg daily every week until TSH = 0.35-5.5mIU/per L

   If TSH ≥ 10 mIU per mL: 1.6 mcg per kg per day
5. **Cardiovascular disease:** start with 12.5 - 25 mcg/day. Increase by 12.5 - 25mcg/day as tolerated.
6. **Paediatric:** 10-15mcg/kg/day

Levothyroxine (L-thyroxine, T4) is the drug of choice for thyroid hormone replacement and suppressive therapy because it is chemically stable, relatively inexpensive,

- Young patients with long-standing disease and patients older than 45 years without known cardiac disease should be started on 50 mcg daily of levothyroxine and increased to 100 mcg daily after 1 month.
- The recommended initial daily dose for older patients or those with known cardiac disease is 25 mcg/day titrated upward in increments of 25 mcg at monthly intervals to prevent stress on the cardiovascular system.
- The average maintenance dose for most adults is about 125 mcg/day, but there is a wide range of replacement doses, necessitating individualized therapy and appropriate monitoring to determine an appropriate dose.
- Levothyroxine is the drug of choice for pregnant women, and the objective of the treatment is to decrease TSH to 1 mIU/L and to maintain free T4 concentrations in the normal range.
- **Liothyronine** (synthetic T3) has uniform potency but has a higher incidence of cardiac adverse effects, higher cost, and difficulty in monitoringwith conventional laboratory tests.
- **Liotrix** (synthetic T4:T3 in a 4:1 ratio) is chemically stable, pure, and has a predictable potency but is expensive.

Treatment of Myxedema Coma [8]

- Immediate and aggressive therapy with IV bolus **levothyroxin,** 300 to 500 mcg, has traditionally been used. Initial treatment with IV **Liothyronine** or a combination of both hormones has also been advocated because of impaired conversion of T4 to T3.
- Glucocorticoid therapy with IV **hydrocortisone** 100 mg every hours should be given until coexisting adrenal suppression is ruled out.

References

1. Stanbury JB, Ermans AE, Bourdoux P, et al. Iodine-induced hyperthyroidism: Occurrence and epidemiology. Thyroid 1998;8:83–100.
2. Singer PA, Cooper DS, Levy EG, et al. Treatment guidelines for patients with hyperthyroidism and hypothyroidism. Standards of Care Committee, American Thyroid Association. *JAMA*. 1995;273(10):808–812.
3. Vanderpump MP, Ahlquist JA, Franklyn JA, Clayton RN. Consensus statement for good practice and audit measures in the management of hypothyroidism and hyperthyroidism. The Research Unit of the Royal College of Physicians of London, the Endocrinology and Diabetes Committee of the Royal College of Physicians of London, and the Society for Endocrinology. *BMJ*. 1996;313(7056):539–544.
4. Igor kravets. Hyperthyroidism: diagnosis and treatment., *am fam physician.* 2016 mar 1 ;93(5):363-370.
5. Kabadi UM. Influence of age on optimal daily levothyroxine dosage in patients with primary hypothyroidism grouped according to etiology. South Med J 1997;90:920–924.
6. Sarlis NJ, Gourgiotis L. Thyroid emergencies. Rev Endocr Metab Disord 2003;4:129–136.
7. Baskin HJ, Cobin RH, Duick DS, et al.; American Association of Clinical Endocrinologists. American Association of Clinical Endocrinologists medical guidelines for clinical practice for the evaluation and treatment of hyperthyroidism and hypothyroidism [published correction appears in *Endocr Pract*. 2008;14(6):802–803]. *Endocr Pract*. 2002;8(6):457–469.
8. Surks MI, Ortiz E, Daniels GH, et al. Subclinical thyroid disease: scientific review and guidelines for diagnosis and management. *JAMA*. 2004;291(2):228–238.

CHAPTER - 14

Geriatrics

Geriatrics or geriatric medicine is a specialty that focuses on health care of elderly people.

It aim's to promote health by preventing and treating diseases and disabilities in older adults. However, geriatrics is sometimes called **medicinal gerontology** specialist "geriatrician". Geriatric patients use more medications compared to young patients because they have more symptoms of disease. Geriatric drug therapy is of concern since increasing age brings about many changes in the blood which influences dosage, pharmacokinetic properties, and physiological changes in the body.

Age Related Changes in the Gastrointestinal Tract, Liver, Kidney Include Reduced (↓) [1]

Gastric acid secretion	Liver size
Gastrointestinal motility	Liver blood flow
Total surface area of absorption	Glomerular filtration
Splanchnic blood flow	Renal tubular filtration

Balance and Gait

Stride length and slower gait, arm swing (↓)

Body Composition

Total body water, lean body mass, body fat, <-> or serum albumin

(↓) CNS Size of the hippocampus & frontal &temporal lobes, no.of receptors all types (↓)&↑ sensitivity of remaining

CVS ↓Cardiovascular response to stress, orthostatic hypotension↑, Cardiac Output C.O↓, ↓ baro receptor activity leading to ↑↓ resting & maximal heart rate.

Endocrine

($\downarrow$) estrogen, testosterone, Thyroid Stimulating Hormone (TSH), Dehydroepiandrosterone (DHEA-s) levels altered insulin signaling.

Immune

Antibody production in response to antigen $\downarrow$, autoimmunity $\uparrow$

Oral

Ability to taste salt, bitter, sweet & sour ($\downarrow$)

Pulmonary

$\uparrow$Residual volume, ($\downarrow$) respiratory muscle strength, chest wall compliance, vital capacity, maximum breathing capacity.

Sensory

Presbyopia, presbycusis, ($\downarrow$) night vision, sensation of smell.

Skeletal

Skeletal bone mass $\downarrow$

Skin/Hair

Langerhans cells, melanocytes & mast cells, depth & extent of the subcutaneous fat layer, thinning of stratum corneum ($\downarrow$)

Risk Factors [2,3]

Over Use

"Poly pharmacy" can be defined as either the concomitant use of multiple drugs or the administration of more medications than are indicated clinically.

According to survey, older patients take avg 2-9 % of non-prescription medication each day. $\uparrow$Use of dietary supplements, such as herbal products, vitamins, minerals. They are taking unnecessary medications; multiple medication use has been strongly associated with ADR's Polypharmacy Increases the Risk of Geriatric Symptoms.

Inappropriate Prescribing

Prescribing medication outside the bonds of the accepted medical standards, 92% of patients taking atleast 1 or more based on (U.S) clinical review applying explicit criteria.

Under Use

Omission of drug therapy i.e indicated for treatment or prevention of disease or condition. Most common problems were the lack of a gastroprotective agent for high risk of non steroidal anti-inflammatory drug users, no angiotensin-converting enzyme inhibitor for patients with diabetes and proteinuria and no calcium/ vitamin D for those with osteoporosis.

Medical Non-Adherence

The WHO defines it as the extent to which a person's behavior taking medication corresponds with agreed recommendations from a health care provider.

It is accosiated with increased health services use & ADR's. older pt's may not adhere to their regiments because of possible ADR's, inability to read product labels, cost, understanding info about prescribed medication, fewer hospitalizations, ↓ cost in patients with certain medication conditions.

Provision of Comprehensive Geriatric Assessment

The term comprehensive geriatric assessment has been applied to geriatric evaluation and management (GEM) in which GEM clinicians & manage the pt. It has become a cornerstone in the care of older adults. It has summarized it's effectiveness in improving suboptimal prescribing &↓ ADR's.

Table 14.1 Age Related Physiological Affecting Pharmacokinetic Parameters.

Absorption	Distribution
Gastric ph↑	C.O↓, Total body wt↓
Absorptive surface↓	↑plasma conc. Of water soluble drugs
Splanchnic blood flow ↓	Lean body mass, serum albumin↓
GI motility↓	α-Acid glycoprotein, body fat↑
Gastric emptying rate↓	Relative tissue perfusion ↓
Dec. first pass metabolism	↓volume of distribution

Metabolism	Excretion
Hepatic mass↓, Hepatic blood flow↓	Renal mass↓
↓clearance	Renal blood flow↓
Hepatic function↓	GFR↓
Phase1 reactions↓, Phase 2 reactions↓	Tubular secretion↓
	↓clearance

Table 14.2 Guidelines for Monitoring Medication Use in Long Term Care Facility Patients [4].

Drug	Monitoring
Acetaminophen (>4g/d)	Hepatic function tests
Aminodarone	Hepatic function tests, TSH levels
Anti epileptic drugs	Drug levels
Angiotensin-converting enzyme inhibitor or angiotensinl receptor blockers	K+ levels
Anti-psychotic agents	Extra pyramidal side effects, fasting serum glucose, seru, lipid panel
Appetite stimulants	Wt, appetite
Digitoxin	Serum blood urea nitrogen, creatinine, through drug level
Diuretic	Serum sodium&potassium levels
Erythropoiesis stimulants	B.P, iron& ferritin levels, CBC
Fibrates	Hepatic function test, CBC
Hypoglycemic agents	Fasting serum glucose levels or glycatedhb level
Iron	Iron & ferrinlevels, CBC
Lithium	Through serum drug levels
Metformin	Serum blood urea nitrogen, creatinine levels
Niacin	Blood sugar levels, hepatic function tests
Statins	Hepatic function tests
Theophylline	Through serum drug levels
Thyroid replacement	TSH levels on tests
Warfarin	Prothrombine time or international normalized ratio

Dosing of Drugs in the Elderly [5]

Drug dose should be reduced in elderly patients because of general decline in body function with age. The lean body mass decreases and body fat increases by almost 100% in elderly persons as compared to adults. Vd of water soluble drugs may decrease and that of lipid soluble drugs like diazepam increases with age. Age related changes in renal and hepatic functions greatly alters the clearance of drugs.

The Cockcroft-Gault formula is sometimes used to estimate renal function in older patients who are to receive potentially nephrotoxic drugs (e.g., aminoglycosides) or drugs that are primarily excreted by the kidneys (e.g., digoxin):

$$\text{Estimated creatinine clearance} = \frac{(140 - \text{age}) \times (\text{Body weight in kg})}{\text{Serum creatinine} \times 72}$$

Dosing of drugs in Hepatic diseases: The influence of Hepatic disorder on the drug bioavailability & disposition is unpredictable because of the multiple effects that liver produces.

The altered response to drugs in liver disease could be due to decreased metabolizing capacity of the hepatocytes, impaired biliary elimination, due to biliary obstruction (e.g. Rifampicin accumulation in obstruction jaundice)

Dosing of drugs in Renal Disease: In patient with renal failure, the half life of the drug is increase and its clearance drastically decreases if it is predominantly eliminated by way of excretion. Hence, dosage adjustment should take into account the renal function of the patient and the fraction of unchanged drug excreted in urine

Guidelines - 2019 American Geriatrics Society Beers Criteria ® for Potentially Inappropriate Medication Use in Older Adults

1. **Anticholinergics:** First-generation antihistamines Brompheniramine Carbinoxamine Chlorpheniramine Clemastine Cyproheptadine
2. Antiparkinsonian agents Benztropine (oral) Trihexyphenidy
3. Antithrombotics Dipyridamole, oral short acting (does not apply to the extended-release combination with aspirin
4. Digoxin for first-line treatment of atrial fibrillation or of heart failure
5. Central nervous system: Antidepressants, alone or in combination Amitriptyline Amoxapine Clomipramine Desipramine Doxepin >6 mg/day Imipramine
6. Nonbenzodiazepine, benzodiazepine receptor agonist hypnotics (ie, "Z-drugs") Eszopiclone Zaleplon Zolpidem
7. Endocrine Androgens Methyltestosterone Testosterone
8. Non –cyclooxygenase-selective NSAIDs, oral: Aspirin >325 mg/day Diclofenac Diflunisal Etodolac Fenoprofen Ibuprofen Ketoprofen Meclofenamate Mefenamic acid Meloxicam Nabumetone Naproxen Oxaprozin Piroxicam Sulindac Tolmetin
9. Skeletal muscle relaxants Carisoprodol Chlorzoxazone Cyclobenzaprine Metaxalone Methocarbamol Orphenadrine

2019 American Geriatrics Society Beers Criteria ® for Potentially Inappropriate Medication Use in Older Adults Due to Drug-Disease or Drug-Syndrome Interactions That May Exacerbate the Disease or Syndrome

1. **Cardiovascular Heart failure Avoid:** Cilostazol Avoid in heart failure with reduced ejection fraction: Nondihydropyridine CCBs (diltiazem, verapamil) Use with caution in patients with heart failure who are asymptomatic; avoid in patients with symptomatic heart failure: NSAIDs and COX-2 inhibitors Thiazolidinediones (pioglitazone, rosiglitazone) Dronedarone Potential to promote fluid retention and/or exacerbate heart failure (NSAIDs and COX-2 inhibitors, nondihydropyridine CCBs, thiazolidinediones); potential to increase mortality in older adults with heart failure (cilostazol and dronedarone)

2. **Central nervous system – Delirium:** Anticholinergics: Antipsychoticsb Benzodiazepines Corticosteroids (oral and parenteral)c H2-receptor antagonists Cimetidine Famotidine Nizatidine Ranitidine Meperidine Nonbenzodiazepine, benzodiazepine receptor agonist hypnotics: eszopiclone, zaleplon, zolpidem

3. **History of falls or fractures:** Antiepileptics Antipsychoticsb Benzodiazepines Nonbenzodiazepine, benzodiazepine receptor agonist hypnotics Eszopiclone Zaleplon Zolpidem Antidepressants: TCAs SSRIs SNRIs Opioids May cause ataxia, impaired psychomotor function, syncope, additional falls; shorteracting benzodiazepines are not safer than long-acting ones. If one of the drugs must be used, consider reducing use of other CNS-active medications that increase risk of falls and fractures (ie, antiepileptics, opioid-receptor agonists, antipsychotics, antidepressants, nonbenzodiazepine and benzodiazepine receptor agonist hypnotics, other sedatives/hypnotics) and implement other strategies to reduce fall risk. Data for antidepressants are mixed but no compelling evidence that certain antidepressants confer less fall risk than others

4. **Kidney/urinary tract - Chronic kidney disease stage 4 or higher (creatinine clearance <30ml/min):** NSAIDs (non-COX and COX selective, oral and parenteral, nonacetylated salicylates) May increase risk of acute kidney injury and further decline of renal function

2019 American Geriatrics Society Beers Criteria® for Potentially Inappropriate Medications: Drugs to Be Used With Caution in Older Adults

1. **Drug:** Aspirin for primary prevention of cardiovascular disease and colorectal cancer
2. **Rationale:** Risk of major bleeding from aspirin increases markedly in older age. Several studies suggest lack of net benefit when used for primary prevention in older adult with cardiovascular risk factors, but evidence is not conclusive. Aspirin is generally indicated for secondary prevention in older adults with established cardiovascular disease.
3. **Drug: Dabigatran Rivaroxaban:** Rationale: Increased risk of gastrointestinal bleeding compared with warfarin and reported rates with other direct oral anticoagulants when used for long-term treatment of VTE or atrial fibrillation in adults ≥75 years
4. **Drug:** Antipsychotics: Carbamazepine Diuretics Mirtazapine Oxcarbazepine SNRIs SSRIs TCAs Tramadol
5. **Rationale:** May exacerbate or cause SIADH or hyponatremia; monitor sodium level closely when starting or changing dosages in older adults

Factors Influencing the Inability to Comply With a Medication Regimen [7]

- Three chronic conditions
- More than five prescription medications;
- Twelve medication dosages per day Medication regimen changed four times during the past 12 months
- Three prescribers involved Significant cognitive or physical impairments (e.g., memory, hearing, vision, color discrimination, child-resistant containers)
- Living alone in the community Recently discharged from the hospital
- Reliance on a caregiver; Low literacy ; Medication cost
- Demonstrated poor compliance history

References

1. Kane RL, Ouslander JG, Abrass IB. Clinical implications of the aging process. In: Essentials of Clinical Geriatrics, 5th ed. New York: McGraw-Hill, 2004:3–15.
2. Masoro EJ. Physiology of aging. In: Tallis R, Fillit H, eds. Brocklehurst's Textbook of Geriatric Medicine, 6th ed. London, Churchill-Livingstone, 2003:291–299.
3. Cusack BJ. Pharmacokinetics in older persons. Am J Geriatr Pharm 2004;2:274–302.
4. Chapron DJ. Drug disposition and response. In: Delafuente JC, Stewart RB, eds. Therapeutics in the Elderly, 3rd ed. Cincinnati, OH: Harvey Whitney, 2000:257–288.
5. Center for Medicaid and Medicare Services Unnecessary Medication Use (Tag F329) 2007, *http://www.cms.hhs.gov/transmittals/downloads/R22SOMA.pdf.*
6. American Geriatrics Society 2019 Updated AGS Beers Criteria® for Potentially Inappropriate Medication Use in Older Adults By the 2019 American Geriatrics Society Beers Criteria® Update Expert Panel*
7. Bero LA et al. Characterization of geriatric drug-related hospital readmissions. Med Care 1991;29:989.

CHAPTER - 15

Pediatrics

- The rate and extent of organ function development and the distribution, metabolism, and elimination of drugs differ not only between pediatric versus adult patients but also among pediatric age groups.
- The effectiveness and safety of drugs may vary among various age groups and from one drug to another in pediatric versus adult patients.
- Concomitant diseases may influence dosage requirements to achieve a targeted effect for a specific disease in children.
- The pediatric medication-use process is complex and error prone because of the multiple steps required in calculating, verifying, preparing, and administering doses.

Absorption from the GI tract is affected by
- Gastric acid secretion
- Bile salt formation
- Gastric emptying time
- Intestinal motility
- Bowel length and effective absorptive surface
- Microbial flora

All these factors are reduced in neonates (full-term and premature) and all may be reduced or increased in an ill child of any age.
- Reduced gastric acid secretion increases bioavailability of acid-labile drugs (eg, penicillin) and decreases bioavailability of weakly acidic drugs (eg, phenobarbital).
- Reduced bile salt formation decreases bioavailability of lipophilic drugs (eg, diazepam). [1]
- Reduced gastric emptying and intestinal motility increase the time it takes to reach therapeutic concentrations when enteral drugs are given to infants < 3 months.
- Drug-metabolizing enzymes present in the intestines of young infants are another cause of reduced drug absorption. Infants with congenital atretic bowel or surgically removed bowel or who have jejunal feeding tubes may have specific absorptive defects depending on the length of bowel lost or bypassed and the location of the lost segment.
- Alterations in intestinal flora that aid metabolism may also affect absorption in the gut.

Injected drugs are often erratically absorbed because of
- Variability in their chemical characteristics
- Differences in absorption by site of injection (IM or SC)
- Variability in muscle mass among children
- Illness (eg, compromised circulatory status)
- Variability in depth of injection (too deep or too shallow)

IM injections are generally avoided in children because of pain and the possibility of tissue damage, but, when needed, water-soluble drugs are best because they do not precipitate at the injection site.

Transdermal absorption may be enhanced in neonates and young infants because the stratum corneum is thin and because the ratio of surface area to weight is much greater than for older children and adults. Skin disruptions (eg, abrasions, eczema, burns) increase absorption in children of any age.

Transrectal drug therapy is generally appropriate only for emergencies when an IV route is not available (eg, use of rectal diazepam for status epilepticus). Site of placement of the drug within the rectal cavity may influence absorption because of the difference in venous drainage systems. Young infants may also expel the drug before significant absorption has occurred.

Absorption of **inhaled drugs** from the lungs (eg, beta-agonists for asthma, pulmonary surfactant for respiratory distress syndrome) varies less by physiologic parameters and more by reliability of the delivery device and patient or caregiver technique.

Distribution [2, 3]

- The volume of distribution of drugs changes in children with aging. These age-related changes are due to changes in body composition (especially the extracellular and total body water spaces) and plasma protein binding.
- Higher doses (per kg of body weight) of water-soluble drugs are required in younger children because a higher percentage of their body weight is water. Conversely, lower doses are required to avoid toxicity as children grow older because of the decline in water as a percentage of body weight.
- Many drugs bind to proteins (primarily albumin, alpha-$_1$ acid glycoprotein, and lipoproteins); protein binding limits distribution of free drug throughout the body. Albumin and total protein concentrations are lower in neonates but approach adult levels by 10 to 12 mo.
- Decreased protein binding in neonates is also due to qualitative differences in binding proteins and to competitive binding by molecules such as bilirubin and free fatty acids, which circulate in higher concentrations in neonates and infants. The net result may be increased free drug concentrations, greater drug availability at receptor sites, and both pharmacologic effects and higher frequency of adverse effects at lower drug concentrations.

Metabolism and Elimination [4]

Drug metabolism and elimination vary with age and depend on the substrate or drug, but most drugs, and most notably phenytoin, barbiturates, analgesics, and cardiac glycosides, have plasma half-lives 2 to 3 times longer in neonates than in adults.

The cytochrome P-450 (CYP450) enzyme system in the small bowel and liver is the most important known system for drug metabolism. CYP450 enzymes inactivate drugs via

- Oxidation, reduction, and hydrolysis (phase I metabolism)
- Hydroxylation and conjugation (phase II metabolism)

Phase I metabolism activity is reduced in neonates, increases progressively during the first 6 mo of life, exceeds adult rates by the first few years for some drugs, slows during adolescence, and usually attains adult rates by late puberty. However, adult rates of metabolism may be achieved for some drugs (eg, barbiturates, phenytoin) 2 to 4 wk postnatally. CYP450 activity can also be induced (reducing drug concentrations and effect) or inhibited (augmenting concentrations and effect) by coadministered drugs. These drug interactions may lead to drug toxicity when CYP450 activity is inhibited or an inadequate drug level when CYP450 activity is induced. Kidneys, lungs, and skin also play a role in the metabolism of some drugs, as do intestinal drug-metabolizing enzymes in neonates. [5]

Phase II metabolism varies considerably by substrate. Maturation of enzymes responsible for bilirubin and acetaminophen conjugation is delayed; enzymes responsible for morphine conjugation are fully mature even in preterm infants.

Drug metabolites are eliminated primarily through bile or the kidneys. Renal elimination depends on

- Plasma protein binding
- Renal blood flow
- GFR
- Tubular secretion

All of these factors are altered in the first 2 yr of life. Renal plasma flow is low at birth (12 mL/min) and reaches adult levels of 140 mL/min by age 1 yr. Similarly, GFR is 2 to 4 mL/min at birth, increases to 8 to 20 mL/min by 2 to 3 days, and reaches adult levels of 120 mL/min by 3 to 5 mo.

Drug Dosing [6]

Because of the above factors, drug dosing in children < 12 yr is always a function of age, body weight, or both. Even within a population of similar age and weight, drug requirements may differ because of maturational differences in absorption, metabolism, and elimination. Thus, when practical, dose adjustments should be based on plasma drug concentration. Unfortunately, these adjustments are not feasible for most drugs.

Factors Affecting Pediatric Therapy

Hepatic Disease

Because most drugs are either metabolized by the liver or eliminated by the kidney, hepatic and renal diseases are expected to decrease the dosage requirements in patients. Because of a lack of specific data on dosage adjustment in hepaticdisease, drug therapy should be monitored closely in pediatric patients to avoid potential toxicity from excessive doses, particularly for drugs with narrow therapeutic indices.

Renal Disease [7]

Serum drug concentrations should be monitored for drugs with narrow therapeutic indices and eliminated largely by the kidney (e.g., aminoglycosides and vancomycin) to optimize therapy in pediatric patients with renal dysfunction. For drugs with wide therapeutic ranges (e.g., penicillins and cephalosporins), dosage adjustment may be necessary only in patients with moderate-tosevere renal failure.

Cystic Fibrosis [8]

These patients require increased doses of certain drugs. Studies have reported higher clearance of drugs such as gentamicin, tobramycin, netilmicin, amikacin, dicloxacillin, cloxacillin, azlocillin, piperacillin, and theophylline in patients with cystic fibrosis compared with patients without the disease. The apparent volume of distribution of certain drugs also may be altered in cystic fibrosis.

References

1. Signer E, Fridrich R. Gastric emptying in newborns and young infants. Acta Paediatr Scand 1975;64:525–530.
2. Kearns GL, Abdel-Rahman SM, Alander SW, et al. Drug therapy: Developmental pharmacology—Drug disposition, action, and therapy in infants and children. N Engl J Med 2003;349:1157–1167.
3. Friis-Hansen B. Body water compartments in children: Changes during growth and related changes in body composition. Pediatrics 1961;28:169–181.
4. Nahata MC, Powell DA, Durrell DE, et al. Effect of gestational age and birth weight on tobramycin kinetics in newborn infants. J Antimicrob Chemother 1984;14:59–65.
5. Rane A. Basic principles of drug disposition and action in infants and children. In: Yaffe JF, ed. Pediatric Pharmacology: Therapeutic Principles in Practice. New York: Grune & Stratton, 1980:7–28.
6. Roberts RJ. Special considerations in drug therapy in infants. In: Drug Therapy in Infants: Pharmacologic Principles and Clinical Experience. Philadelphia: WB Saunders, 1984:25–35.

7. Hogg RJ, Furth S, Lemley KV, et al. National Kidney Foundation's kidney disease outcomes quality initiative clinical practice guidelines for chronic kidney disease in children and adolescents: Evaluation, classification, and stratification. Pediatrics 2003;111:1416–1421.

8. Wallace CS, Hall M, Kuhn RJ. Pharmacologic management of cystic fibrosis. Clin Pharm 1993;12:657–674.

CHAPTER - 16

Pregnancy and Lactation

What is Pregnancy [1]

The period from conception to birth after the egg is fertilized by a sperm and then implanted in the lining of uterus it develops into placenta and embryo and later into fetus. It usually lasts 40 weeks, begining from the first day of the women last menstrual cycle and is divided into 3 trimesters

Pregnancy Stages

First trimester 1 - 12 Weeks
Second trimester 12 - 28 Weeks
Third trimester 29 - 40 Week

First Trimester

- Body undergoes many hormonal changes that effect almost every organ system in the body.
- Period stopping is a clear sign of pregnancy.
- Other changes may include
  - Extreme Tiredness Tender, Swollen Brest / Upset Stomach
  - Craving for certain foods / Mood Swing/ Head ache / Heart Burn

Second Trimester [2, 3]

- The symptoms like nausea and fatigue are going away.
- Abdomen will expand as the baby continuous to grow.
- As body changes to make room for growing baby may have
  - Body aches
  - Stretch make on abdomen, breast, thigh or buttock
  - Darkening of skin around nipple
  - Numb or tingling hand
  - Itching on abdomen, palms and sole of feet.

Third Trimester

- Some of the same discomfort in second trimester will continue
- Some new body change might notice in third trimester include
  - Shortness of breath
  - Heartburn
  - Swelling of the ankle, finger and face
  - Belly button may stick out Trouble sleeping

Lactation

Lactation describes the production of breast milk and its secretion from the mammary gland after delivery.

Physiological and Pharmacokinetic Factors

- The duration of pregnancy is approximately 28 days. Pregnancy is divided into three periods of three calendar months
- Drug absorption during pregnancy may be altered by delayed gastric emptying and vomiting.
- An increased gastric Ph may affect absorption of weak acids and bases.
- Higher estrogen and progesterone levels may alter enzyme activity and increases elimination of some drugs but cause accumulation of others
- Maternal plasma volume, cardiac output, and glomecular filtration increase by 30% to 50% or higher during pregnancy possibly, lowering the plasma concentration of renally cleared drugs may increase
- Plasma albumin concentration decreases.
- The placenta is the organ of exchange between the mother and foetus for drugs.
- Drugs with molecular weight less than 500 Daltons cross readily
- Drugs with molecular weight from 600 to 1000 Daltons cross more slowly
- The drugs with MWT from greater than 1000 Daltons do not cross in significant amounts.
- Lipophilic drugs cross more easily than do water- soluble drugs.

Drugs Selection during Pregnancy [4]

The incidence of congenital malformation is approximately 3% to 6% and it is estimated that less than 1% of all birth defect are caused by medication exposure. Adverse effects on the foetus depend on drug dosage, route of administration and stage of pregnancy when the exposure occurred. Foetal exposure to a teratogen in the first 2 weeks after conception may have on "all or nothing" effect (i.e, could destroy the embryo or have no ill effect). Exposure during organogenesis (18-60 days post conception) may cause structural anomalies.
Principle for drug use during pregnancy include

- Selecting drugs that have been used safely for long time

- prescribing doses at the lower end of the dosing range
- eliminating nonessential medication and discouraging self-medications
- avoiding medications known to be harmful

Preconception Planning

Folic Acid supplementation between 0.4 and 0.9 mg daily is recommended through out the reproduction years to reduce the risk for neural tube (NTD) defects in off spring.

Pregnancy Influenced Issues

1. **Gastrointestinal Tract:** Therapy for gastroesophageal reflux diseases includes lifestyle and dietary modifications. Hemorrhoids during pregnancy are common. Therapy includes high intake of dietary fiber, adequate oral fluid intake. Up to 80% of all pregnant women experience some degree of nausea and vomiting. Pharmacotherapy may include the following: antihistamines (e.g., **doxylamine**), vitamins (e.g., **pyridoxine, cyanocobalamin**), anticholinergics (e.g., **dicyclomine, scopolamine**), dopamine antagonists (e.g., **metoclopramide**).

2. **Gestational Diabetes Mellitus:** It is a first line therapy for all women with Gestational DM which includes
   - Excercise
   - Daily self monitoring of blood glucose is required.
   - Glycemic control is pre-prandial capillary glucose concentration at or below 95mg/dl.

3. **Venous Thrombo Embolism:** For treatment of acute thrombo embolism during pregnancy lower molecular weight heparin is preferred. Duration of therapy should not be less than 3 months.

Acute Care issues in pregnancy

UTI [5]

The principle infecting organism is Escherichia coli. The most commonly used anti biotic for asymptomatic bacteria and cystits are the beta lactam antibiotics (penicillins and cephalosporins).

HeadAche [6]

For tension and migraine headache during pregnancy, first line therapies are non pharmacological including relaxation, Stress management. For tension headache acetaminophen and ibuprofen can be used.

Sexually Transmitted Diseases

Pharmaco therapy for selected Sexually Transmitted Disease Complications of chlamydia trachoma's include pelivic inflammatory diseases and infertility. Neisseria Gonorrhea is risk factor for pelvic inflammatory diseases and pre term delivery.

Table 16.1 Pharmacotherapy in different STD during pregnancy.

STI	Drug Brand Names	Usual Dose	Monitoring
Bacterial Vaginosis	Metronidazole 0.75% gel Alternatives: Clindamycin	500mg by mouth 2 times * 7 days 5g Intravaginally once daily * 5 days	Follow up testing
Genital Herpes	Acyclovir or Valacyclovir	400mg by mouth 3 times a day. 500mg 2 a day	Start Treatment at 36 weeks of gestation
Gonorrhea	Azithromycin	1g by mouth * 1 dose	3 months after treatment
Trichomoniasis	Metronidazole	2g by mouth * 1 dose	Rescreen HIV patients at 3 months after treatment

Chronic illness in pregnancy

Allergic Rhinitis and Asthma [7]

All patients with asthma should have access to short acting inhaled β_2 agonist. Mld persistent asthma-Low medium or high doses of inhaled corticosteroids

Moderate asthma-**inhaled corticosteroid+** β_2 agonist

Severe asthma-high dose **inhaled corticosteroid+systemic corticosteroid**

Diabetics Mellitus

Insulin for type 1 or type 2. Glyburide or metformin can be used.

Epilepsy

Major malformations occur in 4% to 6% of the offspring of women taking **benzodiazepines, carbamazepine, phenobarbital, phenytoin,** or **valproic acid**.

HIV

In women newly diagnosed with HIV or who have not previously received anti- anti-retroviral therapy should be initiated as soon as pregnancy is determined.For ART - use of three drug combination is regimen is recommended.

Hypertension

Antihypertensive drugs may be continued during pregnancy except for **ACEIs** and **angiotensin II receptor blockers**. **Diuretic** use is acceptable for chronic hypertension

Depression

Selective serotonin reuptake inhibitors (SSRIs) are widely used by pregnant women. Lowest possible dose should be used for the shortest possible time to minimize adverse fetal and maternal pregnancy outcomes.

Lactation issues: Drug use during lactation Mediactions enter breast milk via passive diffusion of noniozed and non -protein bound medication. Drugs with high MWT, lower lipid solubility and higher protein bindings are less likely to cross into breast milk.

Re lactation: For Re lactation use metoclopramide, 10 mg three times daily for 7 to 14 days only if non drug therapy is ineffective.

References

1. Namnoun AB, Hatcher RA. The menstrual cycle. In: Hatcher RA, Trussell J, Stewart F, et al., eds. Contraceptive Technology, 17th ed. New York: Ardent Media, 1998:69–76.
2. Polifka JE, Friedman JM. Medical genetics: 1. Clinical teratology in the age of genomics. Can Med Assoc J 2002;167:265–273.
3. Center for Disease Control and Prevention. Preconception care questions and answers. *http://www.cdc.gov/ncbddd/preconception/QandA_providers. htm#1.*
4. Wald A. Constipation, diarrhea, and symptomatic hemorrhoids during pregnancy. Gastroenterol Clin 2003;32:309–322.
5. Le J, Briggs GG, McKeown A, Bustillo G. Urinary tract infections during pregnancy. Ann Pharmacother 2004;38:1692–1701.
6. Silberstein SD. Headaches in pregnancy. Neurol Clin 2004:22:727–756.
7. Blaiss MS. Management of asthma during pregnancy. Allergy Asthma Proc 2004;25:375–376.

CHAPTER - 17

Rational Drug Use

Definition: Prescribing right drug, in adequate dose for the sufficient duration and appropriate to the clinical wards of the patient at lower cost.

The concept of rational drug use is age old, as evident by the statement made by the Alexandrian physician herophilus 300B.C that is "Medicines are nothing in themselves but are the very hands of god if employed with reason and prudence".

Rational drug use attain more significance nowadays in terms of medical, socio economical and loyal aspect.

Factors that have led sudden realization for rational drug use are
- **Drug explosion:** Increase in no. of available has incredibly complicated the choice of appropriate drug for particular indication
- **Efforts to prevent the development of resistance:** Irrational use of drugs may lead to premature demise of highly efficacious and life saving new antimicrobial drug due to development of resistance.
- **Growing awareness:** Today the info about drug development. Its uses and adverse effects travel from one end of the planet to other end with amazing speed through various media.
- **Increase cost of treatment:** Increase in cost of the drug increases economic burden on the public as well as on the government. This can be reduced by rational drug use.
- **Consumer protection act (CPA):** Extension of CPA in medical profession may restrict the irrational use of drugs.

Measures to promote Rational drug use: Medicines cannot be used rationally unless ever one involved in the pharmaceutical supply chain has access to objective information about the drug they buy and use. Knowledge and ideas about drug are constantly changing a clinical expected to know about the new development in drug therapy.

Rational use of injections: Injections are preferred by patients and doctors for variety of health problems even when their administration is not medically justified. The popularity of injections may have its origins in the spectacular uses achieved with injections of quinine in malaria and high public profile of vaccination programs.

In general the use of injections should be restricted to the following situation:
- Oral administration is not tolerated or is not possible.

- ➢ Absorption problem
- ➢ The drug of choice is only formulated as a parenteral product
- ➢ High tissue concentrations are needed and are not achieved by oral administration.
- ➢ Urgent treatment is required due to severe and rapidly progressing illness.
- ➢ The patient is unlikely to comply with oral treatment

Rational use of common OTC drugs in India almost all drugs can be brought over the counter without prescription.

Vitamins and tonics, iron preparations, analgesics NSAID's and cough mixtures are widely used.

Irrational use of injections include using paracetamol injections to bring down fever, multivitamins glucose and calcium injections to improve stamina injections of histamine 2 antagonist or proton pump inhibitors for gastritis and injections given on patient demand. [1,2, 3]

WHO advocates 12 key interventions to promote more rational use [4, 5]
- ➢ Establishment of a multidisciplinary national body to coordinate policies on medicine use.
- ➢ Use of clinical guidelines
- ➢ Development and use of national essential medicines list.
- ➢ Establishment of drug and therapeutics committees in districts and hospitals.
- ➢ Inclusion of problem based pharmacotherapy training in under graduate curricula
- ➢ Continuing in service medical education as a license requirement.
- ➢ Supervision, audit and feedback.
- ➢ Use of independent information on medicines
- ➢ Public education about medicines.
- ➢ Avoidance of perverse financial incentives.
- ➢ Use of appropriate and enforced regulation.
- ➢ Sufficient government expenditure to ensure availability of medicines and staff.

Hazards of irrational use of drugs:
- ➢ Ineffective and unsafe treatment
- ➢ Exacerbation or prolongation of illness.
- ➢ Distress and harm to patient.
- ➢ Increase the cost of treatment.

The pre requisites of rational drug use are
- ➢ Critical assessment and evaluation of benefits and risk of drug used.
- ➢ Compare the advantages disadvantages safety and cost of the drug with existing drug for some indication.

Reasons for irrational use of drugs: [6, 7]
- ➢ Lack of information: Unlike many developed countries we don't have regular facility which provide us up to date unbiased information on the currently used drugs.

- ➤ Faculty and inadequate training and education of medical graduates: Lack of proper clinical training regarding writing a prescription during training periods dependency on a diagnostic aid, rather than clinical diagnosis, is increasing day by day in doctors.
- ➤ Poor communication between health professional and patient.
- ➤ Lack of diagnostic facilities.
- ➤ Demand from the patient: To satisfy the patient expectations and demand of quite relief, clinician prescribe drug for every single complaint.
- ➤ Defective drug supply system and ineffective drug regulation
- ➤ Promotional activities of pharmaceutical industries.

Obstacles exist in Rational drug use:

- ➤ Lack of objective information and of continuing education and training in pharmacology.
- ➤ Lack of well organised drug regulatory authority and supply of drugs.
- ➤ Presence of large no. of drugs in the market.

Steps to improve Rational drug prescribing: [8, 9]

I - Identify the patients problem based on symptoms and recognize the need for action.

II - Diagnosis of the disease. Identify underlying cause and motivating factors. This may be specific as in infectious disease or non specific.

III - List possible intervention or treatment. This may be non drug treatment or drug treatment. Drug must be chosen from different alternatives based on efficacy, convenience and safety of drug including drug interactions and high risk group of patients.

IV - Start the treatment by writing an accurate and complete prescription.

V - Give proper info instruction and warning regarding the treatment given.

VI - Monitor the treatment to check, if the particular treatment has solved the patients problem. It may be passive monitoring or active monitoring by the physician.

Conclusion

Indiscriminate use of drugs not only waste scarce resources that should otherwise by spent on other essential services but also leads to drug induces disease.

The demands of rational drug use are:

- ➤ Availability of essential and life saving drugs and unbiased drug info with generic name.
- ➤ Adequate quality control and drug control.
- ➤ Withdrawal of hazardous and irrational drugs.
- ➤ Drug legislation reform.

References

1. Irrational drug combinations; Need to sensitize undergraduates. Gautam, C.S. Aditya S. Ind. J. Pharmacol; Vol. 38, 3, June 06, 169-170.

2. Essential drugs and Rational Therapeutics Text book of Pharmacology S.D. Seth 1st Ed. 1997, 783-791.
3. Essential drugs and Rational Therapeutics Text book of Pharmacology S.D. Seth 2nd Ed. 2004, 907-916
4. The rational use of drugs, Report on the conference of experts Nairobi, 25-29 Nov. 1985 sponsored by W.H.O. Geneva.
5. https://www.who.int/medicines/areas/rational_use/en/
6. Organization behaviour and community health promoting rational drug use among health professionals Uma Tekur and Isha Gupta Publication from state institute of health and family welfare; Rajasthan 2nd ed. 1998, 273- 276.
7. Rational drug use Organization behaviour and community health promoting rational drug use among health professionals Adesh Mathur. Published by state institute of health and family welfare, Jaipur, 3rd ed. 2001, 95-103
8. Improving drug use Editorial, Action programme on essential drug No. 23 1997
9. Rational use of drugs Gurbani N K., Sharma Rameshwar and Dandiya P.C., Pharma Times, May 2000, 18-33

CHAPTER - 18

Conjuctivitis

Introduction to Conjunctivitis

It is commonly called as pink eye disease.

Definition: Conjunctivitis, or pink eye, is an irritation or inflammation of the conjunctiva, which covers the white part of the eyeball.

The conjunctiva is the thin clear tissue that lies over the white part of the eye and lines the inside of the eyelid. When small blood vessels in the conjunctiva become inflamed the white part of eye appears reddish or pinkish.

Types: Bacterial conjunctivitis- it is uncommon making up 5% of all cases of conjunctivitis. Bacterial conjunctivitis is invariably bilateral and should be suspected when conjunctival inflammation is associated with a purulent discharge.

Viral conjunctivitis: Most cases are caused by virus. This form of conjunctivitis is self limiting. Mainly caused by adenovirus and herpes simplex virus etc.

Allergic conjunctivitis: It affects both eyes and is a response to an allergen causing substance such as pollen.

Conjunctivitis resulting from irritation: Irritation from a chemical splash or foreign object in eye is also associated with conjunctivitis.

Epidemiology [1, 2, 3]

It is most common ocular condition.

Bacterial conjunctivitis is more common in children and viral conjunctivitis is more common in adults.

It is seen in both males and females in equal manner.

It affects all age groups.

135 out of 10,000 adults suffer with conjunctivitis. Conjunctivitis affects many people and imposes economic and social burdens. It is estimated that acute conjunctivitis affects 6 million people annually in the United States.

The prevalence of conjunctivitis varies according to the underlying cause, which may be influenced by the patient's age, as well as the season of the year. Viral conjunctivitis is the most common cause of infectious conjunctivitis both overall and in the adult population and is more prevalent in summer. Bacterial conjunctivitis is the second most common cause and is responsible for the majority (50%-75%) of cases in children; it is observed more frequently from December through April. Allergic conjunctivitis is the most frequent cause, affecting 15% to 40% of the population, and is observed more frequently in spring and summer.

Aetiology

Causes

Bacteria like Streptococcus pneumoniae, staphylococcus, haemophilus influenza, gonococci, moraxella lacunata etc.

Viruses like adenovirus, herpes simplex virus, varicella zoster virus etc.

Allergens like pollen grains.

A chemical splash in the eye.

Foreign object in the eye.

In new born a blocked tear duct.

Risk Factors

Exposure to allergens: IgE mediated hypersensitive reaction precipitated by small airborne allergens. This leads to local mast cell degranulation. There is release of chemical mediators of inflammation i.e histamine, Platelet Activating Factor (PAF) etc. which mediate the immnulogical responses.

Contact or exposure to someone infected with bacterial or viral form of conjunctivitis.

Using contact lenses especially extended wear lenses.

Pathophysiology

Bacterial Conjunctivitis

When the surface tissue of eye is colonized by flora then it results in alteration of host defence mechanism which leads to infection.

Primary defence against infection is epithelial layer covering conjunctiva. Disruption of this layer leads to infection.

Secondary defence against infection includes hematologic immune mechanism which is carried out by rinsing, lacrimation and blinking of eye.

Viral Conjunctivitis

Viruses like adenovirus invades eye through adjacent sides or blood borne Pathways, and replicate in conjunctival mucosa.

Initiation of lymphocytic inflammatory cascade occurs which leads to attraction of white blood cells and red blood cells.

As the WBC reaches to the conjunctival tissue or surface it further leads to accumulation of other WBC through highly permeable capillaries.

Allergic Conjunctivitis

Allergen enters the tear film. When it comes in contact with conjunctival mast cells that bear IgE antibodies, they result in degranulation of mast cells which leads to release of histamine. Histamine further promotes vasodilatation and oedema.

Clinical Manifestations and Features

Signs and Symptoms

Bacterial conjunctivitis - redness of eye, itching, inflammation of eye, lacrimation of eye, yellow colour fluid whoozing out, mild pain.

Viral conjunctivitis - redness of eye, swelling, itching, burning sensation of eye, lot of lacrimation, thick white fluid exudation from eye.

Allergic conjunctivitis - itching, redness, soreness, watery and stringy discharge, swollen eyelids.

Diagnosis with Algorithm

It mainly includes physical examination of eye where redness of eye, inflammation and other symptoms are diagnosed.

Culture test and culture sensitivity test are done to mainly detect the organism and its sensitivity towards antibiotics in case of bacterial conjunctivitis.

RPS adeno detection test, the only test to detect virus in the eye.

Complete blood picture.

Japanese Guidelines for Diagnosis of Allergic Conjunctival Diseases [4]

If there is ocular itching and hyperemia

Absence of conjunctival proliferation-assess if it is seasonal or non-seasonal.

If seasonal-then it is confirmed as: **Seasonal allergic conjunctivitis**

If non-seasonal-

If there is absence of atopic dermatitis – then it is **Perennial allergic conjunctivitis**

If there is presence of atopic dermatitis – then it is **Atopic keratoconjuctivitis**

Presence of conjunctival proliferation – assess if it is without lens or with lens

If without lens- then it is confirmed as **Vernal keratoconjuctivitis**

If with contact lens- then it is confirmed as **Giant papillary conjuctivitis**

Diagnostic Stepwise Approach for Neonatal Conjuctivitis [5]

If the Neonate presents with eye discharge

Take the history and examine the child

If purulent conjunctivitis present –

Treat the baby for gonococcal and chlamydial ophthalmia (AND) treat mother and partner for gonorrhoea and Chlamydia. Educate and counsel. Review the baby in 7 days or sooner if symptoms worsen.

Review in 7 days. If eye infection is cleared, complete treatment course, reinforce education and counselling.

If purulent conjunctivitis is not present- identify the signs of other illness that are present and treat appropriately.

Management

Treatment goals - To improve vision,
To reduce the symptoms,
To control the bacterial load or microbial load.

Pharmacological Treatment

Bacterial Conjunctivitis

Generally antibiotics are prescribed based on the type of organism invaded.

Fluoroquinolone antibiotics - these are mainly helpful in reducing Gram positive bacteria and are the second line drugs to treat.

Their mechanism of action involves inhibition of DNA synthesis by binding to the enzyme DNA complex.

Examples - ciprofloxacin (0.3%) - ointment or solution (one or two drops) QIDfor 7days

Ofloxacin (0.3%) one or two drops Q ID for 7 days

Levofloxacin 0.5% eye drops

Aminoglycoside - they help in reducing Gram Negative bacteria. The mechanism of action includes inhibition of protein synthesis of bacteria by binding to ribosomal units like 50s and 30s and result in inhibition of initiation complex formation.

Examples -   Gentamycin 0.3% eye drops

Tobramycin 0.3% eye drops.

Macrolides - these are the first line drugs used to treat conjunctivitis and they have very broad spectrum of activity. They act by inhibiting Protein synthesis and cell growth of bacteria.

Examples - Erythromycin ointment QID for 7 days

Azithromycin 1% solution or 1 gram orally.

Sulphonamides - These drugs act by inhibiting Folic acid synthesis which is required for DNA synthesis. The mainly in habit the enzyme folate synthase required for formation of dihydrofolate.

Examples - sulphacetamide ointment QID for 7 days or solution 1 – 2 drops every 3 hours for 7 days.

Viral Conjunctivitis

Generally it is self limiting and only support therapy is given like cold compress and use of lubricants to have clear vision.

In civil cases antiviral agents are given.

For herpes simplex virus,

Topical Ganciclovir gel - TID for 7days. It acts by inhibiting replication of viral DNA and potent inhibition of the viral DNA polymerase.

Oral acyclovir-400mg- 5times per day for 7days. It incorporates into and terminates the growing viral DNA chain and inactivates the viral DNA polymerase.

Valacyclovir- 500mg orally- TID for 7days. It is a prodrug of acyclovir.

For Varicella-zoster virus,

Acyclovir- 800mg orally-5times per day for 7days.

Valacyclovir- 1000mg- QID for 7days.

Allergic Conjunctivitis

Mast cell stabilizers agents- these agents prevent degranulation of mast cells and release of histamine.

Example - sodium cromoglycate 2% to 4%

Lodoxamide One drop QID

Nedocromil 2% solution

Antihistamine - these agents block the histamine receptor and also reduce release of histamine from mast cells.

Example - azelastine One drop BD

Emedastine 0.05% QID

Naphazoline 1 to two drops QID

Ketotifen 0.025% B I D or QID.

Olopatadine - it stops mast cells breakdown and release of substances like histamine and leukotrienes (prostaglandins and tryptase).

Used to treat itchy Eyes caused by allergies.

Dose - 0.1% to 0.2% - One drop OD.

Other Drugs in special cases are

Corticosteroids are given when the person is highly resistant to Other Drugs.

Example - prednisolone which is given in CBR conjunctivitis and when there is a decreased vision.

In few cases immunosuppressants are given.

Example - cyclosporine 0.5% BD.

For gonococcal infections pencillin is mainly recommended. Dose of around 6000 units.

Counseling tips for preventing bacterial and viral conjunctivitis transmission [6]

Wash hands frequently with soap and water 20 seconds. Use an alcohol- based hand sanitizer that contains at least 60% alcohol if soap and water are not available.

Wash discharge from around the eyes several times a day with a clean, wet washcloth ot a fresh cotton ball. Clean the washcloth with detergent and hot water, and discard the cotton ball after use.

Avoid touching eyes with hands.

Use a clean towel and washcloth daily, and do not share them.

Do not use a swimming pool until the infection has resolved.

References

1. Udeh BL, Schneider JE, Ohsfeldt RL. Cost effectiveness of a point-of-care test for adenoviral conjunctivitis. Am J Med Sci. 2008;336(3):254-264.
2. Hørven I. Acute conjunctivitis: a comparison of fusidic acid viscous eye drops and chloramphenicol. Acta Ophthalmol (Copenh). 1993;71(2):165-168.
3. Høvding G. Acute bacterial conjunctivitis. Acta Ophthalmol. 2008;86(1):5-17.
4. Etsauko takamura et al., Japanese guidelines for allergic conjunctival diseases Allergology International 2017; 66(2).
5. https://www.clinicalguidelines.scot.nhs.uk/ggc-paediatric-guidelines/ggc-guidelines/emergency-medicine/conjunctivitis-management-in-children/
6. Centers for Disease Control and Prevention. Conjunctivitis (pink eye). https://www.cdc.gov/conjunctivitis/.

CHAPTER - 19

Glaucoma

Introduction to Glaucoma

Glaucoma is a group of ocular diseases, characterized by the damage of optic nerve due to increase in the eye pressure (IOP) and is associated with loss of visual sensitivity.

Normal range of intra ocular pressure (IOP) - 12 to 22 mmHg.

Epidemiology

Glaucoma is the second leading cause of blindness globally. The highest prevalence of Primary Closed Angle Glaucoma (POAG) occurs in Africans, and the highest prevalence of Primary Open Angle Glaucoma (PCAG) occurs in the Inuit, Chinese, and Asian-Indian descent.

Globally, there are an estimated 60 million people with glaucomatous optic neuropathy and an estimated 8.4 million people who are blind as the result of glaucoma.

Etiology

Causes

Blunt (or) chemical injury to the eye

Severe (or) chronic eye infections

Blockade of mesh like channel in the eye (trabecular mesh)

Sometimes, eye surgery to correct other conditions can be a cause to glaucoma.

Risk Factors

Being older than 60 years

Being a particular descent like African- American or Asian

Having a family history of glaucoma

Having elevated IOP

Having poor vision, or other eye disorders or injuries

Having certain medical conditions like, diabetes

Taking certain medications, like corticosteroids for prolonged periods.

Signs and Symptoms

Redness in the eye

Nausea and vomiting

Seeing halos around lights

Eye pain

Blurred vision (hazy eye)

Narrowed vision (tunnel vision)

Loss of vision (shows up in the last stage)

Open Angle Glaucoma

It is also known as wide angle glaucoma. It is the most common form of glaucoma, accounting for at least 90% of all glaucoma cases. In this, the drain structure in the eye looks normal, but the fluid doesn't flow out like normal like it should. Here the angle where the iris meets the cornea is as wide and open hence called as open angle or wide-angle glaucoma.

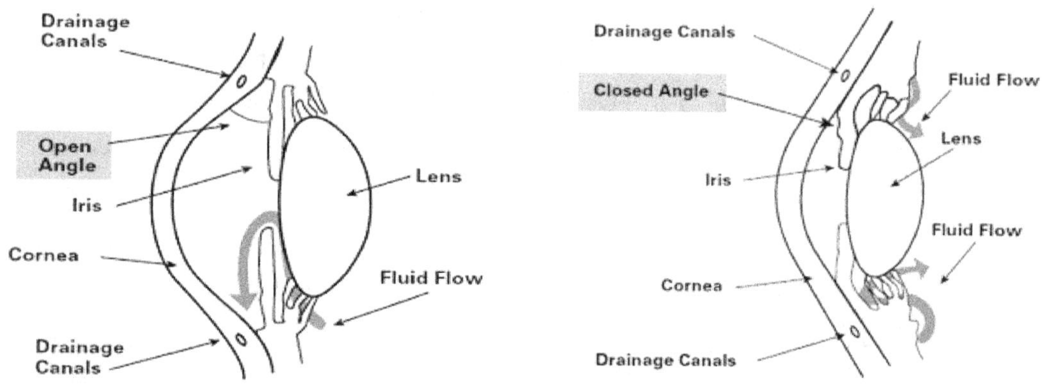

Fig 19.1 Types of Glaucoma.

Source: https://www.sagarbhargava.com/types-of-glaucoma/

Closed Angle Glaucoma

Also called as acute angle or narrow angle glaucoma. It is a less common form of glaucoma. In this the eye doesn't drain out, because the angle between iris and cornea is too narrow and can lead to increase pressure in the eye leading to blurriness or clouding of lens.

Pathophysiology

Normally, the fluid, called aqueous humour flows out of our eye through a mesh like channel. If this channel gets blocked due to any etiological reasons the liquid builds up in the eye and doesn't flow out like it normally should. This leads to the damage of blood vessels and a raised intra ocular pressure which affects the blood flow and perfusion pressure of optic nerve and damage occurs. Thereby, it fails to carry visual information to the brain resulting in loss of vision. If not treated, it may lead to blindness. Very high IOP (>60 mm Hg) may result in permanent loss of visual field within a matter of hours to days.

Table 19.1 Differences between types of Glaucoma.

Open angle glaucoma	Closed angle glaucoma
Is caused by the slow clogging of the drainage canals, resulting in increased eye pressure	Is caused by blocked drainage canals, resulting in a sudden rise in intraocular pressure
Has a wide and open angle between the iris and cornea	Has a closed or narrow angle between the iris and cornea
Develops slowly and is a lifelong condition	Develops very quickly
Has symptoms and damage that are not noticed.	Has symptoms and damage that are usually very noticeable
	Demands immediate medical attention.

Drugs That May Induce or Potentiate Increased Intraocular Pressure

Open-angle glaucoma: Ophthalmic corticosteroids (high risk) Systemic corticosteroids Nasal/inhaled corticosteroids Fenoldopam Ophthalmic anticholinergics Sccinylcholine

Closed-angle glaucoma: Topical anticholinergics Topical sympathomimetics Systemic anticholinergics Heterocyclic antidepressants Low-potency phenothiazines Antihistamines Ipratropium

Diagnosis with Algorithm

Diagnosing glaucoma is not always easy, and careful evaluation of the optic nerve continues to be essential to diagnosis and treatment.

Intra ocular pressure

        Normal range   12-22mmHg

        Open angle glaucoma   <21mmHg (>21mmHg -ocular hypertension)

        Closed angle glaucoma   40-60mmHg

Conditions to be analysed for different types of glaucoma-

POAG & PCAG:

Raised IOP.

Glaucomatous optic nerve changes.

Visual field defects /changes.

Open angle or closed angle of the anterior chamber.

Normotensive (or) low tension glaucoma:

Cupping of disc

Visual field defects

Normal (or)low IOP

Ocular hypertension:

Constantly raised IOP

Without associated glaucomatous damage.

Secondary glaucoma:

Rise of IOP

Associated with primary ocular (or) systemic disease.

Physical examination

Patient presentation

Table 19.2 Symptomatic examination for different types of Glaucoma.

Open angle glaucoma	Closed angle glaucoma
- Asymptomatic	- Severe pain
- Head ache and eye pain	- Emesis associated with pain
- Scotoma (partially/totally diminished visual activity)	- Redness
- Delayed dark adaption	- Photophobia
- Loss of vision and blindness	- H/O intermittent attacks of subacute CAG

Diagnostic Criteria	Name of Test
The inner eye pressure	Tonometry
The shape and colour of the optic nerve	Ophthalmoscopy (dilated eye exam)
The complete field of vision	Perimetry (visual field test)
The angle in the eye where the iris meets the cornea	Gonioscopy (Measure angle between the iris and the cornea)
Thickness of the cornea	Pachymetry (Measure Thickness of the cornea)

Regular glaucoma check-ups include two routine eye tests: tonometry and ophthalmoscopy.

Tonometry: It measures the pressure within the eye using a device called as tonometer. Ocular normotension-12-22mmHg. Most cases are diagnosed with the pressure exceeding 20mmHg.

But few people have glaucoma at pressures between 12-22mmHg.

Opthalmoscopy: This procedure helps the doctor to examine the optic nerve. The eye drops used, dilate the pupil, so that the eye can be easily examined. If the IOP is not within the normal range (or) of the optic nerve looks unusual, other one/two glaucoma tests are to be performed (Perimetry/Gonioscopy)

Perimetry: It provides the complete field of vision of the eye. After glaucoma has been diagnosed, visual field tests are usually done one-two times a year to check for any changes in the vision.

Gonioscopy: The diagnostic exam helps to examine whether the angle where the iris meets the cornea is open and wide (or)narrow and closed. A hand-held contact lens is placed on the eye which has a mirror and shows the angle whether it is closed and blocked [PCAG] (or) wide and open [POAG/chronic glaucoma].

Pachymetry: It is a simple painless test used to measure the thickness of the cornea (clear window at the front of the eye). It takes very less time like about a minute for both eyes.

Management

Goals

To reduce Intra ocular pressure

Protection of eye sight

Treatment

Closure Angle Glaucoma

The goal of initial therapy for acute CAG with high IOP is rapid reduction of the IOP to preserve vision and to avoid surgical or laser iridectomy on a hypertensive, congested eye.

Iridectomy (laser or surgical) is the definitive treatment of CAG; it produces a hole in the iris that permits aqueous humor flow to move directly from the posterior chamber to the anterior chamber, opening up the block at the trabecular meshwork.

Drug therapy of an acute attack typically involves administration of pilocarpine, hyperosmotic agents, and a secretory inhibitor (a β-blocker, α2-agonist, prostaglandin F2α analog, or a topical or systemic Carbonic Anhydrase Inhibitor (CAI).

Open Angle Glaucoma

Medications most commonly used to treat glaucoma are the nonselective β-blockers, the prostaglandin analogs (latanoprost, travoprost, and bimatoprost), brimonidine (an α2-agonist), and the fixed combination product of timolol and dorzolamide.

Algorithm for the pharmacotherapy of open-angle glaucoma.

1. **Start therapy with beta blocker:** If contraindications exist- Alternative first-line agent: prostaglandins or brimonidine If contraindication to first line agents, use topical Carbon Anhydrase Inhibitor (CAI).

2. **Assess response in 2-4 weeks:** If intolerance exists • Reduce concentration if possible or • Change formulations or • Switch to class alternative or • Switch to alternative first-line agent

   Inadequate response: • Ensure compliance • Instruct patient on nasolacrimal occlusion if not currently used • Increase concentration (if possible), or increase dose frequency • Switch to alternative first-line agent if no response, add second first-line agent if partial response

3. **Assess response in 2-4 weeks:** IF Intolerance Exists: • Reduce dose/concentration if possible or • Change formulations or • Switch to class alternatives or • Switch to alternative combination

   Inadequate response to monotherapy • Ensure compliance • If no response, sequentially try alternative first-line topical agents OR • If partial response, add second or third first-line agent or topical CAI, or unoprostone (multidrug regimens containing 2-4 agents may be required)

4. **Assess response in 2-4 weeks:** Intolerance • Reduce dose/concentration if possible • Change formulations • Swicth to class alternatives • Switch to alternative combination

   Inadequate response to first- and second-line topical combination therapy • Ensure compliance • Consider adding direct-acting cholinergic agent (4th line), and if necessary, replace with a cholinesterase inhibitor • Consider adding oral carbonic anhydrase inhibitor in place of topical carbonic anhydrase inhibitor • Mulitiple topical therapies plus oral carbonic anhydrase inhibitor may be necessary

5. **Assess response in 2-4 weeks:** Intolerance or inadequate response to maximally tolerated combination drug therapy, then Laser or surgical procedure is indicated.

Medications

Beta Blockers

1st line agents

Timolol, Betaxolol, Levobetaxolol

Mechanism of Action: They have common a mechanism i.e., they block the beta-adrenergic receptors in the ciliary epithelium of the eye and lower IOP by decreasing the aqueous humour production.

Timolol: Non-selective β1, β2 adrenergic antagonist. It was the first ocular beta-adrenergic blocker marketed. ADRs- decreased pulse rate(5-8bpm), worsening CCF, dyspnoea, airway obstruction, pulmonary failure. Chronic administration- Corneal anaesthesia, pulmonary disease

Contraindications: CHF, Sinus bradycardia, Pulmonary disease, lactation.

Dose: Initial-0.25% sol-one drop-BID

Later-0.5% sol-one drop-BID

Betaxolol and Levobetaxolol: Levobetaxolol is more active than betaxolol, but pharmacological and toxicological effects are similar. -They are selective β-adrenergic antagonists. ADRs- associated with few ocular side effects. Slight decrease in B.P. -It may be the ocular β-blocker of choice in patients with pre-existing CHF (or) pulmonary disease.

Dose: Initial 0.125% one drop- BID; Later 0.5% one drop – BID

Prostaglandin Analouges

They are first line agents, as they are as effective as β-blockers and with minimal side effects.

Latanoprost, Travoprost

Mechanism of Action: Both are $PGF_2\alpha$-prostaglandin agonists. They act by increasing the outflow of intraocular fluid from the eye and are effective at reducing (or)lowering IOP.

Latanoprost: ADRs-Increased pigmentation of iris and eye lid. May cause muscle, joint, back pain, headaches, migraines and skin rashes. Systemic side effects are rare.

Dose: 0.005% one drop -OD (bedtime) [Since BID may be less effective compared to OD at bedtime]

Travoprost-ADRs: Systemic side effects are less but may include cold and upper tract infections.

Increased pigmentation of iris and eye lid.

Dose: 0.004% One drop – OD (bedtime)

α2-Adrenergic Agonists

Brimonidine: Alternative 1st line agent.

Mechanism of Action: It is highly selective for α 2-Adrenergic receptors. They reduce the IOP by increasing the production of aqueous humour and uveoscleral outflow. ADRs- Systemic side effects are more common like dry nose and mouth. It penetrates BBB, thereby may cause, mild systemic hypotension, lethargy and decreased pulse. Contraindications: CVS disorders, depression, renal/hepatic dysfunction, orthostatic hypotension.

Dose: 0.2% one drop – BID-TID

Apraclonidine: It may be used as both preop and postop for preventing an increase in IOP after any laser procedures. ADRs- Doesn't penetrate BBB, may cause mild systemic hypotension, local effects are common, tachyphylaxis. [stinging, burning, oedema of lid, etc.]

Dose: 0.5-1% one drop- preop and postop (or) BID-TID

Topical Carbonic Anhydrase Inhibitors [CAIs]

Brinzolamide, Dorzolamide, **Acetazolamide**

Mechanism of Action: Carbonic anhydrase enzyme occurs in high concentration in ciliary processes and retina of the eye. CAIs lower the IOP by decreasing the flow of bicarbonate, sodium and water production into the posterior chamber of eye and decreases the aqueous humour secretion.

Brinzolamide: Effective long-term monotherapy (or) adjuvant therapy. ADRs- Less systemic side effects. Less burning and stinging compared to Dorzolamide [since pH of Brinzolamide is similar to human tears]. Contraindications- hepatic (or) renal impairment.

Dose: 1% one drop- TID

Dorzolamide: Effective long-term monotherapy (or) adjuvant therapy. ADRs- less systemic side effects. May include ocular burning, stinging, discomfort and allergic reactions. Contraindicatons: hepatic(or)renalimpairment

Drug Interactions: Acetazolamide(oral)+ Dorzolamide(topical)- Toxic effects

Hence, combination of oral and topical CAIs is not recommended.

Dose: 2% one drop- TID

Systemic Carbonic Anhydrase Inhibitors

Acetazolamide: Mechanism of action: decreases aqueous humour production. IOP reduction is 30-40%.

Cholinergic Agonists

Pilocarpine, Carbachol

Pilocarpine: Mechanism of Action: It is a direct acting cholinergic agonist (parasympathomimetic) which causes the contraction of ciliary muscle fibres attached to trabecular work and scleral spur, opening the mesh work to enhance aqueous humour outflow, thereby decreasing IOP.

ADRs: Itching, Irritation, increase tearing, headache, blurred vision

Contraindications: Pregnancy

Dose: Lower concentration-   0.5-1% one drop- QID

0.25-10% 1-2 drops- TID/QID

Laser Surgery

Trabeculoplasty is a laser that is used to increase the outflow of fluid from the eye and reduce the eye pressure. Laser iridotomy is a laser performed that is used to treat narrow angles and Primary Closed Angle Glaucoma (PCAG) that occurs due to the crowding of natural drainage channels of the eye. Cyclophotocoagulation is a non-invasive laser that is used for some types of glaucoma for IOP control.

Glaucoma Surgery

There are number of surgical techniques that are used for controlling eye pressure and the most appropriate technique must be customised for each patient. Minimally invasive glaucoma surgery trabeculotomy creates a new channel to drain fluid from the eye and reduce the pressure that causes glaucoma. Surgeries performed only after mediation and laser procedures have been unsuccessful.

Ophthalmic Corticosteroids

Low Potency: Dexamethasone 0.05% and 0.1%

Intermediate Potency: Clobetasone 0.1%, Loteprednol 0.2% (Lotemax) Loteprednol 0.5% (Alrex) Prednisolone Acetate 0.12% (Pred Mild) Prednisolone Sodium Phosphate 0.125% (Inflamase Mild) Prednisolone Sodium Phosphate 1% (Inflamase Forte)

High Potency: Clobetasone 0.5%, Fluorometholone Acetate 0.1%, Prednisolone Acetate 1%, Rimexolone 1%

Prednisolone acetate 1% and fluorometholone acetate 0.1% have the best anti-inflammatory effects.

Table 19.3 Agents for Glaucoma.

Generic	Brand	Dosage Form	Dosing	Comments
Beta-blockers				
Betaxolol	Generic Betoptic-S	0.5% solution 0.25 suspension	1-2 drops twice daily 1 drop twice daily	MOA: Redice AH production from ciliary body *Beta-selective: Betaxolol Nonselective:* carteolol, levobunolo, netipranolol, timolol
Carteolol	Ocupress	1% solution	1 drop twice daily	
Levobunolol	Betagan	0.25%, 0.5% solution	1-2 drops twice daily	
Metipranolol	OptiPranolo	0.3% solution	1 drop twice daily	
Timolol	Timoptic, Betimol, Istalol	0.25%, 0.5% solution	1 drop 1-2 times daily	
	Timoptic-XE Gel	0.25%, 0.5% gelforming solution	1 drop daily	

Contd...

Generic	Brand	Dosage Form	Dosing	Comments
Prostagladin Analogues				
Bimatoprost	Generic Lumigan	0.03% solution	1 drop at bedtime	MOA: Increase AH outflow through uveoscleral route. Bimatoprost may also improve outflow through trabecleral AH outflow
Latanoprost	Xalatan, generic	0.005% solution	1 drop at bedtime	
Tafluprost	Zioptan*	0.0015% solution	1 drop at bedtime	
Travoprost	Travatan Z, generic	0.004% solution	1 drop at bedtime	
Alpha2 Adrenergic Agents				
Aprachlonidine	Generic iopidine	0.5% solution	1-2 drops 3 times daily	MOA: Both reduce AH production, but brimonidine is also known to increase uveosderal AH outflow
Brimonidine	Generic Alphagan P	0.15%, 0.2% solution 0.1%, 0.15% solution	1 drop 3 times daily	
Direct-Acting Chollnergic Agonists				
Carbachol	Isopto Carbachol	1.5%, 3% solution	1-2 drops 3 times daily	MOA: Increase AH outflow through the trabecular meshwork
Pilocarpine	Isopto Carbachol, generic Pilopine HS	1%, 2%, 4% solution 4$ gel	1 drop 2, 3, or 4 times daily 1 ribbon at bedtime	
Cholinesterase Inhibitors				
Echothiophate	Phsopholine Iodide	0.125% powder for reconstitution	1 drop 1-2 times daily	MOA: Increase AH outflow
Carbonic Anhydrase Inhibitors				
Brinzolamide	Azopt	1% suspension	1 drop 3 times daily	MOA: Reduce AH production by the ciliary body
Dorzolamide	Trusopt, generic	2% solution	1 drop 3 times daily	
Acetazolamide	Generic Diamox Sequels,b generic Generic	125-250 mg tablet 500 mg ER capsule 500 mg powder for injection	125-250 mg 2-4 times daily 500 mg twice daily 500 mg IV; may repeat in 2-4 h	
Methazolamide	Neptazane, generic	25-50 mg tablet	25-50 mg 2-3 times daily	

Contd...

Generic	Brand	Dosage Form	Dosing	Comments
Combination Products				
Brinzolamide-brimonidine	Simbrinza	Brinzolamide 1%-brimonidine 0.2% solution	1 drop 3 times daily	MOA: Varies with each product
Timolol-brimonidine	Combigan	Timolol 0.5%-brimonidine 0.2% solution	1 drop every 12 h	
Trimolo-doezolamide	Cosopt, generic, Cosopt PF[3]	Timolol 0.5%-dorzolamide 2% solution	1 drop twice daily	

[a]Preservative-free.

[b]Extended-release dosage form is not indicated for acute treatment of angle-closure glaucoma.

AH: aqueous humor, ER: extended-release: MOA: mechanism of action.

Pharmacological Treatment for Open Angle Gluacoma

1. Timolol 0.5% or Betaxolol 0.5% eyedrops 1 drop 12 hourly and the morning dose should be as early upon waking as possible.

   Or Latanoprost 0.005% eyedrops given only once at bedtime. (Caution: Maintain constant cold chain)

   Or Bimatoprost 0.03% eyedrops once at bedtime.

   Or Travoprost 0.004% eyedrops once at bedtime. (both do not require cold chain) If initial therapy fails, refer to a higher centre and substitute with another agent preferably belonging to a different group.

2. Dorzolamide 2% eyedrops 2 to 3 times a day.

   Or Brimonidine tartarate 0.2% twice daily

   Or Pilocarpine 1-4% eyedrops 3 times a day or 4% gel once at bedtime.

   If patient is not controlled on 2 topical drugs, then consider alternative treatment with either laser trabeculoplasty or glaucoma filtering surgery.

Pharmacological Treatment for Angle Closure Glaucoma

Angle closure glaucoma – acute Acute pain and blurring of vision along with headache and vomiting, in some cases. Chronic angle closure glaucoma - peripheral synechiae, zipping up of the angle, and persistent rise of IOP with subsequent optic atrophy.

Pharmacological Treatment of Angle Closure Glaucoma – Acute

1. Inj. Mannitol 20%, 1.5-2 g/kg, IV infusion over half an hour.
   Or Glycerol 50%, 1 to 1.5 g/kg in 50% solution orally, mixed with cold lemon or orange juice in 3-4 divided doses. (Caution: It can cause hyperglycaemia in diabetic patients. Do not drink water for 1 hour after ingesting tablet; contraindications include dehydration or cardiac decompensation).
2. Pilocarpine 2% eyedrops every 15 min for 1 hour and thereafter 6 hourly started after IOP has been lowered by hyperosmotics as above.
3. Tab. Acetazolamide 500 mg stat followed by 250 mg every 6 hours and maintained till the definitive treatment of laser peripheral iridotomy relieves the pupillary block.
4. Timolol 0.5% eyedrops 2 times a day (if pressure is still high) to be continued till surgery.

Or Betaxolol 0.5% eyedrops 2 times a day (Preferred in asthmatics and patients with cardiac conduction defects). (Caution: All mydriatics/cycloplegic drugs which dilate pupils are contraindi-cated)

Once the IOP falls to early 20's by the treatment listed above—usually in a day or so, evaluated by gonioscopy, disc cupping and visual field charting. Definitive treatment is iridotomy by laser or surgery depending on the facilities available. Prophylactic laser peripheral iridotomy should be performed on the fellow eyes as soon as possible.

Angle closure glaucoma - chronic IOP is raised due to progressive angle closure or by repeated intermittent subacute attacks secondary to pupillary block. Commonly asymptomatic until significant visual loss has occurred.

Pharmacological Treatment

Timolol 0.5% or Betaxolol 0.5% eyedrops 2 times a day usually required life-long.

Pilocarpine 2-4% eyedrops 4 times a day usually required for life. Laser or surgical iridotomy is done to eliminate any element of pupillary block in affected as well as fellow eye. If the glaucoma is still uncontrolled on maximal tolerable medical therapy (i.e. 2 topical antiglaucoma medications), then glaucoma filtering surgery or trabeculectomy should be performed.

References

1. In: Shield's Textbook of Glaucoma. Allingham, Ramji, Fredman, Moroi, Shafranov and Shields (eds). V Edition, Lippincott William & Wilkins, 2005.

CHAPTER - 20

Acute Renal Failure

Introduction to Acute Renal Failure

Acute renal failure (ARF) is defined as a clinical syndrome characterized by an abrupt decrease in renal functioning over a period of hours to days evidenced by changes in serum creatinine, **BUN and urine output.**

Epidemiology

ARF is a common condition in general population.

Approx 200 cases/ million populations- Annually.

Incidence rate is higher in hospitalized patients in intensive care unit (ICU) (2.25% Patients).

Table 20.1 Incidence & Outcomes of ARF.

	Community acquired	**Hospital acquired**	**ICU acquired**
Incidence	Low (<1%)	Moderate (2-5%)	High (6-23%)
Cause	Single	Single / multiple	Multiple
Survival rate	70-80%	30-50%	10-30%
Prognosis	RRT required	Same as common acquired	Same as hospital acquired
Worsen outcome if	poor pre admission health other failed organ systems	Additionally ischaemic ARF cause	Intrinsic renal disease septic
Better out come if	Non oliguric	Non oliguric Nephrotoxic	Pre renal and post renal cause; non oliguric nephrotoxic hyperglycemia prevented

Staging Systems (or) Classification Schemes for AKI

Based on the criteria - SCr and urine output

   I. RIFLE Criteria

  II. AKIN Criteria

 III. KDIGO Criteria

I. RIFLE Criteria: (Risk; Injury; Failure; Loss stage; End stage)

Risk - SCr ↑50% or GFR↓ 25%   Urine output <0.5ml/kg/hr for >6hrs

Injury: SCr ↑100% or GFR↓ 50%   Urine output <0.5ml/kg/hr for >12hrs

Failure: SCr ↑200% or GFR↓ 75% Urine output >3.0ml/kg/hr 24hrs or anuria for 12hrs

Loss : Persistent ARF for > 4 weeks

ESRD: RRT for > 3 months

II. AKIN Criteria: (Acute Kidney Injury Network)

	SCr	Urine Output
Stage 1	>3.0 mg/kg/hr (1.5-2 folds)	<0.5 ml/kg/hr for > 6hrs
Stage 2	↑ 2-3 folds	<0.5 ml/kg/hr for >12hrs
Stage 3	↑ 3 folds	<0.3ml/kg/hr for >24 hrs Anuria >12 hrs

III. KIDGO criteria (Kidney Disease Improving Global Outcomes)

	SCr	U.O
Stage 1	>0.3mg/dl (1.5-2.9 folds)	<0.5ml/kg/hr 6-12hrs
Stage 2	↑ 2-2.9 folds	<0.5mi/kg/hr >12hrs
Stage 3	↑ 3 folds	Anuria > 12hrs

Etiopathogenesis

Classification of ARF

AKI Type	Common etiology
Pre- renal	Decreased renal perfusion through hypoperfusion
Intra -renal	Renal parenchyma injury
Post -renal	Urinary tract obstruction

A. Renal AKI (Pseudo & Functional): In selected estimations there can be a rise in either BUN (or) the SCr; suggesting presence of renal dysfunction; but GFR is not diminished. In functional ARF, There is a decrease in glomerular hydrostatic pressure (driving force for formation of ultrafilterate). The above can also occur without damage to the kidney. There is decreased glomerular hydrostatic pressure caused due to glomerular afferent arteriole (vasoconstriction) and Glomerular efferent arteriole (vasodilation).

Glomerular afferent vasoconstriction and efferent vasodilation arteriolar conditions are commonly seen in-

1. Individuals who have Reduced effective blood volume (eg: Heart failure, cirrohsis, severe pulmonary disease or hypo albuminemia)
2. Reno vascular disease (eg: Renal artery stenosis)
3. People who cannot compensate for changes in afferent or efferent arteriolar tone.
4. Hepato renal syndrome (leads to further afferent arteriole vasoconstriction)

Drugs those are responsible for alteration of renal hemodynamics

1. **Afferent arteriole vasoconstrictors:**
   Vasodilatory PG inhibitors-NSAIDs;   COX-2 Inhibitors
   Direct afferent Arteriolar vasoconstrictors: Cyclosporine
                                            Amphotericin-B
                                            Radiocontrast media
                                            Vasopressors

2. **Efferent arteriole vasodilators:**
   RAAS: ACEIs/ARBs
   Direct efferent arteriolar vasodilators: CCBs/ diltiazam, verapamil
   Funtional Acute Renal Failure (ARF) is very common in individuals with heart failure receiving ACE Inhibitor (ACEIS) or ARBs inorder to improve their ventricular function. As the decline in efferent arteriole resistance from the inhibition of Angiotensin -II is rapid, if the dose of ARB is increased; it may lead to rise in SCr level and decline or reduced GFR. But if the SCr level rise in mild to moderate (i.e, <30%) medication can be continued.

B. **Pre-Renal acute renal failure:** It is the most common form of AKI (55%). Main reason for pre-renal ARF is decreased blood supply i.e renal hypoperfusion.

Causes of pre- renal ARF

Volume depletion or hypovolemia

(a) **Intravascular hypovolemia** results in arterial hypotension and is caused due to
   - Dehydration: Inadequate fluid intake; Excessive vomiting, diarrhea or gastric suctioning; Increased insensible losses (Fever, burns etc); Diabetes insipidus; glucosuria; Over diuresis
   - Haemorrhage due to decreased cardiac output
   - Hypoalbuminemia: Liver disease; Nephrotic syndrome
     [Albumin helps the body to maintain the intravascular colloidal osmotic pressure and   neutralises toxins and protien binding]

(b) **Arterial hypotension:** Due to Anaphylaxis, sepsis, excessive antihypertensive use

(c) **Decreased cardiac output:** Due to Heart failure, sepsis, pulmonary hypertension, Aorti stenosis

(d) **Isolated renal hypoperfusion**

Causes
- Bilateral arterial (renal arterial) stenosis
- Emboli: Thromboemboli & cholesterol
- Medications - cyclosporine, ACE Inibitor (ACEIS), NSAIDs,
- Radio contrast media.
- Hypercalcemia,
- Hepato renal syndrome.

Mechanisms of pre-renal injury: Because of the predisposing factors like cirrhosis/ liver disease/malnutrition/hormonal disturbances, it leads to decreased albumin synthesis. Nephrotic syndrome, increased albumin catabolism, protein-losing enteropathy conditions lead to increased albumin loss. Systemic inflammation i.e. anaphylaxis, pancreatitis, sepsis causes increased permeability of blood vessels leading to increased albumin extravasation. All these events finally cause hypoalbuminemia. Due to decreased albumin levels in blood, there is decreased plasma osmotic pressure and to maintain osmotic pressure results in fluid extravasation. This finally results in decreased intravascular volume. Because of decreased intravascular volume there is decrease in blood pressure and decrease in stroke volume. Decreased stroke volume leads to decrease in cardiac output which again leads to decreased blood pressure. Because of decreased blood pressure and cardiac output there is decreased renal perfusion, finally leading to pre-renal injury, as kidneys do not receive adequate blood flow to properly carry out their functions.

Other mechanisms of renal hypoperfusion include-

- Vasodilatory drugs cause increased vasodilation, so decreased systemic vascular resistance. Hence decreased blood pressure and renal perfusion leading to pre-renal injury.
- NSAIDs cause decreased prostaglandin synthesis, so decreased afferent arteriole dilation, and so decreased renal perfusion.
- ACIs, ARBs cause decreased Angiotensin-II effects i.e. there is decreased efferent arteriole constriction leading to excessive vasodilatation, decreased blood pressure, decreased renal perfusion.
- Decreased fluid intake/ haemorrhage/ GI loss i.e. diarrhoea. Vomiting, renal loss (osmotic diuretics, diuretics, diabetes insipidus) –all these predisposing factors cause decrease in intravascular volume, so decreased blood pressure, decreased renal perfusion finally leading to pre-renal injury.
- Renal stenosis causes decrease in diameter of renal artery causing renal vasoconstriction. This leads to decreased renal perfusion and renal injury.

C. Intrinsic acute renal failure: 35-40% cases account under intrinsic ARF.

It involves damage or injury within the structure of kidneys.

Acute intrinsic renal failure can be categorized based on structure within the kidney that are injured.

(i) Renal vasculature damage - Renal vasculature

(ii) Glomerular damage - Glomeruli

(iii) Tubular damage (or) Acute tubular necrosis - tubules

(iv) Interstitial damage (or) Acute interstitial nephritis – Interstitium

(i) **Renal vasculature damage:** Possible causes include - vasculitis, hemolytic uremic syndrome, thrombotic thrombocytopenic purpura, atherosclerotic and thrombotic emboli, accelerated HTN.

Occlusion of larger vessels resulting to ARF is not common but can occur if larger emboli occlude in bilateral renal arteries (or) one vessel of the patient with single kidney.

Emboli accumulate in the smaller vessels. These are susceptible to inflammatory processes. Renal capillaries are affected. Undergo microvasculature damage and vessel dysfunction. Neutrophils invade into vessel wall and cause vessel wall damage. This leads to thrombus formation, Tissue infarction and Collagen deposition.

(ii) Glomerular damage:
- Only 5% cases of intrinsic ARF account under glomerular damage.
- Possible causes for glomerular damage include

systemic lupus erythematosus, post streptococcal glomerulonephritis, antiglomerular basement membrane disease.

(iii) Acute tubular necrosis [1,2,3]: Acute Tubular Necrosis (ATN) occurs in part because the renal tubules require high oxygen delivery to maintain their metabolic activity. Consequently, any condition that causes ischemia to the tubules (e.g., hypotension, decreased blood flow) can induce ATN.

(iv) Interstitial damage or acute Interstitial Nephritis: It is the rare causative reason for intrinsic ARF out of which 30% of cases have no identifiable cause. Acute interstitial nephritis is most commonly caused by medications or bacterial or viral infections. Medications such as NSAIDs, certain Antibiotics, Drugs - penicillin's, ciprofloxacin, sulphonamides. Formation of immune complexes within the interstitium, or interstitial infiltration with T cells, will result in an inflammatory reaction. This reaction is triggered by many events, including activation of the complement cascade by antibodies and release of inflammatory cytokines by T lymphocytes and phagocytes. Although the interstitial inflammatory reaction may resolve without sequelae, it sometimes induces interstitial fibroblast proliferation and extracellular matrix synthesis, leading to interstitial fibrosis and chronic renal failure. Cytokines such as transforming growth factor β appear to play a key role in the latter process.

D. Post renal failure: Less than 5% cases of ARF are due to post renal failure.

Causes: Bladder obstruction - Prostatic hypertrophy, infection, cancer, anti cholinergic medication, improperly placed urinary catheter.

Ureteral - cancer with abdomianl mass

Retroperitoneal fibrosis, nephrolithiasis

Renal pelvis / tubules: Nephrolithiasis, oxalate, uric acid, sulphonamides, acyclovir, indinavir.

Clinical Manifestation and Features of Acute Renal Failure (ARF)

General symptoms: Decrease urine out put; decrease BUN, SCr levels

Community dwelling patients are at less risk

Hospitalised patients may develop ARF after either notable reduction in B.P/obstruction (sudden) after catheterization.

Symptoms

Out patient: Change in urinary habits, sudden weight gain; flank pain.

BARF is recognised by physicians, before patient (who may not experience any obvious symptoms).

Signs: Odema, urine coloured / foamy, Orthostatic hypotension - volume depleted patients.

Hypertension - fluid overload patients (or) chronic hypertensive kidney disease.

Diagnosis with Algorithm

Laboratory Tests

Elevation in the serum potassium, BUN, creatinine and phosphorus.

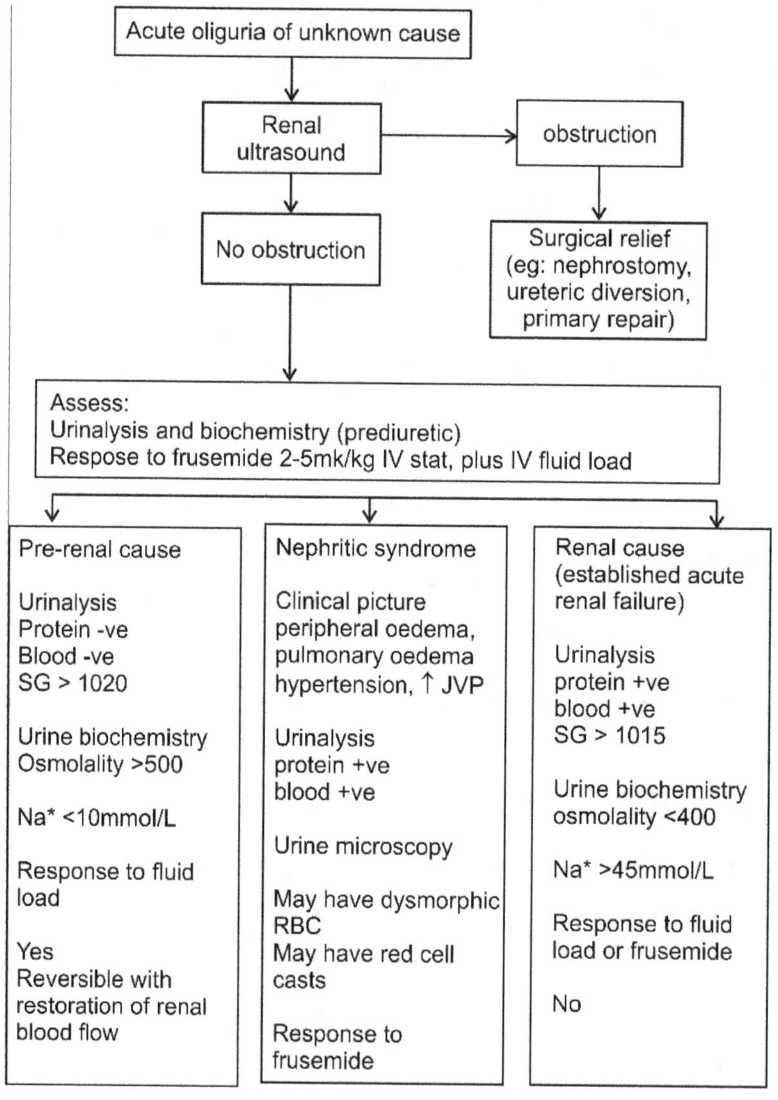

Fig. 20.1 Algorithm for the diagnosis of acute renal failure. Kidney Disease: Improving Global Outcomes (KDIGO) Acute Kidney Injury Work Group. KDIGO clinical practice guideline for acute kidney injury. *Kidney Int Suppl.* 2012;2(suppl 1):1-138.

Reduction in calcium and PH (acidosis) may occur

Clinical findings are different based on the cause of the ARF.

Other diagnostic tests include renal ultrasonography / cytoscopy; renal biopsy (rarely used).

Table 20.2 Diagnostic Parameters for different causes of AKI.

Laboratory test	Pre renal	Intra renal	Post renal
Urine sediment	Hyaline casts, may be normal	Granular casts,cellular debris	Cellular debris
Urinary RBC	None	2-4+	Variable
Urinary WBC	None	2-4+	1+
Urine Na (meq/l)	<20	>40	>40
Fractional excretion of sodium	<1	>2	Variable
Urine/ serum osmolarity	>1.5	<1.3	<1.5
Urine/Scr	>40:1	<20:1	<20:1
BUN/Scr	>20(>80)	~15(~60)	~15(~60)
Urine specific gravity	>1.018	<1.012	Variable

Urinary finding

1. **Urine analysis:** Presence of leucocyte esterases /nitrates-It may indicate pyelonephritis
   Protien mild (<0.5 g/day) indicates Tubular damage
   Moderate (0.5 -3g/day) Glomerulo nephritis, pyelonephritis, tubular damage
   Severe (>3g /day) Glomerulonephritis, Nephrotic syndrome
   Haemoglobin - suggestive of Glomerulo nephritis, pyclonephritis, renal infarction, renal tumors, kidney stones.
   Urine sediment: Presence of Micro organisms-indicates pyelonephritis
   Cells:
   Red blood cells - glomerulo nephritis , pyelonephritis, renal infarction, papillary necrosis , renal tumors, kidney stones.
   White blood cells- pyelonephritis , interstitial nephritis
   Eosinophills - Drug induced interstitial nephritis, renal transplantation rejection
   Casts:
   Granular casts- Tubular necrosis
   Hyaline casts- Pre -renal Azotemia
   White blood cell casts - pyelonephritis , interstitial nephritis
   Red blood cell casts - Glomerulo nephritis , renal infarct, lupus nephritis , vasculitis

Crystals:
Urate- post renal obstruction
Calcium phosphate - post renal obstruction
Serum white blood cell increased - sepsis associated ARF

Contrast Induced Nephropathy [4, 5]

Impairment of kidney function characterised by 25% increase in Scr from base line within 48 - 72 hrs after IV contrast administration.

Mechanism: Increased Concentration of dye usage causes higher penetration of it into blood and tissues (I2 solution/suspension of $BaSO_4$). It results in Oxidative stress mediated Nephrotoxicity   These dyes are used in procedures - CABG, PTCA

Treatment for CIN

Pharmacological therapy

N- Acetyl cysteine - It is a thiol compound. Powerful antioxidant, Anti infective, vasodilator.

Mechanism - It involves in minimizing with vasoconstriction and oxygen free radical generation after radio contrast administration. Hydration is used to prevent contrast induced nephropathy [CIN] which is a common cause of ATN. Use of isotonic crystalloids over colloids and parenteral therapy over oral is preferred in high risk patients, including CKD, Diabetes, volume depletion, concurrent nephrotoxic drug therapy.

KDIGO guidelines recommend either sodium bicarbonate (or) normal saline infusions.

$NaHCO_3$ regimen - 154 m eq / l infused at 3ml/ kg /h for 1 hr - pre procedure

1ml/ kg/hr for 6 hrs - After procedure

Normal saline regimen - 1ml/ kg/ h for 12 hrs - pre and post procedure

Strict glycemic controle with insulin diabetes has also redused the development of ARF.

| Ascoirbic acid | 3g | oral | BD | daily | pre procedure |
| Anti-oxidant | 2g | oral | BD | daily | post procedure |

Prevention of CIN

N-acetylcystiene 600-1200mg oral/every 12hrs/2-3days

KDIGO guidelines for moderate control of blood glucose 110-149mg/dl with insulin and also recommended to limit use of loop diuretics to manage fluid overload.

Management

Goals - To avoid/minimise the degree of insult to the kidney.

To reduce extra renal complications

Restoration of renal functioning to pre-AKI base line.

Treatment of Acute Renal Failure

Treatment Algorithm [6]

> If the Laboratory tests results consistent with acute renal failure (rise of 0.5 mg per dL or a 50 % increase in creatintine above the baseline or a 50% decrease in baseline calculated GFR).
> Take the complete medical history, current mediacations, review of systems to include systemic symptoms (fever, weight loss) and physical exmaination to include vital signs, heart, lung, abdominal, pelvic, rectal and skin examinations.
> If likely cause of acute renal failure is apparent then confirm the diagnosis with appropriate tests to identify the cause and treat the cause.
> If no apparent cause is identified, elctrolytes/ urinalysis with microscopic examination/ renal ultrasound has to be done.
> **Pre-renal failure:** If BUN to creatinine ratio is > 20:1/ FENa < 1 percent/ urine specific gravity > 1.020/Hyaline casts in urine sediment/ no evidence off obstruction
> **Treatment** : hydrate/ eliminate toxins/ treat causes.
> **Intrarenal failure:** If BUN to creatinine ratio is 10: 1 to 20:1/ FENa > 1 percent/ urine specific gravity 1.010 to 1.020/ tubular or granular casts in urine/ultrasound showing medical kidney disease or normal, no obstruction
> **Treatment:** Take CBC/ ESR Consider nephrology consult, kidney biopsy/ eliminate toxins/ treat causes.
> **Postrenal failure:** Ultrasound shows hydronephrosis/ serum and urine tets have simialar results as inrarenal causes.
> **Treatment:** Order CT scan/ relieve obstruction/ consider urology consult.

Non-pharmacological

1. Supportive care goals include maintenance of adequate cardiac output and blood pressure to optimize tissue perfusion
2. Renal Replacement Therapy (RRT) such as hemodialysis and peritoneal dialysis should be done in severe AKI, in order to maintain fluid and electrolyte balance, while removing waste products. medications associated with decrease in renal blood flow should be stopped and nephrotoxins should be avoided in patients with ARF.

Table 20.3 Common Indications for RRT.

	Indications	Clinical setting
A	Acid base abnormalities	Metabolic acidosis resulting from the accumulation of organic and in-organic acids
E	Elecrolyte Imbalance	Hyperkalemia ,hypermagnesia
I	Intoxications	salicylates, lithium, methanol, ethylene glycol, theophyline , phenobarbital
O	Over load of fluid	Post operative fluid over load
U	Uremia	Accumilation of uremic toxins

Forms of renal replacement therapy

The common types of renal replacement therapy used in clinical practice are: • haemodialysis • haemofiltration • haemodiafiltration • peritoneal dialysis

1. **Haemodialysis:** This is placed in a vein (the jugular, femoral or subclavian), which has an arterial lumen through which the blood is removed from the patient and a venous lumen by which it is returned to the patient after passing through a dialyser. Haemodialysis can also be used in patients who have recently undergone abdominal surgery in whom peritoneal dialysis would be ill advised.

   Intermittent haemodialysis- commonly used RRT lasting for 3-4hrs

   Disadvantages - Difficult venous dialysis access in hypotensive patients (rapid removal of large amounts of fluid)

   Continuous hemodialysis

   Advantage: Removes solutes gradually, useful in critically ill patients

   Disadvantage: Limited availibilty of equipment.

2. **Haemofiltration:** Haemofiltration is an alternative technique to dialysis where simplicity of use, fine fluid balance control and low cost have ensured its widespread use in the treatment of AKI. The hydrostatic pressure of the blood drives a filtrate, similar to interstitial fluid, across a high permeability dialyser (passes substances of molecular weight up to 30,000) by ultrafiltration. Solute clearance occurs by convection.

3. **Haemodiafiltration:** Haemodiafiltration is a technique that combines the ability to clear small molecules, as in haemodialysis, with the large molecule clearance of haemofiltration.

4. **Acute peritoneal dialysis:** Acute peritoneal dialysis is rarely used now for AKI except in circumstances where haemodialysis is unavailable. Warmed sterile peritoneal dialysis fluid (typically 1–2L) is instilled into the abdomen, left for a period of about 30 min (dwell time) and then drained into a collecting bag.

Pharmacological Therapy [7]

Diuretics: Diuretics facilitate the management of fluid overload. Continuous infusions of loop diuretics are more effective and have fewer ADRS than intermittent boluses.

(a)   Loop diuretics –Disadvantages: can worsen AKI
      Furosemide; bumetanide; torsemide; ethacrynic acid
      Furosemide   40-80mg   initial   I.V [loading dose]
                    10-20mg/hr   continuous infusion
      Ethacrynic acid is restricted to sulpha allergic pts.
      Metolazone
(b)   Thiazides: Commonly used as it produces effective diuresis at GFR les than 20ml/min
      than ccompared to other thiazides
(c)   Osmotic diuretics
      Mannitol 20% 12.5-25g infused at   rate of over   3-5min.
      Disadvantages: On IV administration-hyposmolarity risk. Need for monitoring
      because mannitol itself can contribute ARF

Treatment algorithm for ICU-acquired oliguric acute renal failure resulting from acute tubular necrosis

1. If ICU-acquired, acute oliguria secondary to suspected acute tubular necrosis is identified.
2. Correct correctible causes Remove as many nephrotoxins as possible Adjust all drug doses for creatinine clearance. Immediately furosemide 80mg to be initiated.
3. If urine output > 1 mL/kg/h with 1 H: adminster furosemide 80mg IV q 6-8 h or 10mg/h/IV. Later Titrate furosemide dose to maintain urine output of >1 mL/kg/h.
4. IF urine output is not > 1 mL/kg/h: administer furosemide 400mg.
5. Measure urine output:
   (a) If it is now > 1 mL/kg/h with 2 h, then administer Furosemide 40 mg/h IV as long as urine output >1 mL/kg/h until euvolemic.
   (b) If still target is not reached, Furosemide 400 mg IV + chlorothiazide 500 mg shoud be administered. Later measure output-if Urine output >1 mL/kg/h within 2 h- Continue chlorothiazide 500 mg q 12h and: Furosemide 40 mg/h IV as long as urine output >1 mL/kg/h until euvolemic.
   (c) Consider renal replacement therapy if: • pulmonary edema • hyperkalemia • acidosis • azotemia

Diuretic Resistance

It is the inability to respond to the administered drug diuretics especially observed in ARF.

Common causes of diuretic resistance in pts with AKI

(a) **Excessive sodium intake:** Sourses - diet, iv fluids, drugs. Potential therapeutic solutions - remove sodium from nut sources and mediccations.
(b) **Inadequate diuretic dose or Inappropriate regimen:** Therapeutic solutions - increase dose, use continuous infusion or combination therapy
(c) **Reduced oral bio availability:** Therapeutic solutions - use parenteral therapy. Switch to oral torsemide or bumetanide
(d) **Nephrotic syndrome:** Therapeutic conditions - increase dose. Switch to diuretics; use combination therapy

(e) **Reduced renal blood flow:** Drugs - NSAIDs, ACEIS, Vasodilators. Therapeutic solutions - discontinue the above drugs if possible

(f) **Heart failure:** Treat heart failure. Increase diuretic dose -Switch to better absorbed loop diuretic

(g) **Cirrhosis:** Therapeutic solutions - High volume paracentesis

(h) **Acute tubular necrosis:** Therapeutic conditions- Higher dose of diuretic, diuretic combination therapy. Add low – dose dopamine

Electrolyte management and nutrition interventions

1. Hyperkalemia is most common and serious electrolyte abnormality in AKI:
   Emergency treatment of hyperkalaemia consists of the following:
   1. 10–30mL (2.25–6.75mmol) of calcium gluconate 10% intravenously over 5–10 min; this improves myocardial stability but has no effect on the serum potassium levels. The protective effect begins in minutes but is short lived (< 1h), although the dose can be repeated.
   2. 50mL of 50% glucose together with 8–12 units of soluble insulin over 10 min. Endogenous insulin, stimulated by a glucose load or administered intravenously, stimulates intracellular potassium uptake, thus removing it from the serum. The effect becomes apparent after 15–30 min, peaks after about 1h and lasts for 2–3h and will decrease serum potassium levels by around 1mmol/L.
   3. Nebulised salbutamol has also been used to lower potassium; however, this is not effective for all patients and does not permanently lower potassium. If used it is seen as a temporary emergency measure.

2. Hypernatremia and fluid retention commonly occur; calculation of daily sodium intake is required. Intravascular fluid overload must be managed by restricting NaCl intake to about 1–2g/day if the patient is not hyponatraemic and total fluid intake to less than 1L/day.

3. Hyperphosphataemia: phosphate-binding agents may be used to retain phosphate ions in the gut.

4. Hypocalcaemia: oral calcium supplementation with calcium carbonate is usually adequate.

5. Infection: Patients with AKI are prone to infection and septicaemia, which can ultimately cause death. Antibiotic therapy should be broad spectrum until a causative organism is identified.

6. Nutrition: There are two major constraints concerning the nutrition of patients with AKI:
   - patients may be anorexic, vomiting and too ill to eat;
   - oliguria associated with renal failure limits the volume of enteral or parenteral nutrition that can be given safely.

Drug dosing considerations

1. We should monitor drug clearance, fluid accumulation in AKI pts.
2. In oedematic conditions, volume of distribution for water soluble drugs is increased.
3. Patients with AKI have higher residual non -renal clearance than those with CKD

Diagnosis, evaluation, and management of acute kidney injury: a KDIGO summary [8]

The six major domains are: (A) definition and staging; (B) risk assessment; (C) evaluation and general management; (D) prevention and treatment; (E) contrast-induced AKI; and (F) RRT for AKI.

1. **AKI is defined as any of the following (not graded):**
   - increase in SCr by $\geq$0.3 mg/dl ($\geq$26.5 µmol/l) within 48 hours; or
   - increase in SCr to $\geq$1.5 times baseline, which is known or presumed to have occurred within the prior 7 days; or
   - urine volume <0.5 ml/kg/hour for 6 hours.

   AKI is staged for severity according to the criteria

2. **Risk assessment:** Causes of acute kidney injury: exposures and susceptibilities for nonspecific acute kidney injury

   Exposures: sepsis, critical illness, burns, trauma, cardiac surgery, nephrotoxic drugs, radiocontarst agents, poisonous plants and animals

   Susceptibility: dehydration or volume depletion, advanced age, female gender, CKD, chronic disease-heart, lung, liver; diabetes mellitus, cancer, anemia

3. **Evaluation and general management:** Evaluate patients with AKI promptly to determine the cause, with special attention to reversible causes (not graded)
   - Monitor patients with AKI with measurements of SCr and urine output to stage the severity
   - Manage patients with AKI according to the stage and cause
   - Evaluate patients 3 months after AKI for resolution, new onset, or worsening of pre-existing chronic kidney disease (CKD)
   - If patients have CKD, manage these patients as detailed in the Kidney Disease Outcomes
   - If patients do not have CKD, consider them to be at increased risk for CKD and care for them as detailed in the Kidney Disease Outcomes Quality Initiative CKD

4. **Prevention and treatment of AKI:**
   - In the absence of hemorrhagic shock, we suggest using isotonic crystalloids rather than colloids (albumin or starches) as initial management for expansion of intravascular volume in patients at risk for AKI or with AKI (Grade 2B)
   - We recommend the use of vasopressors in conjunction with fluids in patients with vasomotor shock with, or at risk for, AKI (Grade 1C)
   - We suggest using protocol-based management of hemodynamic and oxygenation parameters to prevent development or worsening of AKI in high-risk patients in the perioperative setting (Grade 2C) or in patients with septic shock (Grade 2C)

- In critically ill patients, we suggest insulin therapy targeting plasma glucose 110 to 149 mg/dl (6.1 to 8.3 mmol/l) (Grade 2C)
- We suggest achieving a total energy intake of 20 to 30 kcal/kg/day in patients with any stage of AKI (Grade 2C)
- We suggest avoiding restriction of protein intake with the aim of preventing or delaying initiation of RRT (Grade 2D)
- We suggest administering 0.8 to 1.0 g/kg/day protein in noncatabolic AKI patients without need for dialysis (Grade 2D), 1.0 to 1.5 g/kg/day in patients with AKI on RRT (Grade 2D), and up to a maximum of 1.7 g/kg/day in patients on CRRT and in hypercatabolic patients (Grade 2D)
- We suggest providing nutrition preferentially via the enteral route in patients with AKI (Grade 2C)
- We recommend not using diuretics to prevent AKI (Grade 1B)
- We suggest not using diuretics to treat AKI, except in the management of volume overload (Grade 2C)
- We recommend not using low-dose dopamine to prevent or treat AKI (Grade 1A)
- We suggest not using fenoldopam to prevent or treat AKI (Grade 2C)
- We suggest not using ANP to prevent (Grade 2C) or treat (Grade 2B) AKI

A Case Study of Acute Kidney Injury

Summary: A 52 Year old patient was admitted into the hospital with the symptoms which include multiple episodes of vomiting, headache, body pains, generalized weakness and she was suffering with fever since 2 days. She has a past medical history of hypertension and coronary artery disease. By her complete blood picture we find a slight increase in the WBCs by 1200cell/cumm. Urine analysis show turbid appearance of urine, increased albumin presence and including with pus cells. When she had gone through biochemical investigations, serum creatinine and blood urea are found to be raised and also we find that serum electrolyte levels are raised. Urine analysis shows turbid appearance, presence of pus cells, albumin. Biochemical investigations- serum electrolytes increased levels and calculus in the gall bladder, thsesact as diagnostic factors of AKI.

Diagnosis: As the patient has CAD and HTN, they act as stimulating risk factors of AKI.

Treatment:

InjEmset	Ondansetron	4mg
InjProtera	Pantaprazole	40mg
InjOptineuron	Multivitamin	1amp
T. Met XL	Metopolol	25mg OD
T.Lipikind	Atorvastatain	20mg
T.Clopitab	Clopidogrel	75mg OD
InjSpecipime	Cefipime+tazobactum	1.125mg

Daily progress: Patient came on complaints with fever and vomiting which reduced by the next day. On the day three body pains came to an end and day four shows reduced creatinine tissue.

Discharge Medications

T.Doxef	Cefpodoxime	200mg	BD
T.Hoperab	Rabeprazole	20 mg	OD
T.Clopitab	Clopidogrel	75mg	OD
T.Lipikind	Atorvastatain	20mg	OD
T.Met XL	Metoprolol	25mg	OD
T.Neurokind	Multivitamin	1sc	OD

Patient Counselling Measures

1. Decreased fluid intake.
2. Restrict the use of certain drugs.
3. Restricted diet of Na^+, P, K^+.
4. Good nutrition maintenance should be done.

Assignment

1. **How is AKI defined?**

   A sudden loss of kidney function caused by failure of renal circulation or damage to tubules or glomeruli is a reversible condition.

   Urine volume can be variable:

   Anuria- less than 50ml/day

   Oliguria – 100-400 ml /day

   Non-oliguria- greater than 400ml/day.

2. **What are the ocular, cardio vascular, pulmonary, abdominal signs and symptoms of AKI?**

   Ocular: keratitis, iritis, uveitis, dry conjunctivae, auto immune vasculitis, jaundice, band keratopathy, multiple myeloma, signs of DM, HTN and retinopathy.

   Cardiovascular: irregular rythms, thrombo emboli, murmurs, endocarditis, pericardial friction rub, increased jugular venous distentions.

   Pulomonary: pulmonary edema, infectious pulomonary process, hemoptysis, antiglomerular basement membrane syndrome.

   Abdominal: pulsatile mass or bruit, atheroemboli, abdominal or costoverbal angle tenderness, nephrolithiasis, renal artery thrombosis.

   Pelvic and rectal masses: prostatic hypertrophy, distant bladder, urinary obstruction etc

3. **What are the cardiovascular, pulmonary, GI, neurologic complications of AKI?**

   CVS complications: HF, MI, Arrythmias, cardiac arrest, fluid overload, pericarditis, endocarditis, atrial fibrillation with emboli.

Pulmonary complications: good pasture syndrome, granulomatosis with polyangitis, globulinemia, sarcoidosis.

GI complications: nausea, vomiting anorexia, pancreatitis, jaundice, hepatitis

Neurologic complications: SLE, thrombotic thrombocytopenic purpura, hemolytic uresnic syndrome, malignant HTN.

4. **What comorbid conditions increase the risk of AKI?**

   Patient related include male gender, COPD, diabetes, peripheral vascular disease, renal insufficiency, cardiogenic shock, cardiac arrest, previous cardiac surgery, CABG, preoperative creatinine etc

   Procedure related: CPB time, cross clamp time, on pump Vs off pump, heamolysis, pulsatile vs non pulsatile etc

5. **How is volume homeostasis maintained in treatment of AKI?**

   Maintenance of volume homeostasis is one of the primary goals of treatment which includes the following measures:

   Correction of fluid overload with furosemide

   Correction of severe acidosis with bicarbonate administration.

   Correction of hyperkalemia

   Correction of haematological abnormalities like anemia, uremia with measures such as transfusions and administration of desmopressin.

   Dialysis: Volume expansion that cannot be managed with diuretics, hyperkalemia, refractory to medical therapy, Correction of severe acid base disturbances, Severe azotemia, uremia – all these patients should follow volume dialysis.

6. **What is the role of a) furosemide b) vasodilators c) CRTT d) saline e) sodium bicarbonate f) forced diuresis g) N-acetyl cysteine**

   (a) Furosemide: It increases the extraction of water by interfering with the Cl binding co transport system which inhibits sodium and chloride reabsorption.

   (b) Vasodilators:They decrease systemic vascular resistance and increases renal blood flow to cortex and medulla. It improves renal function in patients with severe hypertension.

   (c) Continuous Renal Replacement Therapy (CRTT): It is a slow and continuous extra corporeal blood purification therapy. It mimics the functions of the kidney in regulatory water electrolytes and toxic products by slow continuous removal of solutes and fluids. Used for patients who are haemodynamically unstable.

   (d) Saline: In patients undergoing imaging studies with contrast prophylactic administration of IV saline shows decrease in incidence of contrast nephropathy.

   (e) Sodium bicarbonate: It can be used in patients who are at high risk for volume over load, CHF, left ventricular dysfunction of less than 40% - isotonic sodium bicarbonate should be administered before and after procedure.

   (f) Forced diuresis: It enhances the excretion of certain drugs in urine and used to treat drug overdose or poisoning of these drugs and haemorrhagic cystitis.

   (g) Saline diuresis: enhances renal excretion of alcohols, bromide, chromium, chloride, isoniazid etc

Alkaline diuresis: enhances excretion of chlorpropamide, salicylates, methotrexate etc

(g) N-Acetyl Cysteine: this is administered to high risk patients the day before a contrast study is performed and is continued on the day of procedure. Just provides border line benefit.

7. What is included in long term monitoring of AKI?

When renal recovery is not complete, with the kidneys remaining vulnerable to nephrotoxic effects of all the therapeutic agents . Renal recovery is usually observed within the first two weeks and many nephrologists tend to diagnose patients with end stage renal failure 6-8 weeks after the onset of AKI. It is always better to check these patients periodically, because some patients may regain renal function much later.

8. Which medications of drug class are used in treatment of AKI?

(a) Antidote: N-acetyl cysteine: This drug provides substrate for conjugation with toxic metabolites. It is used for the prevention of contrast induced toxicity in susceptible individuals such as those with DM. The mechanism is presumed by its ability to scavenge free radicals and improve endothelium dependent vasodilation.

(b) Calcium channel blockers: Nifedipine: It relaxes smooth muscle and produces vasodilation which in turn improves blood flow.

(c) Vasodilators: Fenoldopam: It is selective dopamine receptor agonist which acts as arapid acting vasodilator. It is 6 times more potent than dopamine and increases diuresis. Used in HTN and renal compromised patients.

(d) Ionotropic agents: Dopamine: it stimulates adrenergic and dopaminergic receptors and causes vasodilation in small doses.

(e) Loop diuretics: Furosemide: Increases excretion of water by interfering with chloride binding transport system which causes sodium and chloride reabsorption in loop of henle and Distal Convuluted Turbule (DST).

References

1. Robert W Schrier et al., Acute renal failure: definitions, diagnosis, pathogenesis, and therapy. J Clin Invest. 2004;114(1):5-14.

2. Molitoris BA, Sutton TA (2004). "Endothelial injury and dysfunction: role in the extension phase of acute renal failure". *Kidney Int.* 66 (2): 496–9.

3. Fogo A, Cohen AH, Colvin RB et al. Fundamentals of Renal Pathology. Springer 2013. Acute Tubular Necrosis.

4. Pannu N, Manns B, Lee H, Tonelli M. Systematic review of the impact of N-acetylcysteine on contrast nephropathy. *Kidney Int.* 2004 Apr. 65(4):1366-74.

5. Majumdar SR, Kjellstrand CM, Tymchak WJ, Hervas-Malo M, Taylor DA, Teo KK. Forced euvolemic diuresis with mannitol and furosemide for prevention of contrast-induced nephropathy in patients with CKD undergoing coronary angiography: a randomized controlled trial. *Am J Kidney Dis.* 2009 Oct. 54 (4):602-9.

6. Eddie needham. Management of acute renal failure. Am Fam Physician, 2005;7299: 1739-46.

7. Feest TG, Mistry CD, Grimes DS, Mallick NP. Incidence of advanced chronic renal failure and the need for end stage renal replacement treatment. *BMJ*. 1990 Oct 20. 301(6757):897-900.

8. John AK et al., Diagnosis, evaluation, and management of acute kidney injury: a KDIGO summary. Critical care 2013; 17(1): 204.

CHAPTER - 21

Chronic Kidney Disease

Introduction to Chronic Kidney Disease

Generally, kidneys contain 2 million nephrons which under normal conditions work in an organized manner to filter, reabsorb and excrete various solutes and water. Kidney is a 1^0 regulator of sodium-water balance, acid-base homeostasis. Kidney also produces hormones necessary for RBC synthesis and calcium homeostasis. Impairment of kidney function is referred to as kidney disease. Based on the time course of development, kidney disease is mainly classified into two types- Acute renal failure: Rapid loss of kidney function over days to weeks and Chronic kidney disease.

Chronic Kidney Disease

Definition: It is defined as a progressive loss of kidney function occurring over several months to years and is characterized by replacement of normal kidney architecture with interstitial fibrosis. In simple, it is defined as abnormal kidney structure/function present for 3 months or longer with implications for health. CKD is also called as Chronic Renal Insufficiency (or) Progressive Kidney Disease

Classification

- National kidney foundation (NKF) Kidney Dialysis Outcomes and Quality Initiative (KDOQI) has developed a classification based on structural and functional changes in kidney, Glomerular Filtration Rate (GFR).
- According to this NKDQI, CKD is classified into 5 stages
- GFR in adults with normal kidney function is 120ml/min/1.73m^2 (>90ml/min/1.73m^2)
- Along with GFR, CKD patients are also diagnosed to have proteinuria, haematuria.

Table 21.1 Diferrent stges of CKD.

STAGE	GFR (ml/min)	TERMS
1	>90	Normal/High
2	60-89	Mildly decreased
3a	45-59	Mildly to moderately decreased
3b	30-44	Moderately to severely decreased
4	15-29	Severely decreased
5	<15	Kidney failure

Stage 5 is also referred to as End-Stage Renal Disease (ESRD)

Epidemiology

According to United States Renal Data System (USRD's), Around 10.9% of U.S. population (19 million) of age 20 years or older suffer with CKD (with proteinuria, microalbuminuria, increase in serum creatinine). The number of patients entering stage 5 increased by 5% to 10% per year from 1980-2000. CKD has been described as a silent epidemic and is a world wide public health problem

→ The causes and incidence rates include:
- Diabetic nephropathy (150 cases/million)
- Hypertensive nephropathy (80 cases/million)
- Glomerulonephritis (22 cases/million)
- Polycystic kidney disease (5 cases/million)

→ Individuals over 65 years of age and black race are at higher risk of CKD

Etiology

I. **Susceptibility factors** – Advanced stage
Racial/Ethnic minority status
Low birth weight
Family history
Systemic inflammation
Dyslipidaemia

⎫ Main cause for CKD

II. **Initiation factors** – These factors directly result in kidney damage and are modifiable by pharmacologic therapy
- Diabetes mellitus / HTN / Autoimmune disease
- Polycystic kidney disease / Systemic infections
- UTI's/ Urinary stones / Urinary tract obstructions
- Drug Toxicity

Among all these Diabetes, HTN and Glomerular disease are the most common causes for CKD

- **Diabetes mellitus:** Life time risk for developing CKD 40% by type 1DM and 50% by type 2DM
- **Hypertension:** HTN generally develops concomitantly with progressive kidney disease. Elevated BP increases the risk for development of CKD among subjects without initial kidney disease
- **Glomerulonephritis:** Immunoglobulin (Ig) A nephropathy, membranous nephropathy, focal segmental glomerulosclerosis, lupus nephritis etc., are considered causes of CKD

III. **Progression factors:** These factors result in the increase in the rate of decline in kidney function in those who already have damaged kidneys.
- **Proteinuria:** In diabetic patientalbumin excretion rate (>30 mg/day) predicted the development of nephropathy and subsequent loss of kidney function

- **Hypertension:** Improper maintenance of BP leads to further progressions of CKD. Early treatment of HTN and achievement of target values resulted in slowing the rate of progression of CKD
- **Diabetes mellitus:** Hyperglycaemia is an initiation and progression risk factor for CKD. Maintenance of glucose levels especially in type 1 DM reduced the chances for retinopathy, albuminuria.
- **Smoking:** In conditions like diabetes, HTN and Glomerulonephritis, smoking may romote initiation and progression of CKD
- **Hyperlipidaemia:** The prevalence of hyperlipidaemia appears to increase as kidney function declines. Treatment of lipid abnormalities in patients with CKD may slows/reduces the rate of progression
- **Obesity:** Obesity among men and morbid obesity among women is associated with increase in risk for CKD
- Drug Induced CKD- Prolong use of aminoglycosides / NSAIDs

Pathophysiology

Kidney damage can result from heterogenous causes. Initial structural damage depends on the primary disease affecting the kidney. Once half of the total nephrons are lost, CKD progresses similarly regardless of etiology. The remaining nephrons undergo hypertrophy to compensate for the loss of renal function and nephron mass. Initially, this compensatory hypertrophy may be adaptive. Over time, the hyper-trophy can lead to the development of intraglomerular hypertension mediated by angiotensin –II, resulting in increased urinary excretion of albumin and frank proteinuria. Proteinuria alone may promote progressive loss of nephrons as a result of direct cellular damage. Filtered proteins such as albumin, transferrin, complement factors, immunoglobulins, cytokines, and angiotensin II are toxic to kidney tubular cells. Proteins in the renal tubule activates tubular cells which leads to the upregulated production of inflammatory and vasoactive cytokines, such as endothelin, monocyte chemoattractant protein (MCP-1), and RANTES (regulated upon activation, normal T-cell expressed and secreted). Proteinuria is also associated with the activation of complement components on the apical membrane of proximal tubules. These events ultimately lead to scarring of the interstitium, progressive loss of structural nephron units, and reduction in GFR.

Clinical Manifestations and Features

Symptoms: Stage 1&2- Generally asymptomatic

Stage 3&4- Minimal

General symptoms: Oedema, cold tolerance, SOB, palpitations, cramping, muscle pain, depression, anxiety, fatigue, sexual dysfunction

Signs:
- ➤ **Cardiovascular pulmonary:** Oedema, worsening HTN, ECG evidence of left ventricular hypertrophy, arrhythmias, hyper homocysteine, dyslipidaemia

> **Gastrointestinal:** Gastroesophageal reflux disease, weight gain
> **Endocrine:** $2°$ hyperparathyroidism, decreased vitamin D activation, beta 2 – macroglobulin deposition, gout
> **Hematologic:** Anaemia of CKD, iron deficiency, bleeding
> **Fluid/Electrolytes:** Hyponatremia, hyperkalaemia, metabolic acidosis

Diagnosis with Algorithm

Stages of CKD and recommended action plan

Stage 1: Kidney damage with normal or increased GFR- ≥ 90 : diagnose and treat kidney disease and comorbid comorbid conditions, slow progression, reduce cardiovascular risk

Stage 2: Kidney damage with mild decreased GFR- 60-89: estimate progression

Stage 3a: Lid to moderate decreased GFR: 45-59: evaluate and treat complications

Stage 3b: Moderately to severely decreased GFR: 30-44: evaluate and treat complications

Stage 4: Severely decreased GFR: 15-29: prepare for renal replacement therapy

Stage 5: Kidney failure: < 15: renal replacement therapy

- Serum creatinine (0.6-1.4 mg/dl), BUN (7 to 20 mg/dl)
- GFR measurement (120 ml/min/$1.73m^2$)
- Urinalysis (for presence of albumin, protein, pus cells etc.,)
- Imaging studies of kidneys – to know regarding fibrosis/sclerosis
- Proteinuria and Albuminuria (<30 mg/day)
- Kidney biopsy
- Blood test
  1. Haemoglobin (HB) levels (11-16 g/dl)
  2. Vit D levels (20 to 50 ng/ml)
  3. Ca levels (10-10.7 mg/dl)
  4. Parathyroid hormone (10-75 pg/ml)
  5. Phosphorous levels (2.5 to 4.5 mg/dl)
  6. Potassium levels (3.5-5 m eq/l)
  7. LDL (<130 mg/dl)
  8. TG's (<150 mg/dl)
  9. Bicarbonate levels (23-30 m eq/L)
  10. HDL (>60 mg/dl)

Decreased levels are observed for – Creatinine clearance, Bicarbonate, Hb, Vit D, Albumin, Glucose, Calcium, HDL

Increased levels – Serum creatinine, BUN, Potassium, Phosphorous, Parathyroid Hormone (PTH), BP, Glucose, LDL, TG's, T4 levels, Calcium (ESRD)

- **Creatinine clearance:**   Female (88-128 ml/min)
                                Male (97-137 ml/min)

- Random Blood Glucose (70-100 mg/dl)
- T4 levels (4.6-12 ug/dl)

Complications Leading to CKD

I. **Diabetic nephropathy:** Chronic hyperglycemiais thought to be the primary cause of diabetic nephropathy. Unlike other tissues of the body, transmembrane glucose transporters (GLUT) receptors do not facilitate intracellular glucose transport in the kidneys. This effect is mediated via a number of mechanisms including (i) glomerular hyperfiltration, (ii) direct effects of hyperglycemia, and (iii) advanced glycosylation end products (AGE), and (iv) cytokine secretion.

- **Glomerular hyperfiltration:** Glomerular hyperfiltration is mediated mainly via dilatation the afferent arteriole leading to a rise in the GFR and the renal blood flow. This dilatation of the afferent arteriole is mediated by a number of mechanisms in diabetic nephropathy. Hyperglycemia and high insulin-like growth factor-1 (IGF-1) concentrations (observed in diabetic patients) – both are hypothesized to cause a rise in the GFR increasing renal flow. Hyperfiltration of glucose leads to augmented sodium-glucose transport in the proximal convoluted tubule causing enhanced sodium transport
  - Cause expansion of blood volume which leads to a rise in GFR
  - The rise in proximal reabsorption also leads to a reduced distal fluid delivery which activates the tubuloglomerular feedback with the renin-angiotensin system which works to raise the GFR as well.
- **Hyperglycemia and AGE:** Hyperglycemia and Advanced Glycation End Products (AGE) directly induce mesangial matrix production, cellular expansion and apoptosis. The two have also been shown to increase basement membrane permeability to albumin.
- **Cytokines:** Elevations in vascular endothelial growth factor (VEGF), transforming growth factor beta (TFG-β), and profibrotic proteins increase damage to the nephrons at different levels; specific mechanisms are unclear.

II. **Hypertension:** Elevated blood pressure causes a hypertrophic response leading to intimal thickening of the large and small vasculature leading to glomerular damage.

III. **Dyslipidaemia:** There is decrease in HDL, Increase in LDL, TC, Increase in Cholesterol, Apolipoprotein B. this leads to accumulation in glomerular mesangial cells. Later results in lipid peroxidation and release of cytokines. There is Infiltration of macrophages which causes progression of CKD (along c risk factors like HTN, other renal disease)

IV. **Glomerulonephritis:** Excess filtration of glucose and contact with glomerular and tubular cells leads to Increase in cellular osmatic pressure and thickening of capillary basement membrane. There is filtration of proteins-albumin, transferrin, complement factors, Ig, Cytokines, Angiotensin-II. These are toxic to kidney tubular cells. Upregulated production of inflammatory and vasoactive cytokines such as endothelin, Monocyte chemoattractant protein takes place. Activation of complement components on apical membrane of proximal tubules is seen. Progressive protein uric nephropathies are observed. Scaring of interstitial tissue, Progressive loss of nephron mass is observed. Finally decrease in GFR results in ESRD.

Complications of CKD

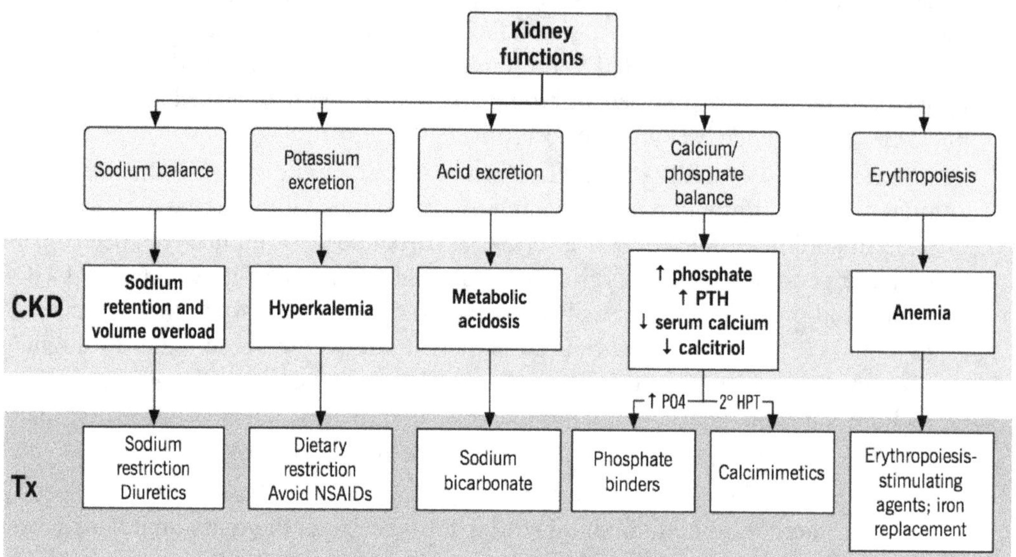

Fig. 21.1 Complications of CKD.

Source: Yashpal S Kanwar [1], Lin Sun, Ping Xie, Fu-You Liu, Sheldon Chen. A Glimpse of Various Pathogenetic Mechanisms of Diabetic Nephropathy. Annu Rev Pathol. 2011;6: 395-423.

Table 21.2 Complications of CKD with mechanism [1,2].

Sign/lab finding	Symptoms	Mechanism
Generalized edema	Swelling	Water retention due to a loss of GFR leading to sodium and fluid retention. Fluid moves into the extravascular space, due to increased hydrostatic pressure, causing pitting edema in the lower extremity (fluid movement could also be due to hypoalbuminemia, in some diseases, leading to a low oncotic pressure).
Pulmonary crackles	Shortness of breath	Fluid accumulation causes pulmonary edema and loss of air space causing ventilation-perfusion mismatch. This leaves less area for oxygen diffusion form the blood vessels.
Anemia	Fatigue, reduced exercise capacity, and pallor	Erythropoietin (EPO), the major erythropoiesis stimulator, is released from the kidneys; with renal failure, there is loss of EPO release.
Weight loss	Loss of lean body mass	Protein-energy malnutrition due to metabolic acidosis. Loss of kidney function results in impaired H+ secretion from the body.

Contd...

Sign/lab finding	Symptoms	Mechanism
Hyperkalemia	Malaise, palpitations	Inability of the kidneys to secrete potassium in the urine leads to life threatening arrhythmias.
Mechanisms of renal osteodystrophy		
Hyperphosphatemia		Damaged kidneys fail to excrete phosphate. Also secondary to high parathyroid hormone levels.
Hypocalcemia		Thought to be secondary to low Vitamin D3 levels. In early stages of CKD, low levels of calcitriol are due to hyperphosphatemia (negative feedback). In the later stages of CKD, low levels are hypothesized to be due to decreased synthesis of 1α-hydroxylase (enzyme that converts calcifediol to calcitriol in the kidneys).
Secondary and tertiary hyperparathyroidism		To compensate for the low calcium due to low Vitamin D levels, the parathyroid glands increase the parathyroid hormone secretion. This leads to a high bone turnover, always attempting to normalize the low calcium levels in the blood. Over time, this becomes maladaptive leading to extraosseous calcification, and parathyroid hyperplasia develops (tertiary hyperparathyroidism).
Complications of uremia		
Urea and other toxins accumulate in the blood and cause life threatening issues.		
Ecchymosis, GI bleeding	Increased tendency to bleed and ecchymosis	Uremia-induced platelet dysfunction
Pericardial friction rub	Chest pain, malaise	Uremic pericarditis
	Headaches, confusion, coma	Uremic encephalopathy; adverse effects of urea on the CNS. Mechanisms unclear.

Treatment

Goals: To delay the progression of CKD, Minimize complications, To improve quality of life

Non – pharmacologic therapy

- Mild dietary protein restriction
- Avoid products with added salts
- Have low potassium foods
- Maintain blood sugar levels and blood pressure levels
- Smoking cessation

Treatment Approach

Pharmacological Management

CKD has no cure but treatment is done to slow its progression. It involves mainly controlling blood sugar, blood pressure and other complications

I. Diabetic CKD

- Progression of CKD can be limited by optimal control of hyperglycaemia
- In type 1 DM – it is achieved by administering Insulin injection (2-3 times/day)
- Type 2 DM – Hypoglycaemic agents are given
    1. **Biguanides:** Metformin: Acts by decreasing hepatic glucose production, increasing Peripheral glucose uptake, improving glucose tolerance & owering fasting and post prandial plasma glucose. Contraindicated in severe CKD where GFR is < 30 ml/min/1.73m^2

       Dose: Stage 3A – 1500 mg/day

                     3B – 1000 mg/day

                     4 – 500 mg/day

    2. **Sulphonyl ureas**

       MOA: These drugs stimulate endogenous insulin secretion by pancreatic P$_0$ cells. These potentially cause hypoglycaemia. Example: Glipizide. Metabolised by liver and its clearance and elimination half life are not affected by reduction in the estimated GFR. Hence, it is considered as drug of choice in CKD patients. Other drugs of this class like glibenclamide, glyburide are eliminated equally in bile and urine and these are contraindicated from stage 3 CKD.

    3. **Glinides:**

       MOA: Stimulate insulin secretion. Have short duration of action

       Example: Nateglinide – Metabolised in liver and active metabolites are excreted renally so contraindicated in renal patients

       Example: Repaglinide – Cautiously used in CKD patients 0.5 mg/ day contraindicated if GFR is < 30 ml/min/1.73m^2

    4. **Alpha glucosidase inhibitors**

       MOA: Reduce rate of digestion and intestinal absorption of Carbohydrates resulting in mild reduction of glycated haemoglobin (ALC)

       Example: Acarbose – Metabolites excreted in urine

       Miglitol – excreted unchanged in urine. Show modest efficiency in glycaemic control, generally, not preferred. Avoided in stage 4 & 5 of CKD

    5. **Glitazones:** Selective agonists of peroxisome proliferator activated receptor.

       MOA: Activation of PPAR nuclear receptors modulates the transcription of number of insulin responsive genes involved in the control of glucose and lipid metabolism.

       These medications may cause fluid retention. Hence, these are used with caution in patients with Heart failure, CKD . Example: pioglitazone

    6. **Dipeptidyl peptidase-4 inhibitors:** MOA: Prevent degradation of incretin hormones by DPP-4, enhancing Glucose – dependent insulin secretion. Example: Linagliptin – mainly eliminated through bile. Other drugs like sitagliptin, alogliptin etc, are mainly excreted through urine. Hence, these are not preferred

II. Hypertension in CKD

Hypertension management algorithm for patients with CKD

- Blood Pressure >130/80 mmHg If Bp > 15-20/10 mmHg Over Goal, Combine Steps 1 And 2 Goal BP = < 125/75 mm Hg for patients with proteinuria
- Step 1 Start ACEI or ARB: BP still not at goal (< 125/75 mm Hg for patients with proteinuria)
- Step 2 Add diuretic: If CrCI $\geq$ 30 ml/min, add thiazide diuretic
  If CrCI < 30 ml/min, add loop diuretic
  BP still not at goal
- Step 3 Add long-acting calcium channel blocker (CCB). May also consider adding low-dose β-blocker instead of CCB at this time if patient has angina, heart failure, or arrhythmia necessitating their use
- BP still not at goal
- Baseline pulse $\geq$ 84:
  Step 4: Add low-dose β-blocker or α/β-blocker (if not already being used) Note: The use of a β-blocker and a nondihydropyridine CCB should be avoided in the elderly and those with conduction abnormalities
- Baseline pulse < 84
  Step 4: Add other subgroup of calcium channel blocker (e.g., a dihydropyridine CCB if a nondihydropine agent is being used). Note: The use of a β-blocker and a nondihydropyridine CCB should be avoided in the elderly and those with conduction abnormalities.
- BP still not at goal
  Step 5 Add long-acting α-blocker, central α-agonist, or vasodilator. Note: Central α-agonists (i.e., clonidine) should not be used with β-blockers due to the high likelihood of severe bradycardia.

Pharmacological Therapy

Adequate BP control can reduce the declination of GFR and albuminuria in patients without diabetes. KDIGO guidelines recommends target blood pressure of 140/90 mmHg or less if urine albumin excretion is < 30 mg/day. If urine albumin excretion is >30 mg/24hr, the target BP is 130/80 mmHg

→ First line drugs: ACE inhibitor
  Angiotensin II receptor blockers (ARB)
  If proteinuria: Add thiazide diuretic with ACEI/ARB
→ When ACEI/ARB – contraindicated, then non dihydropyridine calcium channel blockers are used as a second line anti proteinuric drugs
  ACEI & ARB – contraindicated in hyperkalaemia & rapid decrease in GFR

ACE inhibitors

MOA: These inhibit the formation of angiotensin II and results in Vasodilation. These also blocks the breakdown of bradykinin, increases its levels which can contribute to vasodilator action. Example: Captopril- 25 to 150 mg/day, Enalapril – 10 to 40 mg/day

Ramipril – 2.5 to 20 mg/day

Angiotensin receptor blockers

MOA: These block the action of angiotensin II by preventing Angiotensin II from binding to angiotensin II receptors on the muscles Surrounding blood vessels. As a result, blood vessels dilate and BP is Reduced. Finally, the progress of CKD caused by HTN/Diabetes is solved

Example: Telmisartan – 40 to 80 mg/day; Losartan – 50 to 100 mg/day

Calcium Channel Blockers

MOA: These act by blocking the entry of calcium into the muscle cells of heart and arteries. Thus, reduces electrical conduction within the Heart, decrease force of contraction and dilates arteries.

Dihydropyridines – These primarily used to reduce systemic vascular resistance and arterial pressure. Amlodipine – 2.5 to 10 mg/day, Nicardipine – 60 to 120 mg/day

Non – dihydropyridines: Phenyl alkylamine – verapamil – 40 to 120 mg/day – BD/TID

Benzothiazepine – diltiazem – 30 to 120 mg/day

Diuretics

Especially loop and thiazide diuretics are given in oedematic conditions. These drugs increase the flow of urine. MOA: These work by removing sodium and calcium from body which in turn draws excess water from body. Example: Loop diuretics – furosemide – 90 to 240 mg/day. Thiazides – chlorthalidone – 12.5 to 50 mg/day

Beta - blockers: These are given when ACEI's and ARB's are contraindicated

MOA: They block the action of Nor-epinephrine and epinephrine by Inhibiting their binding to receptors. Especially beta- blockers are used to reduce BP. Example: Propranolol: 40 to 120 mg/day, Metoprolol: 25 to 200 mg/day   Atenolol: 25 to 100 mg/day

Treatment of Secondary Complications

Anaemia: Goals: To increase oxygen carrying capacity, decrease signs and symptoms. KDOQI guidelines suggest a Hb range – 11 to 12 g/dl for all CKD patients, a target transferrin saturation (T sat) of >20%, serum ferritin of greater than 100 ng/ml for CKD Patients not requiring Hemodialysis (HD) and >200 ng/ml for Hemodialysis Patients (CKD). Therapy includes – Erythropoiesis stimulating agents, well tolerated iron supplementation

Algorithm for diagnosis of Anemia of renal origin with management [3]
If the patient is identified with Hb<13 g/dL if male or <12 if female and CKD (eGFR <60ml/min/1.73 m^2) then haematological evaluation is to be completed.

(a) If the cause of anemia is other than CKD: further evaluation of anemia is to be done. Deficits is to be corrected and the cause to be treated. Referral to Internal medicine of Hematology dept, if necessary.

(b) There is no specific cause of anemia and the diagnosis is confirmed as probable renal anemia, the following approach is applicable

(i) If Iron parameters are adequate, then referral to nephrology to evaluate treatment with erythropoiesis stimulating agents is needed if Hb ≤10 g dL and/or iron therapy IV is required.

(ii) If it is identified as iron deficiency anemia- Immediately oral iron therapy is initiated.

- If there is no expected response and if Hb ≤10 g dL, start with erythropoiesis stimulating agents and/or iron therapy by IV route.
- No correction of Iron deficit in 3 months. Then evaluation of Gastrointestinal blood loss and consider referral to the hospital for IV iron therapy.

III. **Erythropoietin Stimulating Agents (ESA): MOA:** Drug binds to protein on cell surface, activation of Janus Kinase/Signal Transducer (JAK/STAT) and Map kinase pathway. There is Proliferation and terminal differentiation of erythroid precursor cells. The therapy has to be Initiated if Hb < 10 g/dl. Do not initiate if Hb is > 10 g/dl. Route of administration is IV/SC. Common adverse effect observed is Hypertension. ESA resistance: Condition when patients do not achieve desired haemoglobin concentration despite higher than usual doses of ESA's. Causes for ESA resistance are Iron deficiency, acute illness, inflammation infection, chronic bleeding, aluminium toxicity, malnutrition, hyperparathyroidism, cancer and chemotherapy

Drugs:

I. Epoetin alfa –   Adult: 50 to 100 units/kg – 3times/week – IV/SC
Child: 50 units/kg – 3times/week – IV/SC

II. Darbepoetin alfa: Adult
- Non-Dialysis – 0.45 mcg/kg – once every 4 weeks
- CKD 5 HD/5 PD – 0.45 mcg/kg – once every week
    Or
    0.75 mcg/kg – once every 2 weeks

Child: 0.45 mcg/kg – once weekly
May give: 0.75 mcg/kg – once every 2 weeks

III. Methoxy PEG – epoetin beta
Adult – initial – 0.6 mcg/kg – every 2 weeks
Once Hb stabilised – double dose is given monthly
Example: 0.6 mcg/kg – every 2 weeks (or)
1.2 mcg/kg – every month

IRON Supplementation: Recommended in non-HD patients and CKD 5HD/5PD patients. Initiated if T sat is <=30%, ferritin <=500ng/ml. Route of administration is Oral (or) IV.

Adverse effects: Oral iron: GI disturbances like conspiration, nausea, abdominal cramps IV Iron: Allergic reactions, hypotension, dizziness, dyspnoea, headache, lower backpain, arthralgia, syncope, arthritis.

IV. Iron preparations:

1. Ferric carboxy maltose – 750 mg per week
2. Ferumoxytol – 510 mg followed by a second dose 510 mg after 3-8 of initial dose
3. Iron dextran – 25 to 1000mg
4. Iron sucrose – 25 to 1000mg
5. Sodium ferric gluconate – 62.5 to 1000mg

Evaluation of Anaemia Therapeutic outcomes:

- Evaluate iron indices before initiating an ESA. Iron status should be reassessed every month
- Monitor Hb until Hb is stable

CKD – Related Mineral and Bone Disorder

- KDOQI guidelines recommended that elemental calcium from calcium containing binders should not exceed 1500mg/day and total daily intake from all sources should not exceed 2000mg. Treatment involves: dietary phosphorous restriction, dialysis and parathyroidectomy and use of phosphate binding agents and vitamin D therapy, calcimimetics.

Phosphate Binding agents:

- These agents decrease phosphorous absorption from the gut and are first line agents for controlling both serum phosphorous and calcium concentrations

Classifications:

1. Calcium based binders – These even acts as calcium supplements
   Example: Calcium acetate (25% elemental calcium) – 1334mg-TID
   Calcium carbonate (40% elemental calcium) – 0.5 to 1 g-TID
2. Iron based binders
   Example: Ferric citrate – 420 mg ferric iron – TID
   Sucroferric oxyhydroxide – 500mg-TID
3. Resin binders
   Example: Sevelamer carbonate – 800 to 1600 mg – TID
   Sevelamer HCL – 800 to 1600mg-TID
4. Other elemental binders
   Example: Lanthanum carbonate – 1500 mg/day
   Aluminium hydroxide – 300 to 600 mg-TID

Adverse effect:

Common for all – GI effects – Constipation, diarrhoea, nausea, vomiting and abdominal pain

Calcium binders – Hypercalcemia

Aluminium binders – CNS toxicity, worsen anaemia $\left.\vphantom{\begin{array}{c}a\\b\end{array}}\right\}$ contraindicated in

Magnesium binders – Hypermagnesemia, Hyperkalaemia $\qquad$ CKD Pt's

Vitamin D therapy:

- Serum calcium and phosphorous should be within normal range before initiation and during continuation of vitamin D therapy. It helps body to take up calcium from diet and use it. Dose depends on CKD stage

Nutritional Vitamin D:

1. Ergocalciferol – (D_2) – 400 to 2000 IU/day
2. Cholecalciferol – (D_3) – 50000 IU/month (or) given weekly

Vitamin D and Analogs (D_3):

1. Calcitriol (D_3) – 0.25 to 5 mcg – directly suppresses PTH synthesis and secretion and upregulates vit D receptors
2. Doxercalciferol (D_2) – 5 to 20 mcg $\left.\vphantom{\begin{array}{c}a\\b\end{array}}\right\}$ Less activity
3. Paricalcitol (D_2) – 1 to 4 mcg

Calcimimetics

Example: Cinacalcet – 30 to 180 mg/day. It reduces PTH secretion by increasing the sensitivity of calcium sensing receptor. It lowers serum calcium and should not be started if serum calcium is less than normal. Common side effect – Nausea and vomiting

Hyperlipidaemia

KDIGO lipid guidelines recommended: Statin treatment in adults age 18 to 49 years with CKD who have one or more of following – coronary disease, DM, Prior ischaemic stroke, estimated 10-year incidence of coronary death or non-fatal MI greater than 10% but these patients are not treated c chronic dialysis or kidney transplantation

Statin treatment or statin/ezetimibe combination in adults >50 years with estimated GFR < 60 ml/min/1.73m^2 but not treated c chronic dialysis or kidney transplantation

Do not initiate statins or statin/ezetimibe combination therapy in adults with dialysis dependent CKD continue these agents if patient is already taking them at time of dialysis initiation

Example: Atorvastatin – 20mg/day

Rosuvastatin – 10mg/day

Lovastatin – 20mg/day

Fluvastatin – 80mg/day

Hypernatremia: Dietary restrictions of sodium intake. Use of diuretics

Hyperkalaemia: Dietary restriction of potassium. Avoid use of NSAID's

Metabolic acidosis: Restrict dietary protein (0.6 g/kg/day). 2. Inj. Sodium bicarbonate IV to maintain an arterial pH of >7.2.

Hypocalcaemia: Tab. Calcium carbonate 1 g/day Or IV Calcium gluconate 10% 10-20 ml given over 20 minutes (if tetany).

Hyperphosphataemia: Restrict dietary phosphate intake (10 mg %. Tab. Allopurinol 100 mg three times a day

Hyperuricaemia: Treatment necessary only if uric acid is >10 mg %. Tab. Allopurinol 100 mg three times a day

Case Study of Chronic Kidney Disease

Summary

A male patient of age 65 years come to hospital with complaints of – shortness of breath +, fever, ulcer over foot. He has a past medical history of type 2 diabetes, hypertension, bronchial asthma. He is on medications T.stamlo – 5mg – OD & on insulin. His vitals showed normal temperature, BP & pulse rate. CBP-WBC – 30,300 cells /cumm – neutrophilic leucocytosis. Lymphocytes – 10% , Urine analysis :   pus cells 2 – 3 /HPF, Albumin - ++, Epithelial cells – 2 – 4 /HPF, LDH – 615 observed for tissue damage especially brain, kidney, lungs etc., Liver function test - serum bilirubin total – 1.3mg/dL, Biochemical investigations (mg/dL) – 1.6 serum creatinine, Blood urea – 85mg/dL, Serum electrolytes- normal, Random blood sugar-150mg/dl ; Culture sensitivity test- kleibsella pneumonia growth; Doppler study of left lower limb venouous system -- chronic various insufficiency; ECG - sinus tachycardia, poor R - wave progression, flattened T- wave; CT of brain- age related cerebral atropy; 2D echo (heart) – AV – scleroid, diastolic dysfunction, mild LV systolic dysfunction; USG . Abdominal. Pelvis –B/L slightly small kidneys; High sensitivity troponin – 78.5mg/L; APTT – 18.5 sec - high chances for clot formation.

Diagnosis: Based on the above obtained subjective and objective data the patient was diagnosed to be suffering with chronic kidney disease with diabetic foot

Progress Chart: From day 1, patient was on antibiotics, anticoagulants, insulin and antacid. From day 1 itself serum creatinine & blood urea levels, serum, electrolytes, vitals and fluid input, output have been mentioned, on day 4, amikacin, dolo, nebulisation were given additionally. Serum creatinine & blood urea levels increased i.e., elevated on day 3,4,5,6 and later have been observed to reduce. Regular mentioning of Sr.Cr, BUN, vitals have been done to know the patient condition.

Drug Treatment Chart

Trade name	Generic name	Category	Route	Dose	Frequney
Inj. Heparin	Heparin	Anti – coagulant	IV	5000 IU	QID
Inj. Dalacin – c	Clindamycin	Anti biotic	IV	600 mg	TID
Inj. Meropenem	Meropenem	Anti biotic	IV	500 mg	TID
Inj. Metrogyl	Metronidazole	Anti infective	IV	100 ml	BD
Inj. Levoflox	Levofloxacin	Fluroquinolone Anti biotic	IV	500 mg	BD
Inj. Pan	Pantoprazole	Antacid	IV	40 mg	OD
Inj. Multivit	Multivitamin	Vitamin supplement	IV	100 ml	OD
Inj. Dexa	Dexamethasone	Corticosteroid	IV	8 mg	HD
Inj. Lantus	Insulin	Anti diabetic	S/C	10units	HD
T. Dytor	Torasemide	diuretic	P/O	10 mg	OD
T. Clopitab	Clopidogrel	Anti platelet	P/O	75 mg	OD
T. Navostat	Rosuvastatin	Anti hyperlipidemic	P/O	10 mg	OD
Inj. Clexane	Enoxaparin	Anti coagulant	S/C	40 mg	BD
T. Chymoral forte	Trypsin, chymotrypsin	Enzyme , blood Supply, swelling	P/O	1 tab	TID
T. Dolo	Paracetamol	Anti pyretic	P/O	650 mg	TID
Inj. Amikacin	Amikacin	Aminoglycoside	IV	500 mg	OD
Neb.Duolin	Salbutamol + ipratropum	Bronchodilator	P/N		SOD
Neb. Budcort	budesonide	Corticosteroid	P/N		SOD

Pharmacist Interventions

Because of patient conditions several drugs have been prescribed but there were few interactions which may worsen situation. Most of the major interactions may result in prolongation of QT – interval, enhance hyperglycemic conditions, risk for ototoxicity, nephotoxicity, and also bleeding complications due to heparin. It is important to regularly mention the patient for these conditions. This can be done by ECG monitoring, prothrombin time, mentioning GRBS along with sr.creatinine & blood urea (even bleeding time). Other minor effects that may occur due to during interactions are dizziness, hypomagnesaemia, fatigue, hyper tension, neuropathy. Therapeutic duplications observed are antiinfective & anti biotics -(3); Blood modifiers- (2); Steroid. (1)

Patient Conselling

- Have plenty of fluids.
- Never miss/skip a dose of any medication.

- If any symptom is observed or any complication immediately inform doctor.
- Should avoid high fat, high salt in Take, limit k+ & phosphorous in take.
- Have a specific diet at regular intervals.
- Avoid high carbohydrate in Take.
- If any social habits are there (Smoking, alcohol) avoid them. Immediately.
- Take rest and try to avoid stressful conditions.
- Maintain hygiene to avoid further infections.
- Do regular small exercises to maintain BP (ex. walking) after discharge
- Regularly consult visit physician to know your condition.
- Stay healthy and happy for a good & peaceful life.
- Try to avoid milk & milk products like butter.
- Regularly check your weight.

Assignment

1. Create a list of Patients drug therapy problems

1. Based on the patients condition several drugs have been prescribed
   Problems due to patient drug therapy are as follows:
   - Amikacin < >   torsemide (major): increased risk for nephrotoxicity
     Especially in patients with renal problems
     RFT should be monitored.
   - Dexamethasone <> levofloxacin (major): corticosteroids may potentiate
     The risk of teniditis & tendon rupture Associated with fluoroquinolone
   - Heparin < > enoxaparin: Potentiate risk of bleeding complications   and also
     therapeutic   duplication
   - Levofoxacin < > insulin (major): quinolones interface with therapeutic
     Effects of insulin and are associated with blood glucose homeostasis
     Apart from these major interactions there are many minor & moderate interactions
     which mainly cause ECG changes, hyperglycemia, electrolyte imbalances,
     neuropathies etc.,
2. Antimicrobials - maximum 3 can be prescribed but in this case 5 were prescribed.
   Blood modifiers – maximum 2, but prescribed are 3.
   Anticoagulants – maximum1 but 2 were prescribed.
   Side Effects (or) adverse drug reactions.
3. Most possible side effects are :
   - Antibiotics – nausea, GI discomfort, nephrotoxicity, ototoxicity, tendon a muscle
     or joint pains etc.,
   - Anticoagulants – excessive bleedings, injection site reactions thrombocytopenia
   - Intravenous corticosteroids – stomach, irritation, rapid heart beat, fluid retention ,
     flushings ,hyperglycemia
   - Diuretics – hypokalemia, headache, hyperglycemia

Most common side effects due to other drugs are nausea, diagnose, vomtings or constipation, lack of appegtite, hepatotoxicity etc.,

4. Drug – food interactions:
    - Mainly avoid alcohol consumption, grape fruit juice, orange juice.
    - Never take antibiotics on empty stomach.
    - As most of drugs interfere with blood glucose hemstasis, avoid high carbohydrate diet.

    Apart from these problems, all drugs prescribed are appropriate for patients condition and symptoms.

2. What information indicate the severity of patients ESRD?

Signs and symptoms :   Shortness of breath
                                        Fever
                                        Ulcer of foot.

Past medical history :   T2 DM on insulin
                                        HTN T.stamlo – 5mg – OD
                                        Bronchial asthma.

Vitals were normal.

Laboratory investigations and other tests
- CBP neutrophilic leucocytosis   WBC – 30,300 cells /cumm) lymphocytes – 10 %
- ESR 120 mm/hr
- Urine analysis – albumin - ++
- Serum creatinine – 1.4mg/dL
- Blood urea – 85 mg/dL
- Lactate dehydrogenase (LDH) - 616 U/L Units
- Culture (sensitivity) test –Klebisella pneumonia growth
- Doppler study of left leg venous system-   chronic venous insufficiency
- Prothrombin test – 1.59 INR
- ECG sinus tachycardia, poor R-wave progression, flattened T- wave
- CT –Brain-   age related cerebral atrophy
- 2D- echo-   AV – sclerosis, GI diastolic dysfunction, mild LV systolic dysfunction
- USG – abdominal pelvic – B/L slightly small kidneys.
- High sensitivity troponin – 78.5 ng/dL   – normal 14ng/dL
- APTT – 18.5 sec – chances for bleedings

Based on the obtained data, the person was diagnosed with CKD and infection and also there are high chances for cardiac failure / heart attack.

3. **What are the goals of pharmacotherapy for each problem listed.**
   - CKD Goals: To delay progression & Improve kidney functioning
     To prevent treat complications
     To improve patients quality of life
   - Hypertension and cardiac problems Goals:
     To maintain blood pressure and GFR
     To prevent heart attack & other complications
     To maintain proper blood circulation
     To maintain proper electrolyte levels & blood volume
   - Diabetes Goals:
     To maintain blood glucose level
     To avoid formation of AGE's
     To avoid further complications due to hyperglycemia
   - Diabetic foot / infection Goals:
     To reduce bacterial growth
     To prevent re occurence
     To avoid systemic infection and other complications
   - Bleedings and clot information Goals :
     Mainly to prevent clot formations
     Avoid clotting complications
     Maintain blood viscosity
     To treat clots formed

4. **What clinical and laboratory parameters would you recommend to evaluate the desired and undesired consequences.**
   - CBP – to know WBC – levels, anemia /thrombocytopenia
   - ESR
   - Blood urea, Sr.creatinine – to know renal function
   - GFR – important to achieve successful therapy & to know stage of CKD
   - RBS – as most of the drugs interface with insulin activity & glucose metabolism
   - Serum electrolytes to know hypo / hyperkalemia (or) natremia
   - Regular ECG monitoring
   - Troponin levels
   - Calcium and phosphorous levels in blood to avoid osteodystrophy & hyperparathyroidism
   - Vitamin D levels
   - Serum lipid profile
   - BP monitoring

5. **What water soluble vitamin supplements to be recommended for ESRD Patients?**
   - Vitamin B1 1.5 mg /day – help to produce energy, proper working of nervous System
   - Vitamin B2- 1.8 mg/day – help to produce energy, normal position, healthy skin

- Niacin B3 - 14 to 20 mg /day – help to produce energy, enzyme functionality
- Vitamin B6 - 5mg /day – produce protein & RBC synthesis 10 mg/day – dialysis
- Vitamin B12 - 2 – 3mg/day – RBC synthesis, maintains nerve cells, help make new cells
- Vitamin C - 60 to 100 mg/day – Iron absorption, immune system healthy, repairs cells
- Vitamin B7-30 to 100 mg/day – produce energy
- Pantothenic acid - 5mg /day - produce energy
- B9 folate-1mg/day

6. What is the pharmacotherapeutic regimen that can be indicated for this patient?

1. Hypertension:

CCB's dihydrophyridine –	Amlodipine- 2.5 to 10 mg /day
	Nifedipine- 30 to 130 mg/ day
	Nicardipine- 60 to 90 mg /day
Non dihydrophyridine –	Diltiazem- 120 to 360 mg/day
	Verapamil- 90 to 480g /day
Advantages of antihypertensive drugs - improves circulation	
	Reduces risk for heart attacks
Disadvantages –	Side effects : dizziness,flushing,tiredness,
	Effect homeostatis, electrolyte imbalance

2. Diabetes:

- Progression of CKD can be limited by optimal control of hyperglycemia
- Patient is already on insulin (10 units)
- It is recommended to continue intake of insulin. if still the blood glucose didn't reach target and there is no charge in proteinuria then add oral anti diabetic drugs

Ex: biguanides–Metformin

Sulphonyl ureas–Glipizide

3. Diabetic foot Infection:

- Antibiotics are to be prescribed
- Empirical antibiotics to Klebsiella pneumonia involve Beta–lactams, Aminoglycosides, Fluroquinolones, Chloromphenicol, Retracyclines, Co-trimoxazole
- But use of aminoglycoside, beta lactum antibiotics results in nephrotoxicity
- Ototoxicity is observed with aminoglycosides, tendinitis joint pains with fluroquinolones
- Careful monitoring is required
  Commonly used antibiotics for K.pneumoniae are-
  Ampicillin – sulbabactam – 2g IV – every day
  Meropenem-500mg – IV –7 days
  (or)
  Levofloxacin – 500mg –IV – 8 days

References

1. Adeline L Y Tan, Josephine M Forbes, Mark E Cooper. AGE, RAGE, and ROS in Diabetic Nephropathy. Semin Nephrol. 2007 Mar;27(2):130-43.

2. Julian Lawrence Seifter[1], Martin A Samuels. Uremic Encephalopathy and Other Brain Disorders Associated with Renal Failure. Semin Neurol. 2011 Apr;31(2):139-43.

3. Aleix Cases et al., Anemia of chronic kidney disease: Protocol of study, management and referral to Nephrology. Nephrologia. 2018; 38(1): 1-108.

CHAPTER - 22

Renal Dialysis

Haemodialysis

Definition: Haemodialysis is the process of purifying the blood of a person whose kidneys are not working normally. It is one of the three replacement therapies.

Principle [1]

It involves diffusion of solutes across semi-permeable membrane. Haemodialysis utilizes counter current flow, where the dialysate is flowing in the opposite direction to blood flow in the extra corporeal circuit. Counter current flow maintains the concentration gradient across the membrane at a maximum and increase the efficiency of the dialysis.

Fluid removal (ultrafiltration) is achieved by altering the hydrostatic pressure of the dialysate compartment, causing free water and some dissolved solutes to move across the membrane along a created pressure gradient.

There are two types of vascular access designed for long term use:
1. Arterio-venous fistula (AV fistula)
2. Arterio-venous graft (AV graft)

A venous catheter is another form of vascular access, recommended for short- term use.

AV Fistula: An AV Fistula is created by directly connecting an artery to a vein, usually in the wrist fore-arm or upper arm. AV fistula causes extra pressure by increasing blood flow into the vein, making it grow larger and stronger and providing easy access to blood vessels.

Types of AV fistula:
1. Radial cephalic fistula
2. Brachial cephalic fistula
3. Brachial basilica fistula

AV Graft

It consists of synthetic tube implanted under the skin, connecting between artery and vein and providing needle placement access for dialysis.

A dialysis catheter is large IV tubing that is inserted into one of the large veins in a persons neck of chest, and placed very close to the heart. The catheter exits from the persons chest and is easily covered up by the clothing. The benefit of catheter over the other options is that it can be used for dialysis as soon as it is successfully placed. However, catheters do not have longevity and are frequently complicated by clotting, insufficient dialysis, and infections. Catheters are recommended only for temporary usage in the order of months, and should be taken out as soon as one of the other options becomes available.

Arteriovenous fistulas (AV fistulas) represent the best option as AV access. Small incisions are done to connect a persons artery to the vein, usually near the wrist or the elbow. Arteries are naturally deep while veins run near the surface. Once the artery is connected to the vein, the robust arterial flow is now running through the superficial vein near the surface. The dialysis technician now has easy access to a lot of blood flow near the surface, and inserts IVs into the fistula to dialyze the person. The AV fistula has been shown to last the longest and has the least infectious and other complications.

Arteriovenous grafts (AV grafts) are created by connecting the persons artery to a large deep vein in his arm or leg. Grafts are reserved for patients whose superficial veins are not suitable for fistula creation. Compared to the catheter, AV grafts have lower risk of complications and can last longer. It typically takes 2-3 weeks for a graft to become ready for dialysis. Like fistulas, it may also take a few procedures to create and maintain a graft in working condition.

Procedure [2]

There are three types of haemodialysis. They are,
1. Conventional haemodialysis
2. Daily haemodialysis
3. Nocturnal haemodialysis

Conventional Haemodialysis

It is usually done three times per week for about 3 – 4 hours for each treatment, during which the patient's blood is drawn out through a tube at a rate of 200-400 ml/min. The tube is connected at 15, 16 or 17 gauge needle inserted in the dialysis fistula or graft or connected to one part of a dialysis catheter. The blood is then pumped out through a dialyzer, and then the processed blood is pumped back into the patient's blood stream through another tube. During this procedure the patient's Blood Pressure is closely monitored and if it becomes low or patient develop any other signs of low blood volume such as nausea, the dialysis attendant can administer extra fluid through machine. During treatment the patient's entire blood volume (about 5000 cc) circulates through machine every 15 min. During this procedure, the dialysis patient is exposed to week's worth of water for the average person.

Daily Haemodialysis

It is typically used by those patients who do their own dialysis at home. It is less stressful but does require more frequent access. This is simple with catheters, but more problematic with fistulas and grafts. The 'button whole technique' can be used for fistulas requiring frequent access. It is usually done for 2 hours, 6 days a week.

Nocturnal Haemodialysis

It is similar to conventional method except it is performed 3-6 nights/ week and between 6-10 hours per session while the patient sleeps.

Advantages and Disadvantages of Haemodialysis

Advantages

1. Higher solute clearance allows intermittent treatment.
2. Parameters of adequacy of dialysis are better defined and therefore under dialysis can be detected early.
3. Technique failure rate is low.
4. Even though intermittent heparinization is required, hemostasis parameters are better corrected with haemodialysis than peritoneal dialysis.
5. In-center haemodialysis enables closer monitoring of the patient.

Disadvantages

1. Requires multiple visits each week to the haemodialysis centre, which translates into loss of control by the patient.
2. Disequilibrium, dialysis hypotension, and muscle cramps are common. May require months before the patient adjusts to haemodialysis.
3. Infections in haemodialysis patients may be related to the choice of membranes, the complement-activating membranes being more deleterious.
4. Vascular access is frequently associated with infection and thrombosis.
5. Decline of residual renal function is more rapid compared to peritoneal dialysis.
6. Restricts independence, as people undergoing this procedure cannot travel around because of supplies' availability.
7. Requires more supplies such as high water quality and electricity.
8. Requires reliable technology like dialysis machines.
9. The procedure is complicated and requires that care givers have more knowledge.
10. Requires time to set up and clean dialysis machines, and expense with machines and associated staff.

Hemodialysis

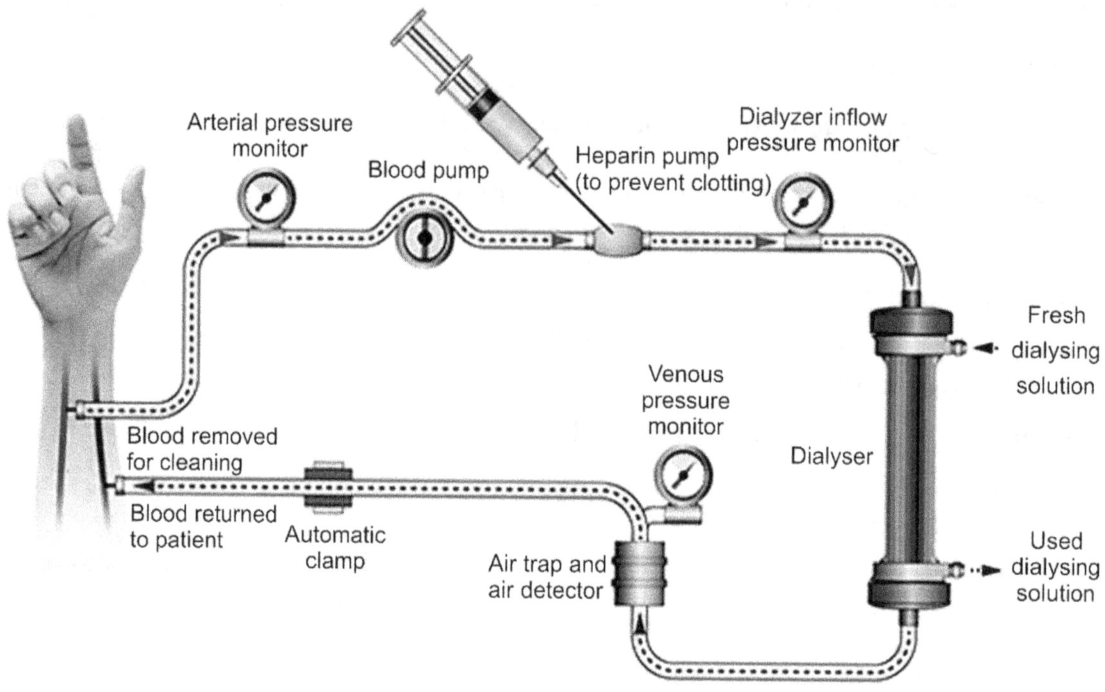

Fig. 22.1 Procedure for Hemodialysis.

Source: https://www.niddk.nih.gov/health-information/kidney-disease/kidney-failure/hemodialysis

Complications [3]

Fluid shifts

Haemodialysis often involves fluid removal (through ultra filtration), because most patients with renal failure pass little or no urine. Side effects caused by removing too much fluid and/or removing fluid too rapidly include low blood pressure, fatigue, chest pains, leg-cramps, nausea and headaches. These symptoms can occur during the treatment and can persist post treatment; they are sometimes collectively referred to as the dialysis hangover or dialysis washout. The severity of these symptoms is usually proportionate to the amount and speed of fluid removal. However, the impact of a given amount or rate of fluid removal can vary greatly from person to person and day to day. These side effects can be avoided and/or their severity lessened by limiting fluid intake between treatments or increasing the dose of dialysis e.g. dialyzing more often or longer per treatment than the standard three times a week, 3–4 hours per treatment schedule.

Access-related

Since haemodialysis requires access to the circulatory system, patients undergoing haemodialysis may expose their circulatory system to microbes, which can lead to bacteraemia, an infection affecting the heart valves (endocarditis) or an infection affecting the bones (osteomyelitis). The risk of infection varies depending on the type of access used (see below). Bleeding may also occur; again the risk varies depending on the type of access used. Infections can be minimized by strictly adhering to infection control best practices.

Anticoagulation-related

Heparin is the most commonly used anticoagulant in haemodialysis, as it is generally well tolerated and can be quickly reversed with protamine sulfate. Heparin allergy can infrequently be a problem and can cause a low platelet count. In such patients, alternative anticoagulants can be used. In patients at high risk of bleeding, dialysis can be done without anticoagulation.

First-use syndrome

First-use syndrome is a rare but severe anaphylactic reaction to the artificial kidney. Its symptoms include sneezing, wheezing, shortness of breath, back pain, chest pain, or sudden death. It can be caused by residual sterilant in the artificial kidney or the material of the membrane itself. In recent years, the incidence of first-use Syndrome has decreased, due to an increased use of gamma irradiation, steam sterilization, or electron-beam radiation instead of chemical sterilants, and the development of new semipermeable membranes of higher biocompatibility. New methods of processing previously acceptable components of dialysis must always be considered. For example, in 2008, a series of first-use type of reactions, including deaths, occurred due to heparin contaminated during the manufacturing process with over sulfated chondroitin sulfate.

Cardiovascular

Long-term complications of haemodialysis include haemodialysis, neuropathy and various forms of heart disease. Increasing the frequency and length of treatments has been shown to improve fluid overload and enlargement of the heart that is commonly seen in such patients. Due to these complications, the prevalence of complementary and alternative medicine use is high among patients undergoing haemodialysis.

Vitamin Deficiency

Folate deficiency can occur in some patients having haemodialysis.

Peritoneal Dialysis

Principle

It involves passage of solution and water across a membrane that separates two fluids containing compartments blood and dialysate.

During dialysis 3 transport processes occur simultaneously-
1. Diffusion
2. Ultra filtration
3. Absorption

Ultra filtration occurs as a consequence of osmotic gradient between the hypertonic dialysate and the relatively hypotonic peritoneal capillary blood.

It is driven by high concentration of glucose in dialysate.
- Types of peritoneal dialysis:
  1. Continuous Ambulatory Peritoneal Dialysis(CAPD)
  2. Automated Peritoneal Dialysis(IPD)

Procedure

The process of filling and then draining the patient's abdomen is called as Exchange. Different methods of peritoneal dialysis have different schedules of exchange. The 2 main are:
1. Continuous Ambulatory Peritoneal Dialysis (CAPD)
2. Continuous Cyclic Peritoneal Dialysis (CCPD)

Continuous Ambulatory Peritoneal Dialysis [4, 5]

It is 3 step process called exchange.
1. FILL- A bag of solution called dialysate put into abdomen through the catheter. This bag holds for about 2 quarts of fluid. It takes about 10-20mins to fill. When the bag is empty, it can be clamped off or tubing can be capped off.
2. DWELL- The solution stays in the abdomen about 4-6 hrs, while the solution is in the abdomen, extra fluid and wastes move from blood and into solution.
3. DRAIN- Using gravity, the solution is then drained out of the body into drain bag. The drained fluid is much like urine and will be clear yellow. It takes about 10-20mins to drain.

When the solution is drained, a new bag of dialysate is connected to catheter and steps are repeated. The 3 steps are done about 4 times each day with meals and at bedtime. Eat cycle takes 20-40 mins.

Continuous Cyclic Peritoneal Dialysis –

With CCPD, there are fill, dwell and drain cycles but dwell time is shorter and machine does the exchange. The dwell time is about 90 mins. The machine is setup and person is connected to this machine for 8-10hrs during the night. The person is unhooked from the machine during day.

Updated KDOQI guidelines for PD adequacy (2006) [6]
1. **Patient with Residual Kidney Function (RKF)-**
   - ✓ Minimal delivered total weekly urea PD+RKF $\geq$1.7.
   - ✓ Total (PD+RKF) solute clearance must be measured after 1month and every 4 months.
   - ✓ 24 hr urine collection for volume and RKF for every 2 months.
2. **Patient without RKF-**
   - ✓ Minimal delivered weekly urea $\geq$1.7.
   - ✓ Total solute clearance must be measured after 1 month and every 4 months.
3. **Increased Intra Abdominal Pressure-**
   - ✓ Hernias
   - ✓ Abdominal and genital leaks.
   - ✓ Hydrothorax.

Clinical presentation of Hernias.
- Lump or swelling that may be tender.
- Bowel Strangulation

Treatment-
- Dialysis around repair depends on renal function and condition of patient.
- Reintroduce PD with low volume, supine position, increase over 2 weeks.

4. **Abdominal wall and Genital edema-**

Clinical presentation-
- Abdominal swelling scrotal or labial edema.
- Weight gain without peripheral edema.
- Pericatheter leak- Wetness or swelling at exit site.

Diagnosis-
- Physical examination.
- Unchanged PET Results.
- CT scan.

Management-
- Reintroduce low pressure PD.

5. **Hydrothorax-** Presence of Peritoneal Dialysis fluids in pleural cavity.

   Pathogenesis- Movement of dialysate under increased intrabdominal pressure, from peritoneal to pleural cavity through congenital or acquired defects in diaphragm.

   Presentation-
   - Shortness of Breath.
   - Right sided pleural effusion.

   Treatment-
   - Thoracentesis.
   - Stop PD.
   - Tetracyclines, Bleomycin.
   - Operative on Pleuroscopic repair.

6. **Hemoperitoneum-** Bloody peritoneal effluent.

   Treatment- IV Heparin.

   Chyloperitoneum- Drainage of chyle into peritoneal cavity.

Peritoneal Dialysis Complications

- ✓ Ultra filtration failure.
- ✓ Biocompatibility- Glucose degradation product and icodextrin related complications.
- ✓ Encapsulating Sclerosing Peritonitis.
- ✓ Mechanical complications.

1. **Biocompatibility of PD fluids:** Glucose related problems-
   Unphysiologic (very high) Glucose content induces cellular and interstitial changes (TGF β VEGF signaling)

Toxic glucose degradation products are formed during heat sterilization.

2. **Sclerosing Encapsulating Peritonitis:**

Etiology - Usually develops after years of PD.

- Associated with high glucose and acetate in Pd fluid.

Diagnosis

- CT scan or MRI.

Treatment-

- Adjust PD regimen for maximum Biocompatibility.
- Transfer patient to HD temporarily or permanently
- Corticosteroids.
- Expert surgical adhesion-lysis.

3. **Peritonitis:**

- Transluminal touch contamination, periluminal, Transvisceral or Hematogenous.
- 1% associated with bacteremia.

Treatment-

- Local antibiotic sensitivity profile.
- Non-nephrotoxic drugs to prevent Residual Kidney Function (RKF).

4. **Mechanical complications:**

(a) Gastro esophageal reflux and delayed gastric emptying.

Treatment-

- Reduce fill volume.
- Motility agents- Metoclopramide, Erythromycin.

(b) Back and Abdominal Pain- Reduce fill volume (or) use biocompatible fluids.

(c) Pleural effusion due to pleuro peritoneal leak.

5. **Others:-**

- ➢ Hypokalemia- Provide liberal potassium diet.
- ➢ Hypomagnesaemia- 0.05mmol/L PD mg level is optimal.

Hypomagnesaemia should be avoided as if may attribute to a dynamic bone disease.

Haemofiltration

Definition

Haemofiltration is a renal replacement therapy which is used in intensive care setting. It is usually used to treat acute kidney injury, but may be of benefit in multiple organ dysfunction syndrome or sepsis. During Haemofiltration, a patient's blood is passed through a set of tubing via a machine to a semi-permeable membrane where waste products and water are removed by convection. Replacement fluid is added and the blood is returned to the patient.

Principle

As in dialysis, in Haemofiltration, one achieves movement of solutes across a semi-permeable membrane. However, solute movement with Haemofiltration is governed by convection rather than by diffusion. With Haemofiltration dialysate is not used. Instead, a positive hydrostatic pressure drives water and solutes across the filter membrane from the blood compartment to the filtrate compartment, from which it is drained. Solutes, both small and big get dragged through the membrane at a similar rate by the flow of water that has been engendered by hydrostatic pressure. Thus convection overcomes the reduced removal rate of larger solutes seen in haemodialysis.

Complications

- Poor vascular access, Clotting, Bleeding, Poor solute clearance.
- Air in extracorporeal circuit, Hypothermia, Hyponatremia.

References

1. Daugirdas J. T., Black P.G., Ing T.S. In "Handbook of Dialysis". 4th ed. Philadelphia, PA: Lippincott Williams & Wilkins, a Wolters Kluwer Business; 2007.
2. Heydari M, Hashempur MH, Zargaran A (2013). "Use of herbal remedies among patients undergoing hemodialysis". Iran J Kidney Dis. 11 (1): 101–12.
3. Birdee GS, Phillips RS, Brown RS (2013). "Use of Complementary and Alternative Medicine among Patients with End-Stage Renal Disease". Evidence-Based Complementary and Alternative Medicine. 2013: 1–6.
4. Vitamin Deficiency Anemia, Mayo Clinic.
5. The Ottawa Hospital (TOH). Guide: Treatment options for chronic kidney disease. Ottawa, Ontario:The Ottawa Hospital Riverside Campus;2008.
6. Updated KDOQI guidelines for PD adequacy 2006; vol 48, 1: S98-129.

CHAPTER - 23

Drug-Induced Kidney Diseases

Introduction to Kidney Diseases

Drug-induced kidney disease constitutes an important cause of acute renal failure and chronic kidney disease in present day. Clinical practical different classes of drugs are non steroidal anti-inflammatory drugs (NSAIDs). Antibiotics, NSAIDs, angiotensin converting enzyme inhibitors (ACEI) and contrast agents are the major culprit drugs contributory to kidney diseases.

Table 23.1 Syndromes of drug-induced nephropathies kidney damage [1].

Syndrome	Drugs
Pre-renal failure	Amphotericin-B, Nor epinephrine,
	NSAIDs, ACE inhibitors, Cyclosporine
Acute tubular necrosis	AMG, Cephalosporin, Rifampicin, Nsaids, Contrast
	Media, Amphotericin B
Acute interstitial nephritis	Methicillin, Ampicillins, Rifampicin, NSAIDs,
	Thiazides,Sulphonamides
Drug- induced crystalluria	Sulfadiazine, Methotrexate, Methoxyflurane,
	Acyclovir, Methysergide, Indinavir, Nelfinavir,
	Acetazolamide, Triamterene
Hypersensitivity angiitis	Penicillin G, Ampicillin, Sulfonamides, Thiazides,
	Metolazone
Isolated proteinuria with nephritic	Gold, Heroine, Captopril, NSAIDs, IFN alpha
Syndrome	Penicillamine
Chronic glomerulopathy	Heroine
Chronic tubulointerstitial disease	NSAIDs, Thiazides, Lithium, Germanium, Chinese herb
	Nephropathy
Retroperitoneal fibrosis	Methysergide Hydralazine, Methyldopa

Individual classes of drug

1. **Aminoglycosides [2]:** AMG are prototype drugs having nephrotoxicity as major side effect. Number of patients developing nephrotoxicity increases with duration of therapy reaching 50% with 14 days or more of therapy.

   Clinical features: Non-oliguric ARF, proximal tubular dysfunction, enzymuria, proteinuria, glycosuria, hypokalemia, hypocalcemia, hypomagnesaemia.

   Mechanisms: Aminoglycosides (AMG) after entering into cytoplasm interferes with the phosphatidyl-inositol pathway. The transport system is a low affinity high capacity system that is not easily saturable. Thus momentary high drug concentrations as achieved immediately after intravenous injection result in saturation of the uptake mechanism.

   Prevention and management: If SCr >1.5 mg/dL stop the drug and consider alternate therapy

   Monitor urine output and start adequate fluid and electrolyte therapy with specific emphasis on K+ and NaCl as well as Ca^{2+} and Mg^{2+} replacement.

2. **β-Lactams and vancomycin [3]:** Nephrotoxicity is rare. Acute interstitial nephritis (AIN) may be seen especially with methicillin. Early formulations of vancomycin had substantial nephrotoxic potential due to impurities but current preparations are free from adverse effect.

   Aminoglycosides (AMG) + Vancomycin combination may have synergistic toxicity.

3. **Sulfonamides:** Use of sulfonamides has increased with advent of AIDS. Sulfadoxine + pyrimethamine combination is used in malaria.

   Spectrum of nephrotoxicity includes

   1. Acute interstitial nephritis (not common)
   2. Necrotizing arteritis
   3. ARF due to massive haemolytic anaemia in G-6-PD deficient patients
   4. ARF due to crystalluria

   Sulfadiazine: Prototype drug causing crystalluria and ARF. The overall incidence is 6%. Renal dysfunction starts after three weeks of commencing treatment in AIDS patients.

   Sulphadiazine has low solubility in acidic urine. Crystals of sulfadiazine and acetyl sulfadiazine are typically recognized by examining the urine sediment where they resemble "sheaves of wheat"

   Patient manifests with asymptomatic crystalluria and microhematuria, gross hematuria, oliguria to anuria and post-renal ARF.

   Risk factors

   Especially in AIDS patients are:

   1. Prolonged duration of therapy than in community acquired pneumonia
   2. Oral fluid intake may be prevented by toxo plasma encephalitis for which it is used
   3. Concurrent diarrhea and volume depletion. Associated presence of HIV associated nephropathy

Prevention and treatment

- Maintain adequate hydration (~3L/day)
- Urinary alkalinization with 6-12 g/day of sodium bicarbonate to ensure urine pH > 7.5.
- Routine urine microscopy 2-3 times a week, to detect gross/microscopic hematuria.
- Perform ultrasonography in all patients of hematuria.

4. **Acyclovir:** Doses > 500 mg/m^2 given i.v. leads to nephrotoxicity. Its low solubility leads to intratubular precipitation with symptoms of obstructive uropathy and hematuria. Urine analysis reveals birefringent needle-shaped crystals. Interstitial inflammation is seen adjacent to areas of intratubular obstruction. Oliguria is very rare.

   Risk factors include: Volume depletion, pre-existing renal insufficiency and rapid bolus infusion. Treatment is prompt withdrawal of therapy, which restores near normal renal function within 10- 14 days. However severe renal failure may occur necessitating

5. **Amphotericin-B [4]:** Disruption of cell membranes leads to endothelial damage with vasoconstriction of afferent and efferent arterioles, causing an acute fall in GFR and an initial oliguric ARF in some patients.

   Clinical spectrum of amphotericin nephrotoxicity

   Azotemia: It is almost universal with Amphoterecin-B. GFR falls to 40% in first 2-3 weeks and stabilizes at 20-60% of normal throughout course of treatment; normalizing on cessation of therapy. Cumulative doses of 3-4g have greater risk; Renal tubular acidosis can occur at cumulative doses of 0.5-1 g but is reversible.

6. **Rifampicin:** Incidence of rifampicin nephrotoxicity varies from 1.8% to 16% of all ARF. Most cases of rifampicin-related renal failure are secondary to drug-induced haemolytic anaemia. However, Acute Interstitial Nephritis (AIN), rapidly progressive glomeru-lonephritis presenting as proteinuria with acute onset deterioration of renal functions and light-chain proteinuria constitute the remaining. Duration of therapy seems important and cases have been reported after two months of therapy; although reactions as early as 13 days have also been seen. Intermittent regimens carry greater risk. The possibility of toxic interaction between isoniazid and pyrazinamide also exists. In most cases prompt withdrawal of therapy and supportive management leads to recovery within three weeks

7. **NSAID [5]:** NSAID-induced hemodynamic deterioration of renal function - Higher than usual dose, volume depletion due to flow loss diarrhoea, congestive heart failure, nephrotic syndrome, cirrhosis particularly with ascites, preexisting renal disease, third space fluid sequestration, diuretic therapy, age > 65 years.

   Syndromes of NSAID nephrotoxicity

   1. ARF - usually oliguric
   2. Acute interstitial nephritis
   3. Hyperkalemia
   4. Sodium and water retention
   5. Hypertension

NSAID-induced tubulointerstitial nephritis-

Clinical Features

- Usually sub acute to chronic course
- Mostly seen with fenoprofen but all NSAIDs till date observed to cause
- Mean period of development 5.4 months
- Associated with heavy proteinuria (> 3.0 day) in 83% of cases
- Fever, rash, Eosinophilia rare (<19%)

Renal sparing NSAIDs: Chronic kidney disease (CKD) and NSAIDs - also known as "analgesic nephropathy".

Consumption of any NSAID for over 20 years. The potential of CKD exists with use of analgesic mixture and is most well studied with aspirin codeine.

Higher risk in female and patient with rhematic disorder and migrane Analgesic cause renal injury

8. **Anti-neoplastic agents [6]:**

   Cisplatin: Major side effects are nephrotoxicity and are irreversible in most cases. Toxicity is cumulative and dose-related (> 25-33 mg/m^2/wk predisposes to nephron-toxicity). Nephrotoxicity is by acute tubular necrosis or tubulointerstitial process with symptoms of azotemia and fluid loss. Biochemical tests usually show tubular proteinuria with prominent tubular casts. High BUN and SCr and low.

   Cyclophosphamide: Although primarily a myelotoxic drug, nephrotoxicity is known. At daily doses of more than 50 mg/kg hyponatremia is seen. Hyponatremia occurs due to impaired water excretion by antidiuretic effect on distal nephron. The effect is transient and dissipates after 24 hrs of discontinuation of therapy. Hemorrhagic cystitis is a more common side effect of cyclophosphamide.

   Methotrexate: Effective chemotherapeutic agent. Nephrotoxicity seen at doses greater than 1.5 g/m2 /week. Mainly due to intratubular deposition of 7- hydroxymethotrexate leading to crystalluria and features of non-oliguric renal failure.

9. **Antihypertensives:** ACE inhibitors - Most common syndrome is reversible ARF seen in cases of hypertension and congestive heart failure and is related to action of angiotensin II on efferent arterioles for maintenance of GFR at time of low perfusion pressure with increasing filtration fraction.

   Hence ACEI cause a sudden decline in GFR due to loss of efferent arteriolar tone.

   Angiotensin receptor blockers (ARBs) -ARBs reduce BP to a degree comparable to ACE inhibitors but propensity to cause renal disease is believed to be less, especially with regard to functional renal failure.

10. **Diuretics:** These cause reduction in GFR by extracellular fluid volume contraction. Other renal diseases induced by the diuretics Hypokalemia nephropathy: all the diuretics expect the potassium sparing diuretics. Polyuria and abnormal concentrating ability. All diuretics (except potassium-sparing) due to chronic hypokalemia.

Interstitial nephritis : thiazides and furosemide

Vasculitis : Thiazides

Prerenal failure : diuretics

Nephrolithiasis : acetazolomide

11. **Gold and D- Penicillamine** – Penicillamine 7% develop nephrotic syndrome with kidney biopsy demonstrating membranous nephropathy. Proteinuria may occur at six months to six years. Gold - Proteinuria occurs in 30% of patient with renal pathology in most being membranous glomerulopathy

    Parenteral gold is more likely to cause proteinuria. Development of proteinuria both with gold and penicillamine is shown to be in HLA-B8 and Human Leukocyte Antigen - B8 (HLA-DRW3) patients.

12. **Poisons masquerading:** Ethylene glycol contamination is recognized by a picture of ethanol-like intoxication, elevated serum osmolality followed by increased anion-gap metabolic acidosis and oxalate crystals in urine.

    Acute tubular necrosis manifested by proteinuria, oliguria and anuria becomes evident in 12 to 24 hours following ingestion. Heavy metals like lead, cadmium, mercury and arsenic are constituents of medicines.

    Interstitial nephritis, tubular damage, decline in GFR and chronic kidney failure.

    Nephrotic syndrome is another manifestation of heavy metal poisonings and arsenic exposure may result in cancer of the bladder and kidneys.

13. **Contrast-induced nephropathy:** It is a condition with impairment in renal function defined as an increase in SCr by more than 25% within three days following intravenous administration of a contrast medium in the absence of an alternative

Risk factors

Renal failure, diabetic nephropathy, severe congestive heart failure, amount of contrast media (> 150 ml) and volume depletion.

Clinical features –

Acute and progressive rise in SCr within 24 hours of i.v. contrast administration is seen. Oliguria is present in 95% of cases

Prevention and management

Minimize amount of contrast administered (< 2 ml/kg or max of 150 mL)

Use of non-ionic contrast iso-osmolar solution for high risk patients is recommended.

Monitor SCr on 2nd and 4th day post procedure in high risk patients.

Patient should be hemodynamically stable

Calcium blockers prevent renal ischemia during initial renal vasoconstrictor phase.

Drug Induced Kidney Structural Functional Alterations

Tubular epithelial cell damage

Acute tubular necrosis	Pentomidine
Amino glycoside antibiotics	Foscamet
Radiographic contrast media	Zoledronate
Cisplatin carboplatin	Osmatic nephrosis
Amphotericin B	Mannitol
Cyclosporine, Tacrolimus	Dextran

Haemodynamically Mediated Kidney Injury

Angiotensin converting enzyme inhibitors	Non steroidal anti inflammatory drugs
Angiotensin II receptor blockers	Cyclosporine

Obstructive Nephropathy

Intratubular obstruction	Nephrolithiasias
Acyclovir	Sulfonamides
Sulfonamides	Triamterene
Indinavir	Indinavir
Methotrexate	Oral sodium phosphate

Tubulo Intestinal Disease

Acute allergic interstitial nephritis	Chronic interstitial nephritis
Penicillins	Cyclosporine
Ciprofloxacin	Lithium
Proton pump inhibitors	Papillary necrosis
Loop diuretics	NSAIDS, Aspirin

Renal Vasculitis Thrombosis & Cholesterol Emboli

Hydralazine	Methamphetamines
Propyl thiouracil	Cyclosporine
Allopurine	Warfarin
Gerncitobine	Thrombolytic agents

Risk factors for amino glycoside nephrotoxicity

Related to amino glycoside: Large total cumulative dose, Prolonged theory, Trough concentration exceeding 2mg/L

Related to synergistic nephrotoxicity: Amino glycosides in combination with Cyclosporine, Amphotericin B, Vancomycin, Cisplatin, NSAIDs

Related to predisposing conditions in patients: Pre existing kidney disease, Diabetes, Increased age, Shock, Gram negative bacteremia, Liver disease, Obstructive jaundice, Hypotension

Prevention of contrast nephrotoxicity: Contrast – minimize contrast volume/dose; Use non iodinated contrast studies, use low or iso osmolar contrast agents

Medications:

Avoid concurrent use of potentially nephrotoxic drugs for eg: NSAIDs, amino glycosides

Isotonic Sodium Chloride:

Initiate infusion 3-12hrs prior to contrast exposure and continue 6-24 hrs post exposure alternative in urgent case initiate infusion at 3ml/kg/h

N-acetyl cysteine:

Administer 600-1200mg by mouth every 12hr, 4 doses beginning prior to contrast exposure

Isotonic sodium bicarbonate:

Initiate and maintain infusion at 3ml/kg/h

References

1. NP Singh, A Ganguli, A Prakash, Drug-induced Kidney Diseases JAPI, VOL. 51: OCTOBER 2003, 970-79.
2. Luft FC. Clinical significance of renal changes engendered by aminoglycosides in man. J Antimicrob Chemother 1984;13(suppl A):23-30.
3. Sorrell TC, Collignon PJ. A prospective study of adverse reactions associated with vancomycin. J Antimicrob Chemother 1985;16:235-41.
4. Wasan KM, Vadiei K, Lopez-Berestein G, Verani RR, Luke DR. Pentoxyphylline in amphotericin B toxicity rat model. Antimicrobial Agents Chemother 1990;34:241-4.
5. Morgenstern SJ, Bruns FJ, Fraley DS, Kirsch M, Borochoitz D. Ibuprofen-associated lipoid nephrosis without interstitial nephritis. Am J Kidney Dis 1989;14:50-2.
6. Feehally J, Walls J, Mistry N, et al. Does nifedipine ameliorate cyclosporin A nephrotoxicity? Br Med J 1987;295:310.

CHAPTER - 24

Systemic Lupus Erythematosus

Introduction to Systemic Lupus Erythematosus (SLE)

It is a fluctuating multi-system disease with a diversity of clinical presentations.

- SLE is the development of autoantibodies to cellular nuclear components that leads to a chronic inflammatory autoimmune disease.
- It has a wide spectrum of symptoms & organ system involvement, making therapy highly patient specific.

Epidemiology: 1.9-5.6/1,00,000 person/ year in adults; Predominant in woman with female to male ratio 10:1 at ages of 15-45 years.

Despite advances in treatment, standardized mortality rates in SLE remain three times higher than in the general population. The risk of mortality is significantly increased for mortality due to renal disease, cardiovascular disease, and infection.

SLE is a risk factor for cervical neoplasia, in particular for premalignant cervical lesions. The risk is highest among patients on immunosuppressants. Treatment-wise, azathioprine was shown to increase the risk of acute myeloid leukemia or myelodysplastic syndrome 7-fold in an autoimmune population, but the study included only a small number of SLE patients.

Lupus nephritis was shown to be an important cardiovascular risk factor with a hazard ratio nine times higher compared to SLE patients without lupus nephritis. SLE doubles the risk of stroke with the highest relative risk for of stroke observed within the first year after diagnosis.

Etiology

- **Genetic Factors:** 1st degree relatives are 20 times more likely to get SLE. Siblings of SLE patients are 30 times more likely to develop SLE.
- **MHC genes** – Human leukocyte antigen genes. Non-MHC genes- Ig receptor genes- contribute to susceptibility.
- Defect in clearance, processing and presenting apoptotic cells and debris to lymphocytes. Increased availability of nuclear debris can provide sufficient self-antigen for induction of self-reactive t cells or activation of immune response.
- **Environmental factors:** chemicals (hydrazine in tobacco); Aromatic amines (hair dyes); diet; environmental oestrogens. Infection (virus – Epstein)-EBV reside in and interact with B cells and promotes IFN alpha production by the dendritic cells suggesting its role

in controlling chronic viral infection, Many drugs may cause drug induced lupus DIL due to hypersensitivity reactions. Sunlight (UV)- may induce breaks in DNA that may alter gene expression or lead to apoptotic or necrotic cell death.

- Hormonal factors

Pathophysiology: Environmental factors, such as infectious organisms, drugs, and chemicals, serve as triggering agents in genetically and hormonally susceptible individuals to induce a state of immune dysregulation. These abnormal immune responses lead to hyperactive T-helper-2 lymphocyte and B-lymphocyte function. Suppressor T-lymphocyte function, cytokine production, faulty clearance mechanisms, and other immune regulatory mechanisms also are abnormal and fail to downregulate autoantibody formation from hyperactive B-lymphocytes. The autoantibodies formed from this immune dysregulation become pathogenic, form immune complexes, and activate complement that leads to damage of host tissue.

Many auto-antibodies are directed against nuclear constituents of the cell- antinuclear antibodies. dsDNA (Double strand); ssDNA (Single strand); RNA

- RNA associated AG's are Smith (Sm) antigen, small nuclear ribonucleoprotein (snRNP), RoSSA antigen and La/SS-B) Antigen.
- Histone is another nuclear component against which Ab are formed.
- Anti-phospholipid antibodies are directed against phospholipid moiety of prothrombin activator complex.

Key events in the pathophysiology of SLE

Innate susceptibility factors like HLA type/immunoregulatory genes/complement levels/ hormonal levels/cytokines/neutrophil activity are responsible for autoimmune proliferation. Environmental stimuli like UV exposure/microbial response/drugs also predispose to autoimmune proliferation and activation of autoimmune antibody production.

1. **Apoptosis:** It is the source of antibodies. In SLE there is an increased spontaneous apoptosis, increased rate of UV-induced apoptosis in skin cells, or impaired clearance of apoptotic peripheral blood cells.
2. **Nucleic acids (DNA & RNA):** their recognition as foreign bodies is prevented in healthy individuals. In SLE they are recognized and served to intracellular sensors (eg Toll like receptors)
3. **Innate immunity:** Toll like receptors now detect DNA as non self-antigen as present for immune responses. Dendrtic cells will produce IFNalpha which further recruits T cells foe further processing. Neutrophils will now get acticated and are responsible for proinflammatory and vascular damage.
4. **Adaptive immunity:** there is activation of T-helper cells by the previous events. B-cells now differentiated into antibody producing plasma cells. Cytokines and chemikines are released by the T and B cells which shape the immune response and promote tissue damage. Excess production of immune complexes, with impaired clearance leads to deposition and tissue damage.

Clinical Manifestation and Features

Constitutional Symptoms

Constitutional symptoms are seen in more than 90% of patients with SLE and are often the initial presenting feature. Fatigue, malaise, fever, anorexia and weight loss are common. While more than 40% of patients with SLE may have lupus flare as a cause of fever, infections must always be ruled out first given the immunocompromised state of these patients. Further, SLE is a very rare cause of fever of unknown origin.

Mucocutaneous Manifestations

SLE skin lesions may be lupus specific, while several non-specific lesions are also seen in SLE. Lupus specific lesions include (1). Acute cutaneous lupus erythematosus (ACLE), which includes localized, malar and generalized, (2). Subacute cutaneous lupus erythematosus (SCLE), which includes annular and papulosquamous, and (3). Chronic cutaneous lupus erythematosus (CCLE), which includes classic discoid lupus erythematosus (DLE), hypertrophic/verrucous, lupus panniculitis/profundus, lupus tumidus, chilblains lupus, mucosal discoid lupus, and lichenoid discoid lupus.

Acute cutaneous lupus erythematosus (ACLE) may be localized or generalized. The hallmark ACLE lesion is the malar rash or the butterfly rash, which is an erythematous raised pruritic rash involving the cheeks and nasal bridge.

The rash may be macular or papular and spares the nasolabial folds. It usually has an acute onset, but may last several weeks, and may cause induration and scaling. The malar rash may also fluctuate with lupus disease activity.

Discoid lupus erythematosus (DLE) is the most common form of chronic cutaneous lupus erythematosus (CCLE). DLE may occur with or without SLE, and can be either localized (only head and neck) or generalized (above and below the neck). The lesions are disk-shaped erythematous papules or plaques with adherent scaling and central clearing.

Hematologic and Reticuloendothelial Manifestations

Anemia is present in more than 50 % of patients with SLE and most commonly is anemia of chronic disease. Other causes of anemia in SLE may include iron deficiency anemia, coomb's positive autoimmune hemolytic anemia, red blood cell aplasia and microangiopathic hemolytic anemia which may be associated with antiphospholipid antibody syndrome.

Leukopenia secondary to neutropenia or lymphopenia is also very frequent and can be severe. Thrombocytopenia can be mild or severe and may be associated with antiphospholipid antibody syndrome and autoantibodies against platelets, glycoprotein IIb/IIIa or thrombopoietin receptor. Pancytopenia is not infrequent and may occasionally be associated with myelofibrosis.

Neuropsychiatric Manifestations

Focal or generalized seizures may be seen, and are associated with disease activity, although they carry a favorable prognosis. Other CNS manifestations include aseptic meningitis, demyelinating syndrome including optic neuritis and myelitis, movement disorders such as chorea and cognitive dysfunction. Patients with SLE are also at high risk for ischemic strokes.

Renal Manifestations

Lupus nephritis is a well-known and common complication of SLE. The involvement may range from mild sub nephrotic proteinuria to diffuse progressive glomerulonephritis leading to chronic kidney damage. Lupus nephritis usually occurs early in the course of SLE. New-onset hypertension, hematuria, proteinuria, lower extremity edema, and elevation in creatinine shall raise suspicion for lupus nephritis.

Pulmonary Manifestations

Pleuritis is the most common pulmonary manifestation, and may not always be associated with pleural effusion. Other pulmonary manifestations include exudative pleural effusions, acute lupus pneumonitis with bilateral pulmonary infiltrates, interstitial lung disease which may be nonspecific interstitial pneumonia (NSIP) or usual interstitial pneumonia (UIP)

Pregnancy Complications

SLE patients with positive antiphospholipid antibodies are at a high risk of spontaneous abortions and fetal loss, pre-eclampsia and maternal thrombosis. Anti-Ro (SSA) and Anti-La (SSB) antibodies can cross the placenta leading to fetal heart block and neonatal lupus presenting with a photosensitive rash, cytopenias, and transaminitis.

American College of Rheumatology criteria for SLE diagnosis Criteria Description

1. Malar rash: Fixed edema, flat or raised, over the malar eminenses
2. Discoid rash: erythematosus circular raised patches with adherent keratotic scaling and follicular plugging; atrophic scarring may occur.
3. Photosensitivity: exposure to ultraviolet light causes rash
4. Oral ulcers: includes oral and nasopharyngeal ulcers, observed by physician
5. Arthritis: non-erosive arthritis of two or more peripheral joints, with tenderness, selling, or effusion.
6. Serositis: pleuritis or pericarditis documented by ECG or rub or evidence of effusion.
7. Renal disorder: proteinuria >0.5g/d or 3+, or cellular casts.
8. Neurological disorder: seizures or psychosis without other causes.
9. Hematologic disorder: haemolytic anemia or leukopenia (<4000/L) or lymphopenia.(<1500/L) or thrombocytopenia (<100,000/L) in thr absence of offending drugs.
10. Immunologic disorder: anti-dsDNA, anti-Sm, and/or anti-phospholipid.

New ACR and Eular Criteria for Classification of SLE

All the patients classified as having SLE must have a serum titer of antinuclear antibody of atleast 1:80 on human epithelial -2 postive cells or an equivalent positive test.

In addition the patient must present atleast 4 ACR criteria.

1. Constitutional domain: Fever
2. Cutaneous domain: Nonscaring alopecia/oral ulcers/subacute cutaneous or discoid lupus/ acute cutaneous lupus
3. Arthritis domain: Synovitis in atleeast 2 joints or tenderness in atleast 2 joints and atleast 30min of morning stiffness
4. Neurologic domain: Delirium/psychosis/seizure
5. Serositis domain: Pleural or pericardial effusion/Acute pericarditis
6. Hematologic domain: Leukopenia/ thrombocytopenia/autoimmune hemolysis
7. Renal domain: Proteinuria>0.5g/24h; class II or V lupus nephritis/class III or IV lupus nephritis
8. Antiphospholipid antibody domain: Anticardiolipin IgG>40 GPL or anti-Beta 2GP1>40 units or Lupus anticoagulant
9. Complement proteins domain: Low C3 or low C4/ Low C3 and low C4
10. Highly specific antibodies domain: Anti-dsDNA antibody/Anti-Smith antibody

https://www.mdedge.com/rheumatology/article/168702/lupus-connective-tissue-diseases/new-sle-classification-criteria-reset

Diagnosis with Algorithm [1, 2]

- If the patient has symptoms from 2 or more of the systems as described above, he is suspected to have SLE.
- If the patient has at least 4 ACR criteria, it is confirmed as SLE.
- ANA is to be estimated and if negative-it indicates very low probability of SLE.
- If ANA test is positive- complete blood count with differential count to be done. Urinalysis, anti-dsDNA, anti-Sm, anti-cardiolipin antibodies have to estimated.
- If all the results are negative it indicates SLE to be unlikely.
- But if High titer to Anti-dsDNA or anti-specific antibodies are detected – it is confirmed as SLE.

Management

Desired Outcomes.

1. Management of symptoms and induction ofremission during times of disease flare
2. Maintenance of remission for as long as possible between diseases flares

General Approach to the Management of SLE

1. If diagnosis of SLE is done, first the patient is counselled- i) about education and psychosocial support, b) balanced diet, c) balanced routine of rest and exercise, d) to avoid smoking.
2. Detection of antiphospholipid antibodies is carried out. If result is positive - consider low-dose aspirin. If result is negative- there is a possibility of symptomatic SLE.
   (a) If it is mild to moderate disease and non organ threatening- then consider NSAIDs or Antimalarials or low dose corticosteroids.

    (b) If the disease is severe, life threatening or organ threatening disease- consider either high dose corticosteroids and/ or cytotoxic drugs.

3. If the disease is controlled and in remission
    (a) If yes-Consider need for continued treatment
    (b) If No-Consider alternative treatment.

Nonpharmacological Therapy

- A balanced routine of rest and exercise, while avoiding overexertion, is essential in managing fatigue
- Avoidance of smoking may be particularly important because hydrazines in tobacco smoke may be an environmental trigger of lupus and likely contribute to accelerated CAD.
- The amount of sunlight exposure limitation should be individualized.

Pharmacological Therapy

Drug therapy for SLE is designed to suppress immune response and inflammation.

NSAIDs

- Anti – inflammatory dose. Main indications in Mild disease, fever, arthritis, Skin rash, serositis.
- Toxicities to monitor: Gi Bleeding, hepatic toxicity, renal toxicity, hypertension
- Baseline evaluation: CBC, Cr, Urinaraly, AST, ALT

Antimalarials

- Hyroxychlorquine (200-400mg *po* daily) Chlorquine (250-500mg *po* daily)
- Main indications: Epericardial inflammation, Mild disease, arthritis, skin rash, serositis, pleuritic, leukopenia
- These are not effective immediately so best used in long term management. Chloroquine (CQ) response occurs within 1-3 months. Hydroxy chloroquine (HCQ) (3-6 months). HCQ is safer than CQ.
- MOA proposed is they interfere with T-lymphocyte activation. Inhibition of cytosine, decreased sensitivity to UV light, anti-inflammatory activity, anti-platelet effects and anti-hyperlipidimicactivity in SLE patients.
- SE include CNS (headache, Insomnia), pigmentation changes in skin.

Corticosteroids

- Goal in SLE with steroids is to suppress and maintain suppression of active disease with lowest dose possible.
- Prednisolone 1-2mg/kg/d *po*< 1mg/kg/d; Initial control of severe disease. Control of mild disease or maintenance after disease suppression with higher doses
- Methyl prednisolone (500-1000mg IV daily 3-6 day); Life threatening diseases.

- Standard Pulse therapy is IV Methyl prednisolone (500-1000mg/3-6 days). Pulse therapy is followed by high dose prednisone 1-1.5mg/kg/d.
- Low dose maintenance therapy for life threatening conditions.
- Toxicities to monitor: Hypertension (HT), Hyperglycemia, hyperlipidemia, hypokalemia, osteoporosis, cataract, weight gain, infections, fluid retention
- Baseline evaluation: BP, Glucose, Potassium levels, TC, LDL, HDL, Triglycerides

Cytotoxic Drugs

- Cyclophosphamide 0.5-1g/m2 IV, monthly for months; then every 3 months for 2 years or for 1 year after remission. Azathioprine (1-3mg/kg *po* daily); Mycophenolate mofetil 1-3g *po* daily.
- Most commonly used in severe lupus nephritis, for other severe disease manifestation
- Azathioprine is used as steroid sparing agent. Allowing for reduction of corticosteroid doses.
- Long term maintenance azathioprine therapy may prevent renal flares after successful cyclophosphamide induction. Adverse effects AE with azathioprine, myelo suppression, opportunistic infections.
- Toxicities to monitor:
- Azathioprine- Myelosuppression, hepatotoxicity, lymphoproliferative disorders,
- Baseline evaluation: Complete Blood Count (CBC), Platelet count, CR, AST, ALT
- Cyclophosphamide: Myelosuppression, secondary infertility, Myelosuppression, hepatotoxicity. Baseline evaluation: Patient count, urinaralysis

Recommendations for the management of patients with systemic lupus erythematosus [3, 4]

Mild SLE with no major organ involvement:
- **Discoid lupus:** sunscreen use; topical corticosteroid/tacrolimus; topical acitretin; with or without systemic glucocorticoids, then add azathioprine or switch to mycophenolate or methotrexate.
- **Uncomplicated digital or cutaneous vasculitis:** systemic glucocorticoids with or without hydroxychloroquine, then add azathioprine or mycophenolate ; then switch to IV cyclophosphamide.
- HCQ is recommended for all patients with SLE, unless contraindicated, at a dose not exceeding 5 mg/kg/real BW.
- In the absence of risk factors for retinal toxicity, ophthalmological screening (by visual fields examination and/or spectral domain-optical coherence tomography) should be performed at baseline, after 5 years, and yearly thereafter.
- Glucocorticoids can be used at doses and route of administration that depend on the type and severity of organ involvement.
- Pulses of intravenous Methylprednisolone (usually 250–1000 mg per day, for 1–3 days) provide immediate therapeutic effect and enable the use of lower starting dose of oral GC

- For chronic maintenance treatment, Gluco Corticoids (GC) should be minimised to less than 7.5 mg/day (prednisone equivalent)

- In patients not responding to HCQ (alone or in combination with GC) or patients unable to reduce GC below doses acceptable for chronic use, addition of immunomodulating/ immunosuppressive agents such as Methotrexate, Azathioprine or Mycophenolate should be considered.

- Cyclophosphamide can be used for severe organ-threatening or life-threatening SLE as well as 'rescue' therapy in patients not responding to other immunosuppressive agents.

- In patients with inadequate response to standard-of-care (combinations of HCQ and GC with or without immunosuppressive agents), defined as residual disease activity not allowing tapering of glucocorticoids and/or frequent relapses, add-on treatment with belimumab should be considered.

Specific manifestations [5]

- **Skin disease**: First-line treatment of skin disease in SLE includes topical agents (GC, calcineurin inhibitors), antimalarials (HCQ, quinacrine) and/or systemic Gluco Corticoids (GC).

- **Neuropsychiatric disease**: Treatment of SLE-related neuropsychiatric disease includes glucocorticoids/immunosuppressive agents for manifestations considered to reflect an inflammatory process, and antiplatelet/anticoagulants for atherothrombotic/aPL-related manifestations.

- **Haematological disease**: Acute treatment of lupus thrombocytopenia includes high-dose GC (including pulses of intravenous methylprednisolone) and/or intravenous immunoglobulin G. For maintenance of response, immunosuppressive/GC-sparing agents such as mycophenolate, azathioprine or cyclosporine can be used. Refractory cases can be treated with rituximabor cyclophosphamide.

- **Renal disease:** Mycophenolate or low-dose intravenous cyclophosphamide are recommended as initial (induction) treatment, as they have the best efficacy/ toxicity ratio. In patients at high risk for renal failure (reduced glomerular filtration rate, histological presence of fibrous crescents or fibrinoid necrosis, or tubular atrophy/ interstitial fibrosis], similar regimens may be considered but high-dose intravenous cyclophosphamide can also be used. For maintenance therapy, mycophenolate or azathioprine should be used.

- Mycophenolate may be combined with low dose of a calcineurin inhibitor in severe nephrotic syndrome or incomplete renal response, in the absence of uncontrolled hypertension, high chronicity index at kidney biopsy and/or reduced GFR

Comorbidities

- **Antiphospholipid syndrome:** All patients with SLE should be screened at diagnosis for antiphospholid antibodies. Patients with SLE with high-risk (aPL) profile (persistently positive medium/high titres or multiple positivity) may receive primary prophylaxis with antiplatelet agents, especially if other atherosclerotic/thrombophilic factors are present, after balancing the bleeding hazard.

- **Alveolitis:** Systemic glucocorticoids plus mycophenolate or IV cyclophosphamide; then add rituximab or IV immune globulin, maintain with azathioprine or mycophenolate.
- **Myocarditis**: Systemic glucocorticoids plus IV cyclophosphamide, with or without hydroxychloroquine, then rituximab, IV immune globulin.
- **Pericariditis**: NSAIDs, then systemic glucocorticoidsn plus hydreoxychloroquin; then add mycophenolate, azathioprine, or methotrexate; then add belimumab or rituximab.
- **Pulmonary artery hypertension**: Systemic glucocorticoids plus IV cyclophosphamide or mycophenolate +then add rituximabs.

Pharmacotherapeutic Complications

- Medication-induced complications are common and require close monitoring. Long-term corticosteroid use in SLE patients frequently leads to osteoporosis which is under-diagnosed and under-treated leading to osteoporotic fractures.
- Other complications of long-term use corticosteroid therapy include avascular necrosis, glaucoma, cataract, weight gain and poor control of Diabetes mellitus. High dose corticosteroid use can also be associated with opportunistic infections and acute psychosis.
- Long term use of hydroxychloroquine may rarely result in maculopathy and retinopathy that is irreversible, and close ophthalmology examinations are recommended.
- Cyclophosphamide use is associated with a significantly high risk of interstitial cystitis and bladder cancer even after drug discontinuation.
- SLE patients are immunocompromised and at a significantly high risk of infections which is one of the major causes of morbidity and mortality in SLE.

Case Study of Systemic Lupus Erethematous (SLE)

Summary

Female patient of age 43 years came to hospital with complaints of fever since 6 months on and off. SOB since 1 month, Butterfly rash, joint pains, Weight loss, No details provided regarding part medical history. These following investigations were done. Physical examination revealed presence of butterfly rash. Vitals showed febrile temperature hypotension & slight increased pulse rate. CBP revealed decreased WBC count (2,700 cells/ cumm). ESR was found to be raised (70mm/hr). Urine analysis showed presence of pus cells. Thyroid levels and blood sugar levels were normal. C-Reactive protein was positive 5.6ng/dL. ECG revealed sinus tachycardia. Antibody testing showed presence of Anti DNA antibody 199.8 lu/mL, Anti nucleus antibody 9.83 lu/mL.

Diagnosis : Based on the obtained subjective and objective data the patient was diagnosed to be suffering with systemic lupus erythematosus

Trade name	Generic name	Category	Route	Dose	Frequency
T. Wysolone	Prednisolone	Corticosteroid	p/o	10 mg	BD
T.Axonal	Hydroxy chloroquine	Anti parasitic	p/o	200mg	BD
T.Aycal C+Z	Calcitriol+CaCo3+elemental mg & Zn	Vitamin & mineral supplement	p/o	1 tab	OD
T. Onfer XTZ	Ferrous ascorbate +folic acid +Znso4	Iron supplement	p/o	1 tab	OD
T.PCM	Paracetamol	Anti pyretic	p/o	650mg	OD
Oint. Zintyl	Salicylic acid	Topical keratolytics	Topical		OD

Progress Chart: On day 1, patient got admitted and was examined. From day 2, regimen for SLE has been started with steroids, Anti parasitic, vitamin & minerals supplements along with salicyclic acid. The same regimen was being continued. No fresh complaints or complications were noted.

Pharmacist Tnterventions

- No major interactions were found
- Use of steroid shouldn't stopped once, dose tempering should be done
- Salicylic acid is only for external use not it internally

Patient Counselling

- This disease doesn't have permanent clue
- Know the disease information & severity of condition
- Should know importance of medications prescribed
- Avoid exposure to heat/ excess sunlight
- Maintain hygiene
- Regularly consult physician & report if any fresh symptoms observed
- Never skip doses , take medicine regularly
- Avoid allergic food & allergic conditions
- Limit use of soaps
- Don't scratch too much in rashes area
- Have plenty of water & and drink boiled water
- Avoid stress

Assignment

1. **What is SLE?**

   Systemic lupus erythematosus is a chronic autoimmune disease that causes systemic inflammation. It is characterised by production of unusual antibodies by body's immune system towards its own cells

Inflammation caused by lupus can affect different body systems including joints, skin, kidneys, blood cells, brain, health & lungs.

2. What signs and symptoms indicate SLE in the patient?

The following symptoms were indicated

Fever since	6 months
SOB since	1 month
Butterfly rash	
Weight loss	
Joint pain	

3. What are the complications of SLE?

Apart from common signs & symptoms like fatigue, fever, joint pains, rashes Etc.,

Inflammation caused by lupus can affect many areas of body

The following complications may occur

- Renal : Serious kidney damage, kidney failure, sr.cr proteinuria
- Neurological: Dizziness, headache, psychosis, depression, seizures, anxiety, Stroke, vision problems
- Hematologic: Anemia, thrombocytopenia, increase risk of bleeding, lymphadenopathy, vascularitis.
- Pulmonary : pleurisy, coughing, dyspnea, lupus pneumonitis, pulmonary hypertension.
- Cardiac : Pericarditis, Myocarditis, Coronary Artery Disease (CAD), heart attack, ECG changes
- GIT : Non specific dyspepsia, abdominal pain, nausea, difficulty in swallowing, bowel haemon
- Musculo Skeletal: Arthralgia, Myalgia, Arthritis.
- Pregnancy Complications: miscarriage, pre eclampsia, premature birth.
- Increase risk of having cancer, weakened immune system

4. What clinical and laboratory tests should be performed to diagnose SLE?

Diagnosing lupus is difficult as the signs & symptoms vary from person to person. The combination of blood, urine tests, symptoms & other tests are done to diagnose SLE

- **Laboratory tests.**
  - *Blood test:* Blood cells count to identity anemia, leucopenia, Erythrocyte Sedimentation rate. (elevated in SLE kidney & liver function assessment (GFR, bilind) anti nuclear antibody test – ANA positive in lupus
  - *Urine analysis:* Presence of RBC, protein in urine

- **Other tests**
  - *ECG:* To detect cardiac abnormalities
  - *Chest x-ray:* To detect pulmonary changes (inflammation)
  - Skin biopsy & other tissue biopsy to detect damage

5. **Which medications in the following drug classes are used for treatment of SLE?**

   (A) Anti malarials   **(B) Corticosteroids**   **(C) Non biological DMARDS**

   (D) NSAIDS   **(E) Biological DMARDS**

(A) Anti malarials	Chloroquine 250 - 500mg - p/o – OD
	Hydroxy chloroquine - 200 to 400 mg – p/o – OD
(B) Corticosteroids	Methyl prednisolone 500 – 1000 mg- IV 3to 6 days
	Prednisolone 1 to 2 mg/kg/day – p/o. (Initial)
	<1mg/kg/day – p/o – (Maintenance)

   (C) Non biological DMARDS

   Cyclophoshamide - 0.5 to 1 g /m2 body surface – IV – monthly for 6 months

   Azathioprine -   1 to 3 mg /kg – p/o – OD

   Mycophenolate mofetil - 1 to 3g – p/o – OD

(D) NSAIDS	Naproxen – 750 mg
	Ibuprofen – 200mg
	Diclofenac – 100 mg
(E) Biological DMARDS	Rituximab (375 mg/m^2)
	Infliximab

6. **What are the patients Counselling Measures?**
   - Take medications without fail
   - Consult doctor regularly
   - Wear protecting clothing to avoid UV light
   - Use sunscreens
   - Regular exercise can help to keep bones stronger
   - Avoid smoking, alcohol consumption
   - Have a healthy diet to boost immune
   - Stay in a healthy environment
   - Avoid stressful conditions
   - Limit sodium in Take, saturated, trans fat
   - Have potassium rich foods

7. What are ACR guidelines for management of SLE with lupus nephritis?

- Goals of treatment include patient survival, long-term preservation of kidney function, prevention of disease flares, prevention of organ damage, management of comorbidities and improvement in disease-related quality of life.
- Kidney biopsy should be considered when there is evidence of kidney involvement, especially in the presence of persistent proteinuria ≥ 0.5 g/24 hours (or urine total protein to creatinine ratio ≥ 500 mg/g in morning first void urine), and/or an unexplained decrease in glomerular filtration rate (GFR)
- Initial treatment for class III–IV Lupus nephritis: Mycophenolate mofetil (MMF) or or low-dose IV cyclophosphamide plus glucocorticoids
- Alternate option for class III–IV Lupus nephritis: Combination therapy of MMF with a calcineurin inhibitor (CNI), especially tacrolimus, particularly in patients with nephrotic-range proteinuria
- To reduce cumulative glucocorticoid dose: Intravenous pulses of methylprednisolone (total dose 500–2500 mg, depending on disease severity), followed by oral prednisone (0.3–0.5 mg/kg/day) for up to 4 weeks, tapered to ≤ 7.5 mg/day by 3 to 6 months
- Initial treatment for pure class V disease with nephrotic-range proteinuria: MMF in combination with methylprednisolone followed by oral prednisone
- Alternate options for pure class V: IV cyclophosphamide or a CNI, especially tacrolimus, as monotherapy or in combination with mMMF/mycophenolic acid (MPA)
- In all Lupus nephritis patients: Hydroxychloroquine (HCQ) should be coadministered at a dose not to exceed 5 mg/kg/day and adjusted for the GFR, in the absence of contraindications
- Patients who improve after initial treatment should receive MMF/MPA (especially if it was the initial treatment) or azathioprine (preferred in women who may become pregnant) in combination with low-dose prednisone when needed to control disease activity
- Gradual withdrawal of treatment (glucocorticoids first, then immunosuppressive drugs) can be attempted after at least 3 to 5 years therapy in patients with complete clinical response. HCQ should be continued long-term.
- Continuation, switching to or addition of CNIs, especially tacrolimus, can be considered in pure class V Lupus nephritis at the lowest effective dose and after considering nephrotoxicity risks
- Patients in whom initial therapy fails should be switched to one of the alternative initial therapies or to rituximab.

8. What are the goals of therapy in this patient?

- Control symptoms
- Improve quality of life
- Prevent further complications
- Maintenance of remission

9. What non drug therapies might be useful?

Acupuncture – may help case the muscle pain associated with lupus life style modifications including dietary changes, quit smoking

Regular exercise

Avoid skin exposure

Avoid stress

Applying sun screen lotion

10. What other medications do you recommend for treating non – renal manifestations of SLE ?

Cycophenolate mofetil 1 to 3 g/day

Azathioprine 2mg /kg/day

Rituximab

Glucocorticoids are also given with above drugs

References

1. Nguyet-cam vu lam, md; maria v. Ghetu, md; and marzena I. Bieniek, md, St. Luke's University Hospital, Bethlehem, Pennsylvania. Systemic Lupus Erythematosus: Primary Care Approach to Diagnosis and Management. Am Fam Physician. 2016 Aug 15; 94(4): 284-294.

2. Seralogic tests: Fluorescent antinuclear Ab (ANA), Ab to native DNA (dsDNA) and to Sm AG are also specific tests.

3. American College of Rheumatology Ad Hoc Committee on Systemic Lupus Erythematosus Guidelines. Guidelines for referral and management of systemic lupus erythematosus in adults. *Arthritis Rheum.* 1999;42(9):1785–1796.

4. Bertsias GK, Ioannidis JP, Aringer M, et al. EULAR recommendations for the management of systemic lupus erythematosus with neuropsychiatric manifestations: report of a task force of the EULAR standing committee for clinical affairs. *Ann Rheum Dis.* 2010;69(12):2074–2082.

5. George Stojan and Michelle Petri. Epidemiology of Systemic Lupus Erythematosus: an update. Curr Opin Rheumatol. 2018 Mar; 30(2): 144–150.

6. Chan TM, Tse KC, Tang CS, Mok MY, Li FK. Long-term study of mycophenolate mofetil as continuous induction and maintenance treatment for diffuse proliferative lupus nephritis. *J Am Soc Nephrol* 2005; 16: 1076– 84.

7. Dooley MA, Jayne D, Ginzler EM, Isenberg D, Olsen NJ, Wofsy D, et al, for the ALMS Group. Mycophenolate versus azathioprine as maintenance therapy for lupus nephritis. *N Eng J Med* 2011; 365: 1886– 95.

CHAPTER - 25

Rheumatoid Arthritis

Introduction to Rheumatoid Arthritis

- Rheumatoid arthritis is an autoimmune disorder. It is the chronic inflammation in the synovial fluid which involves joints.
- Progressive joint damage causing severe disability in young people, demanding considerable resources in terms of doctors, surgery and drugs.
- Severe joint pains and deformities are seen in rheumatoid arthritis patients. Depending upon the type of severity and intensit y the ranges vary.

Epidemiology

- Rheumatoid arthritis affects about 2% of population worldwide and is just common in tropical countries as in cold and damp places. It is about 3 times more common in women as in men. According to stats 5% of cases are seen in women of age groups of 64-74 years in female and 2% cases of men are seen of age groups 55-64 years. There is an increased incidence in those with the family history of rheumatoid arthritis (5-10%).

Etiology

- The main cause of rheumatoid arthritis is unknown; it can be genetic or predisposed due to environmental factors.
- It is the main common systemic inflammatory disease characterized by symmetrical joint involvement including rheumatoid nodules, vasculitis, extra articular symptoms, eye inflammations, neurological dysfunction, lymphadenopathy, splenomegaly are the main reasons.

Risk Factors

Factors that may increase risk of rheumatoid arthritis include:
- **Sex:** Women are more likely than men to develop rheumatoid arthritis.
- **Age:** Rheumatoid arthritis can occur at any age, but it most commonly begins between the ages of 40 and 60.

- **Family history:** If a member of the family has rheumatoid arthritis, there is an increased risk of the disease.
- **Smoking:** Cigarette smoking increases the risk of developing rheumatoid arthritis, particularly if there is a genetic predisposition for developing the disease. Smoking also appears to be associated with greater disease severity.
- **Environmental exposures:** Although uncertain and poorly understood, some exposures such as asbestos or silica may increase the risk for developing rheumatoid arthritis. Emergency workers exposed to dust from the collapse of the World Trade Center are at higher risk of autoimmune diseases such as rheumatoid arthritis.
- **Obesity:** People who are overweight or obese appear to be at somewhat higher risk of developing rheumatoid arthritis, especially in women diagnosed with the disease when they were 55 or younger.

Pathogenesis

RA results from a dysregulation of the humoral and cell-mediated components of the immune system. Most patients produce antibodies called rheumatoid factors; these seropositive patients tend to have a more aggressive course than patients who are seronegative. Immunoglobulins (Igs) can activate the complement system, which amplifies the immune response by enhancing chemotaxis, phagocytosis, and release of lymphokines by mononuclear cells that are then presented to T lymphocytes. The processed antigen is recognized by the major histocompatibility complex proteins on the lymphocyte surface, resulting in activation of T and B cells. Tumor necrosis factor (TNF), interleukin-1 (IL-1), and IL-6 are proinflammatory cytokines important in the initiation and continuance of inflammation. Activated T cells produce cytotoxins, which are directly toxic to tissues, and cytokines, which stimulate further activation of inflammatory processes and attract cells to areas of inflammation. Macrophages are stimulated to release prostaglandins and cytotoxins. Activated B cells produce plasma cells, which form antibodies that, in combination with complement, result in accumulation of polymorphonuclear leukocytes. Polymorphonuclear leukocytes release cytotoxins, oxygen free radicals, and hydroxyl radicals that promote cellular damage to synovium and bone. Vasoactive substances (histamine, kinins, prostaglandins) are released at sites of inflammation, increasing blood flow and vascular permeability. This causes edema, warmth, erythema, and pain and makes it easier for granulocytes to pass from blood vessels to sites of inflammation. Chronic inflammation of the synovial tissue lining the joint capsule results in tissue proliferation (pannus formation). Pannus invades cartilage and eventually the bone surface, producing erosions of bone and cartilage and leading to joint destruction. The end results may be loss of joint space, loss of joint motion, bony fusion (ankylosis), joint subluxation, tendon contractures, and chronic deformity.

Clinical Manifestation and Features

- Rheumatoid arthritis (RA) most typically presents as polyarticular disease and with a gradual onset, but some patients can present with acute onset with intermittent or migratory joint involvement or with monoarticular disease.

- The symptoms of arthritis can affect the patient's capacity to perform the activities of daily living (e.g., walking, stairs, dressing, use of a toilet, getting up from a chair, opening jars, doors, typing) and their ability to do their job.
- Systemic symptoms may also be present in these patients; in up to one-third of patients, the acute onset of polyarthritis is associated with prominent myalgia, fatigue, low-grade fever, weight loss, and depression. Less often, extra articular manifestations such as nodules or episcleritis may also be present.
- **Rheumatoid Nodules:** Rheumatoid factor complexes may be involved in their pathogenesis of granulation tissue, being composed of prominent collections of newly proliferated capillaries in a bed of undifferentiated mononuclear cells and fibroblasts.
- **Rheumatoid Vasculitis:** Dysregulation of cytokine and chemokine networks.
- **Lymphadenopathy:** associated with RA usually demonstrates reactive follicular hyperplasia and polyclonal plasma cell infiltration in the interfollicular area as well as increased GCs with high B cell activity.
- **Neurological dysfunction:** Most neurologic complications are a consequence of articular inflammation and damage that leads to compression of adjacent structures of the central or peripheral nervous system.
- **Felty's syndrome** is a rare, potentially serious disorder that is defined by the presence of three conditions: rheumatoid arthritis (RA), an enlarged spleen (splenomegaly) and a decreased white blood cell count (neutropenia), which causes repeated infections.

Signs

- Swelling, Warmth, tenderness, Limitations to movement, Deformities
- Nodules, Synovial effusions in wrist, knee, hip, feet, Joint deformities

Symptoms

- Severe joint pains, Morning stiffness, General symptoms such as fever, fatigue, malaise
- Disability depends upon changes in individual joints, Non articular symptoms
- Twitching muscles, Sleep disturbances

Extra Articular Involvement

- Rheumatoid Nodules, Vasculitis, Pulmonary complications-pleural effusions
- Ocular Manifestations-include keratoconjunctivitis sicca, inflammation of the sclera
- Pericarditis may occur, resulting in the accumulation of fluid, Lymphadenopathy

Staging of R.A.[1]

- **Stage I:** Early stage RA is notable by the presence of synovial membrane inflammation, which results in joint swelling and pain on motion. Immune cells move to the inflammation site, leading to high cell counts in synovial fluid; however, x-rays are typically negative, other than showing the possible presence of some osteoporosis and soft tissue swelling. Treatment of early-stage RA focuses on joint protection and inflammation control.

- **Stage II:** In moderate stage RA, there is T and B cell proliferation and angiogenesis in the synovium. Synovial tissue starts to grow into the joint cavity, across cartilage, which will be gradually destroyed. The joint begins to narrow because of cartilage loss. There are typically no joint deformities at this stage, though mobility may become limited with adjacent muscle atrophy. There may be mild malaise as well as the presence of nodules. Treatment goals are the same as stage I RA.

- **Stage III:** Also defined as severe RA, this stage is characterized by the accumulation of synovial fluid polymorphonuclear leukocytes (SFPMNs), as well as synovial cell proliferation. The loss of cartilage in the affected joint exposes bone beneath the cartilage. Patients typically have symptoms including joint pain, swelling, limited range of motion, morning stiffness, weakness and malaise. Soft tissue swelling and joint cartilage loss will show on x-ray. Many stage III RA patients have extensive muscle atrophy as well as nodules and deformity. Pain relief and prevention of disability are primary treatment goals.

- **Stage IV:** End-stage RA disease results in a cessation of inflammatory processes. The formation of fibrous tissue and/or bone ankylosing (fusing of bone) results in ceased joint function. MRI will show proliferative pannus (a membrane of granulation tissue). Patient symptoms are much the same as in stage III, i.e. joint pain, swelling, stiffness, weakness and malaise. At this point, treatment goals focus on reduction of pain and halting additional joint damage. Patients with end-stage RA may undergo joint replacement surgery.

Diagnosis with Algorithm [2, 3]

American Rheumatism Association criteria for the diagnosis of rheumatoid arthritis
1. Morning stiffness in and around the joints for at least 6 weeks, lasting at least 1 h before maximal improvement
2. Swelling of three or more joints for at least 6 weeks
3. Swelling of the wrist, metacarpophalangeal or proximal interphalangeal joints for at least 6 weeks
4. Symmetric joint swelling for at least 6 weeks
5. Hand X-ray changes typical of rheumatoid arthritis that must include erosions or unequivocal bony decalcification around the joints
6. Rheumatoid subcutaneous nodules
7. Positive rheumatoid factor

The presence of at least 4 of these indicates a diagnosis of rheumatoid arthritis.

American Rheumatism Association criteria for Complete Clinical Remission in RA
➤ A minimum of five of the following requirements must be fulfilled for at least 2 consecutive months in a patient with RA
1. Morning stiffness not >15 minutes
2. No fatigue
3. No joint pain
4. No joint tenderness or pain on motion

5. No soft tissue swelling in joints or tendon sheaths
6. ESR (Westergren's)

Arthritis profile test includes:

- Positive Antinuclear antibody (ANA-25% of Patients):
- Positive Rheumatoid factor (R.F 60-70% of Patients)
- Designed to detect and measure the level of antibody that acts against the blood components gamma globulin, this test is positive in people with Rheumatoid Arthriris (R.A).
- Positive Anticitrullinated protein antibody (ACPA-50-85% of Patients)
- Elevated ESR
- HLA tissue typing: detects the presence of certain genetic markers in blood. Genetic marker HLA-B27 is always present in people with Rheumatoid Arthritis (R.A).
- Elevated C- reactive protein (CRP)
- Aspirated synovial fluid may reveal turbidity, leukocytosis, reduced viscosity, normal or low glucose concentrations
- Normocytic normochromic anemia is common as is thrombocytosis.
- Joint radiographs may show periarticular osteoporosis, joint space narrowing or erosions.

Treatment

Algorithm for Treatment of Rheumatoid Arthritis

- If Early RA-mild disease: hyroxychloroquine or sulfasalazine +/-NSAID, prednisolone 3-5mg/day for 1-3 months
- If early RA-severe disease: methotrexate or other DMARD with NSAID + prednisolone 5-15 mg/day for 3-4 months
- If the patient is not responding try other DMARD monotherapy if MTX is not used above OR Combination of 2 DMARDs OR Biologic DMARD mono or combo with DMARD
- If still poor response: try other combination, triple drug (DMARD + biologic), add low dose prednisolone for long term, consider second line DMARD.

Management

Goals

- To induce complete remission
- To control disease activity, joint pain
- Slow destructive joint changes
- Delay disability

Non -Pharmacological management

- Adequate rest, weight reduction if obese

➢ Heat and cold electrotherapy given to patient.
➢ Regular physiotherapy and exercise to mobilize the joints and reduce pain.
➢ Maintaining healthy lifestyle.
➢ Surgical treatment such as tenosynovectomy, tendon repair, joint replacements done in severe cases of rheumatoid arthritis.

Classification

I.   NSAIDs including COX-2 inhibitors
II. Disease modifying antirheumatic drugs (DMARDs)
    A. Nonbiological drugs
        1. Immunosuppressants: Methotrexate, Azathioprine, Cyclosporine
        2. Sulfasalazine
        3. Chloroquine or Hydroxychloroquine
        4. Leflunomide
    B. Biological agents
        1. TNFα inhibitors: Etanercept, Infliximab, Adalimumab
        2. IL-1 antagonist: Anakinra
III. Adjuvant drugs
    Corticosteroids: Prednisolone and others
    (Gold and penicillamine are obsolete DMARDs.)

Pharmacological management [4]

- Medications are the cornerstone of treatment for active rheumatoid arthritis. Several classes of drugs are used to treat rheumatoid arthritis: nonsteroidalantiinflammatory drugs (NSAIDs), disease-modifying antirheumatic drugs (DMARDs) (which include both traditional DMARDs and biologic agents), glucocorticoids, and, if needed, pain medications.

I. **NSAIDs** — NSAIDs act primarily by inhibiting prostaglandin synthesis, which is only a small portion of the inflammatory cascade. They possess both analgesic and antiinflammatory properties and reduce stiffness but do not slow disease progression or prevent bony erosions or joint deformity. They should seldom be used as monotherapy for RA; instead, they should be viewed as adjuncts to DMARD treatment.

Aspirin	2.6–5.2 g 60–100 mg/kg	Four times daily
Celecoxib	200–400 mg —	Once or twice daily
Diclofenac	150–200 mg —	Three to four times daily; extended release: twice daily
Fenoprofen	0.9–3 g —	Four times daily
Flurbiprofen	200–300 mg —	Two to four times daily
Meclofenamate	200–400 mg —	Three to four times daily
Meloxicam	7.5–15 mg —	Once daily
Naproxen	0.5–1 g 10 mg/kg	Twice daily; extended release: once daily

| Piroxicam | 10–20 mg — | Once daily |
| Tolmetin | 0.6–1.8 g 15–30 mg/kg | Two to four times daily |

Toxicities to monitor: GI ulceration and bleeding; renal damage

II. DMARDs — DMARDs can substantially reduce the inflammation of rheumatoid arthritis, reduce or prevent joint damage, preserve joint structure and function, and enable a person to continue his or her daily activities. Although some DMARDs act slowly, they may allow you to take a lower dose of glucocorticoids to control pain and inflammation. There are several types of DMARDs:

- Conventional synthetic DMARDs, sometimes termed traditional or small-molecule DMARDs, are produced by traditional drug-manufacturing techniques.
- Biologic DMARDs, sometimes termed targeted biologic agents, are manufactured using molecular biology (recombinant DNA) techniques.

DMARDs [5, 6]:

➤ Methotrexate: 5-25 mg once weekly.

➤ Sulfasalazine: 500mg – 1g. Initial dose is 500 mg and dose is slowly increased to 1g.

Ciclosporine:

➤ It is a cyclic polypeptide containing 11 amino acids. It suppresses humoral immunity and to a great extent, cell-mediated reactions. This action is due to a specific and reversible inhibition of immunocompetent lymphocytes in the G0 or G1 phases of cell cycle. T-helper cells are the main target but T-suppressor cells are also suppressed. Cyclosporine also inhibits lympholine production and release.

➤ Indications: Orally used for prevention of graft rejection after kidney, liver, heart, lung, pancreas. By IV infusion used in bone marrow transplant. Dosage: 2.5 mg/kg/day in two divided doses.

➤ Contra-Indications: Hypersensitivity, lactation.

➤ Special Precautions: Dose should be carefully titrated. Renal and/or hepatic impairment, possibility of hyperkalaemia, hypertension, vaccinations are less effective. Paediatrics: Use with caution. Pregnancy: Safety has not been established. Lactation: Safety has not been established. Elderly: Reduced dose may be necessary.

➤ Side Effects: Kidney damage, convulsions, hypertension, liver damage, tremor, hirsutism, gingival hypertrophy, hyperkalaemia, fluid retention, increased susceptibility to infectons, GI symptoms.

Pencillamine: 250mg -750mg given based on the patient severity and condition of the patient the doses are tapered accordingly.

SE: Nausea, anorexia, myelosuppression, rashes, taste   disturbances

Leflunomide: 10mg-20mg daily.

Combination DMARDs:

1. Methotrexate + sulfasalazine
2. Methotrexate + Leflunomide
3. Methotrexate + Hydroxychloroquine

Methotrexate: MTX inhibits cytokine production and purine biosynthesis, which may be responsible for its anti-inflammatory properties. Its onset is relatively rapid (as early as 2 to 3 weeks), and 45% to 67% of patients remained on it in studies ranging from 5 to 7 years. It is contraindicated in pregnant and nursing women, liver disease and immunodeficient patients. Adverse effects- Myelosuppression, hepatic fibrosis, cirrhosis, pulmonary infiltrates or fibrosis, stomatitis, rash.

Leflunomide: It (Arava) inhibits pyrimidine synthesis, which reduces lymphocyte proliferation and modulation of inflammation. Its efficacy for RA is similar to that of MTX. Dose:

A loading dose of 100 mg/day for the first 3 days may result in a therapeutic response within the first month. The usual maintenance dose of 20 mg/day may be lowered to 10 mg/day

SE: GI intolerance, complaints of hair loss, or other dose-related toxicity. The drug may cause liver toxicity

Contraindications: In patients with preexisting liver disease, GI distress, alopecia.

Hydroxychloroquine: Hydroxychloroquine lacks the myelosuppressive, hepatic, and renal toxicities seen with some other DMARDs, which simplifies monitoring. Its onset may be delayed for up to 6 weeks, but the drug should not be considered a therapeutic failure until after 6 months of therapy with no response.

Dose: 200-400mg daily

Adverse effects- Macular damage, rash, diarrhea

Sulfasalazine: Sulfasalazine, a prodrug, is cleaved by bacteria in the colon into sulfapyridine and 5-aminosalicylic acid. It is believed that the sulfapyridine moiety is responsible for the agent's antirheumatic properties, **Sulfasalazine** use is often limited by adverse effects. Antirheumatic effects should be seen in 2 months. These can be minimized by initiating therapy with low doses and titrating gradually to higher doses, dividing the dose more evenly throughout the day, or using entericcoated preparations.

Dose: 500mg to 3g daily

Adverse effects- Myelosuppression, rash

Other Disease-Modifying Antirheumatic Drugs [7, 8]

These are effective and may be of value in certain clinical settings. However, they are used less frequently today because of toxicity, lack of long-term benefits, or both.

Aurothioglucose (Solganol) (suspension in oil)

Gold sodium thiomalate (aqueous solution) are intramuscular (IM)

Dose: 10 mg test dose, then 50 mg weekly until significant response or total dose of 1000 mg has been given

SE: Rash, oral ulceration, proteinuria, myelosuppression

Auranofin (Ridaura) is an oral gold preparation

Azathioprine is a purine analog that is converted to 6-mercaptopurine and is thought to interfere with DNA and RNA synthesis.

Penicillamine onset may be seen in 1 to 3 months, and most responses occur within 6 months. Early adverse effects include skin rash, metallic taste. Penicillamine is usually reserved for patients who are resistant to other therapies because of induction of autoimmune diseases (e.g., myasthenia gravis).

Cyclosporine reduces production of cytokines involved in T-cell activation and has direct effects on B cells, macrophages, bone, and cartilage cells. Its onset appears to be 1 to 3 months. Cyclosporine should be reserved for patient's refractory to or intolerant of other DMARDs.

Biologic DMARDs [9, 10]

Etanercept (Enbrel) is a fusion protein consisting of two p75-soluble TNF receptors linked to an Fc fragment of human Ig G. It binds to and inactivates TNF, preventing it from interacting with the cell-surface TNF receptors and thereby activating cells. It has been shown to slow erosive disease progression to a greater degree than oral MTX in patients with inadequate response to MTX monotherapy.

Infliximab (Remicade) is a chimeric anti-TNF antibody fused to a human constant-region immunoglobulin G1 (IgG1). It binds to TNF and prevents its interaction with TNF receptors on inflammatory cells. To prevent formation of antibodies to this foreign protein, MTX should be given orally in doses used to treat RA for as long as the patient continues on infliximab.

Anakinra (Kineret) is an IL-1 receptor antagonist (IL-1ra) that binds to IL-1 receptors on target cells, preventing the interaction between IL-1 and the cells. IL-1 normally stimulates release of chemotactic factors and adhesion molecules that promote migration of inflammatory leukocytes to tissues. The drug is approved for moderately to severely active RA in adults who have failed one or more DMARDs.

Rituximab (Rituxan) is a monoclonal chimeric antibody consisting of mostly human protein with the antigen-binding region derived from a mouse antibody to CD20 protein found on the cell surface of mature B lymphocytes. Rituximab is useful in patients failing MTX or TNF inhibitors.

Adalimumab: 40mg every 2 weeks SC route
Etanercept: 25 mg twice weekly or 50 mg weekly
Golimumab 50 mg monthly Subcutaneous
Infliximab 3 mg/kg at week 0, 2 and 6, then every 8 weeks thereafter Intravenous infusion
Rituximab 1 g then 1 g 2 weeks later Max 2 courses/year   Intravenous infusion
Abatacept 750 mg at week 0, 2 and 4, then every 4 weeks thereafter. Intravenous infusion
Anakinra 100 mg daily Subcutaneous

Steroids (glucocorticoids) [11] — Glucocorticoids, also called steroids, have strong anti-inflammatory effects. Drugs in this class include prednisone and prednisolone. Glucocorticoids may be taken by mouth, injected into a vein, or injected directly into a joint. Glucocorticoids quickly improve symptoms of rheumatoid arthritis such as pain and stiffness and also decrease joint swelling and tenderness. Toxicities which require monitoring are hypertension, hyperglycemia and osteoporosis.

1. A daily maintenance dose of prednisolone: 7.5mg given once a day.

2. Methyl prednisolone: 40mg-80mg
3. Triamnicoloneacetonide : 20mg-40mg

Pain relievers — Pain relievers relieve pain, but they have no effect on inflammation. Drugs in this class include acetaminophen, tramadol, and capsaicin cream or ointment. Use of narcotics like codeine, oxycodone, and hydrocodone is generally discouraged because they also have no effect on inflammation and because of the long-term nature of rheumatoid arthritis and the risk of dependence and addiction.

1. Analgesics such as paracetamol or its combinations given to reduce pain .
2. Weak opioids also given to reduce pain.

2015 American College of Rheumatology Guideline for the Treatment of Rheumatoid Arthritis. Recommendations for Patients with Early RA, Established RA, and High-Risk Comorbidities

Recommendations for Early RA Patients

➢ Recommend using a treat-to-target strategy rather than a nontargeted approach, regardless of disease activity level.

➢ For disease-modifying antirheumatic drug (DMARD)-naïve patients with early, symptomatic RA, DMARD monotherapy over double or triple DMARD therapy in patients with low disease activity and conditionally recommend DMARD monotherapy over double or triple DMARD therapy in patients with moderate or high disease activity. Methotrexate should be the preferred initial therapy for most patients with early RA with active disease.

➢ For patients with moderate or high disease activity despite DMARD therapy (with or without glucocorticoids), we strongly recommend treatment with a combination of DMARDs or a (TNF inhibitor) or a non-TNF biologic, with or without methotrexate (MTX) in no particular order of preference, rather than continuing DMARD monotherapy alone. Biologic therapy should be used in combination with MTX over biologic monotherapy, when possible, due to superior efficacy.

➢ For patients with moderate or high disease activity despite any of the above DMARD or biologic therapies, we conditionally recommend adding low-dose glucocorticoids (defined as ≤10 mg/day of prednisone or equivalent). Low-dose glucocorticoids may also be used in patients who need a bridge until realizing the benefits of DMARD therapy. The risk/benefit ratio of glucocorticoid therapy is favorable as long as the dose is low and the duration of therapy is short.

➢ For patients experiencing a flare of RA, we conditionally recommend adding short-term glucocorticoids (< 3 months of treatment) at the lowest possible dose for the shortest possible duration, to provide a favorable benefit-risk ratio for the patient.

Recommendations for Established RA Patients

➢ We strongly recommend using a treat-to-target strategy rather than a nontargeted approach, regardless of disease activity level. The ideal target should be low disease activity or remission, as determined by the clinician and the patient. In some cases, however, another target may be chosen because tolerance by patients or comorbidities may mitigate the usual choices.

➤ For DMARD-naïve patients with low disease activity, we strongly recommend using DMARD monotherapy over a TNFi. For DMARD-naïve patients with moderate or high disease activity, we conditionally recommend DMARD monotherapy over double or triple DMARD therapy and DMARD monotherapy over tofacitinib. In general, MTX should be the preferred initial therapy for most patients with established RA with active disease.

➤ For patients with moderate or high disease activity despite DMARD monotherapy including methotrexate, we strongly recommend using combination DMARDs or adding a TNFi or a non-TNF biologic or tofacitinib (all choices with or without methotrexate) in no particular order of preference, rather than continuing DMARD monotherapy alone. Biologic therapy should be used in combination with MTX over biologic monotherapy, when possible, due to its superior efficacy.

➤ For moderate or high disease activity despite TNFi therapy in patients currently not on a DMARD, we strongly recommend that one or two DMARDs be added to TNFi therapy rather than continuing TNFi therapy alone.

➤ If disease activity is moderate or high despite single TNFi biologic therapy, we conditionally recommend using a non-TNF biologic.

➤ If disease activity is moderate or high despite non-TNF biologic therapy, we conditionally recommend using another non-TNF biologic. However, if a patient has failed multiple non-TNF biologics and they are TNFi-naïve with moderate or high disease activity, we conditionally recommend treatment with a TNFi.

➤ For patients with moderate or high disease activity despite prior treatment with at least one TNFi and at least one non-TNF-biologic (sequentially, not combined), we conditionally recommend first treating with another non-TNF biologic. However, when a non-TNF biologic is not an option (e.g., patient declines non-TNF biologic therapy due to inefficacy or side effects), we conditionally recommend treatment with tofacitinib.

➤ If disease activity is moderate or high despite the use of multiple (2+) TNFi therapies (in sequence, not concurrently), we conditionally recommend non-TNF biologic therapy and then conditionally treating with tofacitinib when a non-TNF biologic is not an option.

➤ If disease activity is moderate or high despite any of the above DMARD or biologic therapies, we conditionally recommend adding low-dose glucocorticoids.

➤ If patients with established RA experience an RA flare while on DMARD, TNFi, or nonTNF biologic therapy, we conditionally recommend adding short-term glucocorticoids (< 3 months of treatment) at the lowest possible dose and for shortest possible duration to provide the best benefit-risk ratio for the patient.

➤ In patients with established RA and low disease activity but not remission, we strongly recommend continuing DMARD therapy, TNFi, non-TNF biologic or tofacitinib rather than discontinuing respective medication.

➤ In patients with established RA currently in remission, we conditionally recommend tapering DMARD therapy, TNFi, non-TNF biologic, or tofacitinib.

> We strongly recommend not discontinuing all therapies in patients with established RA in disease remission

Case Study of Rheumatoid Arthritis

Summary

A patient of age 35 years was admitted in the hospital with complaints of immobility and unable to stand, walk for longer time since 20 days, joint pains radiating to upper arms stimultaneously. Her medical history stated she is suffering from hypothyroidism and is on medication. Her vitals were stable. CBP: Hb- 10.5 [F: 11-14 g/dL]. Peripheral smear RBC- Normocytic Hypochromic. ESR: 25 [F: 0-20 mm/h], Urine analysis: Normal, LFT: Normal, Serum electrolytes: Normal, Antigen test: RA factor- 25, IgM: positive.

Diagnosis

Based on the subjective and objective data the patient is diagnosed with *rheumatoid arthritis*

Drug treatment chart

Generic name	Trade name	Route	Dose	Frequency
Inj.Tramadol	Tramadol	IM	30 mg	OD
Inj. Pan	Pantoprazole	IV	40mg	BD
Inj.Activan	Diclofenac	IM	50mg	OD
T. Buscogast	Hyoscine amine butyl bromide	P/O	30 mg	BD
T.Devim	Dexamethasone	IV	O.5mg	BD
T.Loysolone	Prednisolone	P/O	5mg	h.s.
T.Folvite	Folic acid	P/O	5mg	OD

Progress chart: On day 2 the patients symptoms were slightly relieved and vitals were checked. On further days the patients vitals were normal and she is stable, conscious and coherent.

Pharmacist intervention:

- From the patients drug treatment chart, moderate interaction between drugs was seen.
- Usage of corticosteroids along with NSAIDs in the patient prior peptic ulcer or GI bleeding should be avoided.
- Usage of any prophylactic anti ulcer therapy may be considered.

Patient education:

- Take medication regularly
- Educate about the disease and also for the patient to identify the side effect
- Consult to the physician before starting any exercise program
- Do not take stress and complete bed rest is advisable
- Intake of calcium diet protein food is recommended

Assignment

1. What information indicate the presence and severity of RA?

> About 60% of patients develop symptoms gradually over several weeks- months.

> Patient may present with systemic findings, joint findings or both

Symptoms: A specific symptoms include Fatigue, Weakness, Anorexia, Diffuse Musculoskeletal pain. Pain involved in joints and prolonged morning stiffness.

Signs: Rheumatoid nodules, Limited joint function

Articular signs: Malaise, Warmth, Tenderness, Swelling, Erythema swelling, Low grade fever, Arthralgia

Extra articular manifestations:

Skin: Sub cutaneous nodules

Ocular: Scleritis, keratoconjunctivitis sicca

Pulmonary: Interstitial fibrosis, pulmonary nodules, pleuritic, pleural effusion.

Vasculitis: Ischemic ulcers, skin lesions, leukocytoclastic vasculitis,

Neuralgia: Peripheral neuropathy, Felty's syndrome

Hematologic: Anemia, thrombocytopenia.

Laboratory tests:

- Rheumatoid factor: positive [negative upto 30% patients];
- ESR: erythema sedimentation rate Male - >20 mm/h;   Female->30 mm/h
- C-reactive protein: Elevated CRP-0.7 mg/dl to 7 mg/dl
- Complete blood count: WBC- Slight elevation with a normal differentials, slight
-     anemia, thrombocytopenia.
- Anti-CCP Abs: positive
- Synovial fluid analysis: Synovial fluid- straw colored,
-     slightly cloudy-WBC 2000 – 50000/mm^3)
- Joint X-ray: To identify baseline and evaluate joint damage
- MRI: May detect erosions earlier in the course of disease
  X- rays are not for diagnosis

American council of rheumatology divided RA into 4 stages

Initial	Moderate	Severe	Terminal
Inflammation of synovial fluid Pain: Muscle and body, rheumatism, swelling X- ray: negative	T/B cell proliferation in synovial fluid X- ray: positive	Pores in the cartilage Cartilage erosion X-ray: positive	Bone deformities, joint swollen deformities Bone erosion, X-ray: positive, MRI

2. **What information is needed to assess the patient?**

   Assessing RA can be difficult as many conditions cause joint stiffness and inflammation, there is no definitive test, but most common symptoms include-
   - Stiffness in the joints particularly in the morning
   - Typically effects hands and feet but often the dominant hand is more severely effected
   - Swollen, painful joints (synovitis). The joints are soft and quite different from the square, hard, bony swelling of Osteoarthritis (OA)
   - Fatigue, most people have little energy

   When the disease starts suddenly with the involvement of hands, feet or large joints diagnosis is made quickly.

   Diagnostic tests like ESR, C-reactive protein (CRP), CBC
   - Complete blood count measures blood cells to rule out anemia [cmn in people with , although it doesn't prove RA]
   - Rheumatoid factor and anti-CCP antibodies
   - Almost ½ people with RA have positive Rh factor
   - Positive anti CCP antibodies – RA
   - X-rays, MRI scans

3. **What abnormal lab values in the patient could be used to monitor the efficacy of drug therapy or disease presentation? [12]**

   Various laboratory values include-
   - ESR rate: patient value recording- 25 [F- 0-20 mm/hr]
   - Erythrocyte sedimentation rate is influenced by anemia of chronic disease and by variation in the blood concentration of acute phase proteins
   - RA factor: Rheumatoid arthritis factor in patient – 25
   - IgM (Antibodies) – positive
   - WBC count: 5800 cells/cumm – mild neutrophilia

4. **What non drug therapy should be included in RA management?**
   - Exercise- mild stretching, muscle conditioning should be recommended
   - Diet/ Weight control
   - Rest is advised / splinting (orthotics)
   - Physiotherapy Heat/ cold
   - Electrotherapy/ Emotional support is to be given
   - Adequate sleep is important

5. **What is the role of NSAIDS in RA patient?**
   - NSAIDS interfere with the prostaglandin synthesis through the inhibition of COX enzyme thus reducing the pain and swelling
   - But these are solely not effective in the treatment of RA
   - These are the most widely used agents for the symptomatic treatment in Arthritis

6. **If the patient has aspirin allergy, why should other NSAIDS should also be contraindicated and what are the other alternative therapy for aspirin allergy?**
   - As all NSAIDs work by a common mechanism of inhibiting the cox enzyme, other NSAIDs should also be contraindicated in patients allergic to Aspirin.

- ➤ In patients with Aspirin allergy, if NSAIDS are used they lead to the over production of pro inflammation leucotrienes and that causes variable hypertensive reactions.

Alternative regimen:

- ➤ As per reports, cox -2 inhibitors can be used in aspirin sensitive patients, as they allow cox-1 to continue the production of PG's and decrease pain, inflammation and redness.

7. What renal syndrome is associated with NSAIDS?

NSAIDS are capable of inducing various renal abnormalities.

Respiration in patients with high risk with decrease renal blood perfusion and the abnormalities include-

- ➤ Fluid retention- most common; Electrolyte complications
- ➤ Hyperkalemia is seen frequently in high risk patients
- ➤ Chronic usage of NSAIDs- Increase in serum creatinine levels
- ➤ Permanent complication- Capillary necrosis
- ➤ Nephrotic syndrome with intestinal nephritis- rare and is reversible with cessation of usage of NSAIDs

8. What biological agents are available for the treatment of RA?

1. Infliximab - 3mg/kg-- 0,2,6 wk and then every 8wk; IV
2. Ebanercept- 25mg –twice weekly and 50mg- once weekly by SC
3. Adalimumab – 40mg; SC
4. Certoizumab- initial 400mg, subsequently 200mg every 2 week or 400mg every 4 week by SC
5. Golimumab- 50mg/0.5ml ; evry 4 week by SC
6. Abatacept- Weight based <60 kg-500 mg 60-100: 750 mg >100mg-1000mg by IV
7. Rituximab- Initial- 50mg/h, may increase 30min to max of 400mg/h, Subsequent- 100mg/h, may increase every 30min to max of 400mg/h--- Repeat for 14 days and discontinueby IV

9. What gold preparations are available for treatment and what are the adverse effects possible?

- ➤ Gold therapy was one of the first treatments development for the treatment of RA
- ➤ Gold is a Dmard (disease modifying anti-rheumatic drug)
- ➤ Gold preparations available include
  - Gold sodium thiomalate
  - Myocrisin- 100mg/ml solution for infection

  ADRS: Dizziness, Emesis, Flushing and sweating, Light headedness
- ➤ Kidney/renal disease, Increased joint pain at the initial stage of treatment

References

1. Hingle, Melanie, Renee Kishbaugh, Michael Buchwald, and Lisa High. "Skeletal System and Joint Health", Integrating Therapeutic and Complementary Nutrition, 2006.
2. https://www.cdc.gov/arthritis/basics/rheumatoid-arthritis.html

3. [Guideline] Anderson J, Caplan L, Yazdany J, et al, for the American College of Rheumatology. Rheumatoid arthritis disease activity measures: American College of Rheumatology Recommendations for use in clinical practice. *Arthritis Care Res (Hoboken)*. 2012. 64:640-7.

4. Anderson JJ, Wells G, Verhoeven AC, Felson DT. Factors predicting response to treatment in rheumatoid arthritis: The importance of disease duration. Arthritis Rheum 2000;43(1):22–29.

5. Fries JF. Current treatment paradigms in rheumatoid arthritis. Rheumatology 2000;39(Suppl 1):30–35.

6. Kremer JM. Rational use of new and existing disease-modifying agents in rheumatoid arthritis. Ann Intern Med 2001;134(8):695–706.

7. Pincus T, Ferraccioli G, Sokka T, et al. Evidence from clinical trials and long-term observational studies that disease-modifying anti-rheumatic drugs slow radiographic progression in rheumatoid arthritis: Updating a 1983 review. Rheumatology 2002;41(12):1346–1356.

8. Prakash A, Jarvis B. Leflunomide: A review of its use in active rheumatoid arthritis. Drugs 1999;58(6):1137–1164.

9. Navarro-Sarabia F, Ariza-Ariza R, Hernandez-Cruz B, Villanueva I. Adalimumab for treating rheumatoid arthritis. Cochrane Database Syst Rev 2005(3):CD005113.

10. Adachi JD, Saag KG, Delmas PD, et al. Two-year effects of alendronate on bone mineral density and vertebral fracture in patients receiving glucocorticoids: A randomized, double-blind, placebo-controlled extension trial. Arthritis Rheum 2001;44(1):202–211.

11. Bykerk V, Schieir O, Akhavan P, Hazlewood G, Cheng C, Bombardier C. Emerging issues in the pharmacological management of rheumatoid arthritis: Results of a national needs assessment survey identifying practice variations for the development of Canadian Rheumatology Association Clinical practice recommendations. J Rheumatol 2011;38:1

12. AGREE Collaboration. Development and validation of an international appraisal instrument for assessing the quality of clinical practice guidelines: the AGREE project. Qual Saf Health Care 2003;12:18-23.

CHAPTER - 26

Osteoarthritis

Introduction to Osteoarthritis (OA)

Osteoarthritis is a common, progressive disorder affecting primarily weight bearing diarthrodial joints, characterised by progressive deterioration and loss of articular cartilage, osteophyte formation, pain, limitation of motion, deformity and disability.

Epidemiology

- Symptomatic knee OA occurs in 10% men and 13% in women aged 60years or older.
- OA is more common in United States and 80% in the 75 year or older age groups.
- The number of people affected with symptomatic OA is likely to increase due to the aging of the population and the obesity epidemic. OA has a multi-factorial etiology and can be considered the product of an interplay between systemic and local factors. Old age, female gender, overweight and obesity, knee injury, repetitive use of joints, bone density, muscle weakness, and joint laxity all play roles in the development of joint osteoarthritis, particularly in the weight-bearing joints. Modifying these factors may reduce the risk of osteoarthritis and prevent subsequent pain and disability.

Etiology

It is of primary and secondary origin.

Primary: Idiopathic (unknown reason)

Secondary: Trauma, endocrinal disorder like diabetes, underlying joint disorder like fracture or infection to the joints, obesity, neuropathic disorders, and dysplasia of bones.

Risk Factors [1, 2]

- **Age:** The increase in the prevalence and incidence of OA with age probably is a consequence of cumulative exposure to various risk factors and biologic changes that occur with aging that may make a joint less able to cope with adversity, such as cartilage thinning, weak muscle strength, poor proprioception, and oxidative damage.
- **Obesity:** Obesity increases the risk of bilateral radiographic as well as symptomatic hip

OA. Increased loading on the joint is probably the main, but not only, mechanism by which obesity causes knee or hip OA. Overloading the knee and hip joints could lead to synovial joint breakdown and failure of ligamentous and other structural support.

- **Gender and hormones:** Women not only are more likely to have OA than men. hormonal factors may play a role in the development of OA.

- Congenital/developmental conditions: few congenital or developmental abnormalities (i.e., congenital subluxation, Legg-Calvé-Perthes disease, and slipped capital femoral epiphysis) have been associated with occurrence of hip OA in later life.

- **Injury/surgery:** Severe injury to the structures of a joint, particularly a trans-articular fracture, meniscal tear requiring meniscectomy, or anterior cruciate ligament injury, can result in an increased risk of OA.

- **Occupation:** Repetitive use of joints at work is associated with an increased risk of OA.

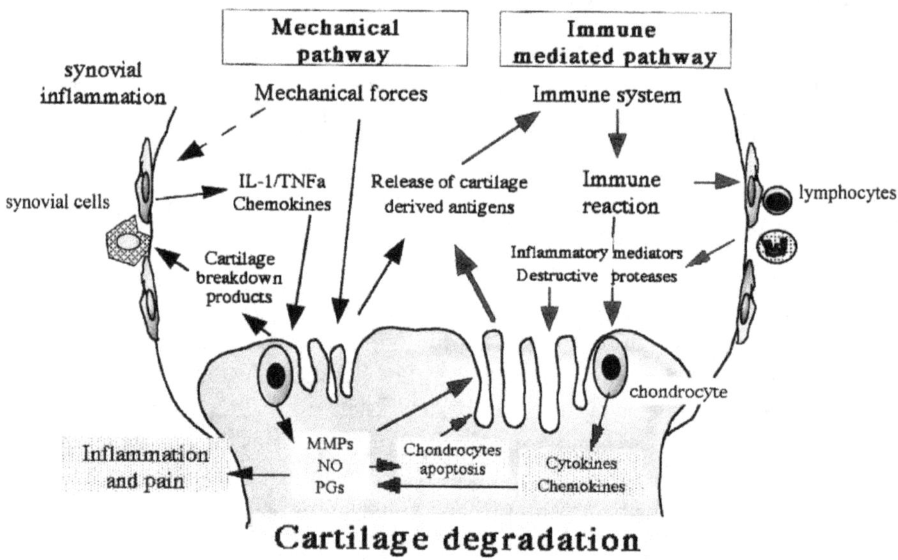

Fig 26.1 Pathophysiology of Osteoarthritic Cartilage.

Source: Guo-Hua Yuan, Kayo Masuko-Hongo, Tomohiro Kato, and Kusuki Nishioka. Immunologic Intervention in the Pathogenesis of Osteoarthritis. ARTHRITIS & RHEUMATISM Vol. 48, No. 3, March 2003, pp 602–611

Pathophysiology of Osteoarthritic Cartilage [3, 4]

Human cartilage is a complex material synthesized and maintained by its living component, the chondrocyte. The biomechanical properties of cartilage are the consequence of interactions between water (which makes up 65% to 80% of cartilage) and matrix proteoglycans, matrix collagens, and other matrix components. These interactions reflect not only the composition of cartilage, but also its biochemistry and organization.

It is in a state of balance between matrix synthesis and matrix degradation. The progressive course of osteoarthritis is the result of sustained imbalance between these two processes, favoring degradation.

The healthy cartilage matrix consists of collagen fibrils through which proteoglycan complexes are intertwined. The backbone of each proteoglycan complex is a long molecule of hyaluronic acid, or hyaluronan, to which large glycosaminoglycan molecules known as aggrecans are attached by link proteins. The complete structure provides cartilage with its most important core biomechanical properties, compressibility and elasticity; the aggrecans are thought to be especially important determinants of these properties [5].

Two families of enzymes are important in matrix degradation, both in healthy cartilage and in osteoarthritis. Matrix metalloproteinases break down collagen, gelatin, and other proteinaceous components of the matrix. Aggrecanases, which degrade aggrecans, are complex proteins. The increased breakdown of aggrecans by enzymes contributes to the loss of cartilage structure and function.

In healthy cartilage, the activity of degradative enzymes is balanced by that of synthetic enzymes; it is also regulated by specific enzyme inhibitors known as tissue inhibitors of matrix metalloproteinases. In the pathogenesis of osteoarthritis, this balance is in favor of degradative activity.

The most important of the mediators are interleukin-1 (IL-1) and tumor necrosis factor (TNFα). Synthesis of IL-1ß and TNF-α, and their membrane-bound receptors, is upregulated in osteoarthritis. These cytokines are potentiators of an inflammatory cascade, stimulating their own production and that of a range of proinflammatory cytokines such as IL-6, IL-8, IL-11 and IL-17. The net effect of these cytokines on chondrocyte metabolism is to increase the synthesis of matrix metalloproteinases and aggrecanases, decrease the synthesis of tissue inhibitors of matrix metalloproteinases and other inhibitors of degradative enzymes, and reduce the rate of matrix synthesis.

IL-1ß and TNF-α activity stimulates the release of nitric oxide. In cartilage, nitric oxide inhibits collagen and proteoglycan synthesis and increase the activity of matrix metalloproteinases. Because chondrocytes are not regenerated, loss of chondrocyte mass and function further accelerates degradative processes.

Chondrocytes respond to the degradative consequences of the inflammatory cascade by increasing the rate at which they synthesize matrix components, and by releasing anti-inflammatory cytokines (IL-4, IL-10, IL-13). However, in osteoarthritis, the increased synthetic and anti-inflammatory activity of chondrocytes loses out to the increased degradative activity. First, increased synthetic activity is confined to deeper layers of cartilage, which allows the imbalance toward degradation to persist in the upper layer, near the synovial boundary. Ultimately, chondrocyte malfunction and apoptosis limit the response potential and hasten the progression of osteoarthritis.

Category of OA Based on Severity According to American College of Rheumatology [6]

Stage 0: normal joint, healthy knee, no signs of OA and no pain.

Stage 1: very minute; small bone spurs growth; usually starts at early 40s and knee hip joints cannot bear weight. This can be relieved by walking and warm up exercise. Bone spur growth is due to obesity.

Stage 2: mild stage. X-ray of knee joints when taken there is an increase in bone spur growth and develops friction and don't subside even with rest.pain is seen. Exercise and rest is indicated.

Stage 3: Moderate OA. The cartilage is damaged. Must be on treatment with NSAIDs. Joint stiffness is seen even at rest. Must be on warming exercise.

Stage 4: severe OA. Great pain and discomfort, joint space between the bones is decreased. Treatment is opting for surgery.

Clinical Manifestations and Features

- Pain at weight bearing joints.
- Pain at distal inter phalangeal , proximal interphalangeal joints.
- Pain at Metatarsophalangeal joints.
- Stiffness of joints.
- Limitation of motion.
- Crepitus, deformities
- Tenderness at the joints is seen
- Bony enlargements at the joints
- Upon arising joint stiffness typically lasts less than 30 mins and resolves with motion.
- Warmth, redness and synovitis is seen.

Diagnosis with Algorithm

- For hip OA, patient must have knee pain and ESR less than 20mm/h; radiographic femoral or acetabular osteophytes; radiographic joint space narrowing.
- For knee OA, age more than 50years, morning stiffness lasting 30mins, crepitus , bony enlargement ,bone tenderness, palpable joint warmth.
- ESR may be slightly elevated if inflammation is present.Rheumatoid factor is negative. Synovial fluid reveals high viscosity and mild leukocytosis (<2000 white blood cells / mm cube)

Management

Goals

1. Educate the patient and family members.
2. Relieve pain and stiffness.
3. Improve the joint stability.
4. Improve the quality of life.
5. Our aim is not to degenerate the cartilage as the patient is geriatric but only aim is to control pain.

Non Pharmacological Treatment

1. Educate the patient about disease process, prognosis and treatment. Promote dietary counselling, exercise and weight loss program for obesity patients.
2. Physical therapy with heat or cold treatment helps maintain range of motion and reduce pain.
3. Assistive and orthotic devices (canes, walker, braces, heel ups) can be used during exercise or daily activities.
4. Surgical procedures like osteotomy, arthroplasty, joint fusion are indicated.
5. Participating in self-management programs.
6. Balance exercises

General Approach to the Management of Patient

1. Combination of Treatment modalities include non-pharmacological and pharmacological therapies is strongly recommended.
2. Step 1: Background treatment

   If symptomatic, paracetamol on a regular basis OR chronic pain- glucosamine sulphate and/or chondroitin sulphate ± as needed paracetamol

   If still symptomatic Add-topical NSAIDs or topical capsaicin. Also walking aids, thermal therapy may be recomended bythe physical therapist.
3. Step 2: Advanced pharmacological management in persistent symptomatic patient.
   - (a) Normal GI risk- nonselective NSAIDs with PPI

     COX-2 selective NSAID
   - (b) Increased GI risk: COX-2 selective NSAID with PPI
   - (c) Increased CV risk: prefer naproxen

     Avoid high dose diclofenac and ibuprofen

     Avoid COX2 selective drugs
   - (d) Increased renal risk: avoid NSAIDs.
   - (e) If still symptomatic : intra-articular hyaluronate

     Intra-articular corticosteroids
4. Step 3: Last pharmacological attempts: short term with opioids; duloxetine
5. Step 4: End stage disease management and surgery:

   If severely symptomatic and poor quality of life- joint replacement;

   if contraindicated – opioid analgesics.

Pharmacological Therapy [7]

A. Oral analgesics

1. Acetaminophen : 1st line treatment
   - Has less risk of serious GIT and CV events.
   - Dose : 325-500 mg   TID
   - MOA: inhibits cox pathway and release of prostaglandins.
2. Tramadol: for hip and knee OA who have failed scheduled full dose acetaminophen and topical NSAIDS or who are not able to receive Intra-articular (IA) corticosteroids.
   - Dose : 25mg in the morning; should be titrated to 50-100mg
   - MOA: Agonist of the μ-opioid receptor and subsides pain centrally.
   - Side effects : hangover effect, dependence, drug abuse, nausea, vomiting dyspepsia etc
3. Hydrocodone/ acetaminophen – 5mg/ 325mg   TID

B. Topical analgesics

- Capsacin – 0.0025% - 0.0075%   3-4 times a day
- MOA: Counter irritant activity by binding to TRPV1 receptors.
- Diclofenac gel – 1%   2-4g   3-4 times a day
- Diclofenac patch 3%   OD

C. Intra Articular Corticosteroids

*Triamcinolone   5-15mg per joint per week

* Methyl prednisolone   10-20mg per joint per week

*IA hyaluronic acid

The following are the six regimens of hyaluronic acid:

- Hylan G-F 20 (Synvisc®), given once weekly for a total of three weeks.
- Hylan G-F 20 (Synvics-OneTM), given once per six months and limited to osteoarthritis of the knee.
- Sodium hyaluronate :
  - Hyalgan®, given once weekly for a total of five injections.
  - Supartz®, given once a week for a total of five weeks.
  - EuflexxaTM, given as a three-injection treatment regimen.
  - Monovisc™, the intra-articular injection is given once.
  - Gel-Syn™, given once weekly for three weeks.
  - GenVisc® 850, treatment cycle consists of five injections given at weekly intervals.

MOA: provides viscoelastic properties to the synovial fluid and acts as shock absorber.

Side effects: Systemic side effects like swelling around the injection site, face, lips etc. Increased pain is also seen.

D. NSAIDs

* Aspirin   - 325 mg TID

*Celecoxib – 50mg   TID

*Diclofenac – 50mg   TID
*Diflunisal   - 250mg BD
*Ibuprofen – 200mg   TID
*Ketoprofen – 75mg   OD
*Indomethacin – 25mg BD
*Mefenamic acid – 250mg TID

Side effects: GIT bleeding, platelet aggregation, bleeding, nausea, vomiting, dyspepsia, dark scaly stools etc.

To counteract the side effects of NSAIDs proton pump inhibitors like pantoprazole is used.

Algorithm for Treatment of HIP and Knee OA

1. If acetaminophen is not contraindicated, 2nd line agents or acetaminophen dose is titrated. If not effective then, 2nd line agents like opioid analgesics or surgery like orthoplasty or knee replacement is advised.
2. If acetamniphen is contraindicated, then oral NSAIDs can be started. Topical NSAIDs can be started to supress side effects or IA corticosteroids can be used. If the patient has resisitance to corticosteroids tramadol can be started.

Algorithm for Hand OA

1. If the patient is greater than 75 years, topical NSAIDs or topical capsacin or tramadol can be initiated.
2. If the treatment id effective continue the treatment. If not effective combination therpay is preferred with 2 first line agents.
3. But if the age of patient is not greater than 75 years- a) Oral NSAIDs or topical NSAIDs or topical capsacin or tramadol can be intiated.
4. If treatment is effective continue. If not effective combination therpay id preferred with 2 first line agents.

American College of Rheumatology 2019 Recommendations for the use of Nonpharmacologic and Pharmacologic Therapies in Osteoarthritis of the Hand, Hip, and Knee

Nonpharmacologic recommendations for the management of Knee, hip and hand OA

We conditionally recommend that health professionals should do the following:

- Exercise, balance exercise, weight loss, self-efficacy and self-management programs, Cognitive behavioral therapy (CBT) is strongly recommended for patients with knee, hip, and/or hand OA

- Cane use is strongly recommended for patients with knee and/or hip OA in whom disease in 1 or more joints is causing a sufficiently large impact on ambulation, joint stability, or pain to warrant use of an assistive device.
- Tibiofemoral knee braces, Patellofemoral braces are strongly recommended for patients with knee OA in whom disease in 1 or both knees is causing a sufficiently large impact on ambulation, joint stability, or pain to warrant use of an assistive device, and who are able to tolerate the associated inconvenience and burden associated with bracing.
- Kinesiotaping, Hand orthoses, modified shoes, Lateral and medial wedged insoles is conditionally recommended for patients with knee and/or first CMC joint OA
- Acupuncture, Thermal interventions (locally applied heat or cold) is conditionally recommended for patients with knee, hip, and/or hand OA
- Paraffin, an additional method of heat therapy for the hands, is conditionally recommended for patients with hand OA.
- Radiofrequency ablation is conditionally recommended for patients with knee OA
- Massage therapy is conditionally recommended against in patients with knee and/or hip OA.
- Iontophoresis is conditionally recommended against in patients with first CMC joint OA
- Pulsed vibration therapy is conditionally recommended against in patients with knee OA.
- Transcutaneous electrical stimulation (TENS) is strongly recommended against in patients with knee and/or hip OA

The optimal management of knee OA requires a combination of non-pharmacological and pharmacological treatment modalities

The treatment of knee OA should be tailored according to:
- Knee risk factors (obesity, adverse mechanical factors, physical activity)
- General risk factors (age, comorbidity, polypharmacy)
- Level of pain intensity and disability
- Sign of inflammation—for example, effusion
- Location and degree of structure damage
  - Paracetamol is the oral analgesic to try first and, if successful, the preferred long term oral analgesic
  - Topical applications (NSAIDs, capsaicin) have clinical efficacy and are safe
  - NSAIDs should be considered in patients unresponsive to paracetamol. In patients with an increased gastrointestinal risk, non-selective NSAIDs and effective gastroprotective agents, or selective COX-2 inhibitors should be used
  - Opioid analgesics, with or without paracetamol, are useful alternatives in patients in whom NSAIDs, including COX-2 selective inhibitors, are contraindicated, ineffective, and/or poorly tolerated
  - Symptomatic slow Acting Drugs for Osteroarthritis (SYSADOA) (glucosamine sulphate, chondroitin sulphate, Avocado Soybean Unsapanifiables (ASU), diacerein, hyaluronic acid) have symptomatic effects and may modify structure

- Intra-articular injection of long acting corticosteroid is indicated for flare of knee pain, especially if accompanied by effusion
- Joint replacement has to be considered in patients with radiographic evidence of knee OA who have refractory pain and disability

Recommendations for the management of hand OA

- Topical treatments are preferred over systemic treatments because of safety reasons. Topical NSAIDs are the first pharmacological topical treatment of choice.
- Oral analgesics, particularly NSAIDs, should be considered for a limited duration for relief of symptoms.
- Chondroitin sulfate may be used in patients with hand OA for pain relief and improvement in functioning.
- Intra-articular injections of glucocorticoids should not generally be used in patients with hand OA, but may be considered in patients with painful interphalangeal joints
- Patients with hand OA should not be treated with conventional or biological disease-modifying antirheumatic drugs
- Surgery should be considered for patients with structural abnormalities when other treatment modalities have not been sufficiently effective in relieving pain. Trapeziectomy should be considered in patients with thumb base OA and arthrodesis or arthroplasty in patients with interphalangeal OA.
- Long-term follow-up of patients with hand OA should be adapted to the patient's individual needs.

Case Study of Osteoarthritis

Summary

A 35 years old female patient was admitted in orthopedics ward with complaints of pain in left hip since 4 months and abdominal pain. Patient has history of trauma 15 years back, radiating to left leg, difficulty in walking. Her vitals were stable. Physical examination: left hip tenderness was seen. Crepts and restricted flexion. CBP: Hb- 10.1 g/dL [F: 11-14 g/dL]. Peripheral smear RBC- Normocytic Hypochromic

ESR: 95 [F: 0-20 mm/h]. Urine analysis: Normal. Other investigations: ECG: Sinus rhythm - second degree AV block (wenckebach type), Poor R wave progression (V3), CT scan of lumbo sacral spine: left hip prosthesis seen insitu. Osteoarthritis of left hip joint. Pneumorrhachis. X-ray: (left hip) cyst seen.

Diagnosis: Based on subjective and objective data the patient was diagnosed with left hip osteoarthritis with secondary Avascular Necrosis (AVN)

Treatment chart

Name	Generic name	Route	Dose	Frequency
T. Dolo	Acetaminophen	Oral	650mg	BD
T. Densical	Calcitriol+Calcium	Oral	1 tab	OD
T.Signoflam	Paracetomol+ Aceclofenac	Oral	1 tab	BD
T.Osteofos	Calcium+VitB3	Oral	70mg	OD
T.Tavopan	Pantoprazole+ Domperidone	Oral	10mg	OD
Inj.Proxime	Cefuroxime	IV	500mg	OD
Inj.Metrogyl	Metronidazole	IV	100mg	TID
T.Amikacin	Amikacin	Oral	500mg	BD
Inj.Dynapur	Diclofenac	IV	75mg	TID
Inj.Pan	Pantoprazole	IV	40mg	OD
Inj.Tramadol	Tramadol	IV	1amp	SOS
T.Ultracet	Tramadol+ Acetaminophen	oral	2 tabs	BD
Inj.Hydrocort	Hydrocortisone	IV	100mg	STAT
Inj. Avil	Pheniramine maleate	IV	1amp	STAT
T.Zerodol	Aceclofenac	Oral	1 tab	BD
Inj.Mecobalamine	VitB12	IV	100mg	OD

Progress chart: Vitals were stable. No improvement of symptoms. X-ray was done, planned for total hip replacement. On day 15th total hip arthroplasty surgery was performed. Patient was stable and conscious.

Patient Counselling

- ➢ Have a balanced diet
- ➢ Manage your body weight
- ➢ Use hot or cold packs for pain relief
- ➢ Take medications regularly
- ➢ Consult doctor before starting any exercise
- ➢ Avoid stress
- ➢ Stay active and stay positive

Assignment

1. ACR recommendations for treatment of OA of hand

A. Pharmacological treatment:

- ➢ OTC, Acetaminophen at dose 3mg/day initially
- ➢ Topical Capsacin 3-4 times a day
- ➢ Oral NSAIDs, including COX-2 selective inhibitors
- ➢ Tramadol 25mg morning; should be titrated to 50-100mg

> If patient age > 75years should use topical rather than oral NSAIDS and topical capsacin or tramadol
> NSAIDs used are

Aspirin 325mg TID	Celocoxib 100mg BD
Diclofenac 50mg TID	Diflunisal 250mg BD
Ibuprofen 200mg TID	Ketoprfen 50mg TID
Indomethacin 25mg BD	Mefenamic acid 250mg TID

B. Non-pharmacological treatment

> Evaluation of ability to perform activities of daily living Activities of Daily Living (ADL).
> Instruct in joint protection technique.
> Provide assistive devices for patient to help in performing (ADL).
> Instruct use of thermal modalities.
> Provide splints for patients with trapeziometacarpel joint OA.

2. ACR recommendations for treatment of OA of knee and hip

Step 1 Nonpharmacologic therapy including
a. patient education
b. self-management programs (e.g., Arthritis Foundation Self-Management Program)
c. personalized social support directly or via telephone contact
d. programs for aerobic exerceis
e. if overweight, weight loss
f. medial taping of the patells for patelofemoral compartment involvement
g. physical therapy involving range of motion exercises, quadriceps strengthening exercises and assistive devises for ambulation
h. occupational therapy involving joint protection and energy conservation, use of splints and assistive devices for daily living activities

Step 2 Pharmacologic therapy (most effective when combined with nonpharmacologic therapy above)

Initial therapeutic approach:
a. For mild-to-moderate pain and symptom control, acetaminophen (up to 4gm qd) should be given. This drug should be used cautiously in patients with existing liver disease and avoided in patients with chronic alcohol abuse. Topical capsaicin or methyl salicylate cream should be considered in patients who do not respond to acetaminophen or do not wish to take systemic therapy.
b. For moderate-to-severe pain and swollen joints, aspiration and intraarticular injection of glucocorticoids (e.g., triamcinolone hexacetonide 40mg) or nonsteroidal anti-inflammatory drug (NSAID) merits consideration.

Alternative approaches when intitial therapy yields inadequate response:
a. Cyclooxygenase 2 (COX-2) specific inhibitors
b. Nonsteroidal anti-inflammatory drugs (NSAIDs) should be started in low analgesic doses and increased to full doses only if lower doses aren't effective. Use of misoprostol or a proton pump inhibitor is recommended if patient has risk factors for upper gastrointestinal (UGI) bleeding or ulcer disease.
c. For patients with moderate-to-severe pain and who have contraindications to COX-2 specific inhibitors and NSAIDs, Tramadol (200-300mg divided evenly, qid)
d. Use of intraarticular therapy such as hyaluronan or glucocorticoids

Step 3 Surgical Management
Referral to an orthopedic surgeon should be considered in patients with severe symptomatic OA who have pain that has failed to respond to medical therapy and who have progressive impairment of activities of daily living.

Fig. 26.2 Treatment recommendations for knee and hip OA according to ACR guidelines Arnett Fc, et al.: Arthritis Rheum 31:315, 1988.

> Acetaminophen 325-500mg TID
> Oral NSAIDS
> Topical NSAIDS

- ➤ Tramadol 25mg morning, should be titrated to 50-100mg
- ➤ Intraarticular corticosteroid injection:
  - Hylantan G F20 (Synvise-R) given once weekly for 3 weeks
  - Hylan G F20 (Synvise One TM) once per 6months
  - Hyalgan® once weekly for a total of 5 injections
  - Supartz® once a week for a total of 5 weeks
  - Euflexxa™3 injection treatment regimen
  - Monovise™ once
  - Gel-Syn™ once a week for 3 weeks
  - Genvise® 5 injections given at weekly intervals

Treatment recommendations for knee and hip OA according to ACR guidelines.

For knee and hip osteoarthritis, the American College of Rheumatology (ACR)/Arthritis Foundation recommends the following regarding nonpharmacologic measures

- Exercise is strongly recommended; balance exercises are conditionally recommended
- Weight loss is strongly recommended for patients who are overweight or obese
- Self-efficacy and self-management programs are strongly recommended
- Tai chi is strongly recommended
- Yoga is conditionally recommended
- Cognitive behavioral therapy is conditionally recommended
- Cane use is strongly recommended for patients in whom disease in 1 or more joints is causing a sufficiently large impact on ambulation, joint stability, or pain to warrant use of an assistive device
- Tibiofemoral knee braces are strongly recommended for patients in whom disease in 1 or both knees is causing a sufficiently large impact on ambulation, joint stability, or pain to warrant use of an assistive device, and who are able to tolerate the associated inconvenience and burden associated with bracing
- Patellofemoral braces are conditionally recommended for patients with patellofemoral knee OA in whom disease in 1 or both knees is causing a sufficiently large impact on ambulation, joint stability, or pain to warrant use of an assistive device.
- Kinesiotaping is conditionally recommended
- Modified shoes and lateral and medial wedged insoles are conditionally recommended *against*
- Acupuncture is conditionally recommended
- Thermal interventions (locally applied heat or cold) are conditionally recommended
- Radiofrequency ablation is conditionally recommended
- Massage therapy is conditionally recommended *against*
- Manual therapy with exercise is conditionally recommended *against* over exercise alone

For pharmacologic treatment of knee osteoarthritis, the ACR/Arthritis Foundation guidelines strongly recommend the following

- Topical NSAIDs; should be considered prior to use of oral NSAIDs
- Oral NSAIDs; however, doses should be as low as possible and treatment should be as short as possible
- Intra-articular glucocorticoid injections

Conditionally recommended agents include the following

- Topical capsaicin
- Acetaminophen
- Duloxetine
- Tramadol

Source: Kolasinski SL, Neogi T, Hochberg MC, et al. 2019 American College of Rheumatology/Arthritis Foundation Guideline for the Management of Osteoarthritis of the Hand, Hip, and Knee. *Arthritis Rheumatol.* 2020 Jan 6

3. **Surgical procedures used in the treatment of OA**
   - ➤ Arthroscopic lavage and debridement: Shaving of rough cartilage smoothening of the degenerated meniscus. Debridement removes torn meniscus fragments and loose cartilage flaps.
   - ➤ Cartilage repair technique:
     Only indicated for focal defects, precursor of OA
   - ➤ Bone marrow stimulating techniques: Abrasion, drilling

   The 2 main surgical treatments for arthritis involve

   (a) Conservative treatment : damaged cartilage is left in place and treated
   (b) Radical treatment : here, the cartilage is replaced by artificial endoprosthesis (Arthroplasty, Arthodesis)

   Hip osteoarthritis

   Conservative treatment:

   (a) Femoral osteotomy: reorientation of femoral head
   (b) Pelvic osteotomy: pelvic reorientation with bone graft addition on top of the hip (provides support and balance).
   (c) Arthroscopy: open or arthroscopic osteochondroplasty of femoral head - neck function (seen in symptomatic cam implingement)

4. **Causes and risk factors of OA**

   Causes :

   - ➤ Age - common in elderly/ Obesity - more weight put stress on joints
   - ➤ injury/ Heridetiry, Muscle weakness/ Scoliosic or other curvature of spines
   - ➤ Birth defects that affect hip joint

Risk factors
- ➢ Overuse of joints/ Posture/ Family history
- ➢ Age / Gender/ Previous history / Certain occupations

5. When should NSAIDs be considered in treatment of OA

NSAIDs are recommended in patients if the first line treatment like acetaminophen and capsaicin do not cause better therapeutic outcomes.

References

1. Lohmander LS, Ostenberg A, Englund M, Roos H. High prevalence of knee osteoarthritis, pain, and functional limitations in female soccer players twelve years after anterior cruciate ligament injury. Arthritis Rheum. 2004;50(10):3145–52.

2. Croft P, Cooper C, Wickham C, Coggon D. Osteoarthritis of the hip and occupational activity. Scand J Work Environ Health. 1992;18(1):59–63.

3. Sun BH, Christopher WW, Kalunian KC. New Developments in Osteoarthritis. Rheum Dis Clin North Am 2007;33:135–148.

4. Sandell LJ, Heinegard D, Hering TH. Cell biology, biochemistry, and molecular biology of articular cartilage in osteoarthritis. In: Moscowitz RW, Altman, RD, Hochberg MC, Buckwalter JA, Goldberg VM, eds. Osteoarthritis: Diagnosis and Medical/Surgical Management, 4th ed. Philadelphia: Lippincott, Williams, & Wilkins, 2007:73–106.

5. Hayami T, Pickarski M, Zhuo Y, et al. Characterization of articular cartilage and subchondral bone changes in the rat anterior cruciate ligament transection and meniscectomized models of osteoarthritis. Bone 2006;38:234–243.

6. Hough AB. Pathology of osteoarthritis. In: Moscowitz RW, Altman, RD, Hochberg MC, Buckwalter JA, Goldberg VM, eds. Osteoarthritis: Diagnosis and Medical/Surgical Management, 4th ed. Philadelphia: Lippincott, Williams, & Wilkins, 2007:51–72.

7. Olivier et al., An algorithm recommendation for the management of knee osteoarthritis in Europe and internationally: A report from a task force of the European Society for Clinical and Economic Aspects of Osteoporosis and Osteoarthritis (ESCEO). Seminars in Arthritis and Rheumatism. Volume 44, Issue 3, December 2014, Pages 253-263.

CHAPTER – 27

Gout and Hyperuricemia

Introduction to Gout

It involves hyperuricemia, recurrent attacks of acute arthritis with monosodium urate crystals (MSU) in synovial fluid leucocytes, deposits of Monosodium Urate (MSU) crystals in tissues in and around joints (tophi), interstitial renal disease, and uric acid nephrolithiasis.
Main joint involved is Toe.

Classification of gout

Normal uric acid levels:

In females: 2.4-6mg/dl

In males: 3.4-7.0mg/dl

Primary gout (90% of cases):
- Increased uric acid production from purines, if normal kidneys are unable to excrete uric acid then causes hyperuricaemia,
- Diet,
- Unknown enzyme defects (80-90%),
- Known enzyme defects Hypoxanthine Guanine Phosphoribosyp Transferase (HGPRT) (Partial HGPRT deficiency),
- Reduced excretion of uric acid with normal production.

Secondary gout (10% of cases):
- May be due to cancer, cellular destruction after chemotherapeutic agents,
- Kidney diseases,
- Endocrine disorders-diabetes, acidosis
- Higher aspirin doses increase uric acid levels.
- Deficiency of hypoxanthine guanine phosphoribosyl transferase (HGPRT) – leads to increased hypoxanthine -increases uric acid (UA) levels.

- Over expression of phosphoribosyl pyrophosphate (PRPP) synthetase – increases IMP – increases inosine – increases hypoxanthine –increases UA levels.
- Under excretion of uric acid.

Epidemiology

The general prevalence of gout is 1–4% of the general population. In western countries, it occurs in 3–6% in men and 1–2% in women. In some countries, prevalence may increase up to 10%. Prevalence rises up to 10% in men and 6% in women more than 80 years old. Annual incidence of gout is 2.68 per 1000 persons. It occurs in men 2–6 folds more than women.

Risk Factors

- Age, increased weight gain, heavy alcohol intake, abnormal kidney function, hypothyroidism, diabetes, some medications.
- Hypertension is known as a risk factor for hyperuricemia and gout. Increased systemic blood pressure results in reduced glomerular filtration rate leading to decreased glomerular blood flow and decreased excretion of UA.
- Diabetes mellitus is also a significant risk factor for hyperuriceamia and gout. Failure of oxidative phosphorylation increases adenosine levels resulting in increased production of uric acid and reduction of its renal excretion.

Etiopathogenesis

I. **Pathogenesis of Hyperuricemia [1, 2]**
   1. **De novo synthesis**: It is for preparation of nucleic acids
   2. **Salvage pathway:** It is a pathway in which nucleotides (purine and pyrimidine) are synthesized from intermediates in the degradation pathway for nucleotides. This pathway is used to recover bases and nucleosides that are formed during degradation of RNA & DNA. This is important in some organs because some tissues cannot undergo denovo synthesis.
   3. **Overproduction of uric acid:** Two enzyme abnormalities resulting in an overproduction of uric acid. First is an increase in the activity of phosphoribosyl pyrophosphate (PRPP) synthetase, which leads to an increased concentration of PRPP. PRPP is a key determinant of purine synthesis and thus uric acid production. Second is a deficiency of hypoxanthine guanine phophoribosyl transferase (HGPRT).
   HGPRT is responsible for the conversion of guanine to guanylic acid and hypoxanthine to inositic acid. These two conversions require PRPP as the co substrate and are reutilization reactions involved in synthesis of nucleic acids. A deficiency in HGPRT enzyme leads to increased metabolism of guanine and hypoxanthine to uric acid and more PRPP to interact with glutamine in first step of purine pathway. A partial deficiency of enzyme may be responsible for marked hyperuricaemia.

4. Underexcretion of uric acid: Uric acid does not accumulate as long as uric acid production is balanced with elimination. It is eliminated in 2 ways. About 2/3rd of uric acid produced is excreted in urine. The rest is eliminated through GIT, after enzymatic degradation by colonic bacteria. A decline in urinary excretion of uric acid to a level below the rate of production leads to hyperuricaemia and an increased miscible pool of sodium urate.

Pathogenesis of acute gouty arthritis

Deposition of UA crystals in the joint cavity is the triggering cause of gout. These crystals initiate the inflammatory process by being engulfed by synovial phagocytic cells leading to release of lysosomal enzymes and production of inflammatory chemokines.

The pathogenesis of gouty arthritis involves initial activation of monocytes and mast cells followed by neutrophils. Before the first attack of gout and in the inter-critical period, macrophages engulf UA crystals and produce abundant amounts of TNF, IL-1, IL-6 and IL-8 along with endothelial activation. This results in increasing vascular permeability and vasodilatation. The chemotactic factors produced by monocytes and mast cells and the local vasodilatation stimulates neutrophilic chemotaxis. Also, endothelial cells activation further aggravates the inflammatory response and migration of neutrophils. This leads to an influx of neutrophils locally.

The chemotactic factors produced by monocytes and mast cells and the local vasodilatation stimulates neutrophilic chemotaxis, activation and exacerbation of acute inflammation. Chronic gout results from chronic inflammation that follows recurrent attacks of gout. Chronic gout manifests by chronic synovitis, bony erosions, cartilage damage and tophi formation. Presence of urate crystals in the synovium leads to stimulation of chondrocytes to produce inflammatory cytokines, nitric oxide and matrix metalloproteases resulting in cartilage damage.

Clinical manifestation and features

Signs and symptoms:

- Fever, rapid onset of excruciating pain, swelling, inflammation, warmth, redness, tenderness (toe, ankles, elbow involved).
- Attack is typically monoarticular – often affecting the first metatarsophalangeal joint (podagra).
- Attacks begin at night with patient awakening with excruciating pain.

Complications:

- Acute gouty arthritis: Deposition of urate crystals in synovial fluid results in an inflammatory process involving chemical mediators that cause vasodilation, increased vascular permeability, complement activation, and chemotactic activity for polymorphonuclear leukocytes. Phagocytosis of urate crystals by leukocytes results in rapid lysis of cells and a discharge of proteolytic enzymes into the cytoplasm. The ensuing inflammatory reaction is associated with intense joint pain, erythema, warmth, and swelling.

- Acute Gouty nephropathy: Crystals deposited in kidney. acute renal failure occurs as a result of blockage of urine flow secondary to massive precipitation of uric acid crystals in the collecting ducts and ureters. This syndrome is a wellrecognized complication in patients with myeloproliferative or lymphoproliferative disorders and results from massive malignant cell turnover, particularly after initiation of chemotherapy. Chronic urate nephropathy is caused by the long-term deposition of urate crystals in the renal parenchyma.
- Nephrolithiasis: Kidney stones or oxalates deposited in kidney. Occurs in 10% to 25% of patients with gout. Predisposing factors include excessive urinary excretion of uric acid, acidic urine, and highly concentrated urine.
- Tophaceous gout: Crystals are bigger and deposited in joints. Untreated disease progresses into destruction of joints with formation of palpable tophi. A tophus is a mass formed of large amounts of accumulated crystals. The most common sites of tophaceous deposits in patients with recurrent acute gouty arthritis are the base of the great toe, helix of the ear, olecranon bursae, Achilles tendon, knees, wrists, and hands.

Diagnosis with Algorithm

Requires aspiration of synovial fluid from affected joints and identification of intracellular mono sodium urate crystals in synovial fluid leucocytes. If joint aspiration not possible then based on signs and symptoms, as well as treatment outcome.

Diagnostic criteria for gout [3]

American College of Rheumatology Diagnostic Criteria for Gout

1. Presence of characteristic urate crystals in the joint fluid OR
2. Presence of a tophus proven to contain urate crystals by chemical means or polarized light microscopy OR
3. Presence of six or more of the following clinical, laboratory, or radiological findings:
   - Asymmetric swelling within a joint on radiography
   - Attack of monoarticular arthritis
   - Culture of joint fluid negative for microorganisms during attack of joint inflammation
   - Development of maximal inflammation within one day
   - Hyperuricemia
   - Joint redness
   - More than one attack of acute arthritis
   - Pain or redness in the first metatarsophalangeal joint
   - Subcortical cyst without erosions on radiography
   - Suspected tophus
   - Unilateral attack involving first metatarsophalangeal joint
   - Unilateral attack involving tarsal joint

Management for Acute Gouty Arthritis

Goals of Treatment:
- To terminate acute attacks
- To prevent recurrent attacks
- To prevent complications associated with chronic deposition of urate crystals in tissues.

Non-Pharmacological:
- Avoid purine rich foods
- Regular exercise
- Take plenty of water to remove stones in kidney
- Local ice application
- Flax seeds and celery root are not recommended.

Treatment with Algorithm [4]

Algorithm for management of an acute gout attack
1. If pain intensity is mild or moderate : initiate monotherapy with NSAIDs or Colchicine or systemic corticosteroid. If treatment outcome is successful, continue the therapy. To prevent recurrent attacks - Recommend diet modifications to prevent hyperuricemia. Educate the patient about uric acid excess in gout attacks. Initiate urate lowering therapy if indicated.
2. If pain intensity is severe: initiate combination therapy
   (a) Colchicine + NSAIDs,
   (b) Colchicine + oral corticosteroids
   (c) NSAIDS + IA corticosteroids
   (d) Colchicine +IA corticosteroids
   (e) Oral corticosteroid + IA corticosteroids

Pharmacological Therapy

Classification of Anti-Gout drugs

These are the drugs which are used in treatment of gout condition which are acts by one of the following mechanism:

By- Inhibiting Uric acid synthesis (Allopurinol).

Increasing Uric acid excretion (Probencid, Sufinpyazone).

Inhibiting leukocyte migration toward joint (Colchicine).

Providing general NSAID's action (Glucocorticoids).

Classification For acute gout: Acute gout is a painful condition that often affects only one joint. Drugs used are Ex- NSAID's, Colchicine, Glucocorticoids. For chronic gout/ hyperuricaemia: Chronic gout is the repeated episodes of pain and inflammation. More than one joint may be affected Ex- Probencid, Sufinpyazone, Allopurinol

1. **NSAIDs:** Therapy started with in 24 hrs, excellent efficacy and minimal toxicity with short term use.
FDA approved drugs:
Indomethacin: 50mg, TID, till complete resolution (5-8 days)
Naproxen: 750mg followed by 250mg every 8hrs until attack subsided.
Sulindac: initial dose -150mg, usual range 150-200mg BD for 7-10 days.
Selective COX-2 inhibitor eg: celecoxib is taken for patients unable to take non-selective NSAID'S. 800 mg followed by 400mg on day 1 then 400mg 2 times daily for 1 week.
Tapering is done only if prolonged therapy is undesirable due to hepatic or renal toxicity.
Others: etodolac, fenoprofen, ibuprofen, ketoprofen, piroxicam

ADRS:

GI: gastritis, bleeding, perforation

Kidneys: renal papillary necrosis, reduced creatinine clearance.

CVS: increased BP, sodium and water retention

CNS: impaired cognitive function, headache and dizziness.

Corticosteroids: Efficacy equivalent to NSAIDS. Route: systemically / intra -articular injection. If attack is polyarticular – go with systemic therapy. Prednisone /prednisolone: 0.5mg/kg orally daily for 2-5 days followed by tapering (reduces risk of rebound attack upon steroid with drawl) for 7-10days. Methyl prednisolone: 6day regimen, IM or oral . Starting 24mg on day 1 and decreasing by 4 mg each day. Triamcinolone: 20-40mg, IA, used if gout is limited to one or two joints involved. IA corticosteroids generally used with oral NSAIDS, colchicine, corticosteroid therapy. Short term corticosteroid is generally well tolerated. Caution in pts with: diabetes, GI problems, bleeding disorders, cardiovascular disease and psychiatric disorders. Avoid long term use: because of risk for osteoporosis, hypothalamic pituitary – adrenal axis suppression, cataracts, muscle deconditioning. Adrenocorticotropic hormone gel: 40-80usp units, IM every 6-8hrs for 2 to 3 days and then discontinued.

Colchicine

- Highly effective in acute gouty arthritis when started with in 24hrs of onset of attack
- **Mechanism of action:** Anti-inflammatory - Reduces mobility, adhesiveness, and chemotaxis of polymorphonuclear cells. - Interferes with ICAM, selectins, thus inhibiting T-lymphocyte activation and its adhesion to endothelial cells. - Impairs cellular secretion of procollagen and increases collagenase production that promotes a larger collagenolytic action.
- **Pharmacokinetics:** Pale to greenish yellow crystals or powder. Oxidizes into a dark color, {different photoisomers} When exposed to UV radiation, Hence, it must be shielded. Rapidly absorbed when taken orally; peak plasma levels are reached 30 - 120 min after ingestion. 50% of the drug circulates and links to plasma proteins. Metabolized in the liver, and the majority is eliminated through bile in the feces. Also distributed in spleen and kidney. Overall, 10-20% of the dose is eliminated unchanged in the urine. Dose: 0.6mg, oral, 2tabs or BD.

Dose dependent adverse effects: GI: nausea, vomiting, diarrhea; Non-GI: neutropenia, axonal neuropathy. Do not use with p-glycoprotein or strong cyp450 3A4 inhibitors (eg: clarithromycin) Decreases biliary excretion increases plasma colchicine levels leads to toxicity. Caution in patients with renal or hepatic insufficiency. Colcrys is FDA approved product 0.6mg oral tablets. 1.2mg initially followed by 0.6mg 1 h later

Hyperuricemia in Gout

- Recurrent gout attacks can be prevented by maintaining uric acid levels.

Non-pharmacological

- Promote weight loss by caloric restriction
- Exercise to enhance renal urate excretion
- Alcohol restriction by American College of Rheumatology (ACR) guidelines
- Limiting consumption of high fructose corn syrup and purine rich foods (organ meats and sea foods)
- Encouraging consumption of vegetables and low fat dairy products.
- Eliminate urate elevating medications if necessary lke diuretics, niacin, calcineurin inhibitors
- Plenty of water
  Goal: To maintain serum uric acid levels less than 6mg/dl.

Pharmacological

Xanthine oxidase inhibitors: first line therapy

MOA: Inhibits conversion of hypoxanthine to xanthine and then to uric acid

Eg: Allopurinol, febuxostat.

Allopurinol: lowers UA levels dose dependent manner

Dose no greater than 100mg daily gradually titrating every 2-5 weeks up to max. 800mg/day until serum urate target is achieved.

Pt with CKD: no greater than 50mg/day.

Adv. effect: Skin rash, GI problems, headache and urticaria

Allopurinol hypersensitivity syndrome: Fever, eosinophilia, dermatitis, vasculitis, (renal or hepatic dysfunction) rarely 20% mortality rate.

Febuxostat: (uloric), lowers Uric Acid (UA) dose dependent manner.

Dose: 40mg OD, if serum urate levels not achieved then increase the dose to 80mg OD after 2wks.

Adv. Effect: Nausea, arthralgia, minor hepatic transaminases elevation.

No dose adjustment in hepatic or renal dysfunction.

- Give concomitant therapy with colchicine or NSAIDS for atleast the 1st 8wks of therapy to prevent acute gout flares.

Uricosurics: MOA: increases renal clearance of UA by inhibiting the post secretory renal proximal tubular reabsorption of uric acid. Dose: 250mg BD daily for 1 to 2 wks, then 500mg twice daily for 2wks. Maxi dose of 2g/day

Adv. Effect: GI irritation, rash and hypersensitivity, precipitation of acute gouty arthritis, stone formation.

Contraindicated: impaired renal function and over production of Uric Acid (UA). Start at low dose to avoid stone formation.

Pegloticase: Pegloticase – is a pegylated recombinant uricase that converts (UA) to allantoin (water soluble). Dose: 8mg, IV infusion over at least 2hrs every 2wks. Because of infusion related allergies patient must be pre-treated with antihistamines and corticosteroids. Expensive than 1st line urate lowering agents.

Anti-Inflammatory Prophylaxis During Initiation of Urate Lowering Therapy

The ACR guidelines recommend:

1st line therapy- low dose oral colchicine (0.6mg BD)

Low dose NSAIDs (naproxen- 250mg BD)

Patient on long term NSAIDs prophylaxis – a proton pump inhibitor or acid suppressing therapy indicated to avoid gastric problems.

If lack of response to first line or intolerance or contraindications – go with

Lose dose corticosteroid (prednisone less than or equal to 10mg/day)

- Continue prophylaxis for atleast 6mon or 3 months after achieving target serum uric acid whichever is longer.
- For patient with one or more tophi: continue prophylactic therapy for 6months after achieving the serum urate target.

2018 Eular Recommendation for the Management of Patients with Gout

1. Optimal treatment of gout requires nonpharmacologic and pharmacologic modalities tailored to specific risk factors Serum Uric Acid (SUA) (SUA levels, prior attacks); clinical phase of gout; and general risk factors (age, comorbidity, drug interactions)
2. Patient education and lifestyle modifications (e.g., weight loss if obese, reduced beer and other alcohol consumption) are important.
3. Associated comorbidity and risk factors (e.g., hyperlipidemia, HTN, hyperglycemia, obesity, smoking) should be addressed.
4. Oral NSAIDs or colchicine are first-line agents for systemic treatment of acute gout. In the absence of contraindications, an NSAID is a convenient and well accepted treatment.

5. High doses of colchicine cause side effects and low doses (e.g., 0.5 mg TID) can be sufficient.

6. Intra-articular aspiration and injection of a long-acting steroid is an effective and safe treatment for an acute attack.

7. Urate lowering therapy is indicated in patients with recurrent acute attacks, arthropathy, tophi, or radiographic changes of gout.

8. The therapeutic goal of urate lowering (i.e., Serum Uric Acid (SUA) less than the saturation point for MSU of 6 mg/dL) is to promote crystal dissolution and prevent crystal formation.

9. Allopurinol, an appropriate long-term urate-lowering agent, should be initiated at 100 mg/day and increased by 100 mg every 2–4 weeks, if required. The dose must be adjusted in patients with renal impairment. If toxicity occurs, options include other xanthine oxidase inhibitors, a uricosuric agent, or allopurinol desensitization (in mild rash).

10. Uricosuric agents (e.g., probenecid, sulfinpyrazone) can be alternatives to allopurinol in patients with normal renal function, but relatively contraindicated in patients with urolithiasis. Benzbromarone can be used in patients with moderate renal insufficiency, but carries a small risk of hepatotoxicity.

11. Prophylaxis against acute attacks during the first months of urate lowering therapy can be achieved by colchicine (0.5–1 mg/day) and/or NSAID (with gastroprotection, if indicated).

12. When gout is associated with diuretic therapy, discontinue the diuretic if possible.

13. Switching to a second XOI over adding a uricosuric agent is conditionally recommended for patients taking their first XOI, who have persistently high SU concentrations (>6 mg/dl) despite maximum-tolerated or FDA-indicated Xanthine Ozidase Inhibitor (XOI) dose, and who have continued frequent gout flares (>2 flares/year) or who have nonresolving subcutaneous tophi

14. Switching to pegloticase over continuing current Urate Lowering Therapy (ULT) is strongly recommended for patients with gout for whom XOI treatment, uricosurics, and other interventions have failed to achieve the SU target, and who continue to have frequent gout flares (≥2 flares/year) OR who have nonresolving subcutaneous tophi.

2020 American College of Rheumatology
Guideline for the Management of Gout [5]

Gout flare management

1. Using colchicine, NSAIDs, or glucocorticoids (oral, intraarticular, or intramuscular) as appropriate firstline therapy for gout flares over IL-1 inhibitors or adrenocorticotropic hormone (ACTH) is strongly recommended for patients experiencing a gout flare.

2. Given similar efficacy and a lower risk of adverse effects, low-dose colchicine over high-dose colchicine is strongly recommended when colchicine is the chosen agent.

3. Using topical ice as an adjuvant treatment over no adjuvant treatment is conditionally recommended for patients experiencing a gout flare.

4. Using an IL-1 inhibitor over no therapy (beyond supportive/analgesic treatment) is conditionally recommended for patients experiencing a gout flare for whom the above antiinflammatory therapies are either ineffective, poorly tolerated, or contraindicated.
5. Treatment with glucocorticoids (intramuscular, intravenous, or intraarticular) over IL-1 inhibitors or ACTH is strongly recommended for patients who are unable to take oral medications.

Management of lifestyle factors

1. Limiting alcohol intake is conditionally recommended for patients with gout, regardless of disease activity.
2. Limiting purine intake is conditionally recommended for patients with gout, regardless of disease activity.
3. Limiting high-fructose corn syrup intake is conditionally recommended for patients with gout, regardless of disease activity.
4. Using a weight loss program (no specific program endorsed) is conditionally recommended for those patients with gout who are overweight/ obese, regardless of disease activity.
5. Adding vitamin C supplementation is conditionally recommended against for patients with gout, regardless of disease activity.

Management of concurrent medications

1. Switching hydrochlorothiazide to an alternate antihypertensive when feasible is conditionally recommended for patients with gout, regardless of disease activity.
2. Choosing losartan preferentially as an antihypertensive agent when feasible is conditionally recommended for patients with gout, regardless of disease activity.
3. Stopping low-dose aspirin (for patients taking this medication for appropriate indications) is conditionally recommended against for patients with gout, regardless of disease activity.
4. Adding or switching cholesterol-lowering agents to fenofibrate is conditionally recommended against for patients with gout, regardless of disease activity

References

1. C.F. Kuo, M.J. Grainge, W. Zhang, M. DohertyGlobal epidemiology of gout: prevalence, incidence and risk factors. Nat Rev Rheumatol, 11 (11) (2015), pp. 649-662
2. G. Kosmadakis, M. Viskaduraki, S. MichailThe validity of fractional excretion of uric acid in the diagnosis of acute kidney injury due to decreased kidney perfusion Am J Kidney Dis, 54 (6) (2009), pp. 1186-1187.
3. Wallace SL, Robinson H, Masi AT, Decker JL, McCarty DJ, Yü TF. Preliminary criteria for the classification of the acute arthritis of primary gout. *Arthritis Rheum.* 1977;20(3):895–900.
4. P. Richette, M. Doherty, E. Pascual, V. Barskova, F. Becce, J. Castaneda-Sanabria, *et al.*2016 updated EULAR evidence-based recommendations for the management of gout. Ann Rheum Dis, 76 (1) (2017), pp. 29-42.
5. John et al., 2020 American College of Rheumatology Guideline for the Management of Gout. Arthritis Care & Research; 2020; 0: 1-17.

CHAPTER – 28

Spondylitis

Introduction to Spondylitis

Spondylitis is an inflammation of vertebra. It is a form of spondylopathy. In many cases spondylitis involves one or more vertebral joints as well, which itself is called spondylarthritis.

It is autoimmune or auto inflammatory disease [inflammation to our own cells].

The pain is usually concentrated around the cervical region of the neck, shoulder and lower spine, with downward moving stinging pain.

Types of Spondylitis

Cervical Spondylitis: Which affects the cervical spine, causing pain to spread the back of the neck.

Lumbar Spondylitis: Which causes pain in the lumbar region (Hip)

Ankylosing Spondylitis: Which is a primarily a disease that affects the sacroiliac joints, causing stiffness in the neck, jaw, shoulders, hips and knees.

Epidemiology

- It is a disorder with many possible etiologies and many definitions.
- 25 years and greater are more prone to spondylitis; rarely > 18yrs are affected.
- The incidence of lumbar spondylitis is 27%-35% of the asymptomatic lower back pain population.
- However, men and women are likely to experience different symptoms, which can affect diagnosis and treatment methods. While condition is most prevalent in men than women.

Etiology

- Genetic: About 90% of people with spondylitis have a specific gene, HLA-B27. Individuals with this gene are at a greater risk for developing spondylitis.
- Age: Most people with spondylitis developed the spine condition between the ages of 17 and 45. When people get older, discs dehydrate, become thinner and become harder. Then they provide less support to the vertebrae resting on the dics.

- Gender: Males develop spondylitis much more frequently than females.
- Environmental factors and Food habits.

Pathophysiology

HLA-B27 Antigen genotype (inherited gene), Auto antibodies are developed against them. There is activation of inflammatory mediators TNF-α and IL-1. Inflammatory cascade is initiated. Inflammation of spinal cord and spinal nerves which leads to Spondylitis.

Ankylosing Spondylitis

Long term Inflammation of the joints of the spine. Spinal cord is highly inflamed at ileac sacral Joints.

Clinical Presentation

- Stiffness and pain in the back.
- Pain that runs from the lower back down one or both legs.
- Pain and stiffness is more in the morning and subsides gradually as physical activity is done.
- Chronic pain and discomfort when standing, sitting or walking.
- Flexion and extension of lumbar spine is decreased, inability to twist and turn or to do so without pain.
- Weightloss, fatigue, fever.
- 40% of Alkylosing spondylitis have chance to develop eye redness, uveitis, eyepain, sensitivity of light.
- Some people also have CV complications.

Diagnosis

- Physical examination.
- X-Ray of spine- bone spurs, thickening of joints and narrowing of intervertebral discs are identified.
- MRI, CT Scan and SPECT (Single-Photon emission Computed Tomography)
- Presence of Auto antibodies.
- Positive family history of axial spondylitis
- Elevated 'C' reactive protein and ESR.
- Schober's Test- Lumber flexion.

Diagnosis Algorithm

Modified New York Criteria for the Diagnosis of Ankylosing Spondylosis

1. **Clinical**
   - Low back pain and stiffness > 3months, which improves with exercise and not relieved by rest
   - Limitation of lumbar spine in both saggital and frontalplanes
   - Limitation of chest expansion relative to normal for age and sex

2. Radiological

Bilateral sacrolitis > grade 2; Unilateral sacrolitis > grade 3 or 4

Grade 0=normal; Grade 1= suspicious;

Grade 3= severe erosions, widening of the joint space, some ankylosis

Grade 4=complete ankylosis

3. AS is present if the radiological criterion is associated with atleast one clinical criterion

Management

Box : Overview of treatment modalities in spinal disease of AS	
Benefits	**Risks**
Exercise	
Maintain spinal mobility Maintain good posture Delay disease progression Quality of life	Time management Lack of motivation Injury
NSAIDs	
Readily avaialbe first-line agent Effectively reduce joint pain and stiffness by at least 20%[24] Promote sleep efficacy Ability to maintain exercise regime Improve quality of life	Gasrointestinal side effects Cardiovascular disease May cause wheezing or worsen asthma symptoms Skin reactions Interaction with warfarin Antagonism/synergism with aspirin
Corticosteriods	
Supression of inflammation Symptom relief Allows full benefit of rehabilitation programmes	Short term side effect include headache, insomnia. Mood changes Long-term use results in osteoporosis, acne, water retention, hypertention, diabetes mellitus, adrenal suppression
TNF blockade	
Reduce inflammation and symptoms Improve quality of life Maintain/improve work capacity Generally well-tolerated	Side effects: Skin irritation, allergic reaction nausea Lymphoma Systemic and local infections, especially TB Heart failure (Contraindication) Induction of auto-antibodies Possible demyelinating disease
Surgery	
Correct deformities Increase functional ability (regain use of joints) Relieve pain Improve quality of life Improved self-confidence	Anaesthetic risk Post-op complications such as pain, infection, technical failure Paralysis in spinal surgery

Fig. 28.1 Nonpharmacological approaches for ankylosing Spondylitis. Maksymowych WP, Jhangri GS, Leclercq S, et al. An open study of pamidronate in the treatment of refractory ankylosing spondylitis. J. Rheumatol 1998; 25(4): 714-7.

Treatment Goals

- ✓ To prevent and hault the symptoms.
- ✓ To prvent progression of disease.
- ✓ To increase the quality of life.

Non-Pharmacological Therapy

- Regular basic exercise.
- Maintaining a healthy weight, eating nutrious food.
- Apply either ice (or) heating pad at the affected area for reducing the pain.
- In severe case bed rest is required, long term bed rest is avoided as it puts patient at risk for Deep Vein Thrombosis (DVT).

Pharmacological Therapy

The first line of drugs is NSAID'S, DMARD'S and Steroids.

1. **NSAID's**
   - (a) Ibuprofen- Adults : 400-800mg/dose 3-4 times/ day (max. dose 3200mg/day) Children: 20-40mg/kg divided dose every 8 hr.
   - (b) Phenylbutazone- 100mg/dose 2times/day.
   - (c) Naproxen- 250-500mg orally twice a day.
   - (d) Diclofenac- 150 -200m orally in 2-4 divided doses.
   - (e) Celecoxib – 200mg twice daily.
   - (f) Rofecoxib- 50 mg orally once daily.
2. **Opioid Relievers** – for intense pain.
   - (a) Fentanyl- 100-150mcg IV/day.
   - (b) Tramadol- 50 to 100mg orally every 4 to 6 hours.
3. **DMARD'S**
   - (a) Sulfasalizine- 500mg twice a day.
   - (b) Methotrexate- 2.5mg orally every 12 hrs for 3 doses in a week (max. weekly dose is 20mg)
     - **Tumor Necrosis Factor-α Inhibitors**
       - (a) Infliximab 5mg/kg given at 0,2,6 weeks. Maintenance dose- 5mg/kg IV Every 6 weeks.
       - (b) Golimumab 50mg S.C once a month. 2mg/kg IV over 30min at weeks 0 and 4, every eight weeks there after.
       - (c) Adalimumab- 40mg S.C every other week.
     - **Interleukin-6 Inhibitors**
       - (a) Tocilizumab- 4mg/kg IV 60min once every 4 weeks.
       - (b) Rituximab 1000mg IV infusion separated by 2 weeks.

- **Interleukin -17 A Inhibitors**
    (a) Secukinumab- 150mg S.C at 0, 1, 2, 3, 4 weeks and every 4 weeks thereafter.
4. Local injection with Corticosteroid can be used for certain people with Peripheral Arthritis.

Cervical Spondylitis

- Cervical spondylitis is a chronic degeneration of the bones (vertebrae) of the neck (cervical spine) and the cushions between the vertebrae (discs), the condition usually appears in men and women older than 40 and progress with age.
- Cervical spondylitis affects both sexes equally, men usually develop it at a earlier age than women do. The degeneration in cervical spondylitis most likely is a result of wear and tear on the neck bones as aging.
- The changes that accompany the degeneration, such as developing abnormal growths (bone spurs) on the spine, can lead to pressure on the spinal nerves and sometimes, the spinal cord itself.
- Mild cases of cervical spondylitis often require no treatment or may respond to conservative treatment, including wearing a neck bone and taking pain medication.

Predisposing Factors

- As ageing, the discs of the spine become drier and less elastic.
- Degeneration can cause some of the discs to bulge and, in some cases, cause the central cartilage of the discs to protrude through a crack in the ring that surrounds the disc (Herniate).
- The surrounding ligaments become less flexible, and the vertebrae may develop bone spurs.
- These degenerative changes may be a result of wear and tear throughout the life.
- An earlier injury to the neck may predispose to degeneration.
- Some occupations or hobbies involve repetitive or heavy lifting. such as construction work, they put extra pressure on spine.

Clinical Manifestation and Features

Signs and Symptoms

- Neck pain and stiffness that gets progressively work may be an indication of cervical spondylitis.
- The pain may range from mild to severe and debilitating.
- Neck pain that radiates to the shoulders and arms.
- Numbness or weakness in the arms, hands and fingers.
- Headache that radiates to the back of the head.
- Loss of balance.

- Numbness or weakness in the legs, if the spinal cord is compressed.
- Loss of bladder or bowel control, if the spinal cord is compressed.

Diagnosis with Algorithm

- Physical examination- typical examinations testing your reflexes, checking for muscle weakness or sensory defects.
- X-Rays can be used to check for bone spurs and other abnormalities.
- CT scan can provide more detailed images of your neck.
- MRI, which produces images using radio waves and a magnetic field, helps to locate pinched nerves.
- Electro myogram (EMG) checks whether nerves are functioning normal when sending signals to your muscles. EMG measures "Nerves Electrical Activity".
- A nerve conduction study is used to check the speed and strength of the signals sent by nerves.

Differential diagnosis of cervical spondylosis [1]

- ➤ Lesions of the bones of the upper cord cervical spine, Myeloma, Osteomyelitis
- ➤ Metastatic tumor, Erosive inflammatory disease, eg. Rheumatoid arthritis, Paget's disease

Management

Treatment Goals

- To relieve pain and symptoms.
- To prevent permanent injury to Spinal cord and nerves.
- To improve quality of life.

Non-Pharmacological Therapy

- Exercise regularly to help you recover faster.
- Use a heating pad or cold pack on your neck to provide pain relief for sore muscles.
- Wear a soft neck brace or collar to get temporary relief.
- Physical therapy helps you stretch your neck and shoulder muscles. This makes them stronger and ultimately relieves pain.

Pharmacological Therapy

1. **Muscle Relaxants**- to treat muscle spasms.
   (a) Cyclobenzaprine- 5mg orally TID.
2. **Narcotics**- for pain relief.
   (a) Hydrocodone- 2.5mg – 10mg (every 4-6)

3. **Antiepileptic Drugs**- to relieve pain caused by nerve damage.
   (a) Gabapentine- 300mg orally [max- 1800mg/day – 600mg orally TID]
4. **Steroid Injections**- to reduce tissue inflammation and subsequently lessen pain.
   (a) Prednisone- 5mg-10mg orally.
5. **Skeletal Muscle Relaxants**
   (a) D-Tubocurarine- 6mg-9mg followed by 3-4.5mg.
   (b) Succinyl choline- 20mg/ml-100mg/ml IV.

Surgery

Surgery is rarely necessary for cervical spondylosis. This can involve getting rid of bonespurs, parts of neck bones or herniated discs to give your spinal cord and spinal nerves.

2019 Update of the American College of Rheumatology/Spondylitis Association of America Recommendations for Adults with Active Ankylosing Spondylitis

1. We strongly recommend treatment with NSAIDs over no treatment with NSAIDs
2. We conditionally recommend continuous treatment with NSAIDs over on-demand treatment with NSAIDs.
3. We do not recommend any particular NSAID as the preferred choice.
4. In adults with active AS despite treatment with NSAIDs, we conditionally recommend treatment with sulfasalazine, methotrexate, or tofacitinib over no treatment with these medications. Sulfasalazine or methotrexate should be considered only in patients with prominent peripheral arthritis or when TNFi are not available.
5. In adults with active AS despite treatment with NSAIDs, we conditionally recommend treatment with TNFi over treatment with tofacitinib
6. In adults with active AS despite treatment with NSAIDs, we strongly recommend treatment with TNFi over no treatment with TNFi.
7. We do not recommend any particular TNFi as the preferred choice.
8. In adults with active AS despite treatment with NSAIDs, we strongly recommend treatment with secukinumab or ixekizumab over no treatment with secukinumab or ixekizumab.
9. In adults with active AS despite treatment with NSAIDs, we conditionally recommend treatment with TNFi over treatment with secukinumab or ixekizumab.
10. In adults with active AS despite treatment with NSAIDs, we conditionally recommend treatment with secukinumab or ixekizumab over treatment with tofacitinib.
11. In adults with active AS despite treatment with NSAIDs and who have contraindications to TNFi, we conditionally recommend treatment with secukinumab or ixekizumab over treatment with sulfasalazine, methotrexate, or tofacitinib

References

1. Sandanha GJ. Headache and facial pain. In: Fillit HM, Rockwood K, Woodhouse K, eds. *Brocklehurst's Textbook of Geriatric Medicine and Gerontology*. 7th ed. Philadelphia, PA: Saunders Elsevier; 2010:466-477.
2. Miceli-Richard C, Dougados M. NSAIDs in ankylosing spondylitis. Clin. Exp. Rheumatol 2002; 20(6 Suppl 28): S65–6 27. Braun J, Pincus T. Mortality, course of disease and prognosis of patients with ankylosing spondylitis. Clin. Exp. Rheumatol. 2002; 20(6 Suppl).

CHAPTER – 29

Osteoporosis

Introduction to Osteoporosis

The word osteoporosis, osteon is bone, porosis is hole in Greek.

Osteoporosis is a systemic skeletal disorder characterized by low bone mass, micro architectural deterioration of bone tissue leading to bone fragility and consequent increase in fracture risk. It is a disorder where the bone is with low density and high fracture risk.

Etiology

- Neurological disturbances, Gonadal dysgenesis, Age, Postmenopausal condition,
- Idiopathic, Nutrition problems, Gastrointestinal disease, Malignancy,
- Endocrine disorders, Sedentary lifestyle, Inflammatory Arthritis, Fracture.

Risk factors

- Age, Cigarette Smoking, Alcohol intake, Family history, Gender,
- Low calcium intake, Oestrogen deficiency, Low sun exposure, Immobility,
- Medications - immunosuppressant, diuretics.

Pathophysiology

Bone is continuously changing. New bone is formed and old bone is broken down, a process called bone remodelling or bone turnover. It has two main functions:
1. To repair micro damage within skeleton, tomaintain strength,
2. To supply calcium to maintain serum calcium levels.

In young, the body makes newer bones faster than it breaks down old bones and thus bone mass increases. Thus it reaches the peak bone mass in mid 30s. As the age passes, again imbalance between formation and resorption occurs but here resorption rate increases. This leads to increased bone loss.

- ❖ Factors responsible for such resorption of bones are :-
    - ➢ Excessive bone loss can be due to increased osteoclastic or osteoblastic activity.
    - ➢ Oestrogen deficiency during Menopause increases osteoclast activity which results in increased bone resorption than formation.

> Calcium deficiency leads to decreased serum calcium, hence in order to maintain Calcium balance, bone resorption occurs.
> Hormone, vitamin D deficiency lead to increased bone turnover and reduced osteoblast formation.
> Glucocorticoidglucocorticoids - Increase osteoclastogenesis,
>> Decrease apoptosis of osteoclasts,
>> Decrease osteoblast agenesis,
>> Increase eclecticism osteoblast,
>> Finally bone resorption increases.
> Other medications like anticonvulsants, immunosuppressant.
> Vitamin D deficiency causes hyperparathyroidism leading to osteoporosis.
> Cigarette smoking effects osteoblast, modify oestrogen metabolism resulting in detrimental effect on human bone mass.

Clinical manifestation and features

Signs and symptoms

- Fractures occur after bending, lifting, falling,
- Pain,
- Immobility,
- Discoloured skin (bruising),
- Depression,
- Shortened stature,
- Bone pain or fractures,
- Kyphosis(curvature of spine causing hunching of back),
- Lordosis (inward curvature of spine).

Diagnosis with algorithm [1]

Algorithm for the Management of Postmenopausal Osteoporosis

1. After the clinical assessment is made, general measures like calcium intake, physical activity have to be assessed. In the elderly-Vitamin D + calcium levels have to be estimated.
2. If patients are with risk factors but no fracture-FRAX ¼ Fracture Risk Assessment Tool, is advised.

   Bone mineral density assessment has to be done.

   > If T score $\geq$ -1: It is considered normal, monitor and reassess with BMD after 2 years
   > If T score < -1 to -2.5: It is considered as Osteopenia. If multiple risk factors are present then treatement options are- SERM's Selective estrogen receptor modulator/ Alandronate / hormonal therapy/ STEAR ¼ Selective tissue estrogenic activity regulator. If no risk facors are present, reassess with BMD after 2 years. If BMD deteriorates then treatment has to be initiated.

➢ If T score ≤ -2.5 : It is considered as Osteoporosis. Treatment options are Bisphosphonates/ Selective estrogen receptor modulator/ activated Vitamin D/ Storcium renolate. Follow up after 2 years.

3. If the patients are with prior low trauma fracture- It is diagnosed as Osteoporosis-
Treatment options are
Bisphosphonates/ Selective estrogen receptor modulator/ activated Vitamin D/ Storcium renolate. Follow up after 2 years.

Diagnostic tests

1. Physical examination: Bone pain, postural changes, loss of height.
2. Laboratory testing:
    CBP, Creatinine levels, BUN, calcium levels, TSH levels, Phosphorus levels, alkaline phosphate, free testosterone, 2, 5 hydroxyvitamin D, and 24 hour urine calcium measurement.
3. The best screening is Dual Energy X-ray Absorbimetry (DEXA)
    It measures the density of bones in spine, hip, wrist. It is used to accurately follow changes in bones overtime.
4. Bone mineral density :
    It is the most common test.
     Results are reported using T- score (how much higher or lower your bone mass density is compared to that of a healthy individual)
    T- Score:Category:

-1.0 or above	Normal.
-1.0 or 2 – 2.5	Osteopenia (low bone mass).
-2.5 or less	Osteoporosis.
-2.5 or less with	

One or more fragility fractures severe osteoporosis.

Management

Goals

1. Primary goal is prevention,
2. Optimising peak bone mass when young, reduces the future incidence of osteoporosis,
3. In osteoporosis condition - stabilize or improve bone mass and strength and prevent fractures,
4. In osteoporosis condition patient with fractures- Reducing pain and deformity,
5. Improving function and quality of life, Reducing fall and fractures.

Non pharmacological therapy

1. Balanced diet with adequate intake of calcium and Vitamin D
2. Controlled alcohol consumption
3. Caffeine intake decreased

4. Smoking cessation
5. Weight bearing aerobic and strengthening exercises - improves muscle strength, balance, mobility and decrease the fractures.

Algorithm for management of Osteoporosis in post menopausal women.

Consider the following risk factors in post menopausal women: Age over 70 years, multiple risk factors, low-trauma fracture or prevalent vertebral deformity, radiographic evidence of osteopenia, medical conditions or medications known to increase the risk for bone loss and fracture (hypogonadism and glucocorticoid use). Check for bone marrow density (BMD) testing.

(i) Normal: If T score is $\geq$ -1.0. The following therapy can be adviced. Calcium 1000-1500 mg/day. Vitamin D 400-800IU/day. Exercise. Fall prevention strategies. Lifestyle modifications. Reevaluate in five years or as appropriate.

(ii) Osteoporosis: If T score is $\leq$ -2.5 or T score -2.0 to -2.4 with $\geq$ one major risk factor for fracture. Then investigate for secondry cause.

 (a) If the secondary cause is not identified: Calcium 1500 mg/day. Vitamin D $\geq$ 800IU/day. Exercise. Fall prevention strategies. Lifestyle modifications.

 Drug therapy: First line: Alendronate 70mg p.o. weekly or Risendronate 35mg p.o. weekly. Second line: Teriparatide 20 µg s.c. daily. Third line: Testosetone therapy. Reevaluate in five years or as appropriate.

 (b) If the secondary cause is identified- Treat underlying cause. Calcium/Vitamin D supplementation. Exercise. Fall prevention strategies. Lifestyle modifications. Reevaluate bone marrow density BMD in one or two years.

(iii) Osteopenia: If T score -1.1 to -1.9 or T score -2.0 to -2.4 without $\geq$one major risk factor for fracture. Then investigate for secondry cause.

 (a) If the secondary cause is identified- Treat underlying cause. Calcium/Vitamin D supplementation. Exercise. Fall prevention strategies. Lifestyle modifications. Consider drug therapy. Reevaluate bone marrow density BMD in one or two years.

 (b) If the secondary cause is not identified- Calcium 1000-1500 mg/day. Vitamin D 600-800IU/day. Exercise. Fall prevention strategies. Lifestyle modifications. Testosterone therapy. Reevaluate bone marrow density BMD in one or two years.

Pharmacological therapy [2, 3]:

Antiresorptive therapy

1. **Calcium supplementation:**
 (a) Calcium: Increase bone mass density - but less effective.

It should be combined with Vitamin D and osteoporosis medication when needed.
Elemental calcium - maximum dose 600mg or less is recommended

(b) Calcium carbonate:
Salt of choice as it contains high concentration of elemental calcium (40%)
Least expensive. Ingested with meals to enhance absorption in a medium.

(c) Calcium citrate: Absorption is acid independent. Fewer side effects as calcium carbonate.

(d) Tricalcium phosphate- 38% calcium
Calcium-phosphate complexes limits calcium absorption
Side Effects: constipation (common) kidney stones (rarely) flatulence or stomach upset.

2. Vitamin D supplementation:

- It maximises intestinal calcium absorption and BMD.
- non-prescription cholecalciferol (Vitamin D3) products ,higher dose prescription ergocalciferol (vitamin D2) regimens - weekly monthly quarterly
- through food and supplementation – 2,5 hydroxyvitamin D concentration at 30ng/ml or more maintained
- T1/2 of vitamin D is 1 month; hence check the concentration for every 3 month.

3. Bisphosphonates:

- They inhibit bone resorption, increase BMD, and reduce the fracture risks.
- For the first 6-12 months of therapy – BMD increases.
  After discontinuation – levels are sustained.
- E.g. Alendronate, Risedronate, IV Zoledronic acid –are used in post-menopausal women, males and in glucocorticoid induced osteoporosis patients.
  IV and oral bandronate is used only in postmenopausal women
- Administered carefully in order to optimise clinical benefits and minimise adverse GI effects. Each oral tablet – morning – 30 minutes before consuming food with 6oz of plain water
  Exception is Risedronate – after breakfast with 4oz of plain water.
  Patient should remain upright for 30 minutes to 1 hour to avoid oesophageal irritation.
- Adverse effects of oral tablets: - nausea, abdominal pain, dyspepsia, oesophageal, gastric, duodenal irritation, perforation, ulceration, bleeding.
- Adverse effects due to IV medications:-fever, flu like symptoms, local reaction.

4. Denosumab:

- It is a Receptor Activator of Nuclear Factor KB (RANK) ligand inhibitor – it inhibits osteoclast formation and increases its apoptosis.
- Recommended for women and men at higher risk for fracture.
- Dose: 60 mg given subcutaneous route for every 6 months.
- Adverse effects: flatulence, dermatitis, Eczema, Rash.
- Contraindication: hypocalcaemia patient.

5. **Mixed oestrogen agonist/ antagonist:**
   - Raloxifene oestrogen antagonist in breast and uterine tissueand oestrogen agonist in bone.
   - Used in postmenopausal osteoporosis women.
   - Action: increases Spine and hip bone mass density, decrease vertebral fractures.
   - Adverse effects: hot flushes, leg cramps, muscle spasms.
   - Contraindications: women with history of venous thromboembolic disease.

6. **Calcitonin:**
   - Endogenous hormone released from thyroid gland when serum calcium level is elevated.
   - Salman calcitonin- clinically used.
   - Indicated in women at least five years past Menopause last line therapy.
   - Action: decrease vertebral fractures, pain relief in acute vertebral fractures.
   - Dose: intranasal- 200 units per day; subcutaneous route- 100 units rarely used.
   - Adverse effects: - Nausea, local infection at injection site, rhinitis, epitaxis when given through nasal route.

7. **Oestrogen therapy - FDA indicated:**
   - In women and patients for whom other osteoporosis medications are not used.
   - Action: - increases bone mass density.

8. **Testosterone - not FBA indicated:**
   - In men with low level of testosterone. Increase bone mass density in men.

Anabolic therapy

Teriparatide

- Recombinant product representing first 34 amino acids of human parathyroid hormone.
- Dose: 20 mcg given subcutaneously once daily.
- Used in postmenopausal women, glucocorticoid induced osteoporosis patient, men with idiopathic or hypo gonadal osteoporosis, men and women in tolerant to other medications.
- Action: reduce fracture, lumbar spine bone mass density increases.
- Adverse effects: transient hypercalcemia, nausea, headache, dizziness, muscle cramps, pain at injection site.
- Contraindications: osteosarcoma.

Recommendations to Postmenopausal Women and Men Age 50 and Older

Universal recommendations

- Counsel on the risk of osteoporosis and related fractures.

- Advise on a diet that includes adequate amounts of total calcium intake (1000 mg/day for men 50–70; 1200 mg/day for women 51 and older and men 71 and older), incorporating dietary supplements if diet is insufficient.
- Advise on vitamin D intake (800–1000 IU/day), including supplements if necessary for individuals age 50 and older.
- Recommend regular weight-bearing and muscle-strengthening exercise to improve agility, strength, posture, and balance; maintain or improve bone strength; and reduce the risk of falls and fractures.
- Assess risk factors for falls and offer appropriate modifications (e.g., home safety assessment, balance training exercises, correction of vitamin D insufficiency, avoidance of central nervous system depressant medications, careful monitoring of antihypertensive medication, and visual correction when needed).
- Advise on cessation of tobacco smoking and avoidance of excessive alcohol intake.

Diagnostic assessment

- Measure height annually, preferably with a wall-mounted stadiometer.
- Bone mineral density (BMD) testing should be performed:
  - In women age 65 and older and men age 70 and older
  - In postmenopausal women and men above age 50–69, based on risk factor profile
  - In postmenopausal women and men age 50 and older who have had an adult age fracture, to diagnose and determine degree of osteoporosis
  - At dual-energy X-ray absorptiometry (DEXA) facilities using accepted quality assurance measures
- Vertebral imaging should be performed:
  - In all women age 70 and older and all men age 80 and older if BMD T-score is ≤-1.0 at the spine, total hip, or femoral neck
  - In women age 65 to 69 and men age 70 to 79 if BMD T-score is ≤-1.5 at the spine, total hip, or femoral neck
  - In postmenopausal women and men age 50 and older with specific risk factors:
    - Low-trauma fracture during adulthood (age 50 and older)
    - Historical height loss (*difference between the current height and peak height at age 20*) of 1.5 in. or more (4 cm)
    - Prospective height loss (*difference between the current height and a previously documented height measurement*) of 0.8 in. or more (2 cm)
    - Recent or ongoing long-term glucocorticoid treatment
  - If bone density testing is not available, vertebral imaging may be considered based on age alone.
- Check for secondary causes of osteoporosis.
- Biochemical markers of bone turnover can aid in risk assessment and serve as an additional monitoring tool when treatment is initiated.

Pharmacologic treatment recommendations

- Initiate pharmacologic treatment:
  - In those with hip or vertebral (clinical or asymptomatic) fractures
  - In those with T-scores ≤-2.5 at the femoral neck, total hip, or lumbar spine by DXA
  - In postmenopausal women and men age 50 and older with low bone mass (T-score between -1.0 and -2.5, osteopenia) at the femoral neck, total hip, or lumbar spine by DXA and a 10-year hip fracture probability $\geq 3\%$ or a 10-year major osteoporosis-related fracture probability $\geq 20\%$ based on the USA-adapted WHO absolute fracture risk model (Fracture Risk Algorithm (FRAX®); www.NOF.org and www.shef.ac.uk/FRAX)
- Current FDA-approved pharmacologic options for osteoporosis are bisphosphonates (alendronate, ibandronate, risedronate, and zoledronic acid), calcitonin, estrogen agonist/antagonist (raloxifene), estrogens and/or hormone therapy, tissue-selective estrogen complex (conjugated estrogens/bazedoxifene), parathyroid hormone 1–34 (teriparatide), and receptor activator of nuclear factor kappa-B (RANK) ligand inhibitor (denosumab).
- No pharmacologic therapy should be considered indefinite in duration. After the initial treatment period, which depends on the pharmacologic agent, a comprehensive risk assessment should be performed.

References

1. Swan et al., A summary of the Malaysian Clinical Guidance on the management of postmenopausal and male osteoporosis, 2015. Osteoporosis and Sarcopenia 2 (2016) 1-12.
2. Richard Eastell, Clifford J Rosen, Dennis M Black, Angela M Cheung, M Hassan Murad, Dolores Shoback. Pharmacological Management of Osteoporosis in Postmenopausal Women: An Endocrine Society* Clinical Practice Guideline. *The Journal of Clinical Endocrinology & Metabolism*, Volume 104, Issue 5, May 2019, Pages 1595–1622.
3. Follin SL. Update in osteoporosis. In: Mueller B, Bertch K, Dunsworth T et al., eds. Pharmacotherapy self-assessment program, 4th ed. Men's health module. Kansas City, MO: American College of Clinical Pharmacy; 2003:350.

CHAPTER - 30

Psoriasis

Introduction to Psoriasis

Psoriasis is a common chronic inflammatory disease characterized by recurrent exacerbations and remissions of thickened, erythematous, and scaling plaques.

Psoriasis is a chronic skin disease result in patches of thick red skin covered with the silvery scales. These patches are referred as plaque which usually occurs on the elbow, knees, legs, scalp, lower back, face, palm and sole of the feet, nails too.

Definition

Psoriasis is defined as a persistent skin disease, causes cell to build rapidly on the surface of the skin, forming thick silvery scales, itchy, dry and red patches.

Epidemiology

- 1-3% in America and western countries
- Lower rates are found in Japanese and psoriasis is rare in West Africans
- Psoriasis first appears during two peak age ranges: The first peak occurs in persons aged 16-22 years, and the second occurs in persons aged 57-60 years.

Etiology

Idiopathic cause. Some of the factors that may trigger psoriasis are: Genetic Autoimmune reaction, Infection, Injury to skin, Stress, Obesity, Smoking.

Medication: Lithium, Antimalarial Medications, Indomethacin,

Pathogenesis [1, 2]

Genetic and environmental factors act in conjuction to produce immune dysregulation in the presence of a defective skin barrier. Interaction of damage associated molecular patterns (DAMP) and the pathogen associated molecular patterns (PAMP) with their receptors, such as Toll Like receptor (TLR) and Nucleotide-bindingolimerization domain (NOD) like receptors, causes the activation of keratinocytes and the epidermal innate immune system and thus, increased secretion of antimicrobial proteins. This interaction between DAMP/PAMP with TLR/NOD like receptors is also followed by liberation of inflammatory cytokines such as TNF-α, IL-8 and IL-1β, all of which are potent chemoattractants.

Once the APCs engulf the inciting antigen, they migrate to the local lymph nodes where they interact with naïve T-cells, resulting in T-cell activation. This process requires interaction between the major histocompatibility complex antigens on APCs with the T-cell receptors. In addition, costimulatory interactions between receptors and ligands on APCs and TCR are important. These include interaction of lymphocyte function antigen (LFA)-3 and CD2; between intercellular adhesion molecule-1 and LFA-1; and between B7 and CD28. Activation of such naïve T cells to pathogenic T cells is facilitated by the presence of polymorphisms in IL-23 genes and HLA-C*06. Sustained activation of HLA-C*06 restricted immunodominant epitopes could lead to antigen specific activation of CD8+ T cells, further amplifying the production of TNF-α and IFN-γ, although such a subtype of T cells has not been identified. Once the T cells are activated, both CD4+ and CD8+ T cells infiltrate the skin and secrete Th1 and Th17 cytokines which activate the keratinocytes. Together with IL-1 and TNF-α from keratinocytes, Th17 cytokines and IFN-γ increase expression of antimicrobial peptides (AMPs). This leads to a vicious positive feedback cycle where initial activation of keratinocytes promotes immune system activation, which in turn activates the keratinocytes and is responsible for the chronic nature of the disease.

Clinical Manifestations and features

It will vary according to types of psoriasis. Intially the first sign of psoriasis is often red spots on the body. The patches of skin: Dry, swollen and inflamed. Covered with silver white flakes raised and thick skin. Other symptoms of psoriasis includes: Pain, itching and burning. restricted joint motion or pain, cracked and bleeding skin, dandruff on scalp, pus filled blisters, genital lesions in males. Pitting, small depression on the surface of the nail, yellow, discolored nail, Koebner phenomenon Arthritis.

Classification: There are several types of psoriasis include [3, 4]:
- Plaque psoiasis
- Guttate psoriasis
- Inverse psoriasis
- Pustular psoriasis
- Erythrodermic psoriasis
- Nail psoriasis
- Psoriatic arthritis

Plaque Psoriasis

It is the most common type of psoriasis. It is also known as psoriasis vulgaris. It is appear as raised, inflamed, red skin covered by silvery patches or scales. Sites: Elbows, Knees, sacrum, Scalp, lower back, Hands and Feet.

Guttate Psoriasis (Latin Gutta = drop)

Characterized by eruption of small (0.5 to 1.5 cm in diameter) papules over the upper trunk and proximal extremities. Manifests at an early age. Streptococcal throat infection frequently precedes or is concomitant with the onset or flare.

Inverse Psoriasis

Localized in the major skin folds, such as the axilla, the inguinal and inflammatory areas and sweating areas. Scaling is usually minimal or absent, and the lesions appear glossy, smooth and bright red. It is commonly seen in obese people.

Pustular Psoriasis

It is usually uncommon but mostly appears in adult. It appears as pus filled lesion surrounded by red skin. It appears mostly at hands and feet. It is the serious condition so immediate medical attention is required.

Erythrodermic Psoriasis

The disease affects all body sites. Erythema is the most prominent feature with superficial scaling / peeling that may appear like burning. Causes: sun burn, allergic reaction, strong coal product use.

Nail Psoriasis

Commonly seen along with psoriatic arthritis. It appear as a pitting small bit nail, yellow-brown nail, tender and painful nail with chalk like debris build up under nails. Treated by steroid injected into nail or light therapy

Psoriatic Arthritis

This is the condition which involves both psoriasis and joint inflammation.

Diagnosis with Algorithm [5]

Collect history - Physical examinations -Skin biopsy: under local anesthesia -Blood and radiography test done to rule out psoriatic arthritis

Classification criteria for psoriatic arthritis
1. **Established inflammatory articular disease +**
2. **Score of 3 or more based on the following clinical findings**
   Psoriasis
   - Current active psoriasis (2 points)
   - Negative test for rheumatoid factor (1 point)
   - Personal history of psoriasis (1 point)
   - Typical psoriatric nail dystrophy (1 point)

Dactylitis
- Current swelling of an entire digit (1 point)
- History of dactylitis confirmed by a rheumatologist (1 point)
- Plain radiography of hand or foot showing juxta-articular new bone formation (1 point)

Management of Psoriasis [6, 7]

Goals of therapy

Interrupt the cycle that cause an increased production of skin cells thereby reducing inflammation and plaque formation. Remove scales and smooth skin, which is particularly removed by topical treatment.

General Approach to Treatment of Psoriasis

1. Determine the severity of psoriasis
2. If it is Mild to moderate (<5% of body surface area) and a candidate for intermittent therapy- inititate corticosteroids, vitamin D analogs, tazorotene.
3. If he is a candidate for continuous therapy-go with Calcineurin inhibitors
4. If the person is with severe psoriatic symptoms (5% or more body surface area) and is less than 20% BSA which is affected- treat with Vitamin D analogs and or phototherapy.
5. If BSA is > 20 % start systemic therapy and or phototherapy, referral to dermatologist.

Topical Agents for Treatment of Psorissis (Mild-Moderate; < 20% Body Involvement)

1. Emollients: advantages are-basic adjuncts for all treatments. Safe, inexpensive, reduces scaling, itching, and related discomfort. Disadvantage is providing minimal relief alone.
2. Keratolytics (salicylic acid, urea, α-hydroxy acids [i.e., glycolic and lactic acids]): Reduce hyperkeratosis; enable other topical modalities to better penetrate; inexpensive but disadevantages are- Provide minimal relief individually; nonspecific; salicylism (tinnitus, nausea, vomiting) with salicylic acid if applied extensively.
3. Topical corticosteroids: Rapid response; control inflammation and itching; best for intertriginous areas and face; convenient, not messy; mainstay topical treatment modality for psoriasis. Disadvantages are-Temporary relief; less effective with continued use.
4. Coal tar: Particularly effective for "flaky" scalp lesions; new preparations "pleasant"; efficacy enhanced in combination with UVB (i.e., Goeckerman regimen). Disadvantage - Effective only for mild psoriasis or scalp psoriasis.
5. Calcipotriene (Dovonex): As effective as topical corticosteroids, although slower onset, without long-term corticosteroid adverse effects; convenient, well tolerated. Disadvantage- Slow onset; expensive; potential effects on bone metabolism.

6. Tazarotene (Tazorac): Extended response; convenient (applied daily, in gel formulation); maintenance therapy; effective on scalp and face; used in combination with topical corticosteroids. Disadvantage- Slow onset; local irritation and pruritus.
7. Ultraviolet B (UVB): Effective as maintenance therapy; eliminates problems of topical steroids. Disadvantage - Expensive (insurance reimburses); office-based therapy; sunburn (exacerbates psoriasis); photoaging; skin cancer.

Agents for the Treatment of Severe Psoriasis (>20% Body Involvement)

1. UVA and psoralen (PUVA) 80% efficacy; "suntan" cosmetically desirable. Disadvanatge - Time-consuming; expensive, sunburn (exacerbates psoriasis); photoaging
2. Acitretin (Soriatane) Not as effective as other systemic agents; efficacy enhanced if given with PUVA or UVB. Disadvantage-Teratogenic
3. Methotrexate: Effective for skin lesions and arthritis as well as psoriatic nail disease. Disadvantage: Hepatotoxicity (periodic liver biopsy); bone marrow toxicity
4. Cyclosporine: Toxicities and short-lived remissions; used in patients with extensive disease—not responsive to other agents, but disadvantage is renal toxicity.
5. Immunomodulators (alefacept, efalizumab, etanercept, infliximab): Specific, targeted therapy; effective for moderate to severe both skin lesions and arthritis; maintains remission. Disadvantage- Expensive, ; increased risk of serious infections

Pharmacological approaches for patients with Psoriasis and Psoriatic arthritis.

1. Patients with Psoriasis only
   (i) Mlid: Topical therapies – corticosteroids; Vitamin –D; anlagesics; topical immunomodulators such as tacrolimus, tazorolene; salicylic acid; coal tar; anthralin; emollients.
   (ii) Moderate-severe:
   - Topicals+phototherapy/photochemothrapy
   - Topicals+systemic agents (Methotrexate, cyclosporine, acetretin,, azathioprine, mycophenolate mofetil, JAK kinase inhibitor)
   - Topicals+biologic agents (TNF inhibitors, anti IL-17 agents)

2. Patients with Psoriatic arthritis only
   (i) Peripheral arthritis: Intra-articular corticosteroids
       Mild: NSAIDs
       Moderate-severe:DMARDs-Methotrexate, cyclosporine, sulfasalazine, Biologic agents (TNF inhibitors, anti IL-17 agents)
   (ii) Dactylitis: Intra-articular corticosteroids
        Biologic agents (TNF inhibitors)
   (iii) Nail disease: Topicals
         DMARDs: cyclosporine
         Biologic agents (TNF inhibitors
   (iv) Axial disease: Mild-moderate: NSAIDs, physiotherapy
        Moderate –severe: Biologic agents (TNF inhibitors)

3. Patients with Psoriasis and Psoriatic arthritis
   (i) Mild: Topicals+NSAIDs
       Topicals+ intraarticular corticosteroids
   (ii) Moderate-Severe:
       Topicals+systemic agents (Methotrexate, cyclosporine, leflunomide)
       Above+phototherapy
       Topicals+biologic agents

Psoriasis treatment is divided into three main types:
- Topical treatment
- Light therapy
- Systemic medications

1. Topical corticosteroids
- They are commonly first-line therapy in mild to moderate psoriasis and in sites such as the flexures and genitalia, where other topical treatments can induce irritation and skin folds.
- Improvement is usually achieved within 2 to 4 weeks.
- They slows the cells turnover by suppressing the immune system which reduce inflammation and relieves associated itching
- Strong corticosteroids use for smaller area of skin like hands and feet.
- Long term use may cause thinning of skin and resistance too.
- Low potency steroids are usually recommended for sensitive area and treating wide spread patches damage skin.

Topical Steroids [8, 9]
- To avoid systemic effects of class I glucocorticoid, a maximum of 50 g ointment may be used per week
- For small plaques (< 4cm), triamcinolone acetonide aqueous suspension 10 mg/mL diluted with normal saline is injected into the lesion

Vitamin D Analogues [10]

Calcipotriene (calcipotriol)"Betdaivonex". Potent topical corticosteroids are superior to calcipotriene. But calcipotriene was more effective than coal tar or anthralin. The efficacy of calcipotriene is not reduced with long-term treatment. Calcipotriene is applied twice daily. Salicylic acid inactivates calcipotriene. Hypercalcemia is the only major concern. Other vitamin D analogues are tacalcitol and maxacalcitol. Used as first-choice therapies in the topical treatment of mild to moderate psoriasis.

Coal Tar

The use of tar to treat skin diseases dates back nearly 2000 years. Tar is the dry distillation product of organic matter heated in the absence of oxygen. Coal tar, in concentrations 5- 20% in creams, ointments, shampoos and in pastes. It is often combined with salicylic acid (2-5%), which by its keratolytic action leads to better absorption of the coal tar. Disadvantages include: allergic reactions, folliculitis, it has foul smell and appearance and can stain clothing and other items. Coal tar is carcinogenic.

Tazarotene (zar, Zarotex)

It is a third-generation retinoid. It reduces mainly scaling and plaque thickness, with limited effectiveness on erythema by normalize the DNA activity. It is available in 0.05 percent and 0.1 % gels, and a cream. When used as a monotherapy, a significant proportion of patients develop local irritation(especially with the 1% formulations). It will use along with sun screen lotion.

Topical Calcineurin Inhibitors [11, 12] "Tarolimus" Pimecrolimus. They inhibit activation of T-cells which inturn reduces inflammation and plaque build up. They are not effective in plaque psoriasis. However, for treatment of inverse and facial psoriasis, these agents appear to provide effective treatment

Emollients: Between treatment periods, skin care with emollients should be performed to avoid dryness. Emollients reduce scaling, may limit painful fissuring, and can help control pruritus. They are best applied immediately after bathing or showering. The use of emollients in combination with topical treatments improves hydration while minimizing treatment costs

2. **Light Therapy:** Ultraviolet light is a wavelength of light in a range too short for human eye to see. When exposed to the UV light, the activated T-cells in the skin are destroyed which lead reduces scaling and inflammation. Sun exposure should be for brief duration of time to improve psoriasis.

Ultraviolet Boardband Phototherapy: Control dose of Ultraviolet B (UVB) light from an artificial light source may improve mild to moderate psoriasis symptoms. UVB phototherapy is also called "Broadband UVB" can be used to treat to single patches and psoriasis resistant to topical treatment.

Side effect: Redness, dryness and itching which can be minimized by using moisturizer.

Photochemotheraphy/Psoraien Plus Ultraviolet-A: Photochemotheraphy involves taking light sensitizing medication (psoralen) before exposure to UVA light. UVA light penetrate deeper in skin and psoralen make more responsive to UVA exposure

Side effect: Nausea, headache, burning and itching, wrinkle skin or skin cancer.

Eximer Laser: A controlled beam of UVB light of a specific wavelength is directed to the psoriasis plaque to control scaling and inflammation. It does not harm healthy skin More powerful UVB light is used

Side effect: Redness and blistering

Pulse Dye Laser Pulse dye laser used dsifferent form of light to destroy the tiny blood vessel that contribute to psoriasis plaque. Side effect : Bruising, Scarring,

Combination Light Therapy Combine UV light with other treatment such as retinoids frequently improve phototherapy effectiveness. [13]

Table 30.1 Management of Psoriasis by Phototherapy.

Candidate for phototherapy	Psoriasis patients who have inadequate response to topical agents (75%)

UVB	• nbUVB according to local data (100%)
	  - Starting dose: 180-350 mJ/cm^2.
	  - Increasing by 10-20% each time or a fixed increment of 50-100 mJ/cm2.
	  - Usually, the final dose should be 5-10 times higher than the initial starting dose to achieve clinical remission.
	  - Receiving treatment at least twice per week is required to induce clinical remission
	• If psoriasis has improved by nbUVB
	  - Maintain the same dose & start long-term once-a-week treatment.
	• Pregnancy (95.7%)
	  - Pregnancy is not a contraindication to the use of UVB
	  - nbVUB therapy has been used successfully in the treatment of psoriasis in pregnancy.
	  - nbVUB should be considered as 1st- line therapy in pregnant patients with plaque & guttate psoriasis who need a systemic approach.
	• Children (100%)
	  - Although there are no studies documenting the long-term safety of UVB phototherapy in childhood psoriasis, judicious use is reasonable for appropriately selected patients.

PUVA	• Systemic psoralen plus UV according to local data (100%)
	  - 8-Methoxypsoralen, 10-40 mg, taken 1-2 h prior to exposure to UVA.
	  - Avoid sunlight exposure for 12 h after ingestion of psoralen the use of UV protective eyewear & sunscreen being recommended in daytime when there is risk of UV exposure.
	  - Starting dose: 1-2 J/cm^2
	  - Increasing: 0.5-1 J/cm^2 each time.
	  - Receiving treatment at least twice per week is required to induce clinical remission.

nbVUB – narrow-band UVB: PUVA = psoralen UVA.

3. Systemic Medications [14]

Cyclosporin A: Neoral 100mg/ml Suspension and 100 mg capsules. Action- Binds cyclophilin producing a complex that blocks calcineurin, reducing the effect of the Nuclear Factor of Activated T-Cells) NFAT in T cells, resulting in inhibition of interleukin 2

Dosage -High-dose method: 5 mg/kg daily, then tapered. Low-dose method: 2.5 mg/kg daily, increased every 2-4 wk up to 5 mg/kg daily, then tapered

Side effect: Nephrotoxicity, Hypertension, Immuno-suppression, Neurotoxicity, Increased risk of malignancy.

Contraindication: Prior bone marrow depression, Pregnancy, Lactation, Renal abnormalities.

Methotrexate: Methotrexate 2.5 mg tab & 50 mg/ml vial. Action- Blocks dihydrofolate reductase leading to inhibition of purine and pyrimidine synthesis. Leading to accumulation of anti-inflammatory adenosine

Dosage: Start with a test dose of 2.5 mg and then gradually increase dose until a therapeutic level is achieved (average range, 10-15 mg weekly; maximum, 25- 30 mg weekly

Side effect: Chronic use may lead to hepatic fibrosis. Fetal abnormalities or death. Pulmonary fibrosis.

Contraindication: Liver toxicity, Pregnancy

Acitretin: Acitretin 25 mg cap. Action: Binds to retinoic acid receptors. May contribute to improvement by normalizing keratinization and proliferation of the epidermis.

Dosage: Initiate at 25-50 mg daily.

Side effect: Hepatotoxicity, Lipid abnormalities, Fetal abnormalities or death, Alopecia.

Contraindication: Severe infections, Malignancy.

Complications: Infection, Fluid and electrolyte imbalance, Low self esteem, Depression, Stress, Metabolic syndrome, Hypertension, Joint damage.

Combinational, Rotational, and Sequential Therapy

- If monotherapy with a systemic agent does not provide optimal outcomes, combining systemic therapies with other modalities may enhance benefit. The dose of each agent may often be reduced, resulting in lower toxicity.

Combinations include:

✓ Acitretin + UVB light

✓ Acitretin + photochemotherapy using UVA light (PUVA)

✓ Methotrexate + UVB light

✓ PUVA + UVB light

✓ Methotrexate + cyclosporine

Table 30.2 Biologic Agent Mechanism and Efficacy.

Generic (Brand)	Mechanism	Dose & Route
Adalimumab (Humira®)	Human monoclonal antibody against TNF to neutralize its effects.	80 mg SC on day 1, then 40 mg every other week beginning on day 8 for moderate to severe plaque psoriasis
Etanercept (Enbrel®)	Human fusion protein of the TNF receptor to Fc portion of IgG1. Binds TNF to neutralize its effects.	50 mg SC twice weekly for 3 month then maintenance 50 mg weekly for moderate to severe plaque psoriasis
Infliximab (Remicade®	Chimeric (murine-human) antibody against TNF-α. Binds TNF to neutralize its effects.	IV infusion, 5 mg/kg over 2-3 hours at 0, 2 and 6 weeks, then every 8 weeks for moderate to severe plaque psoriasis

Contd...

Generic (Brand)	Mechanism	Dose & Route
Secukinumab (Cosentyx®)	Human monoclonal antibody against TNF to neutralize its effects	150 or 300 mg SC for moderate to severe plaque psoriasis
Ustekinumab (Stelara®)	Immunomodulator, Human monoclonal antibody against the p40 subunit of IL-12 & IL-23 from human immunoglobulin transgenic mice. Blocks the actions of IL-12 and IL-23.	45 mg at week 0 & 4 if weight is ≤100 kg, 90 mg at week 0 & 4 if weight is >100 kg, then every 12 week afterward for moderate to severe plaque psoriasis
Golimumab (Simponi)	Human monoclonal antibody against TNF to neutralize its effects	50 mg SC once monthly for psoriatic arthritis

ACR = American College of Rheumatology Criteria, IL = Interleukin, IV = intravenous, MTX = Methotrexate, PASI = Psoriasis Area and Severity Index Score, TNF = Tissue Necrosis Factor, SC = subcutaneously, *Designed to take continuously to maintain improvement

Treatment of Psoriasis in problem areas:

1. Scalp: Hair-bearing areas are not receptive to ointment vehicles. A topical corticosteroid and/or topical calcipotriene (Dovonex) in a solution vehicle are recommended, along with daily use of a tar shampoo.

2. Nails: The thick keratin of the nail blocks absorption of topical agents. For onycholysis, a topical corticosteroid in a solution vehicle may be used under the nail. Systemic therapy may be required to improve severe disease.

3. Genitalia: The thin skin of the genitalia is highly sensitive to the adverse effects (atrophy) of topical corticosteroids. A low-potency topical corticosteroid ointment is recommended. Topical calcipotriene, which is not associated with a risk of atrophy, may be used.

4. Palms and soles: The thick stratum corneum of palms and soles is a barrier to penetration of topical agents. A highest-potency topical corticosteroid is recommended. Methotrexate (Rheumatrex) or acitretin (Soriatane; a systemic retinoic acid analog) may be needed.

Joint American academy of Dermatology- National Psoriais Foundation guidelines of care for the manegement and treatment of psoriais in pediatric patients [15]

1. Topical corticosteroids with Vitamin D are commonly used as an off label treatment for pediatric psoriasis. However, caution should be used regarding ultra-high and high potency corticosteroids. Topical tazarotene is used in combination with topical corticosteroids for skin or nail psoriasis. Psoriasis treatment of the face and genitalia is effective with off-label topical calcineurin inhibitors either as monotherapy or in combination with topical corticosteroids.

2. Phototherapy is effective for moderate to severe plaque as well as guttate psoriasis and is often used in conjunction with anthralin or coal tar as adjuvants.

3. Among non-biologic systemic drugs, methotrexate is most commonly used for moderate to severe psoriasis with good efficacy and should be supplemented with folic acid. Cyclosporine is effective for moderate to severe pediatric psoriasis particularly for patients with pustular or erythrodermic psoriasis

4. Etanercept and Ustekinumab are FDA approved for four years and older and twelve years and older respectively. Other biologic drugs are used off-label. Biologics can be used in combination with systemic and topical therapies.

Case Study of Psoriasis

Summary

A 14 year old male patient was admitted in the hospital with chief complaints of hypo pigmented patches all over since 6 years associated with black patches over left malleoulus and right and left knee associated with itching sensation. No history of fever. Blood pressure: 120/80 mmHg and pulse: 80bpm. CBP showed relative lymphocytosis (46%). Liver Function Test (LFT) showed increase in alkaline phosphatase (453IU/L). Mantoux test: No erythema and no induration seen at site after 48hours.

Diagnosis: By above data the patient was found to be suffering with hypertrophic psoriasis with palpular follicles

His therapy includes:

Drug	Route	Dose	Frequency
Light liquid paraffin	Topical		BD
Moisturex soft cream	Topical		OD
T. Talmega	Oral		OD
T. Atarax	Oral	10mg	OD
T. Xyzal	Oral	5mg	OD
Fucidin cream	Topical		BD

Daily Progress: Day 1 patient was admitted with complaints of patches all over associated with itching. Day 3 complaints of itching. Rx given. Day 6 vitals stable, no fresh complaints.

Patient Counselling:

- Take daily baths.
- Use moisturizer.
- Expose your skin to small amount of sunlight.
- Avoid psoriasis triggers.
- Avoid alcohol intake.
- Follow your doctor's recommendations.
- Use covers ups when necessary.

Assignment

1. **What physical findings are characteristics of psoriasis?**

   Physical findings include: scaling, papules, plaques, erythematous macules,

   Macules are seen first and progress to maculopapules, itching, and dry skin.

2. **What lab studies should be performed prior to initiating systemic therapy for psoriasis?**

   The following lab tests are performed:

   Complete blood count, blood urea nitrogen, serum creatinine, liver function tests, hepatitis panel, tuberculosis screening, pregnancy test, uric acid level may be elevated in psoriasis.

3. **Which medications are used in treatment of psoriasis?**
   - Topical corticosteroids: they relieve itching and used with other treatments.
   - Vitamin D analogues: these synthetic forms of vitamin D slow skin cell growth.
   - Anthralin: helps slow skin growth.
   - Topical retinoids: these are vitamin A derivatives that may decrease inflammation.
   - Calcineurininhibitors: Ex: tacrolimus – reduce inflammation and plaque builds up.
   - Salicylic acid : promotes sloughing of dead skin cellsand reduces scaling,
   - Coal tar: reduces scaling, itching and inflammation.
   - Moisturizers: reduces scaling, itching and dryness.
   - Light therapy: uses natural or artificial UV light.the simple and easiest form of phototherapy involves exposing of skin to contolled amount of natural sunlight.
   - Methotrexate: helps by decreasing the production of skin cells and reducing inflammation.
   - Cyclosporine: suppresses the immune system and reduces skin cell production.
   - Other medications: thioguanine, hydroxyurea can be used when other drugs can't be given.

4. **What are the treatment guidelines for moderate-severe plaque psoriasis? [16,17]**
   - Expert dermatologists from across the globe released a consensus report on the treatment optimization and transitioning for mod-sev plaque psoriasis:
   - Methotrexate can be used as long as it remains effective.
   - Cyclosporine is generally used intermittently for inducing a clinical response with one more courses over 3-6 months.
   - Transition from conventional systemic therapy to a biological agent may be done directly or with an overlap if transitioning is needed because of lack of efficacy.
   - Combination therapy may be helpful.
   - Continuous therapy for patients receiving biologicals is recommended.

- Switching biological because of lack of efficacy should be performed without a washout period while switching biological for safety reasons may require a treatment free interval.

5. What are the non pharmacological treatment options for psoriasis?

- Daily sun exposure/Sea bathing/Moisturizing/Relaxation/Do not itch or scratch/ Aloevera may reduce redness, scaling, itching and inflammation.
- Bathing daily.

6. When is surgery indicated in the treatment?

Ocular manifestations such as trichiasis (ingrowth of eyelashes) and cicatricialectropion (sagging of lower eyelid) usually require surgical treatment. Progression of corneal melting, inflammation and vascularization may require lamellae or penetrating keratoplasty.

7. Which environmental factors exacerbate psoriasis?

Stress, cold, trauma, infections (streptococcal, staphylococcus etc), alcohol, drugs (aspirin, lithium, beta blockers etc). Patients with history of severe gingivitis, injury to skin.

8. What is the role of genetics?

Patients with psoriasis have a genetic predisposition for the disease. Psoriasis is associated with certain human leucocyte antigen (HLA) alleles. The strongest being human leucocyte antigen Cwb. In some families psoriasis is an autosomal dominant trait. Additional HLA antigens that have shown association with psoriasis and geriatric subtypes include HLA-B27, HLA-B13, HLA-B17 and HLA-DR7.

If one of the parents has psoriasis, there is 10% chance of getting it.

If both parents have psoriasis, there is 50% chance of getting it.

About 1/3rd of people diagnosed with psoriasis have a relative with it.

9. What are the guidelines on psoriasis biologic therapy?

Guidelines on psoriasis biologic therapy from British association of dermatologists. Patients who are starting the biologic therapy, the opportunity to participate in longterm safety registries. Biologic therapy to people with psoriasis requiring systemic therapy if methotrexate and cyclosporine have failed or not tolerated or contraindicated.

If the patient has a large impact on physical, physiological or psychological functioning and one/more of the following disease severity criteria apply.

- If psoriasis is extensive.
- The psoriasis is severe at localized sites and is associated with significant functional impairment and high levels of distress.

  Consider biologic therapy, earlier in treatment pathway in people with psoriasis that fulfills disease severity criteria and who also have psoriatic arthritis or for perisistant psoriasis.

Review of Biologic Therapy

- Assess intital response of biologic therapy at times appropriate for drug and then on a regular basis during therapy.

- Review response to therapy by taking into account the consideration like adherence to treatment, benefits and risks of treatment, impact of psoriasis on patient, agreed treatment goal etc.
- Assess whether the minimal response has been met.
- 50% or more reduction in the baseline severity and
- Clinically relevant improvement in patient's physical, social and psychological functioning.

Consider a change for alternative for therapy including another biological therapy if patient

- Psoriasis doesn't achieve the minimum response.
- Initially responds to treatment but subsequently loses response.
- Current therapy becomes non tolerable or contraindicated.

Choice of Biologic Therapy

1st Line (Adults)

Ustekinumab – For patients who fulfill the criteria for biologic therapy.

Adalimumab – For adults particularly when psoriatic arthritis is a consideration.

Consider Secukinumab in adults without/with psoriatic. arthritis.

2nd Line: Offer any of the licensed biologic therapies if patient doesn't respond to first line therapy.

Consideration: reverse infliximab for use in patients with very severe disease condition or whether other agents have failed or contraindicated.

Consider escalating the dose in adults, when adequate primary response maybe due to sufficient drug dosing but this might also increase risk of infection, depending on the drug.

Biological agent	Suggested dose escalation
Ustekinumab 45mg every 12 weeks(<100kg)	90mg every 12 weeks
(>100kg) 90mg every 12 weeks	90mg every 8 weeks
Adalimumab 40mg every other week	40mg weekly
Etanercept 50mg once weekly	50mg thrice weekly
Infliximab 5mg/kg every 8 weeks	5mg/kg every 6 weeks

References

1. Martin BA, Chalmers RJ, Telfer NR. How Great is the Risk of Further Psoriasis following a Single Episode of Acute Guttate Psoriasis. Archives of Dermatology. 1996;132(6):717-8.

2. O'Doherty CJ, Macintyre C. Palmoplantar Pustulosis and Smoking. British Medical Journal (Clinical Research Ed). 1985; 291:861-4.

3. Krueger J, Bowcock A. Psoriasis Pathophysiology: Current Concepts of Pathogenesis. Annals of the Rheumatic Diseases. 2005; 64:30-6.

4. Nancy Weigle M, Duke. Psoriasis. American Family Physician. 2013; 87:626-33.

5. Taylor W, Gladman D, Helliwell P, Marchesoni A, Mease P, Mielants H; CASPAR Study Group. Classification criteria for psoriatic arthritis: development of new criteria from a large international study. *Arthritis Rheum.* 2006;54(8):2665–2673.

6. Brown AC, Hairfield M, Richards DG, McMillin DL, Mein EA, Nelson CD. Medical Nutrition Therapy as a PotentialComplementary Treatment for Psoriasis-Five Case Reports. Alternative Medicine Review. 2004; 9:297-307.

7. Menter A, Korman NJ, Elmets CA, Feldman SR, Gelfand JM, Gordon KB, et al., Guidelines of Care for the Management of Psoriasis and Psoriatic Arthritis: section 6. Case-based Presentations and Evidence-based Conclusions. Journal of the American Academy of Dermatology. 2011; 65:137-74.

8. Lebwohl M, Ali S. Treatment of Psoriasis. Part 1. Topical Therapy and Phototherapy. Journal of the American Academy of Dermatology. 2001; 45:487-502.

9. Brown BD. Management of Psoriasis: An Update. Bulletin on Drug & Health Information Foundation for Health Action. 2006; 13:1.

10. Huynh N, Cervantes-Castaneda RA, Bhat P, Gallagher MJ, Foster CS. Biologic response modifier therapy for psoriatic ocular inflammatory disease. *Ocul Immunol Inflamm.* 2008 May-Jun. 16(3):89-93.

11. [Guideline] Menter A, Korman NJ, Elmets CA, Feldman SR, Gelfand JM, Gordon KB, et al. Guidelines of care for the management of psoriasis and psoriatic arthritis: section 4. Guidelines of care for the management and treatment of psoriasis with traditional systemic agents. *J Am Acad Dermatol.* 2009 Sep. 61(3):451-85.

12. [Guideline] Smith CH, Jabbar-Lopez ZK, Yiu ZZ, Bale T, Burden AD, Coates LC, et al. British Association of Dermatologists guidelines for biologic therapy for psoriasis 2017. *Br J Dermatol.* 2017 Sep. 177 (3):628-636.

13. Tsen-fang tsai et al.,. Taiwanese Dermatological Association consensus statement on management of psoriasis. Dermatologica Sinica. 2017; 35(2): 66-77.

14. Emily Tiping Gan et.al., Therapeutic Strategies in Psoriasis Patients with Psoriatic Arthritis: Focus on New Agents. BioDrugs (2013) 27:359–373.

15. Kaushik S.B. and Lebwohl M.G. Psoriasis: which therapy for which patient: focus on special populations and chronic infections. *J Am Acad Dermatol.* 2019; 80: 43-53

16. Hsu S, Papp KA, Lebwohl MG, et al.; National Psoriasis Foundation Medical Board. Consensus guidelines for the management of plaque psoriasis. *Arch Dermatol.* 2012;148(1):95–102.

17. Lebwohl M. Psoriasis. Lancet 2003;361:1197-204.

CHAPTER – 31

Scabies

Introduction to Scabies: Scabies is a contagious skin infection by mite *sarcoptus scabiei*. It is also called as the seven-year itch.

Epidemiology: Scabies affects about 100 million people around the world as of 2010 and is equally common in both genders. It infects all ages and races equally.

Etiology: Scabies is caused by infection with the female mite *sarcoptusscabieivor hominis*. The mite burrows into the skin to live and deposit eggs. Often only 10-15 mites are involved in an infection.

Mode of transmission:
- Direct skin-skin contact
- Crowded living condition
- Sexual contact

Pathogenesis: There is direct person-person transmission of *Sarcoptes scabiei var. homonis* to new host. Fertilized females secrete proteolytic enzymes that allow them to burrow through the stratum corneum (2mm/day). After that females lay 2-3 ova/day which hatch in the stratum cornuem in pockets after 3 days. The larvae molt and mature for 2 weeks and mate within the pockets in the stratum corneum. Following mating, male mites die and female begin burrowing.

Cycle is propagated as new female mites create more burrows in stratum corneum. At this stage there is increase in IgG abd IgE and peripheral eosinophilsare seen in blood circulation. There is inappropriate immune response by T-helper cells, following which there is delayed Type IV hypersensitivity reaction in 2-4 weeks following initial contact to antigens. Now the person is presented with urticarial crusted papules, eczematous plaques, and uncontrollable itch. This is followed by secondary infection and skin breakdown.

Clinical manifestations and features

Signs and symptoms: The symptoms of scabies are due to reaction to the mites. Once infected the patient will usually develop the symptoms in between 2 and 6 weeks. If person has second exposure symptoms may begin within as little as 24 hours.

The signs and symptoms are:
- Itching/Redness/Superficial burrows/ Rashes/Burning sensation/Stinging

Diagnosis with algorithm [1]

Four points to diagnose a case of scabies:
- **Types of lesion** - Burrow, a linear tunnel in which the mite lives. Other skin manifestations include papules, blisters, nodules and eczematous changes.
- **Sites of involvement**: The skin lesions commonly involve web spaces, flex surface of wrists, axillae, waist, feet and ankles. Facial and palm oplantar involvement is unique ti infantile spasms.
- **Symptoms**: Itching, most severe at night
- Other members: Itching takes 4-6 weeks to develop in others.

Table 31.1 Summary of 2018 IACS criteria for the diagnosis of scabies [2].

A	Confirmed scabies	Atleast one of:
	A1	Mites, eggs or faeces on light microscopy of skin samples
	A2	Mites, eggs or faeces visualized on individual using high-powered imaging device
	A3	Mite visualized on individual using dermoscopy
B	Clincical scabies	At least one of:
	B1	Scabies burrows
	B2	Typical lesions affecting male genitalia
	B3	Typical lesions in a tyhpical distribution and two history features
C	Suspected scabies	One of:
	C1	Typical lesions in a typical distribution and one history feature
	C2	A typical lesions or atypical distribution and two history features
		History features:
	H1	Itch
	H2	Close contact with an individual

Source: David J. Chandler Lucinda C. Fuller. A Review of Scabies: An Infestation More than Skin Deep. Dermatology. Dec 2018.

Management

Goal: The aim of treatment for scabies is to suppress the discomfort due to the disease, to limit the risk for secondary infection and related complications such as (heart and kidney disease), and to limit the dissemination of the disease in the family and more widely in the community.

Prevention:
- Avoiding direct contact with the patient.
- Lounder the clothes of the patient.
- All family members are recommended for the treatment.

Treatment with algorithm [2, 3]

European Guideline for the Management of Scabies

1. **Recommended treatments:**
   Permethrin 5% cream, repeat once after 7-14 days OR
   Ivermectin p.o. 200mg/kg repeat after 7 days   OR
   Benzyl benzoate lotion 10-25% on days 1, 2 and repeat after 7 days.
2. Alternative treatments
   Malathion-0.5% aqueous lotion   OR
   Ivermectin 1% lotion OR
   Sulphur 6-33% as cream, ointment or lotion on 3 successive days or
   Synergized pyrethrine foam
3. Crusted scabies
   A typical scabicide daily for 7 days then 2 times weekly until cure and
   Ivermectin p.o. 200µg/kg on days 1, 2, 6

Classification of Antiscabietic drugs

1. Topical agents'
   - Permethrin 5% cream
   - Lindane 1% lotion or cream
   - Benzyl benzoate 10% and 25% lotion or emulsion
   - Malathion 0.5% lotion
   - Monosulfiram 25% lotion
   - Crotamiton 10% cream
   - Precipitated sulphur 2%-10% ointment
2. Oral drug: Ivermectin

Topical agents: [4, 5]

Sulphur: It is the oldest Antiscabietic in use.

It is available as an ointment (2%-10%) andusually 6% ointment is preferred.

Usage: The ointment is applied and thoroughly rubbed into the skin over the whole body for 2-3 consecutive nights.

It should be used only in situations where adults cannot tolerate lindane, permethrin or ivermectin as it is to all these agents.

Advantages: Economical

Disadvantages: It is messy and malodourous. It stains clothing in a hot and humid climate conditions may lead irritant dermatitis.

Benzyl benzoate: It is an ester of benzoic acid and benzyl acid and benzyl alcohol. It is obtained from balsam of tolu and peru.

It is available as 25% emulsion.

It is neurotoxic to the mites.

In young adults or children, the dosage can be reduced to 12.5%.

Usage: It should be applied below the neck three times within 24 hours without an intervening bath.

Crotamiton: Crotamiton (crotomyl-N-ethyl-O-toluidine) is used as 10% cream or lotion.

Usage: Applied twice daily for 5 consecutive days after bathing and changing clothes.

Monosulfiram: It is tetraethyl thiuram monosulphide.

It is available as 25% lotion.

Usage: It is applied all over the body after a bath and it should be rubbed well once a day on 2-3 consecutive days.

Malathion: It is available as 0.5% lotion.

It is an organophosphate insecticide that irreversibly blocks the enzyme acetylcholinesterase. It is not recommended now-a-days due to severe adverse effects.

Lindane: It is also known as gamma benzene hexachloride. It is an insecticide.

It acts on CNS of insects and leads to increased excitability, convulsions and death.

It is available as 1% cream or lotion.

Usage: It should be applied on cool and dry skin.

Apply for 6 hours.

Wash after 6 hours with soap and water.

Advantages: Non-irritating.

Dis advantages: CNS toxicity.

Permethrin: It is a synthetic pyrethoid and potent insecticide.

It is available as 5% cream.

It is effective against mites with low mammalian toxicity.

It is metabolised by skin esterase's and excreted in urine.

Usage: Applied overnight once a week for 2 weeks to the entire body including head in infants.

Advantages: No allergic side effects.

Disadvantages: Most expensive.

Oral Antiscabietic agent: [6, 7]

Ivermectin: It is dihydro derivative of Ivermectin B_1.

It acts via the suppression of conduction of nerve impulses in the nerve muscle synapses of insects by stimulation of gamma amino butyric acid from presynaptic nerve endings and enhancement of binding to presynaptic receptors.

Dose: 0.2 mg/kg in a single dose.

It is relatively safe with side effects such as headache, pruritis, pains in joints and muscles, fever, rash, lymphadenopathy.

Contraindication: Allergy to ivermectin, CNS disorders.

Other agents:

Allethrin: Used as an insect repellent. Effective when used as spray. It is neither irritant nor sensitizer.

Thiobendazole: 5% cream.

Management of special forms of scabies: [8]

Scabies in infants: Sulphur-2%-10%

Permethrin – 5% cream is used only in infants older than 2 months.

Ivermectin and lindane are contraindicated in infants

Scabies in children: Permethrin – 5% cream

Benzyl benzoate – 12.5% cream

Scabies in pregnant and lactating women:

Precipitated sulphur – 6% is recommended

Ivermectin, permethrin and lindane are contraindicated.

Nodular scabies: It a chronic form of scabies characterised by nodules on the covered parts of the body particularly on male genitalia, groin and axillary region. It is treated with anti-scabietics followed by intralesional steroids.

Crusted scabies: It needs prolonged and persistant treatment. Oral ivermectin is effective. The hyperkeratosis is treated with keratolytic agent (5-10% salicylic acid in petroleum). Nails are short and brushed with scabicidal agent. Cure is obtained after a mean treatment of 3 weeks.

Problems encountered in treatment:

Persistent itching: Itching usually persists for 1 week after treatment but if it persists for longer time it should be taken to the prescriber notice.

Patient counselling
- Start with warm water bath and dry thoroughly afterwards.
- The medication provided must be rubbed into the skin. All parts of the body whether involved or uninvolved should be treated.
- Treatment is best done at night before going to bed.
- Avoid touching your mouth or eyes with your hands.
- Lounder the clothing after treatment.

- Everyone in the house should be treated at the same time.
- You may itch for few days but do not repeat the treatment without prescriber suggestion.
- Report your doctor regularly.

Case Study of Scabies

Summary

A female patient of age admitted in hospital with chief complaints of generalized itching all over the body since one week. History of aggregation of itching. She has no past medical surgical history and family history. CBP: Eosinophils 10%, WBC: Eosinophilia ESR: 10mm/hr. Urine analysis: pus cells: 1-2/High Power Field (HPF); Epethilial cells: 2-3\HPF. CRP; positive -2.4 mg\dL. IgE-1882.1IU\ml. cutaneous examination: wide spread excoriation over the trunk fore arm chest lateral and inner aspects of thighs. Skin punch biopsy; epidermis shows parakeratosis and mild elongation of rete ridges.dermis shows mild lymphotic infiltration around blood vessels and few and focal melanism incontinence. Lichenoid eruption

Diagnosis: Based on the subjective and objective data patient is diagnosed with SCABIES

Trade name	Generic name	Category	Route	Dose	Freq
T.Iver	Ivermectin	Anti parasitic	p\o	12	Stat
T.Xyzal	Levocetrizine	Antihistamine	p\o	15	OD
T.Atarax	Hydroxyzine	Anihistamine	p\o	10	OD
Nulon	Paraffin +stearates	Emollient	Topical		BD
T.Pantop	Pantoprazole	Antacid	p\o	40	OD
T.Omnacoctil	Omnicoctil	Steroid	p\o	40/30	OD
T.Augmetin	Amoxicillin+clavulnate	antibiotic	p\o	625	BD

Progress Chart: From day 1 vitals were checked regularly no fresh complaints are noted

Patients in medication and was getting stabilized. On day 4 antibiotic course for 6 days. Therapy was being continued since 15 days

Pharmacist Intervention

No interactions found

Therapeutic duplication for antihistamines was noted

No adverse effects

Patient Counselling

Avoid allergic food

Take medication regularly

Maintain hygiene

Wash clothes bed sheets pillow covers of the patient regularly

Don't scratch too much in infected areas

Limit the use of soap

Assignment

1. **What are the signs of scabies, which areas of body commonly affected?**

   Scabies is an itchy condition caused by a burrowing mite called sarcoptes scabie. It is contagious and can spread through physical contact after infestation by mite; it takes, four to six weeks for skin to react

   Symptoms:

   Intense itching at nighttime; A pimple like rash

   Scales and blisters; Sores

   Scabies can be found any part of body

   Between the finger; in the armpits, around waist; inner elbows soles of feet around breast; around male genital area on knees buttocks, scalp and palms of the hands

2. **Clinical appearance of scabies?**

   Scabies rash-causes little bumps which look like hives tiny bites knots under skin

   Scaly patches

   Scratching itchy rash causes sores

   Crust form when a patient develops severe scabies.

3. **What is presentation of (a) Nodular scabies (b) crusted scabies?**

   (a) Nodules in 7-10%patients with scabies

   Children-pinkish brown nodules ranging from 2-20 mm

   General signs: itchy skin, raised bumps, persistent nodules

4. **How scabies diagnosed?**

   Physical and local examination to identify rash nodules, cutaneous examination

   Skin punch biopsy, Skin scrapping observed under the microscopy

   PCR: but it is difficult to do.

5. **How pruritis in scabies are treated?**

   Anti histamines – Levocetrizine, Loratidine hydroxyzine

   Promaxine lotion

   Steroid creams - Hydrocortisone

   Applying wet cloth on skin to minimize itching

6. **What are the risk factors?**

   People living in crowded areas

   Age: young children

   Older adults because of weakend immune system

   Living with scabies patient sexual partners

   Immuno compromised patients like HIV, cancer

7. Therapeutic regimen available for treatment of scabies?

Group weight	Base line therapy (day 1 to 3)	Treatment after 10-42 days
<3.5kg	Topical 10% Crotamiton-OD for 3 days	Topical 10% Critamine –OD for 3 days
3.5 to < 6kg	Topical 5% Permethrin	Topical 5% Permethrin
6 to < 15kg	Topical 5% Permethrin and oral Albendazole 200 mg or 400 mg –OD for 3 days	Topical 5% Permethrin
<15 kg and non pregnant	Oral Ivermectin -200micro gm \mg	Oral Ivermectin 200 micro gm\kg
Pregnant	Topical 5% Permethrin	Topical 5% Permethrin

The following medication:

1. Permethrin cream –synthetic parathyroid kills mites and eggs
2. 10%cromiton cream –antibacterial
3. 5-10%sulphur ointment
4. Lindane lotion -1% oraganochloride
5. Ivermectin-oral anti parasitic agent
6. Benzyl benzoate- alternative to permethrin

8. How is benzyl benzoate used in scabies treatment?

It is lethal to scabies mites

It exerts toxic effects on nervous system of parasite. It is also toxic to mite ova.

It is alternative to permethrin lotion.

9. What are the CDC guidelines for treatment of scabies?

Medications

Produces used to kill scabies mites are called scabicides. No "over-the-counter" (non-prescritpion) products have been tested and approved to terat human scabies.

The following miedications for the treatment of scabies are available only by precrition.

Classic scabies: one or more of the following may be used

1. **Permethrin cream 5%** Brand name product: Elimite* Permethrin is approved by the US Food and Drug Ad ministration (FDA) for the treatment of scabies in persons who are at least 2 months of age. Permethrin is a synthetic pyrethroid similar to naturally occurring pyrethrins which are extracts from the chrysanthemum flower. Permethrin is safe and effective when used as directed. Permethrin kills the scabies mite and eggs. Permethrin is the drug of choice for the treatment of scabies. Two (or more) applications. each about a week apart. may be necessary to eliminate all mites. Children aged 2 months or older can be treated with permethrin.

2. **Crotamltonlodon 10% and Crotamlton cream 10% Brand name products:** Eurax*; Crotan*Crotamiton is approved by the US Food and DrugAdministration(FDA) for the treatment of scabies in adults; it is considered safe when used as directed. Crotamiton is not FDA-approved for use in children. Frequent treatment failure has be•en reported with crotamiton.

Contd...

3. **Sulfur (5%-10%) ointment (multiple brand names)** Sulfurin an ointment base (petrolatum) is safe for topical use inchildren. including infants under 2 monthsof age. The odor and cosmeticquality may make it unpleasant to use.

4. **Lindane lotion 1%** Brand name products: None availablelindane is an organochloride. Although FDA-approved for the treatment of scabies, lindane is not recommended as afirst-line therapy. Overuse, misuse, or accidentally swallowing lindane can be toxic to the brain and other parts of the nervous system; its use should be restricted to patients who have failed treatment with or cannot tolerate other medications that pose less risk. Lindane should not be used to treat premature infants, persons with a seizure disorder. women who are pregnant or breast-feeding, persons who have very irritated ski nor sores where the lindane will be applied, infants. Children, the elderly, and persons who weigh less than 110 pounds.

5. **Ivermectin** Brand name product: Stromectol*Ivermectin is an oral antiparasitic agent appro.,ed for the treatment of worm infestations. Evidence suggests that oral ivermectin may be a safe and effective treatment for scabies; however, ivermectin is not FDA-approved for this use. Oral ivermectin should be considered for patients who have failed treatment with or who cannot tolerate FDA-approved topical medications for the treatment of scabies. If used for classic scabies. two doses of oral ivermectin (200µg/kg/dose) should be taken with food, each approximately one week apart. The safety of ivermectin in children weighing less than 15kg and in pregnant women has not been established.

Note that although ivermectin guidelines recommend taking on an empty stomach, scabies experts recommend taking with a meal to increase bioavai l ability.

References

1. Hogan DJ, Schachner L, Tanglertsampam C. Diagnosis and treatment of childhood scabies. Pediatr Clin North Am 1990;38:941–56.
2. Behl PN, Taplin D. Eradication of scabies with a single treatment schedule [letter and response]. J Am Acad Dermatol 1985;12(1 pt 1):117–18.
3. Hurwitz S. Scabies in infants and children. In: Orkin M, Maibach HI, Parish LC, et al, eds. Scabies and pediculosis. Philadelphia: Lippincott, 1977:31–9.
4. Lin A, Reamer R, Carter D. Sulfur revisited. J Acad Dermatol 1988;18:553–8.
5. Percival CH. Organized treatment of scabies. Br J Dermatol 1941;53:346–350.
6. Alberici F, Pagani L, Ratti G, et al. Ivermectin alone or in combination with benzyl benzoate in the treatment of human immunodeficiency virus associated scabies. Br J Dermatol 2000;142:969–72.
7. Hernandez-Perez E. Resistance to antiscabietic drugs. J Am Acad Dermatol 1983;8: 121–3.
8. Roth WI. Scabies resistant to lindane 1% lotion and crotamiton 10% cream. J Am Acad Dermatol 1991;24:502–3.

CHAPTER – 32

Eczema

Introduction to Eczema

Eczema is an itchy erythematous (red) eruption consisting of ill-defined erythematous patches or papules. The skin surface is usually scaly and as time progresses, constant scratching leads to thickened, 'lichenified' skin.

Rather than a specific health condition, eczema is a reaction pattern that the skin produces in a number of diseases. It begins as red, raised tiny blisters containing a clear fluid atop red, elevated plaques. When the blisters break, the affected skin will weep and ooze.

In older eczema, chronic eczema, the blisters are less prominent and the skin is thickened, elevated, and scaling. Eczema almost always is very itchy.

Types of eczema

1. Atopic dermatitis
2. Contact eczema
3. Seborrheic eczema
4. Nummular eczema
5. Neurodermatitis
6. Stasis dermatitis
7. Dyshidrotic eczema

Etiology

1. **Irritants:** Soaps, detergents, disinfectants (Chlorine),
   Contact with juices from fresh fruits, meats, vegetables, chemicals, fumes
2. **Microbes:** Certain bacteria, viruses, fungi
3. **Allergens:** House dust mites, pets, pollens, molds, dandruff
4. **Others:** hot or cold temperatures, foods, stress, hoemones

Clinical Manifestations and Features

Acute eczema is an inflammatory process leading to edema in the epidermis. Edema manifests as fluid that collects into tiny blisters which may then coalesce. Tightly packed keratinocyte cells in the epidermis usually prevent transepidermal fluid loss and the entry of pathogens. This barrier function of the skin is lost in eczema. In the chronic form of eczema, prolonged rubbing and scratching results in a thickened epidermis and an increase in the upper horny cell layer of keratin, termed hyperkeratosis. Clinically, the skin appears thick, leathery, scaly and 'lichenified' with exaggerated skin markings. Both acute and chronic stages are accompanied by a heavy chronic inflammatory cell infiltration of the dermis and epidermis. The main consequent symptom of these pathological processes is itch.

Atopic Eczema

Atopic eczema is the commonest skin disorder of childhood. This health condition has a genetic basis. Atopy is a special type of allergic hypersensitivity that is associated with asthma, inhalant allergies (hay fever), and a chronic dermatitis.

Epidemiology [1, 2]

The cumulative incidence of Atopic dermatitis varies between 11% and 21% depending on age and region. In a clinicoepidemiological study in a north Indian pediatric population, the mean age at onset and mean duration of the disease were 4.2 and 3.3 months, respectively, in the "infantile Atopic Dermatitis" group, and in the "childhood Atopic Dermatitis" group, the corresponding figures were 4.1 and 1.9 years, respectively. Patients from urban areas significantly outnumbered those from rural background.

Pathogenesis [3, 4]

A genetic defect in the filaggrin protein is thought to cause atopic dermatitis by disrupting the epidermis. This disruption, in turn, results in contact between immune cells in the dermis and antigens from the external environment leading to intense itching, scratching, and inflammation. Scratching can then lead to further disruption and inflammation of the epidermal skin barrier; this has been described as the itch scratch cycle.

Clinical Manifestations

Signs and Symptoms

Dry sensitive skin, intense itching, red and inflamed skin, recuuring rash,

Scaly areas, rough and leathery patches

Oozing or crushing, areas of swelling, dark colored pateches of skin

Diagnosis with Algorithm [5, 6]

Revised Criteria for the Diagnosis of Atopic Dermatitis

Must have pruritus/ itching+ 3 of the following
- (a) History of flexural dermatitis (front of elbows, back of knees, front of ankles, neck, around the eyes) or involvement of cheeks and / or extensor surfaces in children aged > 18 months.
- (b) Visible flexural dermatitis involving the skin (or the cheeks and / or extensor surfaces in children aged >18 months)
- (c) History of a dry skin in the past year
- (d) History of asthma or hay fever
- (e) Onset < 2years

Differential Diagnosis of Atopic Dermatitis

Seborhoeic dermatitis/ discoid dermatitis/ allegic contact dermatitis/ HIV dermatitis/Psoriasis/ scabies/ insect bite/ filariasis

Assessment of Severity of Atopic Dermatitis

1. Mild: If < 5% body surface involved/ no acute changes/ no significant impact on quality of life.
2. Moderate: 5-30% body surface involved/ mild dermatitis with acute changes/ mild dermatitis with significant impact on quality of life
3. Severe: > 30% body surface involved/ moderate dermatitis with acute changes/ moderate dermatitis with significant impact on quality of life

Management of atopic dermatitis [7]

Nonmedical Treatment in atopic dermatitis
- Clothing should be soft next to the skin. Cotton is comfortable and can be layered in the winter. Wool products should be avoided.
- Cool temperatures, particularly at night, are helpful because sweating causes irritation and itch.

Moisturization
- Depending on the climate, patients usually benefit from 5-minute, lukewarm baths followed by the application of a moisturizer such as white petrolatum.
- Frequent baths with the addition of emulsifying oils (1 capful added to lukewarm bath water) for 5-10 minutes hydrate the skin. The oil keeps the water on the skin and prevents evaporation to the outside environment.
- In infants, 3 times a day is not a great burden; in adults, once or twice a day is usually all that can be achieved. Leave the body wet after bathing.

Pharmacological management [8]

Treatment algorithm for atopic dermatitis

- **Initial** assessment of disease history, extent, severity and activity is to be done.
- Mild or moderate AD: moisturizers & emollients as first line therapy. Topical corticosteroids to be avoided in face and genitalia and beyond 3 weeks. Cyclosporine as second line therapy. Azathioprine, phototherapy, methotrextae can be used as third line therapy. Biologics and apremilast can be used as 4th line therapy if still not controlled.
- Severe Atopic dermatitis: moisturizers & emollients as first line therapy + short course (2 weeks and taper) of oral steroid. Cyclosporine as second line therapy. Azathioprine, phototherapy, methotrextae can be used as third line therapy. Biologics and apremilast can be used as 4th line therapy if still not controlled.
- **Adjuvant therapy:** Identification and avoidance of triggers. Oral antihistamines if required. For control of infection-short course of topical or systemic antibiotics can be used.

Topical steroids [9]

- Topical steroids are currently the mainstay of treatment. In association with moisturization
- Ointment bases are preferred, particularly in dry environments.
- Initial therapy consists of hydrocortisone 1% powder in an ointment base applied 2 times daily to lesions on the face and in the folds.
- A midstrength steroid ointment (triamcinolone or betamethasone valerate) is applied 2 times daily to lesions on the trunk until the eczematous lesions clear.
- Steroids are discontinued when lesions disappear and are resumed when new patches arise.

Immunomodulators [10]

- Tacrolimus (topical FK506) is an immunomodulator that acts as a calcineurin inhibitor.
- Tacrolimus is available in 2 strengths, 0.1% for adults and 0.03% for children
- Tacrolimus is an ointment and is indicated for moderate-to-severe Atopic Dermatitis (AD). It is indicated for children older than 2 years.
- Pimecrolimus 1% is also an immunomodulator and calcineurin inhibitor
- Pimecrolimus is produced in a cream base for use twice a day; it is indicated for mild Atopic Dermatitis (AD) in persons older than 2 years and is particularly useful on the face.
- These agents are much more expensive than corticosteroids and should only be used as second-line therapy.

Other treatments [11]

- Probiotics have recommended as a therapeutic option for the treatment of AD.
- The rationale for their use is that bacterial products may induce an immune response of the Th1 series instead of Th2 and could therefore inhibit the development of allergic IgE antibody production

- UV-A, UV-B, a combination of both, psoralen plus UV-A (PUVA) or UV-B1 (narrow-band UV-B) therapy may be used. Long-term adverse effects of skin malignancies in fair-skinned individuals should be weighed against the benefits.

Contact Eczema/Contact Dermatitis

Contact eczema (contact dermatitis) is a localized reaction that includes redness, itching, and burning where the skin has come into contact with an allergen (an allergy-causing substance) or with an irritant, such as an acid, a cleaning agent, or other chemical. Other examples of contact eczema triggers include washing powder and liquids, nickel (present in jewellery and clothing buckles), cosmetics, fabrics, clothing, and perfume. The condition is sometimes referred to as allergic contact eczema (allergic contact dermatitis) or irritant contact eczema (irritant contact dermatitis) depending on what is involved in triggering the reaction

(a) **Allergic Contact Dermatitis (ACD)**

ACD is a delayed type IV hypersensitivity reaction that develops in response to an antigen to which the host immune system has been previously sensitised. As a consequence, symptoms rarely develop on first exposure to the stimulus and may only manifest months or years later following repeated re-exposure.

Many common compounds can lead to ACD. The most common compounds implicated are:

- Metals, for example nickel and cobalt
- Neomycin, a topical antibiotic found in over-the-counter
- Fragrance ingredients, for example Balsam of Peru
- Rubber compounds
- Hair dyes, for example p-phenylediamine
- Plants, for example poison ivy.

Diagnosis relies heavily on a detailed patient history as well as recognizing the pattern and distribution of the eczematous rash.

The standard confirmatory investigation is patch testing and is used to differentiate allergic from Irritant Contact Dermatitis (ICD). This involves application of a standard, with or without a specialized range of compounds, to the patient's back over 72 h. This is followed by examination for a cutaneous reaction at day 2 and day 4. Identification of relevant compounds allows the patient to avoid the substance in the future, and this will hopefully reduce symptoms.

Non pharmacological Treatment:

- The first intervention involves identification, withdrawal, and avoidance of the offending agent.
- The second treatment is symptomatic relief while decreasing skin lesions. Cold compresses help soothe and cleanse the skin
- They are applied to wet or oozing lesions,
- If affected areas are already dry or hardened, wet dressings applied as soakswill soften and hydrate the skin

- Soaks should not be used on acute exudating lesions.
- Calamine lotion or Burrow solution (aluminum acetate) may also be soothing.

Pharmacological management

Localized acute allergic contact dermatitis lesions are successfully treated with mid- or high-potency topical steroids, such as triamcinolone 0.1% or clobetasol 0.05%. If allergic contact dermatitis involves an extensive area of skin (greater than 20 percent), systemic steroid therapy is often required and offers relief within 12 to 24 hours. Five to seven days of prednisone, 0.5 to 1 mg per kg daily, is recommended. Emollients, moisturizers, or barrier creams may be instituted as secondary prevention strategies to help avoid continued exposure.

(b) **Irritant Contact Dermatitis (ICD)**

This is the most common form of occupational dermatitis and the commonest cause of hand eczema. Unlike ACD, ICD is not immunologically mediated. The mechanism involves disruption of the epidermal permeability barrier and a direct cytotoxic effect depending on the irritant. Patients with pre-existing epidermal barrier dysfunction such as atopic eczema are at higher risk. The occupation of the individual may also be a risk factor, especially those workingas builders, hairdressers, gardeners, healthcare workers and chefs. Irritants include detergents, oils, water, inorganic acids, alcohols and plastics. Preventative skin care is key and this includes the use of barriers such as emollients or cotton gloves in addition to avoiding suspected irritants.

Nummular or Discoid Eczema

Discoid eczema - also called nummular eczema or nummular dermatitis - is characterized by coin-shaped patches of irritated skin, most commonly located on the arms, back, buttocks, and lower legs, that may be crusted, scaling, and extremely itchy. Middle-age males are most commonly affected. Nummular eczema is usually a long-term (chronic) condition. A personal or family history of atopic eczema, asthma, or allergies increases the risk of developing the condition. Relatively uncommon

Stasis Eczema

- Stasis eczema is also called stasis dermatitis, gravitational dermatitis or varicose eczema.
- It is a clinical component of chronic venous insufficiency seen in addition to other features which include varicose veins, skin discoloration, peripheral edema, leg discomfort and non-healing ulcers.
- Clinical features include scaly eczematous plaques confined to the lower legs. Multiple topical medicines and dressings often lead to a secondary ACD. Stasis dermatitis occurs as a direct consequence of venous insufficiency.
- Disturbed function of the 1-way valvular system in the deep venous plexus of the legs results in a backflow of blood from the deep venous system to the superficial venous system, with accompanying venous hypertension

Seborrhea Dermatitis

- Seborrhea dermatitis is a chronic inflammation of skin that typically waxes and wanes. It causes red scaling, occasionally with weepy, oozy eruption.
- Commonly involves portions of the scalp, brows, mid-face, ears, mid-chest, and mid-back. It is not unusual for it to affect the skin of infants and young children where it often involves the scalp and the diaper area.
- Seborrhea dermatitis is also known as seborrhea. It is usually confined to areas with high sebum production. The likely etiological mechanism is overgrowth of the communal yeast *Malassezia furfur* (Pityosporumovale). Extensive and severe seborrhoeic dermatitis can be seen in patients with underlying HIV infection or Parkinson's disease. Treatment usually includes topical imidazoles.
- The distribution of this rash is often of great help in making the diagnosis.Although in both adults and children the rash may have no symptoms; it commonly causes itching, especially in the scalp.

Treatment for Eczema

First-line treatment of eczema should include an emollient and soap substitute for washing. Topical steroids are used for anti-inflammatory effect. Systemic treatments for adult atopic eczema include oral prednisolone, cyclosporine and azathioprine.

If there is a secondary bacterial infection, then this should be treated with oral antibiotics.

The antibiotic(s) should be chosen based on sensitivity determined by wound swab.

OTC Products

- Some OTC eczema treatments are used for moisturizing skin
- Some are used to help skin symptoms such as rash, redness and itch and some are for gently cleaning skin to prevent infection.

Emollients

Emollients, topical hydrating agents consisting of fat or oil to soften the skin, are the mainstay of eczema management.

Emollients are effective first-line treatments for all types of eczema, and regular, liberal use will reduce topical steroid requirements.

The greasier products have more emollient effect

Dry skin is aggravated by soap and bath products, and therefore an emollient soap substitute for washing is advisable

Topical corticosteroids

- Topical steroids act as anti-inflammatory agents and are extremely useful and important in managing eczema. Overuse of topical steroids causes long-lasting side effects, to high levels of anxiety regarding possible side effects concerning their use. This can commonly lead to under treatment in children.
- Patient education regarding appropriate topical steroid use is a crucial part of eczema management.
- They are classified into four main groups according to potency: mild, moderately potent, potent and very potent.
- The choice of topical steroid is dependent on the site and severity of skin disease. Potent and very potent steroids should be avoided on delicate sites such as the face, genitals and flexures.
- Side effects are mainly local and include stretch marks, telangiectasia (visible dilated small blood vessels), epidermal thinning, purpura (bruising), acne and perioral dermatitis.
- Lower frequency side effects include poor wound healing, spread or worsening of untreated infections and hypertrichosis.
- Hypopigmentation is a temporary side effect of long-term topical steroid
- Rarely, adrenal suppression or Cushing's syndrome due to systemic absorption may occur.
- Local and systemic side effects are extremely rare with appropriate use and duration of topical steroid treatment.
- Patients should be advised to spread preparations thinly either once or twice daily
  Allergies
  o Both immediate and delayed hypersensitivity reactions to topical corticosteroids can occur, although not commonly. These can be reactions to either the steroid molecule itself or the vehicle in which it is found. Allergic reactions to one topical steroid may cross-react to others. Therefore, allergy testing is mandatory for such patients. Betamethasone may be less likely to cause allergic reactions than other topical preparations.
  Antibiotics and steroid combinations
  o Combination preparations can be useful in treating mild bacterial infection of eczematous skin. Long-term use should be limited due to the risks of sensitisation and antibiotic resistance

Calcineurin inhibitors

- These non-steroid immunomodulators inhibit calcineurin phosphatase which is important in T-lymphocyte activation. The main side effect is burning or stinging on initial application, but this usually improves after a few days
- Calcineurin inhibitors should not be used on infected skin and are generally not very useful in severely inflamed eczematous skin. Their greatest value appears to be in maintenance therapy.

- Tacrolimus ointment is a calcineurin inhibitor. The 0.1% and 0.03% preparations are indicated in the treatment of moderate to severe atopic dermatitis in adults and children over the age of 2 years.
- Pimecrolimus 1% cream is indicated for short-term or intermittent long-term use in mild to moderate atopic dermatitis.
  Studies have shown that it is effective, well tolerated and has minimal adverse effects in the long-term control of eczema in children aged over 2 years

Antihistamines

- Pruritis is the most distressing feature of eczema. Oral antihistamines have no direct effect on pruritis in eczema; their main effect is sedation. Sedating antihistamines may cause day time drowsiness, and caution should be taken when driving and also if prescribed to school age children.

Topical imidazoles

- Ketoconazole as a shampoo or cream is effective in reduction of *Pityosporumovale*on the skin and is therefore useful in the treatment of seborrhoeic dermatitis.

Coal tar preparations

- Tar creams and ointments can be used in the management of hyperkeratotic, lichenified eczema. Coal tar is an effective anti-pruritic.

Systemic therapies

Systemic steroids

Oral prednisolone can be used as a short-term treatment in the management of severe acute eczema that needs rapid control. Long-term treatment with oral steroids is now rarely used due to the risk of side effects including hypertension and osteoporosis.

Ciclosporin: Ciclosporin is a systemic immunosuppressant that blocks activation of T-lymphocytes. Intermittent courses at doses of 2.5–5 mg/kg/ day are useful, but dose-related renal nephrotoxicity is inevitable. During treatment with ciclosporin, patients also require close monitoring of renal function and blood pressure.

Azathioprine: Azathioprine is a purine analogue that inhibits DNA synthesis and can be effective as monotherapy in adult eczema. Bone marrow suppression and toxicity are the major side effects. Patients with borderline thiopurinemethyltransferase (TPMT) levels require a lower dose of azathioprine. Patients with low levels of TPMT should not be offered this treatment.

Methotrexate: Methotrexate is occasionally used in unresponsive adult atopic eczema. Can be used as a second-line therapy for the treatment of moderate to severe atopic eczema in adults

Mycophenolat emofetil: Mycophenolatemofetil is an oral systemic agent that prevents T- and B-cell proliferation, thereby reducing inflammatory cytokine release. This can be used as an alternative in severe adult atopic dermatitis where azathioprine or ciclosporin are contraindicated. Side effects are gastro-intestinal upset, bone marrow suppression and an increased risk of infection

Phototherapy

- Phototherapy can be effective in select cases of atopic dermatitis.
- Narrow-band UVB is the therapy of choice
- Side effects include burning, premature ageing and a small increased risk of skin cancer.
- A small proportion of patients have photosensitive eczema which should be considered
- A treatment course requires a patient to attend two or three times a week for at least 6 weeks.

Non- pharmacologic measures for infants and children:
- Give lukewarm baths, Apply lubricants/moisturizers immediately after bathing
- Use scent-free moisturizers liberally each day, Keep fingernails filed short
- Select clothing made of soft cotton fabrics
- Consider sedating oral antihistamines to reduce scratching at night
- Keep the child cool; avoid situations that cause overheating
- Learn to recognize skin infections and seek treatment promptly
- Identify and remove irritants and allergens

Patient counselling

Provide patients with information regarding causative factors, avoidance of substances that trigger skin reactions, and potential benefits and limitations of nondrug and drug therapy.
- Evaluate patients with chronic skin conditions periodically to assess disease control,the efficacy of current therapy, and the presence of possible adverse effects

Case Study of Dermatitis

Summary

A 50 years male patient came to hospital with complaints of itching. Dry scaly lesions over face, dorsum of both hands & feet since 6months. Itching over scalp. He has no medical history and surgical history, no known allergies. His vitals were normal and other investigations done showed the following-

1. CBP-Normal;
2. Urine analysis-pus cells 4-5/HPF, Epithelial cells 1-2/HPF, Reaction 6.5;
3. Liver function test-total proteins-8.4g/dl [6-8gm/dL],
4. Lipid profile-within normal limits,
5. BUN & serum creatinine-normal,
6. RBS-93mg/dl,

7. Skin examination-hyper pigmentation with scaling, thickening, Present over dorsum of both hands and palms and dorsum of feet. Multiple fissures present over soles. Diffuse scaling present over face and neck.

Diagnosis: Based on the data obtained the patient was diagnosed to be suffering with dermatitis.

Drug chart:

Trade name	Generic name	Category	route	Dose	Frequency
T. Xyzal	Levocetrizine	Anti-histamine	P/O	5mg	OD
Liq.Paraffin	Liq.Paraffin	Emollient	E/A		TID
Moisturex Soft cream	Light liq. Paraffin +white soft paraffin	Emollient	E/A		OD
T.Hcq	Hydroxy chloroquine	DMARD	P/O	200mg	BD
T.Nicoglow	Niacin	Vitamin B3	P/O	1tab	OD

Progress chart: On this day of admission, patient was conscious and stable. He was given with emollient and anti-histamine. No ADRs were observed. On day 2 & day 3, no fresh complaints were noted and the medications were continued.

Patient counseling:
- Avoid exposure to excess heat/sunlight. Avoid scratching.
- Apply moisturizers, medicated creams. Limit the use of soaps. Stay hygiene.

Assignment

1. **What is allergic contact dermatitis?**

   Allergic contact dermatitis is a skin condition characterized by red and itchy rash that occurs when skin comes into contact with an allergen.

   Many substances can cause such reaction like soaps, cosmetics, pollen, plant etc. and also use of certain medicines may also result in allergic dermatitis.

2. **Differentiate atopic and allergic dermatitis?**

Atopic Dermatitis	Allergic Dermatitis
*It is a chronic eczematous skin condition that usually begins in childhood	*It a skin conditionthat occurs when allergen or chemicals come into contact causing a reaction
*It may be inherited from parents	*May be caused by antibiotics, chemicals, rubber products, dyes, sunscreens etc
*common symptoms are dry, itchy red skin, scratchings , dry scaly brownish grey skin	*common symptoms incude itching, red skin, scaly, sun sensitivity
*It may result in asthama or allergic rhinitis	*It is a localized condition
*It is a type1 hypersensitivity reaction	*It is a type4 hypersensitivity reacion

3. **Write the signs & symptoms.**

   Symptoms & signs of allergic contact dermatitis are- skin reddish/ dry, scaly areas of skin/ Burning sensation of skin/sunsensitivity/itching/fever/blistered areas that may ooze.

4. **What are the risk factors?**

   Certain jobs & hobbies put people at higher risk for contact dermatitis. They are as follows-

   *health care, dental employees/mental works/construction workers/cosmetologists

   *hair dressers/swimmers/ cleaners/gardeners and agricultural workers/cooks

   Other risk factors include- use of dyes/using different soaps/creams/having allergic food/ over exposure of sunlight.

5. **Write the procedures used to diagnose it.**

   *Patch test; during this test, small amounts of potential allergens are applied to adhesive patches, which are placed on skin. The patches remain on skin for 2 to 3days. Then the doctor checks skin reactions under these patches.

   *Skin biopsy is also done where tissue is isolated and examined.

   *Di methylglyxime test; It is a useful and practical way to identify metallic objects that contain enough nickel to provoke allergic dermatitis.

   *Repeat open application test; It is most useful when an individual has a if reaction to a chemical found in a consumer product if dermatitis develops after few days of repeated application of suspected product then the weak patch test reaction is highly relevant.

6. **What pharmacological treatments are available to manage the disease?**

   Goals: To improve quality of life/ To reduce allergy/ To relieve symptoms

   To prevent further complications

   Pharmacological treatment:

   The following drug classes are used-

   1. Corticosteroids:

      *These topically applied creams or ointments help soothe the rash.

      *For severe allergic dermatitis- class1 topical corticosteroids in a 3-week course.

      Ex: Diflorasone diacetate- ointment, 0.05%

      Clobetasol propionate- cream, 0.05%

      *For acute severe allergic dermatitis- a week course of systemic corticosteroids.

      Ex: Prednisolone- 40mg to 60mg initial dose & tapered over a 2week period.

      Triamcinolone acetonide- 40 to 60mg-IM- can be used in place of oral prednisolone

      *For dermatitis of intertriginous areas of face, class 6/class 7 topical corticosteroids are used.

      Ex: Betamethasone valerate- lotion, 0.05%

      Desonide- cream, 0.05%

      Dexamethasone sodium phosphate- cream, 0.1%

      Hydrocortisone acetate- cream, 1%

2. Topical Immunomodulators: These are prescribed for cases of allergic contact dermatitis when they offer safety advantages over topical corticosteroids
Ex: Tacrolimus-0.1% ointment- for hands
Topical tacrolimus- can be used even for eyelid dermatitis
Pimecrolimus- dermatitis of face

3. Phototherapy: *used for chronic allergic contact dermatitis that is not controlled by corticosteroids. Eg. Psoralen plus ultraviolet- A treatment

4. Immunosupressive agents: Used for severe chronic widespread dermatitis
Ex: Azathioprine- 1.5 to 2.5mg/kg/day or 10 to 22.5mg/wk
Mycophenolate- 1g/day
Cyclosporine- 2.8 mg/kg/day

5. Disulfiram: Chelating effect is helpful in reducing the nickel burden in body

6. Anti-histamines: To relieve symptoms like itching.
Ex: Diphenhydramine
Cetrizine- 10mg OD
Loratadine-10mg OD

7. What patient education has to be given to ensure successfully therapy?

*Take medications without fail especially steroids/ avoid allergic food.

*Avoid over exposure to sun/ Do not skip dose or double the dose of medicines prescribed/ Apply given creams/lotions/ Take oat meal baths/ wearing protective clothing.

*Applying cool, wet compresses.

8. What is pathogenesis of allergic contact Dermatitis?

Cosmetics, fragrances, occupational hapten, metals, antiseptics, plants, act as predisposing factors and start the sensitization phase. In this phase haptens penetrate the epidermis and activate langerhans cells which travel to regional lymph nodes and activate naicve T-cells.

Next phase is elicitation phase in which re-exposure to offending hapten leads to Type 4 hypersensitivity reaction. Sensitized T-cells circulate in blood and arrive at skin sites where antigen is present. There is activation of mast cells, eosinophils, CD4+/CD8+ T cells and inflammatory cytokines. Mast cells release leukotrienes which cause fever. CD8+ T cells cause keratocyte apoptosis which is presented as papule, vesicles, bullae, erythema, burning, and pruritus. The process continues and later is presented as scaling, lichenification.

9. What is the role of phototherapy/PUVA in the treatment?

Phototherapy, also called light therapy is treatment with a special kind of light. It is used to treat dermatitis, eczema that is all over body or for localized eczema that has not gotten better with topical treatments. The most commonly used is narrow band UV-B. this uses a special machine to emit UVB light. Broad band UVB phototherapy, psoralen& UVA, UVA light are other forms of phototherapy.

It helps to reduce itch / calm inflammation/ increase vit D production. Overall, it is safe but few known risks include- skin aging, sun burn, headache & nausea, melanoma, cataracts.

10. **Role of UV light in development of dermatitis**

    Apart from various chemicals, substances, it is also possible to have an allergy to UV light, called sun allergy or photosensitivity which is linked to faulty immune system. Exposure to UV rays triggers an inflammatory response in the skin, same as that of normal allergens. This allergy can be inherited. Symptoms involve bumps, blisters, blotchy red patches on skin. Treatment involves oral antihistamines, oral/topical steroids etc.

11. **Role of immunosuppressants in treatment?**

    In dermatitis/eczema, the immune system overacts and produces inflammation leading to various symptoms. Immunosuppressants are the drugs that control/ suppress the immune system to slow down the symptoms. Immunosuppressants help to stop the itch scratch cycle, allow skin heal reduce the risk of skin infection.

    Ex; Azathioprine/ Cyclosporine/ Mycophenolate mofetil

References

1. Spergel JM. Epidemiology of atopic dermatitis and atopic march in children. *Immunol Allergy Clin North Am.* 2010;30(3):269-280.

2. Dhar S, Kanwar AJ. Epidemiology and clinical pattern of atopic dermatitis in a North Indian pediatric population. Pediatr Dermatol 1998;15:347-51

3. Wolff KL, Johnson RI. Atopic dermatitis. In: Wolff K, Johnson RA, Fitzpatrick TB. *Fitzpatrick's Color Atlas and Synopsis of Clinical Dermatology.* 6th ed. New York, NY: McGraw-Hill Medical; 2009:34–36.

4. Maintz L, Novak N. Getting more and more complex: the pathophysiology of atopic eczema. *Eur J Dermatol.* 2007;17(4):267-283.

5. Williams HC, Burney PG, Hay RJ, et al. The UK Working Party's diagnostic criteria for atopic dermatitis. I. Derivation of a minimum set of discriminators for atopic dermatitis. Br J Dermatol 1994;131:383-396.

6. Werfel T, Heratizadeh A, Aberer W, Ahrens F, Augustin M, Biedermann T, *et al.* S2k guideline on diagnosis and treatment of atopic dermatitis – Short version. Allergo J Int 2016;25:82-95

7. Ring J, Alomar A, Bieber T, Deleuran M, Fink-Wagner A, Gelmetti C, *et al.* Guidelines for treatment of atopic eczema (atopic dermatitis) Part II. J Eur Acad Dermatol Venereol 2012;26:1176-93

8. Hanifin JM, Cooper KD, Ho VC, et al. Guidelines of care of atopic dermatitis, developed in accordance with the American Academy of Dermatology (AAD)/American Academy of Dermatology Association "Administrative Regulations for Evidence-Based Clinical Practice Guidelines" [published correction appears in *J Am Acad Dermatol.* 2005; 52(1):156]. *J Am Acad Dermatol.* 2004;50(3):391-404.

9. Green C, Colquitt JL, Kirby J, Davidson P. Topical corticosteroids for atopic eczema: clinical and cost effectiveness of once-daily vs. more frequent use. *Br J Dermatol.* 2005;152(1):130-141

10. Reitamo S, Ortonne JP, Sand C, et al.; European Tacrolimus Ointment Study Group. A multicentre, randomized, double-blind, controlled study of long-term treatment with 0.1% tacrolimus ointment in adults with moderate to severe atopic dermatitis. *Br J Dermatol.* 2005;152(6): 1282-1289.

11. Friedmann PS, Arden-Jones MR, Holden CA. Atopic dermatitis. In: Burns T, Breathnach S, Cox N,Griffiths C, eds. Rook's Textbook of Dermatology. 8th ed. Chichester, UK: Wiley Blackwell Publishers, 2010:24.27-24.28.

CHAPTER – 33

Impetigo

Introduction to Impetigo

Impetigo is a bacterial infection that involves the superficial skin. The most common presentation is yellowish crust on the face, arms or legs; less commonly there may be large blisters which affect the groin or armpits.

Epidemiology:

- The bullous form is most frequently affects neonates & accounts for approx. 10% of all cases.
- Low-middle income countries estimate the global population of children suffering from impetigo.

Predominantly in tropical, resource-poor countries

Causative organism

Staphylococcus aureus and *Staphylococcus pyrogenes* which spreads by contact.

- Children between the ages of 2-5 years are at greater risk. Impetigo is also known as Infantigo.
- There are 2 ways an initial infection occurs-
    1. Primary Impetigo: It is when bacteria invades the skin through a cut, insect bite or other injury.
    2. Secondary Impetigo: It is where bacteria invades skin because the skin barrier has been disrupted by another skin infection such as scabies or eczema.
        - **Types – (A) Bullous Impetigo (B) Non-Bullous Impetigo**
            - ➢ **Bullous Impetigo:** It is caused by staphylococcus bacteria that produce a toxin that cause a break between the top layer and the lower levels of skin forming blisters.

                Blisters can appear in various skin areas, especially the buttocks, though these blisters are fragile & often & leave red, raw skin with ragged edge.
            - ➢ **Non-Bullous Impetigo:** This is the most common form, caused by both staphylococci and streptococci bacteria.

It appears as small blisters or scabs, which then form yellow or honey-colored crusts. They start around the nose, on face & also may affect arms and legs.

Etiology:
- It is most common during hot, humid weather which facilitates microbial colonization of the skin.
- Minor trauma, such as scratches or insect bites then allow entry of organisms into superficial layers of skin and infection ensues.
- On exposed skin, mainly on face.

Pre-disposing factors:
- Age (childhood)
- Crowded environment
- Poor sanitary practices
- Exposure to persons with current infection
- Daily hygiene routine

Pathophysiology

There is infection of superficial epidermis. Then proteolytic cleavage of extracellular domain of desmoglein -1 protein within leratinocytes in granular layer takes place. It results in impetigo which is of two types. Non-bullous impetigo (70% cases) is caused by S.aurues and group A streptococci. Then there is local production of exfoliative toxins which are responsible for ulcerative penetrating epidermis into dermis. It is presented as ecthyma. If the infection is by Group A streptococci the infection is presented as acute post streptococcal glomerulonephritis. 2nd type of impetigo is bullous impetigo caused exclusively by S.aureus and there is local production of exfoliative toxins A ans B. If the infection is by staphylococci it is presented as scalded skin syndrome.

Clinical manifestations and features

Signs:
- Lesions rapidly develop into pus- filled blisters that rupture readily.
- Purulent discharge from lesions dries to form golden yellow crusts.
- Regional lymph nodes may be enlarged.
- Lesions begin as vesicles & turn into bullae containing clear yellow fluid.

Symptoms:
- Pruritis(severe itching), scratching of lesions may further spread the infection through excoriation of skin.
- Weakness, fever, diarrhea
- Itchy rashes
- Skin lesions
- Swollen lymph nodes
- Painful blisters

Diagnosis with Algorithm [1]:
- Diagnosed by physical examination by looking at the sores.
- Culture Sensitivity tests are done to identify the type of bacteria causing lesions.
- A complete blood count is performed.

Management [2]:
- ➤ Goals
  - Impetigo may resolve spontaneously, antimicrobial treatment is indicated to relieve symptoms, prevent formation of new lesions & prevent complications.
  - Mild cases can be handled by gentle cleaning, removing crusts & applying prescription strength antibiotic ointment.

Table 33.1 Pediatirc Impetigo Treatment Regimens.

Drug	Dosing
	Topical Agents
Mupirocin 2% ointment	Children ≥2 mo: Apply 10 lesions 2-3 times daily few 7-10 days
Retapamutin 1% ointment	Children ≥9 mo: Apply to affected areas twice daily few 5 days
	Oral Agents
Amoxteillin ctavulanic acic[a]	Infants <3 mo: 30 mg/kg/day po divided q12h x 10 days Children ≥ 3 mo and <40 kg: 30-90 mg/kg/day po divided q8-12h × 10 days Children ≥40 kg: 250-500 mg po q8h or 875 mg q12h × 10 days
Cefuroxime[b]	Infants and children 3 mo-12 y: 30 mg/kg/day (max 1 g/day) divided q12h × 10 days (suspension) Children ≤ 12 y: 250 mg q12h × 10 days (tablet) Adolescents: 250-500 mg q12h × 10 days (tablet)
Cephalexin	Children ≥ 1y:25-100 mg/kg/day in divided doses every 6-8 h × 10 days; max 4 g/day
Oicloxacillin	Neonates: Not recommended Children <40 kg: 12.5-100 mg/kg/day divided q6h × 5-7 days Children ≥40 kg: 125-250 mg q6h × 5-7 days
Erythromycin[c]	Erythromycin base: 30-50 mg/kg/day in 2-4 divided doses × 5-7 days; max 2 g/day Erythromycin ethylsuccinate: 30-50 mg/kg/day in 2-4 divided doses × 5-7 days; max 3.2 g/day Erythromycin stearate: 30-50 mg/kg/day in 2-4 divided doses × 5-7 days; max 2 g/day

[a]Dosing based on amoxicillin component.

[b]Cefuroxine axetil film-coated tablets are not bioequivalent to the oral suspension and therefore cannot be substituted on an mg/mg basis.

[c]Due to differences in absorption, 250 mg of erythromycin base or state will produce serum levels equilent to 400 mg ethylsuccinate may maximum. Source Reference 24

- ➤ Pharmacological Therapy: More severe or widespread cases, especially of bullous impetigo, may require oral antibiotic medication for impetigo.

❖ Penicillinase resistant penicillins

Ex: Dicloxacillin

Dose: 12.5mg/kg orally in 4 divided doses for children

MOA: Bactericidal activity- Blocks transpeptidase cross-linking of bacterial cell wall. Beta-lactum ring of penicillin binds to and competitively inhibits the transpeptidase enzyme.

❖ First generation cephalosporins

> Cephalexin

Dose: 25-50mg/kg orally daily in 2 divided doses for children.

> Cefadroxil

Dose: 30mg/kg orally daily in 2 divided doses for children.

> Penicillin - Administered as either as single intramuscular dose of benzathine penicillin G

Dose: 3, 00,000 – 6, 00,000 units in children

1.2 million Units in adults

> Clindamycin

Dose: Adults: 150 – 300mg orally every 6-8hrs

Children: 10 – 30 mg/kg per day in 3-4 divided doses

Duration of therapy: 7-10 days

MOA: Bactericidal activity- It disrupts the synthesis of peptidoglycan layer forming cell wall which is responsible for cell structural integrity.

❖ Mupirocin

• Topical ointments are used to prevent complications. Mupirocin ointment applied 3 times daily for 7 days. It is used to treat non-bullous impetigo.

MOA: Mupirocin reversibly binds to bacterial isoleucyl t-RNA synthetase, an enzyme. It promotes conversion of isoleucine & t-RNA to isoleucyl t-RNA. Prevention of these enzymes from functioning properly results in inhibition of bacterial protein & RNA synthesis.

Patient Counselling

• Cool sterile saline dressings initially to reduce pain.
• Warm, moist heat to aid in localization and allow spontaneous drainage.
• Elevation and immobilization may reduce the edema and swelling.
• Topical dressings provide a protective barrier against infective organism.

References

1. Holly Hartman-Adams, Christine Banvard, Gregory Juckett (2014): Impetigo: Diagnosis and Treatment. *American Family Physician 90 (4): 229-235.*
2. Impetigo. *Lexi-Drugs Online.* Hudson, OH: Lexi-Comp, Inc; 2013. http://online.lexi.com.

CHAPTER - 34

Basic Principles of Cancer Therapy

Introduction to Cancer

Cancer is a group of more than 100 different diseases that are characterized by uncontrolled cellular growth, local tissues invasion and distant metastases. The four most common cancers are prostate, breast, lung and colorectal cancer, skin cancer.

Neoplasm (New growth) & Tumour (Swelling)

Benign tumours enlarge but do not invade surrounding tissue. They are generally much less dangerous than malignant tumours, which invade local tissue and spread the distant sites. Tumours of brain or endocrine glands do not invade.

Etiology of Cancer

In both sexes – lung cancer is more common.

Cancer incidence generally increases with age.

Occupation: scrotal cancer among chimney sweeps, bladder cancer among azo dye workers and bone cancer among watch workers, painting walls etc

Geographic and ethnic variation: stomach cancer is more in japan; less incidence of colon cancer in Asia and Africa; skin cancer is common in Australia.

Carcinogenesis

It is a multi-stage process that is genetically regulated. The first step is

1. **Initiation** which requires exposure of normal cells to carcinogenic substances. These carcinogens produce genetic damage that if not required results in irreversible cellular mutation.
2. During the second phase **Promotion**, carcinogens or other factors alter the environment to favour growth of the mutated cell population over normal cells. The difference between initiation and promotion is that promotion is a reversible process. So a target for many chemotherapeutic agents.
3. **Conversion or transformation:** On the type of cancer 5-20 years may elapse between carcinogenic phase and development of a clinically detectable cancer.

4. **Progression:** Involves genetic changes leading to increased cell proliferation.

Drugs/ Hormones	Types of cancer
Alkylating agent	Leukemia
Anabolic steroids	Liver
Steroidal	Endometrium, breast, liver
Analgesics containing phenacetin	Rectal, urinary bladder

5. **Physical agents that act as carcinogens:** Ionising radicals UV light. These induce mutations by forming free radicals that damage DNA and other cellular components.

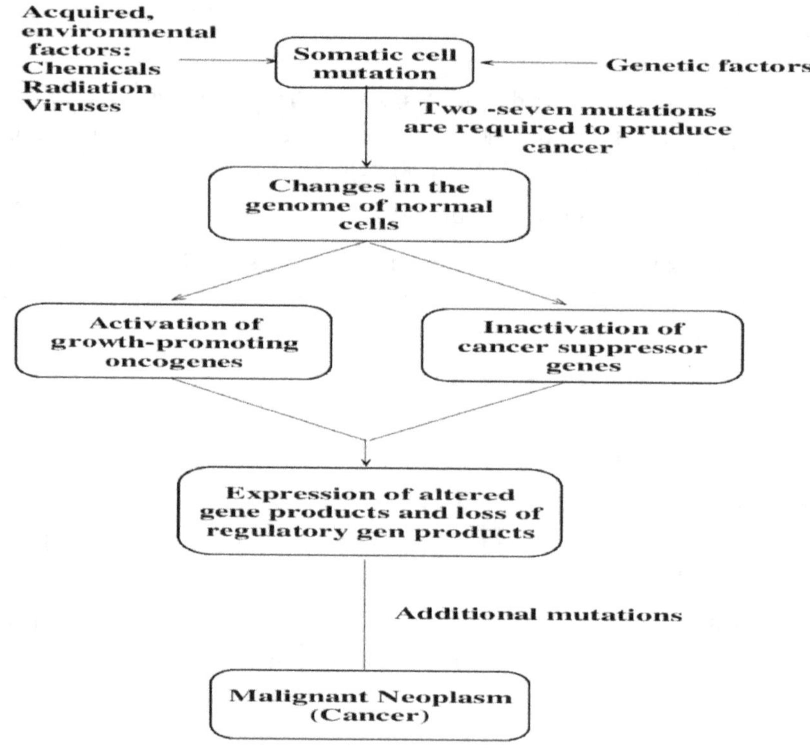

Fig. 34.1 Molecular mechanism of cancer.

Source: https://www.slideshare.net/reshma14695/other-mechanisms-of-molecular-pathogenesis-of-cancer

Genetic and Molecular Basis of Cancer [1]

Functional capabilities acquired by cancer cells:
1. Sustained angiogenesis
2. Self- proliferation
3. Insensitivity to antigrowth signals

4. Tissue invasion and metastasis
5. Anti – apoptotic effects
6. Limitless growth potential

- Proto- oncogenes convert to oncogenes. They are present in all cells and are essential regulators of normal cellular functions. Genetic alteration of proto oncogenes through point mutations oncogenes. These genetic alterations may be casually by radiation, chemicals, or viruses or they may be inherited once oncogenes are activated they cause dysregulation of normal cell growth and proliferation.
- Tumour suppressor genes regulate and inhibit inappropriate cellular growth and proliferation. Gene loss or mutations results in loss of control over normal cell growth.
- DNA repair genes repair DNA that is damaged by environment factors or errors in DNA that occur during replication. If not corrected these errors can result in mutations that activate oncogenes or inactivate tumour suppressor genes.
- Oncogenes and tumour suppressor genes provide the stimulating and inhibitory signals that ultimately regulate the cell cycle through cyclin and cyclin dependant kinases.
- When the normal regulatory mechanism for cellular growth fails back up defence systems may be activated i.e. Apoptosis and cellular senescence (aging). Over expression of Bcl2 anti-apoptotic protein is seen. Once a cell population has undergone a present number of doubling growth stops and cells die. This is known as senescence, a process regulated by telomeres.
- Telomeres are DNA segments or caps at the end of chromosome with each replication the length of telomeres are shortened and senescence is triggered. In cancer cells, telomeres length is protected by telomerases. These enzymes protect the telomeres from degrading and permitting an infinite number of cell doubling.
- Tumour cells may be either benign or malignant. Benign tumours are non- cancerous growths that are often encapsulated localised and indolent. Cells of benign tumours resemble the cells from which they are developed. These masses seldom metastasize and once removed they rarely occur. In contrast malignant tumours invade and destroy the surroundings tissue. Malignant cells lose the ability to perform their usual functions. This loss of structure and function is called anaphasia.

Invasion and metastasis

- Metastasis is the spread of neoplastic cells from primary tumour site to distant sites. The two pathways of metastasis are hematogenous and lymphatic. Other fewer modes include dissemination via CSF and Trans abdominal spread within the peritoneal cavity.

Table 34.1 Types of cancer.

Tissue of origin	Benign	Malignant
Epithelial		
Surface epithelium	Papilloma	Carcinoma
Glandular tissue	Adenoma	Adenocarcinoma

Contd...

Tissue of origin	Benign	Malignant
Connective tissue		
Fibrous tissue	Fibroma	Fibrosarcoma
Bone	Osteoma	Osteosarcoma
Smooth muscles	Leiomyoma	Leiomyosarcoma
Striated muscles	Rhabdomyoma	Rhabdomyosarcoma
Fat	Lipoma	Liposarcoma
Bone marrow elements		
Lymphoid tissue		Hodgkins and non hodgkins lymphoma
Plasma cells		Multiple myeloma
Neural tissue		
Glial tissue	Gliomas	Glioblastoma, astrocytoma
Nerve sheath	Neurofibroma	Neurofibrosarcoma
Melanocytes	Pigmented (mole)	Malignant melanoma
Mixed tumours		
Gonadal tissue	Teratoma	Teratocarcinoma

Warning signs of cancer

1. A new or unusual lump or swelling anywhere on your body.
2. A sore that will not heal, anywhere on your body or in your mouth
3. A change in the shape, size or colour of mole
4. Blood in your urine or bowel motions.
5. A cough, croaky voice or difficulty swallowing that lasts longer than 4 weeks.
6. A change to looser or more frequent bowel motions longer than 4 weeks.
7. Difficulty passing urine
8. Unexplained weight loss
9. Bleeding from vagina, after menopause
10. Unexplained pain or ache for more than 4 weeks.

Cancer warning signs in children

➢ Continued unexplained weight loss
➢ Headaches with vomiting in the morning
➢ Increased swelling or persistent pain in bones or joints
➢ Lump or mass in abdomen, neck or elsewhere
➢ Recurrent fevers not caused by infections
➢ Exercise bruising or bleeding
➢ Prolonged tiredness

Hierarchy of aims in cancer management

o Prevention
o Cure – Eradication of tumour and metastasis
o Remission –Significant reduction in tumour loads/ increased survival

o Symptomatic/ Palliation–Treatment of secondary compliments

o Terminal care –Improve QOC, Optimize symptom control

Factors governing the choice of treatment in cancer

1. Surgery –well defined solid tumour/ non-vital region eg. Mastectomy
   Nonmutilating result eg. Unsuitable for haed and neck tumors
2. Radiotherapy: Diffuse but localised tumour. E.g.: lymphoma
   Vital organ/region eg. Head and neck, CNS
3. Pharmacotherapy: Firm evidence base, combination with radiotherapy, diffuse tumour
   eg.leukaemia, some primary tumours – Hodgkin's lymphoma

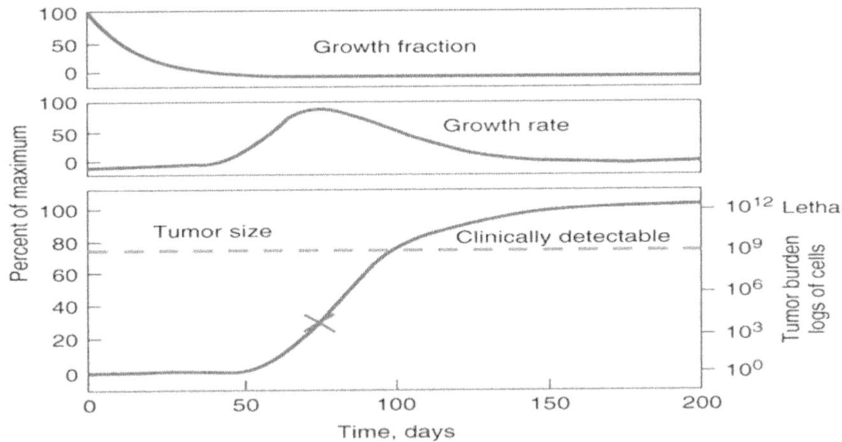

Fig. 34.2 Tumor growth curve.

Source: http://pathalamus.blogspot.com/2012/10/tumor-growth-and-mets.html

The growth of most tumours is illustrated by gompertzian tumour growth curve. In early stages, tumour growth is exponential which means that the tumour takes a constant amount of time to double its size. During, this phase large portion of tumour cells is actively dividing called growth fraction. Doubling time is short. Anti cancer agents are effective in this phase. As the tumour grows doubling in time is slowed may due to tumour outgrowing its blood and nutrient supply or the inability of blood and nutrients to diffuse through out the tumour mass.

Doubling time for solid tumour – 2- 3 months. Some tumour doubling time is few days. It takes about 10^9 cancer cells (1g mass 1cm area) for tumour to be clinically detectable by radiography. Such a tumour has undergone about 30 doubling in cell. It takes 10 additional doubling for this 1g mass to reach 1kg size. A tumour with 10^{12} cells is lethal. Thus a tumour is clinically undetectable for most of its lifespan.

Tumour burden also impacts response to chemotherapy. Tumour has 1000 cancer cells and chemotherapy regimen kills 90% of the cells, then 10% or 100 cells remain. The 2nd chemotherapy course kills 90% of cells and again only 10% or 10 cells remain. Tumour burden will never reach zero. Tumours of greater than 10^4 cells are to be eliminated by host immunologic mechanisms.

References

1. Joseph Dipiro. Pharmacotherapy: A Pathophysiological Approach. 7th Edition. Patrick J. Medina And Chris Fausel Chapter 130, Copyright © 2008, 2005, 2002 By The Mcgraw-Hill Companies, Inc.2085-91.

CHAPTER - 35

Cancer Chemotherapeutic Agents

Classification of Anti-cancer Agents

I.   Alkylating agents
   A. Nitrogen mustards: Mechlorethamine hydrochloride (nitrogen mustard), Cyclophosphamide, Chlorambucil, Melphalan, Ifosfamide
   B. Alkyl sulfonates: Busulfan
   C. Nitrosoureas: Carmustine , Lomustine, Semustine, Streptozocin
   D. Ethylenimines: Thiotepa
   E. Triazenes: Dacarbazine

II.   Antimetabolites
   A. Folate antagonist: Methotrexate
   B. Purine analogues: Thioguanine, Mercaptopurine (6-MP), Fludarabine, Pentostatin, cladribine
   C. Pyrimidine analogues: Cytarabine (cytosine arabinoside), Fluorouracil (5-FU)

III. Antibiotics
   A. Anthracyclines: Doxorubicin   hydrochloride   (Adriamycin),   Daunorubicin (daunomycin), Idarubicin
   B. Bleomycins: Bleomycin sulfate
   C. Mitomycin
   D. Dactinomycin (actinomycin D)
   E. Plicamycin

IV.   Plant-derived products
   A. Vinca alkaloids: Vincristine, Vinblastine
   B. Epipodophyllotoxins: Etoposide, Teniposide
   C. Taxanes: paclitaxel

V.   Enzymes: L-Asparaginase

VI.   Hormonal agents

    A. Glucocorticoids

    B. Estrogens, antiestrogens: Tamoxifen citrate, Estramustine phosphate sodium

    C. Androgens, antiandrogens: Flutamide

    D. Progestins

    E. Luteinizing hormone–releasing hormone (LH-RH) antagonists: Buserelin, Leuprolide

    F. Octreotide acetate

VII.   Miscellaneous agents: Hydroxyurea, Procarbazine, Mitotane, Hexamethylmelamine, Cisplatin, Carboplatin, Mitoxantrone

VIII. Monoclonal antibodies

IX.   Immunomodulating agents: Levamisole

    B. Interferons: Interferon alfa-2a, Interferon alfa-2b

    C. Interleukins: aldesleukin (interleukin-2, IL-2)

X.   Cellular growth factors: Filgrastim (G-CSF); Sargramostim (GM-CSF)

II.   Classification based on cell cycle phase specific agents:

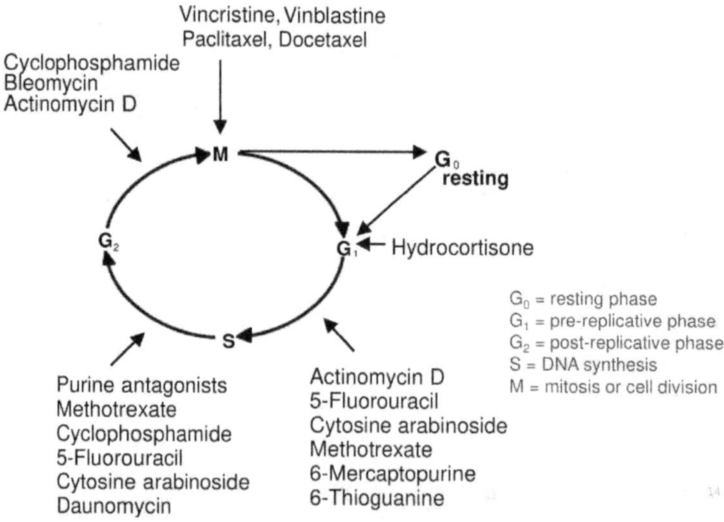

Fig. 35.1 Classification based on cell cycle phase specific agents.

III. Classification based on mechanism of action of drugs

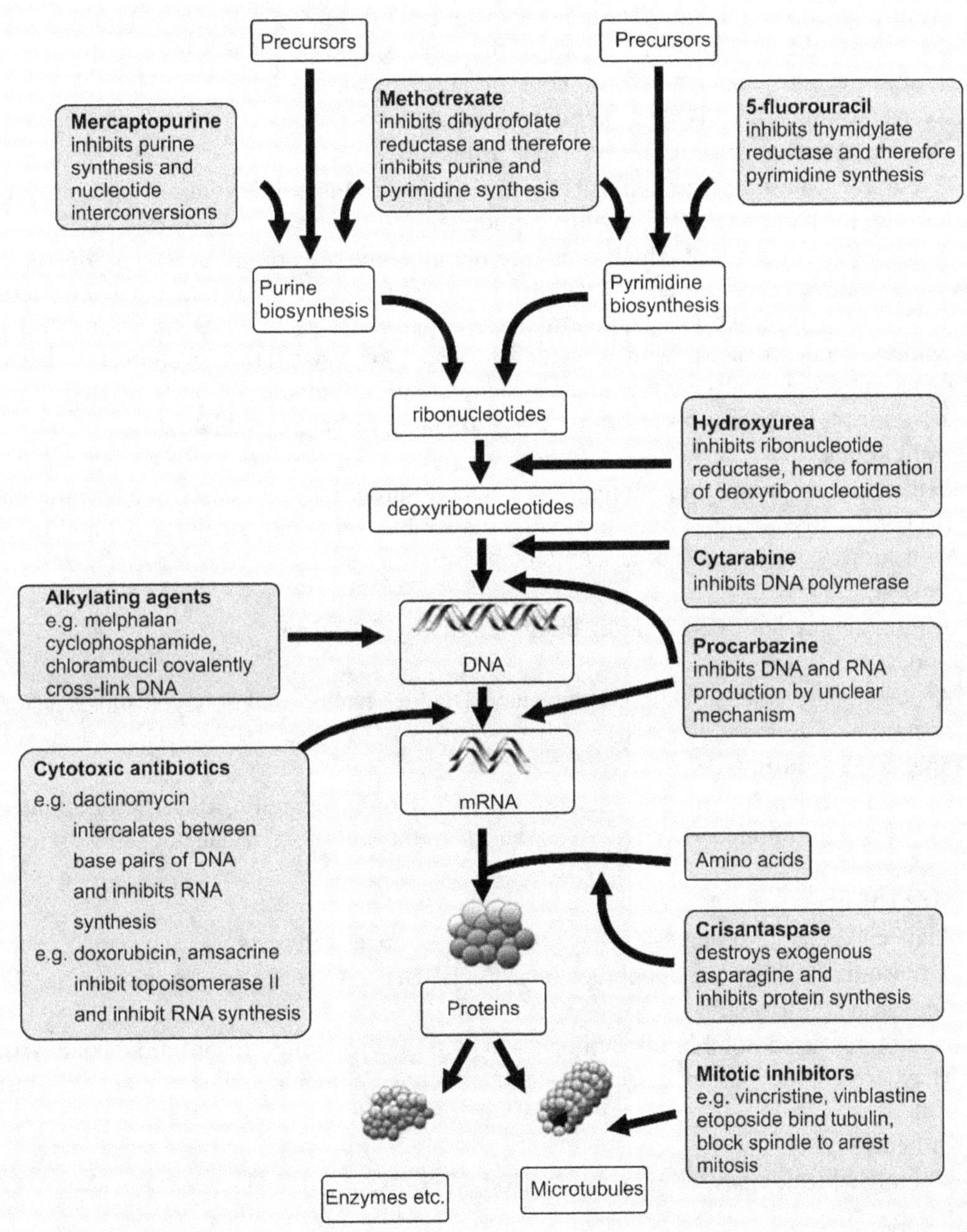

Fig. 35.2 Classification of Anti-cancer drugs based on mechanism of action.

Source: https://basicmedicalkey.com/cancer-8/

Clinical Pharmacology of chemo-therapeutic agents: [1]

I. **Alkylating agents**: The most common binding site for alkylating agent is the seven nitrogen group of guanine. These covalent interactions result in cross linking between 2 DNA strands or between 2 bases in the same strand of DNA. DNA replication is inhibited as interlinked strands do not separate as required.

Resistance: Increased DNA repair capabilities,

Decreased entry into or accelerated exit from cells.

Cyclophosphamide/Ifosfamide: They are nitrogen mustard derivatives phosphamide mustard (Active metabolite) and Ifosfamide mustard (Active)

It is an alkylating agent which produces highly reactive carbonium ion intermediates which transfer alkyl groups to cellular macromolecules by forming covalent bonds. This results in cross linking/abnormal base pairing/scission of DNA strand. Cross linking of nucleic acids with proteins can also take place. Transformtion into active metabolites occurs in the liver and a wide range of antitumour action is exerted. It has a prominent immunosuppressant property. It is less damaging to platelets.

Indications

Leukaemias, lymphogranulomatosis, lymphosarcoma, reticulum cell sarcoma, Hodgkin's disease, multiple myeloma. Inoperable solid malignancies. Combination with surgery, radiation & other hemotherapeutics drugs.

Dosage

2-3 mg/kg/day oral; 12-15 mg/kg body wt IV evey 7-10 days.

Contra-Indications

Acute Urinary tract infection. Pregnancy. Bladder haemorrhage. Myelosup-pression. Lactation.

Special Precautions

Chloramphenicol retards the metabolism of cyclophosphamide. Elderly, debilitated, diabetes. Discontinue if WBC. Count is less than 3000. Cardiac, hepatic or renal disease.

Side Effects

Alopecia, gonadal suppression, cardiotoxicity. ulmonary fibrosis

Nitrosoureas: They are lipophilic and cross BBB. Eg: Carmustine/ Lomustine

Lomustine (Nitrosoureas)

It is highly lipid soluble alkylating agent with a wide range of antitumour activity. They cross blood brain barrier and are effective in meningeal leukemias & brain tumours.

Indications

Meninigeal leukemias, brain tumours, Hodgkin's disease.

Dosage

100-130mg/sqm body surface area single oral dose every 6 wks.

Contra-Indications

Pregnancy, lactation, Hypersensitivity.

Special Precautions

Renal impairment. C.N.S disturbances, Monitor blood counts. Paediatrics: Not recommended in infants. Pregnancy : Safety not established. Lactation : Safety not established. Elderly : Use with caution.

Side Effects

Nausea, vomiting, seizures, Bone marrow depression is delayed for 6 wks. Visceral fibrosis and renal damage.

Decarbazine/ Temozolamide: undergo methylation to same active intermediate (monomethyl triazeno- imidiazole- carboxamide) that interrupts DNA replication by causing methylation of guanine. Decarbazine is poorly absorbed and should be given IV, Temazoloamide is rapidly absorbed after oral administration.

II. **Anti- metabolites:**

1. **Fluorinated pyrimidines**: Fluorouracil (prodrug) converted into fluorodeoxyuridine monophosphate. In this presence of folate it binds tightly to and interferes with function of thymidylate synthase. This enzyme is required for synthesis of thymidine one for blocks of DNA.

   Another metabolite of 5FU triphosphate nucleotide is incorporated into RNA as a false base and interferes with its function. Capecitabine is an orally active pyrimidine analog of uracil and a prodrug 5FU. It is converted to 5FU and shares the same MOA. It generates higher levels of 5FU selectively within some tumours than healthy tissues.

   ### 5-FLUOROURACIL

   It is pyrimidine analogue and is converted in the body to the corresponding 5 fluoro-2-deoxyuridine monophosphate, which inhibits thymidylate synthetase and blocks the conversion of deoxyuridilic acid to deoxythymidylic acid. Selective failure of DNA synthesis occurs due to non-availability of thymidylate: thymidine can partially reverse its toxicity.

   ### Indications

   Malignant neoplasms of breast, colon, urinary bladder, liver, pancreas, adjuvant to surgery, radiotherapy & other chemotherapeutic drugs. Topical application in cutaneous basal cell carcinoma.

   Dosage

   12 mg/kg body wt once daily for 4 successive days i.v. Max daily dose: 800 mg.

   Contra Indications

   Pregnancy Depresed bone marrow function. Serious infections. Poor nutritional state.

   Special Precautions

   Careful care at some Hospital or nursing home must for 1st course of treatment. Paediatrics: Should not be used. Pregnancy: Should not be used. Lactation: Should not be used. Elderly: May increase the adverse effects.

   Side Effects

   Toxicity on bone marrow & G.I.T. Nausea, vomiting, Skin pigmentation.

2. **Cytidine analogs**

   Cytarabine is an arabinose analog of cytosine. It inhibits DNA polymerase and enzyme responsible for strand elongation. It is also incorporated directly into DNA where it inhibits the replication of DNA and acts as chain terminator to prevent DNA elongation. Cytotoxic concentration is maintained in CNS for several hours after intrathecal administration and for more than 2 weeks following administration of depot formulated cytarabine intrathecally. Toxicity is dose dependant.

   Gemcitabine: It is a fluorine substituted deoxycytidine analogue related structurally to cytarabine. MOA is same. It achieves intracellular concentration 20 times higher than cytarabine.

   Acacytidine (Decitabine): Approved in 2004/2006 used for treatment of patients with myelodysplastic syndrome. Direct incorporation into DNA and inhibition of DNA methylase transferase which cause hypomethylation of DNA.

3. **Purine and purine anti-metabolite:**

   6-mercapto purine and 6–thioguanine: They are rapidly converted to ribonucleotide of 6– MP that inhibits purine biosynthesis. They also undergo purine interconversion reactions needed to supply purine precursor for synthesis of nucleic acids.

   Fludarabine monophosphate: It is an analogue of purine adenine. It interferes with DNA polymerase causing chain termination. It is also incorporated into RNA resulting in inhibited transcription.

   Mercaptopurine

   It is a highly effective antineoplastic drug. It is converted in the body to corresponding monoribonucleotides which inhibits the conversion of inosine monophosphate to adenine and guanine nucleoties. There is also feed back inhibition of de novo purine synthesis.

   Indications

   Childhood acute leukemia, choreocar-cinoma. Chronic granulocytic leukaemia.

   Dosage

   2.5 mg/kg/day, half dose for maintenance.

   Contra Indications

   Lactation.

   Special Precautions

   Renal or hepatic dysfunction. Monitor blood count, hepatic function, uric acid levels. Paediatrics: Reduced dose necessary. Pregnancy: Not usually prescribed. Lactation: The drug passes into breast milk. Elderly: Reduced dose may be necessary.

   Side Effects

   Bone marrow depression, nausea, vomiting, Hepatotoxicity, rash, fever, intestinal ulcers, hyperuricaemia.

4. **Antifolates**: Folates vitamins are essential co-factors in DNA synthesis. They carry one carbon in transfer reactions that are required for purine and thymidine acid synthesis, and in turn for formation of DNA and for cell division.

Dietary folates in presence of DHFR (Dihydro folate reductase) forms Tetrahydroforms to be active which inhibits purine synthesis and prevents DNA synthesis.

Methotrexate: It is transported intracellularly by active transport system. Resistance to MTX a) Amplification of DHFR b) Slow rates of thymidylates synthase c) decreased affinity of DHFR to MTX d) Lack of poly-glutamation with tumour cells.

Therapeutic drug monitoring is also an effective means of increasing the likelihood of therapeutic success.

Mechanism: It has a cell cycle specific action-kills cells in S phase; primarily inhibits DNA synthesis, but also affects RNA and protein synthesis. It blocks the conversion of a essential coenzyme required for one carbon transfer reaction in de novo purine synthesis and amino acid inter conversions.

Indications

Lymphoblastic leukaemia. Choriocarcinoma.

Dosage

Lymphoblastic leukaemia: 20-40 mg/sqm. body surface area twice weekly i.v or i.m. Maint dose: 15-30 mg/sqm 1-2 times weekly. Choriocarcinoma: 15-30 mg daily for 5 days.

Contra-Indications

Severe leucopenia or thrombocytopenia. Serious anaemia

Special Precautions

Use of folinic acid rescue has permitted much higher doses of methotrexate. Hepaticand renal dysfunction. C.N.S. disturbance. Bone marrow depression. Paediatrics: Use only in cancer treatment. Pregnancy: Contraindicated due to its teratogenic effects. Lactation: Should not be used. Elderly: Use with caution.

Side Effects

Megaloblastic anaemia, pancytopenia, Desquamation and bleeding may occur in GIT.

III. **Microtubules targeting agents:**

  1. **Vinca alkaloids:** Vincristine, Vinblastine are natural alkaloids from vinca plants. They act as mitotic inhibitors or spindle poison. Vinorelbino, Vinblastine – myelosuppression.

    (a) Vincristine – myelosuppressive, neurotoxic

    (b) They bind to tubulin, protein that polymerise to form microtubules. They disrupt the normal balance between polymerisation and depolymerisation of microtubules inhibiting assembly of microtubules which interfere with formation of mitotic spindle and cause cells to accumulate in mitosis.

Indications

Inducing remission in childhood acute leukemia, lymphosarcoma. Hodgkin's disease, Wilm's tumour. Ewing's sarcoma and carcinoma lung.

Dosage

Children : 2mg/sq.m. body surface. Adults: 1.4 mg/sq.m. body surface.

Contra-Indications

Pregnancy.

Special Precautions

Acute uric acid neuropathy may occur. Reduce bone marrow reserve, impaired liver function, bronchospasm and jaundice. Paediatrics: Adjust dose according to body weight. Pregnancy: Should not be used. Lactation: Use with caution. Elderly: Use with caution.

Side Effects

Peripheral neuropathy, alopecia, Bone marrow depression.

2. **Taxanes** – Paclitaxel and docetaxel are taxanes plant alkaloids with anti-mitotic activity.

   (a) Act by binding to tubulin. They induce tubulin polymerisation resulting in formation of inappropriately stable, non-functional microtubules. The stability of microtubules damage cells, because microtubules dependant structure required for mitosis and other cellular functions are disrupted. They also inhibit angiogenesis.

   Resistance – Alteration in tubulin or tubulin binding sites, P- glycoprotein mediated MDR.

IV. Topoisomerase inhibitors:

1. **Camptothecin derivatives:** Camptothecin a plant alkaloid from camptotheca acuminate is a potent inhibitor of DNA topisomerase-I. Irinotecan, topotecan are analogues were synthesised to reduce toxicity and improve therapeutic effects.

2. **Etoposide/ Teniposide:** They are semi synthetic podophyllotoxin derivatives. Podophyllin is extracted from Mayapple plant. It binds to tubulin and interferes with microtubules formation. They are cell cycle phase specific and arrest cells in S/G_2 phase. So, activity is much greater in divided doses than large single doses.

Etoposide:

Indications

Small cell lung cancer. Malignant lymphomas. Acute leukaemias, Testicular tumours. Bladder cancer & trophoblastic diseases.

Dosage

Dose in combination with other chemoth erapeutic agents: 50-100 mg/sqm body surface area/daily on days 1through 5 to 100 mg/sqm BSA/daily on days 1, 3, 5. Give a gap of 3-4 wks to recover from toxicity before repeating.

Contra-Indications

Hypersensitivity, severe liver dysfunction.

Special Precautions

Renal disease, infections, avoid contact with the skin, mucosa and eye. Paediatrics: Safety not established. Pregnancy: Should not be used. Lactation: Should not be used. Elderly: Safe.

Side Effects

Alopecia, GIT. disturbances, nausea, vomiting, diarrhoea, thrombophlebitis, neuritis, myelosuppression.

3. **Anthracene derivatives**: Doxorubicin, Daunorubicin, Idarubicin.
    (a) Mechanism: They are anti-tumour antibiotics, they are topoisomerase
    (b) Inhibit by producing double strand DNA breaks that can damage DNA and cell membranes
    (c) Resistance: P-glycoprotein dependant Melti Drug Resistance (MDR), Altered topoisomerase 2 activity.

Indications

Malignant lymphoma. gastro-intestinal tract carcinoma. Bronchogenic, bladder, breast & ovarian carcinoma. Wilm's tumour. Acute myeloblastic leukaemia. soft tissue & bone sarcomas.

Dosage

1.2-2.4 mg/kg body wt or 60-75 mg/sq metre of body surface given as a single dose every 3 weeks by slow i.v. inj.

Contra-Indications

Cardiac disease. Hepatic dysfunction.

Special Precautions

ECG changes, arrhythmias, hypotension, or be delayed congestive heart failure. Paediatrics: Reduced dose necessary. Pregnancy: Not usually prescribed. Lactation: Not prescribed. Elderly: Reduced dose may be necessary.

Side Effects

Cardiotoxicity, alopecia, Marrow depression, cardiomyopathy, stomatitis, vomiting and local tissue damage.

V. Heavy metals compounds: Cisplatin, Carboplatin, Oxyplatin:

They bind to DNA and form an intrastrand crosslines or aduction by neighbouring guanines. These intrastrand links cause a major binding of DNA. They may cause cellular damage by distorting the normal DNA conformation and preventing bases that are normally paired from lining up with each other.

Resistance: Ability to repair platinum induced DNA damage is increased and agents are inactivated by increasing levels of GSH. Altered uptake into the cells.

Side effects: Cisplatin is highly toxic anti-cancer agents – Nephrotoxicity, Ototoxicity, Peripheral neuropathy, emesis, anaemia.

VI. Miscellaneous:

Bleomycin: It is an anti-tumour antibiotic. It is a mixture of peptide from fungal Streptomyces one unit is roughly equal to 1mg of polypeptide protein.

Mechanism – DNA strand breakage via free radical formation. The bleomycin complex then reduces molecular O_2 to free oxygen radicals that cause primarily single- strand breaks in DNA. It has great effect on cells in G_2 phase of cell cycle and in mitosis. It is inactivated within cells by enzyme aminohydrolase.

Indications

Testicular tumour, squamous cell carcinoma of skin, head & neck, genito-urinary tract & oesophagus, Hodgkin's lymphoma. Malignancy o lungs & cervix.

Dosage

30 mg twice weekly in average cases, otherwise dose can be varied between 15 mg daily to 15 mg weekly. Total dose: 300-400 mg.

Contra Indications

Dot not mix glutathione with bleomycin. Pre-existing lung diseases.

Special Precautions

Paediatrics: Safety not established. Pregnancy: Should not be used. Lactation: Should not be used. Elderly: Dose adjustment is necessary.

Side Effects

Mucocutaneous toxicity, pulmonary fibrosis, Dermatitis, Nephrotoxicity. Hepatic toxicity.

L–Asparaginase- It is an enzyme produced by E.coli and other bacteria. L- Asparagine is a nonessential amino acid that can be synthesized by most mammalian cells, except for those of lymphoid human malignancies which lack or have very low levels of synthetase enzyme required for l–asparagine formation. L-asparagine is degraded by enzyme l-asparaginase, which depletes existing supplies and inhibits protein synthesis.

Indications

Acute leukaemia. Malignant lymphoma..

Dosage

50-200 k.u/kg body wt. daily or every alternate day by i.v infusion.

Contra Indications

Hypersensitivity.

Special Precautions

Anaphylaxis can occur, allergic reaction (being a foreign protein). Paediatrics: Safe. Pregnancy: Should not be used. Lactation: Should not be used. Elderly: Use with caution.

Side Effects

Liver damage, pancreatitis & C.N.S symptoms (due to defective protein synthesis)

VII. Monoclonal Antibodies

Two main classes of MOAB's are used in the treatment of cancer unconjugated or naked MOAB's and immunoconjugates which are MOAB's conjugated to a toxin, chemotherapy agent or radioactive particles

The letter o, u, xi and zu before the – mab suffix indicate a murine, human, chimeric and humanised source.

Mono Clonal Antibodies (MOA): Unconjugated that target antigens on the cell surface of cancer cells may directly mediate cell killing through complement activation, signalling the cascade of events that lead to tumour cells apoptosis, antibody dependant cellular toxicity. Finally Ab binding may result in transmission of signals that induce apoptosis in the targeted cells.

In addition, to mechanisms of cell death, immunoconjugates deliver a chemotherapy agent or radioactive peptide to site of disease. Once, internalised by target cells and kills tumour cells through traditional mechanism of action.

MoAB's conjugated to radiation deliver radiation targeting to site of tumor involvement resulting in cell death.

1. MoAB's that target cell surface glycoproteins

Gentuzumab Ozogamicin: It is a recombinant humanized anti–CD33 MoAB conjugated to calicheamicin derivative N- acetyl gamma calicheamicin, a cytotoxic antitumor antibiotic by the linker ozogamicin myeloid cell surface antigen-33 is expressed on surface of leukemic blasts. The binding of Fab fragment to CD33 antigen result in formation of complex that is internalized into CD33 cells. Upon internalization the calicheamicin derivative is cleaved from Ab and released inside the cell. The released earlier derivative binds to DNA in minor groove resulting in DNA double strand breaks and cell death. Indicated in CD33+ acute myelogenous leukaemia. SE: Myelosuppression, Hepatotoxicity

Rituximab:

It is a chimeric Monoclonal antibodies (MoAb's) directed against CD20 antigen found on surface of malignant B cells. Fragment Antigen Binding Region (Fab) domain of rituximab binds to CD20 Ag on B lymphocytes and Fc domain recruits immune effector functions to mediate B cells lysis.

Indications:

- Relapsed/refractory, low grade, follicular CD20 positive, B-cell non-Hodgkin's lymphomas
- First line therapy for non- Hodgkin's lymphomas (NHL) along with chemotherapy
- Chronic lymphocytic leukemia
- Refractory rheumatoid arthritis
- Immune mediated diseases-aplastic anemia

Dosage

Intravenous infusion only. For NHL=375mg/nv; for CLL=375mg/square meter body surface area the day prior to initiation of FC chemotherapy, then 500mg/m^2 on day 1 of cycles 2-6 (every 28 days).

Contra Indications

Hypersensitivity, severe active infection

Special Precautions

If infusion reaction accurs, interrupt infusion or slow the rate of infusion.

SE-Transient fever, chills, Nausea (N), headache.

2. Agents that target growth factor receptors and ligands:

Human epidermal growth factor receptor family: (HER follows tyrosine kinase receptor mechanism).

Cetuximab and Panitumumab: Cetuximab is a chimeric moab'sthat binds to extracellular domain of EGFR on both normal and tumor cells. It competitively inhibits the binding of Epidermal Growth Factor (EGF), transforming growth factor. Binding of cetuximab to Epidermal Growth Factor Receptor (EGFR) results in inhibition of cells growth and induction of apoptosis. Given as monotherapy or in combination for metastatic colorectal cancer, Head and neck cancer.

Side Effects: Acne like reactions, infusion related reactions, Trastuzumab and Erlotinib

3. **Vascular endothelial growth factor (VEGF)**

   Process of angiogenesis is regulated by proangiogenic growth factor, fibroblast growth factor, platelet derived growth factor, TNF-alpha, anti- angiogenic GF – IL-12, INF-r, Platelet Activating Factor-4 (PAF-4) and tissue inhibitor of metalloproteinase.

   Bevacizumab: It is a humanized Monoclonal Antibody (MOAB) directed against circulating Platelet Activating Factor-4 (VEGF). It binds to all biologically active circulating isoforms of VEGF and prevents the activation and of promotion of angiogenesis.

   Indications: With 5-Fluorouracil for metastatic colorectal cancer. First line treatment with carboplatin and paclitaxel for lung cancer.

   Dosage

   Intravenous infusion: 5-15mg/kg variable dose.

   Adverse effects: Hypertension, bleeding episodes, thrombotic events.

Miscellaneous Biologic Targeting Agents

Imatinib, Dasatinib

Imatinib is a selective inhibitor of tyrosine kinase activity of BCR- ABL fusion gene, the product of Philadelphia chromosomes. It binds to kinase binding site of BCR- ABL gene competitively blocking access to ATP. This prevents tyrosine kinase phosphorylation of gene and downstream activation of cellular proliferation. It also causes apoptosis of hematopoietic cells expressing BCR-gene.

Uses: Newly diagnosed Philadelphia chromosomes positive (Ph+), chronic myeloid leukaemia, C-KIT positive GI stromal tumours

Dosage: Chronic Phase CML: 400mg-600mg/day.

Contra Indications: Hypersensitivity.

AE- fluid retention, superficial oedema, increased liver enzyme, muscle cramps.

Temsirolimus and Everolimus

Mammalian target of rapamycin (MTOR) is a composed of intracellular signalling pathway involved in growth and proliferation of cells. MTOR receives input from upstream signalling pathway GF, hormones once activated MTOR stimulates protein synthesis by phosphorylation translation regulators. MTOR also contributes to protein degradation and angiogenesis.

Temsirolimus binds to FKBP – 12 and protein drug complex inhibits the activity of MTOR by blocking kinase activity. MTOR inhibitionalso results in reduced levels of cells GF's involved in angiogenesis such as VEGF.

Uses: Metastatic renal cell carcinoma.

SE: Rash, fatigue, mucositis, edema, loss of appetite.

Interferons

They are a family of proteins produced by nucleated cells and by rDNA technology.

IFN increases activity of cytotoxic cells within the immune system. Prolong cell cycle and apoptosis.

References

1. Joseph Dipiro. Pharmacotherapy: A Pathophysiological Approach. 7th Edition. Patrick J. Medina And Chris Fausel Chapter 130, Copyright © 2008, 2005, 2002 By The Mcgraw-Hill Companies, Inc.2092-2109.

CHAPTER - 36

Chemotherapy Induced Nausea & Emesis

- Nausea is defined as inclinations to vomit or as a feeling in the throat epigastric region altering an individual that variating is imminent.
- Vomiting is defined as ejection or explusion of gastric contents through the mouth and is often a forceful event.

Nausea and vomiting is due to GI, CVS, infection, neurologic, metabolic disease processes. It is also due to pregnancy, operative procedures. It is also seen with certain medications for treating cancer.

Anticipatory N/V: a learned conditional or psychological response to a poor outcome from a previous event. Triggered by tastes, odours, light, thoughts or anxiety associated with chemotherapy.

Emetics risk (if no prophylactic medication is administered)

High (>90%) – Cisplatin, cyclophosphamide.

Medium – (30- 90%) –doxorubicin, carboplatin

Low (10-30%) –5FU, paclitaxel

Minimal – Bleomycein, vincristine, busifan.

Pathogenesis

- ➤ Any stimulus from sensory input (i.e. pain, sight, smell) sends the message to higher cortical centres which relays the information to vomiting centre to induce vomiting.
- ➤ Any stimulus initiated due to treatment with chemotherapeutic drugs or radiation therapy, stimulates the sensory receptors present in GIT ie serotonin receptors which relay the impulse from GIT to CTZ. It relays the information to vomiting centre which upon activation induces vomiting.
- ➤ It consists of 3 phases:
    1. Nausea- imminent need to vomit is associated with gastric statis and a separate and singular symptom

2. Retching- laboured movement of abdominal and thoracic muscle before vomiting.
3. Vomiting- Forceful expulsion of gastric content caused by GI retro peristalsis.

➢ Act of vomiting requires coordinated contractions of abdominal muscles, pylorus, antrum, a raised gastric cardia, diminished lower oesophageal sphincter pressure and esophageal dilatation.

Presentation of N & V

General: Depending on severity of symptoms, points may present in mild, severe, distress.
Symptoms: Simple – self limiting, resolves spontaneously, require only symptomatic therapy
Complex: Not relieved after administration of anti-emetics, progressive deterioration of patient secondary to fluid & electrolyte imbalance
Signs: Simple – patient complaint of discomfort
       Complex – weight loss, fever, abdominal pain
Laboratory tests: Simple – none
          Complex – Serum electrolyte concentrations, upper/lower GI evaluation.

Chemotherapy induced Nausea & Vomiting (CINV)

Five categories

- Acute – N&V that occurs within 24hrs of chemotherapy administration
- Delayed - 24hrs after chemotherapy administration
- Anticipating N&V – Emesis occurring during previous chemotherapy,
- Breakthrough N&V –Emesis occurring despite prophylactic administration of anti–emetics
- Refractory N&V – poor response to multiple anti–emetic regimens.

Factors to consider for selecting an anti- emetic for CINV

- Emetic risk of chemotherapeutic agents or regimens
- Patient specific factors
- Patterns of emesis after administration of specific chemotherapy agents or regimens.

Prophylaxis of Acute CINV (one dose administered prior to chemotherapy)[1, 2]

Emetic risk of chemotherapeutic agents is the primary factors to consider an anti – emetics
Patients with emetic:
(i) Patients with emetic risk high
    (a) 5HT3 Receptor antagonists: Dolasetron 100 mg orally/ 100mg IV/ 1.8 mg/kg
        Granisteron–2mg orally/1mg IV/ 34.3 mg transdermal patch.
        Ondansteron–16-24mg orally/ 8-12 mg IV max 32 mg
        Palanosteron – 0.25mg IV.
        and
        B.Dexamethasone –12mg orally / IV

      and C.Substance P/Neurokinin 1 receptor antagonists like
      Fasoprepitant–115mg IV or Aprepitant 125mg orally

(ii)   Patients with moderate risk

    (a)   5HT3 Receptor antagonists: Dolasetron 100 mg orally/ 100mg IV/ 1.8 mg/kg and

    (b)   Dexamethasone 8-12 mg orally/IV and

    (c)   In selective patients who have been given anthracycline antiobiotics, cyclophosphamide, carboplatin, doxorubicin, ifosfamide etc.

    Aprepitant 125mg orally / Fosaprepitant – 115mg IV.

(iii)   Patients with Low risk- Dexamethasone 8-12mg orally/ IV
      Prochlorperazine/metoclopramide/lorazepam

(iv)   Patients with minimal risk- None
      Low risk – dexamethasone 8-12mg orally/ IV

Prophylaxis of delayed CINV

- Aprepitant, dexamethasone, metoclopramide are effective in delayed CINV, 5HT$_3$RA receptor antagonsists are inconsistent.

- But patient receiving cisplatin 3 days regimen it is prescribed

    (i)   High Risk – Palanosetron 0.25mg IV+Dexamethasone 8-12mg orally on 2-4 days+Aprepitant 80mg orally on days 2 and 3 after chemotherapy

    (ii)   Moderate Risk – 5HT3 RA –Dolasetron 100mg orally daily;   Ondasetron 8mg orally daily
      Granisetron 1-2mg orally daily or Dexamethasone 8-12mg orally daily or
      Aprepitant – 80mg orally on day 2 & 3.

    (iii)   Low risk – none

    (iv)   Minimal risk – None

References

1. Herrstedt. J. (2008). Antiemetics: An update and the MASCC guidelines applied in clinical practice. Nature clinical practive Oncology, 5(1),32-42.

2. Kris, M.G., Hesketh, P.J., Somerfield, M.R., Feyer, P., Clark-Snow, R., Koeller, J.M.m et al., (2006). American society of clinical oncology guidelines for antiemetics in oncology. Update 2006. Journal of clinical oncology, 24(18), 2932-2947.

CHAPTER - 37

Breast Cancer

Introduction to Breast Cancer

Breast cancer is a malignancy originating from breast tissue. Disease confined to a localised breasts lesion is referred to as early primary, localised or curable. Disease detected clinically or radially in sites distant from the breast is referred to as advanced or meta-static breast cancer, which is usually curable.

Epidemiology

Breast cancer is more common in females. Male genders are also at risk for developing cancer.

Etiopathogenesis and risk factors [1]

Breast cancers can start from different parts of the breast. Most breast cancers begin in the ducts that carry milk to the nipple (ductal cancers). Some start in the glands that make breast milk (lobular cancers). Two variable most strongly associated with occurrence of breast cancer are gender and advancing age. Additional risk factors include endocrine factors (eg: early menarche, nulliparity, late age at first birth, hormone replacement therapy, genetic factors, personal, family history, mutations of tumor suppressor genes BRCA 1 and BRCA 2), environmental and lifestyle factors (eg: radiation exposure)

Breast cancer cells often spread undetected by contiguity, lymph channels and through blood early in course of disease, resulting in metastatic disease after local therapy. Common metastataic sites are lymph nodes, skin, bone, liver, lungs & brain.

Breast cancer can occur mainly in women, but men can get it too. Many people do not realize that men have breast tissue and that they can develop breast cancer. Here we talk about breast cancer in women.

- For men life time risk of getting breast cancer is about $1/10^{th}$ of 1% (1 in 1000)
- IDC and ILC are the most common type of breast cancer which are also known as acquired mutations
- Inherited gene mutations are in every cell of the body and can be passed on to children. (BRCA gene (BRCA 1 and BRCA 2) are tumour suppressors genes).

- Mutations in these genes can be inherited from parents. When they are mutated they no longer suppress abnormal growth and cancer is more likely to develop.

Women who as children or young adults had radiation therapy to the chest areas as treatment for another cancer (such as Hodgkins disease or non – Hodgkins lymphoma) are at much higher risk for breast cancer.

Risk of developing breast cancer can appear to be highest if the radiation was given during adolescence when the breast was still developing.

Post Menopausal Hormone Therapy (PHT) is used to help relieve symptoms of menopause and to help prevent osteoporosis (thining of the bones).

These are 2 main types of PHT: estrogen and progesterone (known as combined PHT) and estrogen alone (known as estrogen therapy (ET)).

- Use of combined PHT increases the risk of breast cancer. The increased risk is seen after as little as 2 years of use.
- Using oral contraceptives or the injectable contraceptives Depo-Provera increases breast cancer risk.
- Having the first full term pregnancy before 30 and having many term pregnancies reduce breast cancer risk.
- Women who have had more menstrual cycles because they have started menstruation at an early age and/or went through menopause at a later age have slightly higher risk of breast cancer with hormones like estrogen and progesterone.
- Before menopause the ovaries produce most estrogen and fat tissue produce a small amount. After menopause most of a woman estrogen comes from fat tissue. Having more fat tissue after menopause can increase estrogen levels and increase the likelihood of developing breast cancer.
- Compared to non- drinkers, woman who consume 1 alcoholic drink a day have very small increase in risk. Those who have 2-3 drinks daily have 20% higher risk than women who don't drink alcohol.

MRI is recommended for women who:
- ✓ Have a known BRCA 1 or BRCA 2 gene mutations
- ✓ Have a first- degree relative (parent, brother, sister or child) with a BRCA1 or BRCA2 gene mutation but have not had genetic testing themselves.

For most women, at high risk, screening with MRI and mammograms should begin at the age of 30 years and continue for as long as is in good health.

Other Risk factors

- ❖ Primary cousins: due to gene transfer and should undergo diagnosis once in a year.
- ❖ People having pregnancy less than 30 years of age have less risk on getting breast cancer.
- ❖ People having pregnancy greater than 30 years of age are more prone to breast cancer.
- ❖ Progesterone hormonal therapy in post menopausal women.
- ❖ Late stage menopause.

❖ Mutations in genes from parent to progeny, which is expressed in progeny but not in the parent.
❖ People menstruating at early age.
❖ Greater the menstrual cycles, greater is the risk.
❖ People using oral contraceptives for 2 years.
❖ Women having alcohol and women smoking tobacco.
❖ Children with leukemia, non Hodgkin's / Hodgkin's lymphoma and children who have undergone chemotherapy with radiations are at high risk.
❖ Obesity and lack of physical exercise.

Clinical manifestation and features

General

The patient may not have any symptoms, as breast cancer may be detected in asymptomatic patients through routine screening mammography.

Signs and symptoms

❖ Painless palpable lump in the initial stages.
❖ Malignant mass is solitary, unilateral, irregular, non mobile, hard to feel, palpable.
❖ Change in colour or appearance of areola.
❖ Discharge or bleeding.
❖ Redness or pitting over the skin of breast [like the skin of orange]
❖ Lumps also observed in the axillary region
❖ Morphology of nipple changes. [Dimpling, retraction].

Signs and symptoms of systemic metastases

Depends on the site of meta- states, but many include bone pain, difficulty breathing, abdominal pain, or enlargement, jaundice, mental stress pronges.

Diagnosis with Algorithm

Algorithm for newly diagnosed breast cancer

1. If the patient has Palpable mass or abnormal mammogram, initial workup has to be done.
2. History and physical examination, diagnostic mammaogram, ultrasound of breast has to be done
3. Then sample is sent for biopsy-stereotactic core biopsy and ultrasound guided core biopsy
4. If the patient is newly diagnosed of invasive breast cancer
   (a) Then pathologic type, nuclear grade, differentiation, estrogen/progesterone receptor status/ proliferation indices/ HER2 status to be checked
   (b) Then routine serum studies/ assignment of clinical stage and Tumor Node Metastasis (TNM) stage to be evaluated

5. The patient is categorized as
   (a) Stages I and II: additional tests if indicated by symptoms or abnormal serum studies/ multidisciplinary treatment to be initiated
   (b) If the ptient is Stage III: staging studies to rule out disease in liver, lung and bone/ multidisciplinary treatment to be initiated

Laboratory tests:

1. Tumour markers such as cancer antigen or carcinoembryonic antigen may be elevated.
2. Alkaline phosphatase or liver function tests may be elevated in meta-static disease.
3. Testing for tumor cells for Hormone receptors.
4. FISH Test (Fluorescence Insitu Hybridization).
5. Blood tests.

Other diagnostic tests

Mammogram (with or without ultrasound, breast MRI or both)

Biopsy for pathology review and determination of tumour estragon/ progesterone receptor status or HER2 status.

Systemic staging tests – chest X-ray, chest CT, bone scan, abdominal CT or bone scan, abdominal CT or ultrasound or MRI.

Staging

Stage (anatomical extent of disease) is based on primary tumor extent and size, presence and extent of lymph nodes involvement and presence or absence of distant metastates (mo-1). The staging system determines the prognosis and assists with treatment decisions.

Early Breast cancer

Stage 0 - Carcinoma in -site or disease that has not invaded the basement membrane.

Stage 1 - Small primary invasive tumour without lymph nodes involvement.

Stage 2 – Involvement of regional lymph nodes.

Locally advanced breast cancer:

Stage 3 - A large tumour with extensive nodal involvement in which the node or tumour is fixed to the chest wall also includes inflammatory breast cancer which rapidly progressive.

Advanced or Meta-static breast cancer

Stage 4 – Metastases in other organs, distant from primary tumour.

Table 37.1 TNM staging classification for breast cancer.

	TNM Staging classification for breast cancer
	Primary tumour (T)
T_0	No evidence of primary tumour
T_{is}	Carcinoma in – situ non-infiltrating intraductal carcinoma or Paget's disease of nipple with no evidence of tumour
T_{b1}	Tumor of 2cm or less in its greatest dimension T T1a – No fixation to underlying pectoral fascia or muscle. T2a – Fixation to underlying pectoral girdle fascia or muscle
T_{b2}	Tumour of > 2cms but NMT 5 cmsin its greatest dimension T2a – No fixation to underlying pectoral fascia and or muscle T2b –Fixation to underlying pectoral fascia.
T_{b3}	Tumour of >5cms in its greatest dimension
T_{b4}	Tumour of any size with direct extension to chest wall or skin T4a – Fixation to chest wall T4b- Edema, ulceration of skin of breast T4c –Both of above T4d- inflammatory carcinoma

Node involvement (N)

N_0	No palpable homolateral axillary nodes
N_1	Movable homolateral axillary nodes
N_2	Homolateral axillary nodes containing growth
N_3	Homolateral supraclavicular nodes

Distant metastasis (M): -

M_0 – No evidence of distant metastasis

M_1 – Distant metastasis present

Classification of Drugs for Treatment of Breast Cancer

1. **Chemotherapy drugs:**
   (a) **Doxorubicin** – Anthracycline derivatives. They are anti– tumour antibiotics. They are topoisomerase inhibitors producing double strand breaks. Damage DNA.
   (b) **Cyclophosphamide**–alkylating agent belongs to nitrogen mustard derivatives. They cause DNA double strand cross linking. DNA replication is inhibited.
   (c) **5-fluorouracil**–Antimetabolites – Inhibits thymidylate synthatase
   (d) **Methotrexate** –Antifolates inhibits folic acid synthesis. No purine and thymidine synthesis – no DNA formation
   (e) **Paclitaxel/Docetaxel:** Taxanes – inhibit microtubule formation binding to tubulin and induce polymerization – inhibit mitosis.

2. **Endocrine therapy:**

   (a) **Aromatase inhibitors-Nonsteroidal** – **Anastrozole, letrozole** Steroidal-Examestane

   Mechanism of action:

   They are a class of drugs used in treatment of breast cancer in postmenopausal women and gynaecomastia in men. Aromatase is the enzyme **that** synthesises estrogen. As breast and ovarian cancers require estrogen tp grow, Aromatic inhibitor (AIs) are taken to either block the production of estrogen or block the action of estrogen on receptors.

   AIs work by blocking the conversion of androstenedione and testosterone into estrone and estradiol by process aromatisation.

   (b) **Anti estrogens (SERM's)** –Tamoxifen, Toremifene

   Mechanism of Tamoxifen in breast cancer: Tamoxifen is a selective estrogen receptor. It is a prodrug having relatively little affinity for its target protein-estrogen recptor. Metabolised to 4 hydroxy tamoxifen (4OHT) which have 30-100 times more affinity with ER than tamoxifen itself. These active metabolites compete with estrogen in the body for binding to ER. In anscription of breast 4OHT acts as ER antagonist so that transcription of estogen responsive genes is inhibited.

   4OHT binds to ER competitively in tumor cells and other tissue targets, producing a nuclear complex that decreases DNA synthesis and inhibits estrogen effects. It is nonsteroidal agent with potent anti-estrogenic properties.

   Tamoxifen causes cells to remain in G_0 and G_1 phases of cell cycle. Because it prevents cancerous cells from dividing but does not cause cell death, it is cytostatic rather than cytocidal.

   (c) **LHRH agonist** Goserelin, Leuprolide.

   MOA of LHRH analogs in breast cancer: inhibition of pituitary and gonadal function. Continuous treatment with LHRH agoinists causes a downregulation LHRH receptors and an uncoupling of LHRH signal transduction mechanism. This results in desensitisation of gonadotrophins and a marked reduction in the secretion of bioactive LH&FSH. This state is reversible and is called selective medical hypophysectomy.

   Decrease in circulating LH & FSH together with downregulation of gonadal hormones for LH&FSH produces a complete inhibition of testicular or ovarian function and a fall in sex-steroid levels. This state is called medical castration.

   (d) **Progestins** –Megasterol acetate, medroxy progesterone

   (e) **Androgens:** Fluoxymesterone

   (f) **Estrogens**–Ethinyl estradiol.

3. Biologic or Targeted therapy:
  (a) **Anti HER-2 agents** –Trastuzumab, Lapatinib and Pertuzumab

Management of Breast Cancer

Goals of Treatment

- ❖ Adjuvant therapy for early and locally advanced breast cancer is administered with curative intent.
- ❖ Treatment of MBC is done to improve symptoms and quality of life and prolong survival.
- ❖ Treatment can cause substantial toxicity which differs depending on the individual administration method and combination regimens.

Treatment Options

- ❖ Surgery
- ❖ Chemotherapy
- ❖ Hormonal Therapy
- ❖ Radiation Therapy
- ❖ Targeted Therapy

Table 37.2 Surgical approach for the management of Breast cancer.

Surgical Options in Treating Carcinoma of Breast	
Radical Mastectomy	Removal of entire breast, overlying skin, pectoral muscles, major or minor, axillary lymph nodes and fat
Extended radical mastectomy	As above, plus internal mammary nodes
Modified radical mastectomy	Removal of entire breast, overlying skin, leaving pectoral muscle intact
Simple mastectomy	Removal of breast, some fat, axillary nodes
Subcutaneous mastectomy	Removal of mammary tissue, preserving overlying skin
Lumpectomy	Removal cancerous mass

Radiation: Radiotherapy is usually given after surgery to the region of tumour bed and regional lymph nodes, to destroy Microscopic tumour cells that may have escaped surgery.
Radiation therapy can be delivered as:
1. External beam
2. Internal radiotherapy (Brachytherapy)
Radiation therapy can reduce the risk of recurrence by 50-66%
  1. Early Breast Cancer
    (i) **Local-regional therapy**: Surgery can cure those with stage-II cancers. Radiation therapy is administered for over 4-6 weeks to eradicate residual disease.

(ii) Adjuvant Chemotherapy: Early administration of effective combination chemotherapy at a time of low tumor burden should increase the likelihood of cure and minimize emergency of drug resistance cell clones.

(a) Anthracycline containing regimens:

Eg: Doxorubicin and Epirubicin

They occur as glycosides of the anthracyclinone. The glycosidic linkage usually involves 7-hydroxyl group of anthracycline and beta enantiomer of sugar with usually has anti-neoplastic activity and reduces the rate of recurrence and death.

(b) Alkylating Agents:

Cyclophosphamide : Mechanism: Binds to N-7 terminal of guanyl derivative (guanine) residue. Forming covalent Bonds alkylates the 7th Nitrogen and results in abnormal base pairing. Damaged DNA is formed.

(c) Antimetabolites:

1. Methotrexate: Mechanism: Inhibits dihydrofolate reductase which converts the dihydrofolic acid to tetrahydrofolic acid. No formation of folic acid and Nitrogen base.

   Inhibition of cell proliferation.

2. Fluorouracil: Mechanism: It is converted into 5- Fluoro-2 deoxy uridine monophosphate. Inhibits the thymidilate synthetase and blocks the conversion of deoxy uridic acid to deoxy thymidilic acid. No formation of pyimidines. No cell proliferation.

(d) Taxanes: Docetaxel, Paclitaxel

Mechanism: This stabilizes the polymerization of Tubulin and the depolymerization is prevented .Microtubule are not formed and cell proliferation is inhibited.

❖ Initiate chemotherapy within 12 weeks of surgical removal of the primary tumor optimal duration of adjuvant treatment is unknown but appears to be 12 – 24 weeks, depending on the regimen used.

❖ Concominant or sequential administration of a taxane with an anthracycline, standard care in node positive breast cancer.

Regimens:

(a) AC :- Doxorubicin 60mg/m^2 IV, day 1 cyclophosphamide 600mg/m^2 IV, day1 repeat cycles every 21 days for 4 cycles.

(b) AC :- Paclitaxel :- Doxorubicin:- 60mg /m^2 IV, Cyclophosphamide:- 600mg/m^2 IV day 1, repeat cycles every 21 days for 4 cycles followed by Paclitaxel 80mg/m^2 IV weekly, repeat cycle every 21 days – 6 cycles.

(c) CEF : - Cyclophosphamide :- 75mg/m^2 per day orally on 1 – 14 days.

Epirubicin :- 60mg/m^2 IV on days 1 – 8.

Fluoromacil :- 600mg/m^2 IV, days 1-8 days

Repeat cycle every 21 days - 6 cycles.

(iii) Adjuvant biologic therapy: Trastuzumab in combination with adjuvant chemotherapy is indicated in early stage.

(iv) Adjuvant endocrine therapy: Tamoxifen, tormifene, oophorectomy, ovarian ablation, LHRH agonists and aromatase inhibitors are used in primary stages.

2. **Locally Advanced Breast Cancer (STAGE-III)**

Neoadjuvant or primary chemotherapy is treatment of choice. Anthracycline and taxane regimens is recommended. Trastuzumab is preferred for HER-2 positive tumors. Cure is the goal of therapy.

3. **Metastatic Breast Cancer**

   (a) Endocrine therapy:

   Preferred for hormone receptor positive metastases in soft tissue, bone, pleura of viscera.

   1. Aromatase inhibitors: First line therapy for post menopausal women.

      Eg: Anastrazde: 1mg orally daily.

      Exemestane: 25mg orally daily

      Letrozole: 2.5mg orally daily

      SE: hot flushes, myalgias, headaches, diarrhea

   2. Anti-estrogens:

      (a) Selective Estrogen Receptor Modulator (SERMs) Toremifene: Also a SERM, has similar efficacy and   tolerability as tamoxifen and is an alternative therapy in post menopausal patients.

      (b) Selective Estrogen Receptor Downregulators (SERDs) Fulvestrant: 2nd line intramuscular agent with similar efficacy   and safety when compared to anastrazole.

         Tamoxifen: 20mg orally daily.

         Fulvestrant: 500mg IM every 28 days.

         SE: Hot flashes, vaginal discharge, nausea, thromboembolism, endometrial cancer

   3. Leutinising Hormone Releasing Hormone (LHRH) analogs: Medical castration with an LHRH analogue (Goserelin, Leuprolide) is reversible alternative to surgery.

      Goserelin: 3.6mg SC every 28 days.

      Leuprolide: 3.75mg SC every 28 days.

      SE: Hot flashes, amenorrhea, menopausal symptoms

   4. Progestins: Megestrol acetate, medroxyprogesterone

      Medroxymogesterone: 400mg IM / week

      SE: Weight gain, hot flashes, vaginal bleeding, edema,

   5. Androgens: fluoxymesterone 10mg orally twice a day

      SE: alopecia, fluid retention

   6. Estrogens: diethylstilbestrol, ethinyl estradiol

      Ethinyl Estradiol: 1mg orally TID

      Diethylstilbestrol: 5mg orally TID

      SE: Nausea/vomiting, fluid retention, anorexia,

(b) Chemotherapy: Used as initial therapy for women with hormone receptor-negative tumors, with rapidly progressive lung, liver or bone marrow involvement.

Single agent chemotherapy

1. Anthracyclines and taxanes produce response rates of 50 – 60% used as first line therapy. Single agents Capecitabine, vinorelbine, gemcitabine have response rates of 20-25%, when used after a taxane.
2. Ixabepilone: A Microtubule stabilizing agent given as Monotherapy or in combination with Capecitabine.
3. Eribulin: "Anti Microtubule" approved as a Monotherapy.
   Paclitaxel 175mg/m2 IV over 3 hours, day 1 repeat cycles every 21 days.

Combination chemotherapy Regimens

(a) Paclitaxel + Gemcitabine: P: 175mg/m2 IV over 3 hours, day 1.
    G :- 1250mg/m^2 IV on day 1 and 8 :- Repeat every 21 days.
(b) Ixabepilone + Capecitabine
    Ixabepilone: 40mg/m2 IV over 3 hours day 1.
    Capecitabine: 1750 – 2000mg/m2 / day orally divided for 14 days.
    Repeat cycles every 21 days.
(c) **Biologic or targeted therapy:** Three anti-HER2 agents –Trastuzumab, lapatinib and pertuzumab are available. Trastuzumab produced response rates of 15-20%. It is well tolerated.
(d) **Radiation therapy:** Radiation is commonly used to treat painful bone metastases or other localized sites of disease including brain and spinal cord lesions. Pain relief is seen in approximately 90% of patients who receive RT.

Prevention of Breast Cancer

The most clinical information is available for the SERM's (tamoxifen) which reduces the rates of invasive breast cancer in female at high risk for developing it.

Exemestane: Taken for 5 years significantly reduces the rates of invasive breast cancer with tolerable ADR's.

Breast Cancer Screening Guidelines for Women (American Cancer Society)[4] [2]

1. Women aged 40 to 49 years with average risk: Women aged 40 to 44 years should have the choice to start breast cancer screening once a year with mammography if they wish to do so. The risks of screening as well as the potential benefits should be considered. Women aged 45 to 49 years should be screened with mammography annually
2. Women aged 50 to 74 years with average risk: Women aged 50 to 54 years should be screened with mammography annually. For women aged 55 years and older, screening with mammography is recommended once every two years or once a year. Women aged 55 years and older should transition to biennial screening or have the opportunity to

continue screening annually. Among average risk women, clinical breast examination to screen for breast cancer is not recommended.

3. Women aged 75 years or older with average risk: Women should continue screening with mammography as long as their overall health is good and they have a life expectancy of 10 years or more

4. Women with dense breasts: Evidence is insufficient to recommend for or against yearly MRI screening.

Treatment of HER2-Positive Breast Cancer [3, 4]

Evidence-based guidelines from the American Society of Clinical Oncology (ASCO) for treatment of *HER2* -positive breast cancer, which are largely adapted from the 2015 Cancer Care Ontario (CCO) clinical practice guidelines, are as follows:

- Trastuzumab +chemotherapy for all patients with *HER2*-positive, node-positive breast cancer and for patients with *HER2*-positive, node-negative breast cancer (>1 cm)
- Trastuzumab plus chemotherapy may be considered in small (≤1 cm), node-negative tumors in patients with *HER2*-positive T1a-b N0 disease
- In high-risk *HER2*-positive disease, the recommended regimen is sequential anthracycline and taxanes given concurrently with trastuzumab; or docetaxel, carboplatin, and trastuzumab for six cycles
- For lower-risk node-negative *HER2*-positive disease, an alternative regimen is paclitaxel and trastuzumab in combination once weekly for 12 weeks, with trastuzumab then given for 1 year
- In patients with high-risk disease and when a taxane is contraindicated, the optimal dose of an anthracycline three-drug regimen that contains cyclophosphamide is recommended, with a cumulative dose of doxorubicin ≥240 mg/m² or epirubicin ≥600 mg/m², but no higher than 720 mg/m²; the cumulative dose of doxorubicin in two-drug regimens should not exceed 240 mg/m²
- Docetaxel and cyclophosphamide for four cycles is an acceptable non-anthracycline regimen
- For patients in whom anthracycline-taxane is contraindicated, cyclophosphamide-methotrexate-fluorouracil (with oral cyclophosphamide) is an acceptable chemotherapy alternative to doxorubicin-cyclophosphamide
- Concurrent administration of trastuzumab with the anthracycline component of a chemotherapy regimen is not recommended because of the potential for increased cardiotoxicity, but trastuzumab should be preferentially administered concurrently (not sequentially) with a non-anthracycline chemotherapy regimen
- Second-line treatment, for patients whose disease progresses during or after first-line treatment with *HER2*-targeted agents, is with ado-trastuzumab emtansine (T-DM1)
- T-DM1 can be used as third-line treatment if the cancer progresses during or after second-line treatment, in patients who have not previously received the drug

References

1. Ashford A. Chapter 16: Inherited genetic factors and breast cancer. In: Harris JR, Lippman, Morrow M, Osbourne CK, eds. Diseases of the Breast. 5th ed. Philadelphia, Pa: Lippincott Williams & Wilkins; 2014.

2. Oeffinger KC, Fontham ET, Etzioni R, Herzig A, Michaelson JS, Shih YC, Walter LC, Church TR, Flowers CR, LaMonte SJ, Wolf AM, DeSantis C, Lortet-Tieulent J, Andrews K, Manassaram-Baptiste D, Saslow D, Smith RA, Brawley OW, Wender R; American Cancer Society. Breast cancer screening for women at average risk: 2015 guideline update from the American Cancer Society. JAMA 2015;314(15):1599–1614.

3. [Guideline] Giordano SH, Temin S, Kirshner JJ, Chandarlapaty S, Crews JR, Davidson NE, et al. Systemic therapy for patients with advanced human epidermal growth factor receptor 2-positive breast cancer: American Society of Clinical Oncology clinical practice guideline. *J Clin Oncol*. 2014 Jul 1. 32 (19):2078-99. [Medline].

4. [Guideline] Denduluri N, Somerfield MR, Eisen A, Holloway JN, Hurria A, King TA, et al. Selection of Optimal Adjuvant Chemotherapy Regimens for Early Breast Cancer and Adjuvant Targeted Therapy for Human Epidermal Growth Factor Receptor 2-Positive Breast Cancers: An American Society of Clinical Oncology Guideline Adaptation of the Cancer Care Ontario Clinical Practice Guideline. *J Clin Oncol*. 2016 Apr 18

CHAPTER - 38

Leukemia

Introduction to Leukemia

The leukemias are heterogeneous hematologic malignancies characterized by unregulated proliferation of the blood-forming cells in the bone marrow. These immature proliferating leukemia cells (blasts) physically "crowd out" or inhibit normal cellular maturation in bone marrow, resulting in anemia, neutropenia, and thrombocytopenia. Leukemic blasts may also infiltrate a variety of tissues such as lymph nodes, skin, liver, spleen, kidney, testes, and the central nervous system.

It is a broad spectrum disease affecting bone, bone marrow, lymphoid system and spleen. They are divided into four groups:

1. Acute myeloblastic leukemia (AML)
2. Acute lymphoblastic leukemia (ALL)
3. Chronic myelocytic leukemia (CML)
4. Chronic lymphocytic leukemia (CLL)

Epidemiology [1]

Despite the low incidence rate, the acute leukemias are the most common malignancy in persons younger than 15 years of age, accounting for approximately 30% of all childhood malignancies.

- Haematological malignancies account for 5% of all cancers. Of these, CLL is the most common (90% are elderly)
- CLL occur at age 50-60 years, males are more prone.
- CML occurs at middle age 40-50 years.
- Acute leukemia's accounts for 4 cases per 100,000 populations.
- AML accounts for 75%, it rarely occurs in children.
- ALL predominantly occurs in children, with the peak incidence at the age of 3-5 years.

Etiology

It is not fully understood. Leukemia is thought to result from combination of factors that induce genetic mutations which allow cells to proliferate faster than normal cells.

General Risk factors:

1. Radiation causing mutations.
2. Exposure to chemical and cytotoxic drugs.
3. Viruses (T-cell leukemia).
4. Genetic factors (Down's syndrome).
5. Haematological disorders.

Risk factors for AML:

- Age/ Sub type (FAB- M_2)/ Chromosome status such as t (8; 21) or inversion (16).
- Among children male gender is more prone/ Platelets count less than $20*10^3/\mu L$
- Hepatomegaly/ Myelodysplastic syndrome.

Risk factors of ALL:

- Age, WBC count/ Cytogenic abnormalities.
- Ploidy, leukemic cell immunophenotype.
- Translocation of MLL gene occurs in infant ALL.
- Degree of initial response to therapy
- Translocation of chromosome 12&21 (TEL-AML 1 fusion).

Risk factors of CML:

- Older age/ Splenomegaly/ High percent blasts in blood/ High platelet count.

Risk factors of CLL:

- Lymphocytosis with accompanying anemia (Hb<11g/dL).
- Thrombocytopenia (platelets $<100*10^3/\mu L$, 110 g/L)/ ZAP-70 mutations.

Pathophysiology

Haematopoiesisis defined as the development and maturation of blood cells and their precursors. It occurs in liver, spleen and bone marrow in utero haematopoiesis. After birth occurs in bone marrow.

Pathogenesis of acute myeloid leukemia

In AML a single myeloblast genetic changes which freeze the cell in its immature state and prevent differentiation. When such a differentiation arrest is combined with other mutations which disrupt genes controlling proliferation, the result is uncontrolled growth of an immature clone of cells, leading to AML.

The growth of leukemic clone cells, which tends to displace or interfere with the development of normal cells in the bone marrow. This leads to neutropenia, anemia and thrombocytopenia.

Pathogenesis of acute lymphoid leukemia

Damage to DNA leads to uncontrolled cellular growth and spread in the body. Malignant neoplastic proliferation and accumulation of immature and nonfunctional lymphoid line of blood cells in the bone marrow.

Pathogenesis of chronic myelogenous leukemia

Philadelphia (Ph) chromosome translocations of the genetic material between long arms of chromosomes 9 and 22. Results in apposition of BCR gene (chromosome-22) and ABL gene(chromosome-9). Leads to overactivity of tyrosine kinase which encodes a protein fusion. So there is Uncontrolled growth characteristic of leukemia cells.

Pathogenesis of chronic lymphoid leukemia

- There is accumulation of genetic abnormalities in more mature lymphoid B-cells which leads to clonal division of neoplastic B lymphocytes within lymph nodes. This is a slow process of neoplastic cell division and the patients are most commonly aymptomatic at initial presentation. With continued cell division, b-cell spill over into the peripheral blood.
- Multifactorial causes with unclear mechanisms are responsible for this. At this stage the patient will have weight loss, malaise, fever, chills, night sweats.
- Now B-cells excessively proliferate and are non-functional which decrease body's ability to produce antibodies for immune response. At this stage it is presented in the patient as Lymphocytosis and hypogammaglobulinemia. Because of this there is risk for infection. In the next stage-Neoplastic B-cells fail to die and continue to divide within lymph nodes over time. It is presented as lymphadenopathy.
- Neoplastic B cell precursors infiltrate the spleen and the bone marrow, which is presented in the patient as spleenomegaly. In spleen sequestration of RBC's happen causing decrease in RBC's and presenting as anaemia in the patient.
- A small % of CLL patients undergo transformation, in which their disease evolves into diffuse age B-cell lymphoma. There is abundance of B-cell precursors in circulation; there is decrease in platelets-thrombocytopenia. The patient has easy bleeding tendencies.

Cell of origin

CLL is characterized by small, relatively incompetent B-lymphocytes that accumulate in blood and bone marrow over time. The exact cell of origin is controversial but has been described as an antigen activated B- lymphocyte.

Clinical course:

- Low risk disease is asymptomatic and median survival exceeds to 10 years.
- Intermediate is associated with lymphadenopathy and has median survival about 7 years.
- High risk patients with anemia has median survival of 3 yrs.

Classification (French-American-British)

Morphologic "FAB" classification of AML:

MO = Acute myeloblastic leukemia without maturation.

M1= Acute myeloblstic leukemia with minimal maturation.

M2 = Acute myeloblastic with maturation.

M3 = Acute promyeloblastic leukemia.

M4 = Acute myelomonocytic leukemia.

M5a = Acute monoblastic leukemia, poorly differentiated.

M5b = Acute monoblastic leukemia, well differentiated.

M6 = Acute erythroleukemia.

M7 = Acute megakaryoblastic leukemia.

FAB classification of ALL

Subtype	Cell of origin
L1	Early pre-B cell, Pre-B cell, B cell, T cell.
L2	Early pre-B cell, Pre-B cell, B-cell, T-cell.
L3	B-cell

Clinical manifestations and features

Symptoms of AML:

AML is due to translocation of genetic material between chromosome 15 and 17 leading to disseminated intravascular coagulation (DIC).

Weakness, malaise, bleeding, weight loss, lymphadenopathy, massive hepatosplenomegaly, bone pain , hypertrophy,chloromas. Less commomlyhypermetabolism, hyperuricaemia.

Symptoms of ALL:
- Fever, fatigue pallor, malaise, bleeding, weight loss.
- Neutropenic patients often febrile and susceptible to infections.
- Patients with thrombocytopenia present with petechiae,bruising,ecchymosis.
- Adenopathy,hepatomegaly,splenomegaly.

Symptoms of CML:
- Malaise, night sweats, enlarged spleen, bone pain.
- Hepatomegaly, neutropenia, thrombocytopenia.

Symptoms of CLL:
- Lymphadenopathy,fatigue, chills, bleeding.

- Chronic infections owing to immature lymphocyte.
- Organomegaly mainly spleenomegaly and hepatomegaly.
- Decreased serum gammaglobulin leading to bacterial and viral infections.

Diagnosis with Algorithm [2]

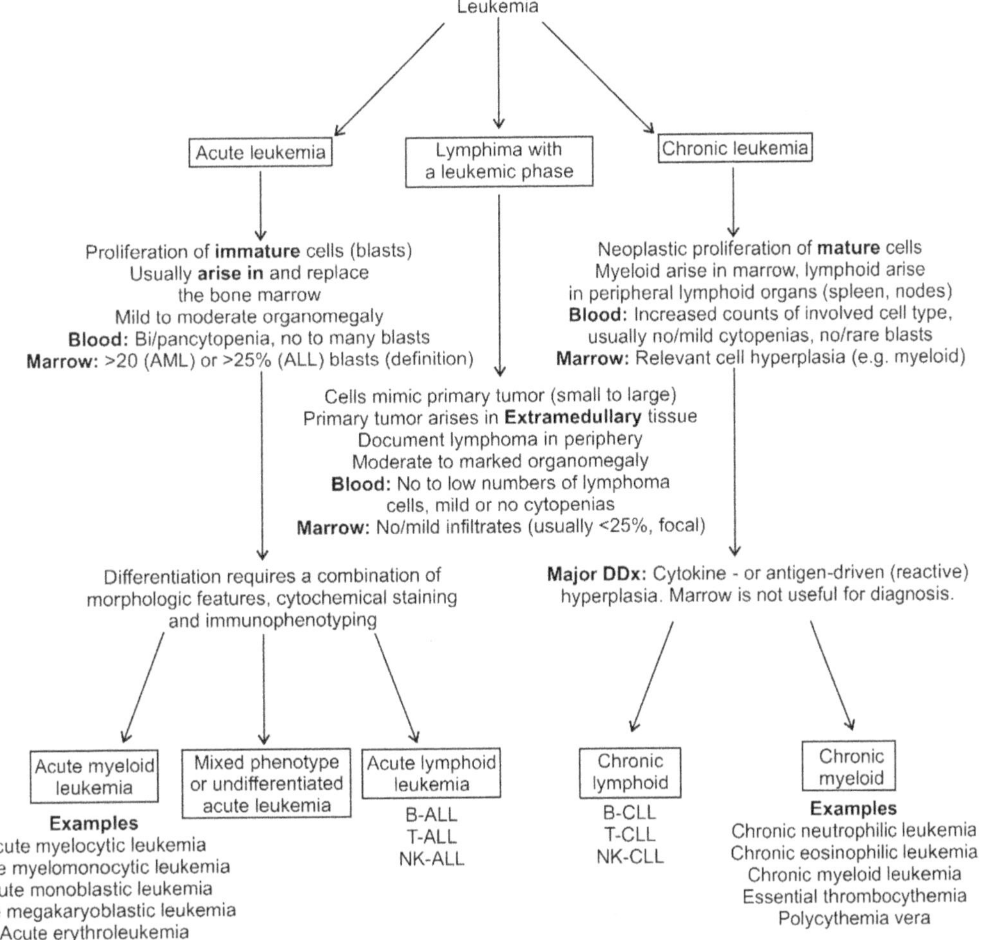

Fig. 38.1 Algorithm for the diagnosis of Leukemia.

Source: http://eclinpath.com/hematology/leukemia/leukemia-types/leukemia-aligorithm-3/

- Lab tests: CBP, RBC (Normocytic, Normochromic)
- Blood count – 250,000 cells/cubic mm.
- Increased uric acid levels (uricemia).
- Electrolytes are disturbed K^+ and P^+ increased, Ca^{+2} decreased.
- Increased prothrombintime, thromboplastin time, hypofibronemia.

- Flow cytometric analysis, bone marrow aspiration.
- Leukocytosis (WBC >100 × 10^4/μL).
- Presence of blasts with hypercellularity in bonemarrow.
- Hypo gamma globulinemia in CLL patients.

Management

Goal of therapy:

- Prophylaxis treatment of CNS by the physician.
- Improve quality of life.
- Stop the progression of disease.

Management of ALL divided into 3 phases.

1. Remission induction (control): Remission is defined as the absence of all clinical & microscopic signs of leukemia, less than 5% of blast cells. Goals include
   - Control of over proliferation.
   - Allow the normal cells to mature.
   - Cut down the blast cells.
2. Intensification (consolidation): goal of intensification is to administer dose-intensive chemotherapy to further reduce the burden of residual leukemic cells.
3. Maintenance (continuation): purpose is to further eliminate leukemic cells and produce enduring regimen.

Table 38.1 Pharmacological regimen for the management of ALL.

Remission (4 weeks)	Dose	Route	Regimen
Vincristine	1.5 mg/m^2	IV	Weekly for 4 weeks
Prednisolone	40 mg/m^2	Oral	Daily for 4 weeks
L-Asparginase	6000 μ/m^2	IM	3* for 3 weeks
Daunorubicin	45 mg/m^2	IV	Daily for 2 days
Intensification (1 week)			
Vincristine	1.5mg/m^2	IV	1 dose
Etoposide	100mg/m^2	IV	Daily for 5 days
Cytarabine	100mg/m^2	IV	BD, daily for 5 days
Thioguanine	80mg/m^2	Oral	Daily for 5 days
Maintenance Therapy (2 YRS)			
Methotrexate	20mg/m^2	Oral	Weekly
6.Mercaptopurine	75mg/m^2	Oral	Daily
Prednisolone	40mg/m^2	Oral	5days/month
Vincristine	1.5mg/m^2	IV	Monthly
CNS prophylaxsis (3 weeks)			
Cranial irradiation	24 Gy	-	-
Methotrexate	10mg/m^2	Intrathecal	Weekly for 3 weeks

Treatment for Pediatric ALL:

1. Induction (1 month):
   - Intrathecalcytarbine ,oral.
   - Prednisolone, 40mg/m^2, OD, for 28 days.
   - Intathecalmethotrexate , weekly 2-4 doses.
   - Vincristine.

2. Consolidation (1 month)
   - Mercaptopurine.
   - Vincristine.
   - Methotrexate weekly, 1-3 doses.

3. Maintenance (2 months)
   - Methotrexate 20 mg/m^2, orally.
   - Mercaptopurine,orally,daily for 49 days.
   - Vincristine, 1.5mg/m^2
   - Dexamethasone, 6mg/m^2 per day orally on days 0-1 and 28-32.

4. Delayed Intensification (2 months)
   - Thioguanine, 60mg/m^2 orally on 28-41 days.
   - Mtx-intrathecal,
   - Vincristine, 1.5mg/m^2 iv for 3 doses.
   - Doxorubicin, 25mg/m^2 iv on 0, 7, 14 days.
   - Cytarabine, 75mg/m^2 iv.

5. Maintenance (12 weeks cycle)
   - MTX, 20mg/m^2 orally
   - Vincristine 1.5mg/m^2 iv.
   - Mercaptopurine, 75mg/m^2 orally.
   - Vincristine 1.5mg/^{m}2 iv.
   - Dexamethasone, 6mg/m^2 orally.

Management of AML

Aim: Blast in bone marrow with new population cells. Blast cells in blood circulation have to be killed. Management includes Remission induction and maintenance.

Regimen for Remission induction:

Starts at 3 & 7 days.

- Cytarabine (1-7 days)
- Daunorubicin (for 3 days)

If response is better then go with maintenance therapy.

Maintenance:

- L-Asparginase 100mg/m^2/day (5 days, continuous infusion)

- Mitoxantrone, it is a standard arm.
- L-Asparginase 400 mg/ m^2/day (intermediate arm)
- Mitoxantrone 3g/m^2/2 days over 3 hours.

Again response of patient is taken, if not responding go with HSCT.

Haemopoeitic stem cell therapy (HSCT):

(a) **Allogenic Haemopoeitic stem cell therapy (HSCT):** it is used in pediatric AML in first complete remission. Hematopoiesis is restored by the infusion of stem cells harvested from an HLA compatible donor, rescuing the patient from consequences of total aplasia.

(b) **Autologous Haemopoeitic stem cell therapy (HSCT):** Since the majority of the patients lack a HLA identical donor, patients own bone marrow, obtained while in CR, is used as a source of hematopoietic regeneration.

AML in elderly: older patients are not as tolerant as younger patients. Anthracycline and cytarabine has been used.

Treatment approach for the management of AML patients

1. **Favourable risk cytogenetics:** Standard dose cytarabine 100-200 mg/m^2 continuous infusion x 7 days with Idarubicin 12mg/m^2 or Daunorubicin 60-90mg/m^2 x 3 days.

   or

   Standard dose cytarabine 200 mg/m^2 continuous infusion x 7 days with Daunorubicin 60mg/m^2 x 3 days and Gemtizumab 3mg/m2 on day 1.

2. **Intermediate –risk cytogenetics and CD33+:** Standard dose cytarabine 200 mg/m^2 continuous infusion x 7 days with Daunorubicin 60mg/m^2 x 3 days and Gemtizumab 3mg/m2 on day 1.

   or

   Standard dose cytarabine 200 mg/m^2 continuous infusion x 7 days with Daunorubicin 60mg/m^2 x 3 days and oral Midastaurin 50mg every 12 hours, days 8-21.

3. **Therapy related AML other than Core binding factor acute myelogenous leukemia (CBF-AML):** Standard dose cytarabine 100-200 mg/m^2 continuous infusion x 7 days with Idarubicin 12mg/m^2 or Daunorubicin 60-90mg/m^2 x 3 days.

   or

   Dual drug liposomal encapsulation of Daunorubicin 44mg/m2 and cytarabine 100mg/m2 IV over 90min on days 1, 3, and 5 x 1 cycle.

4. **Other recommended regimens for intermediate or poor risk disease:** High dose cytarabine 2 g/m2 every 12 hours X 6 days or 3 g/m2 every 12h x 4 days with idarubicin 12mg/m2 or Daunorubicin 60mg/m2 x 3 days.

   or

   Fludarabine 30mg/m^2 IV days 2-6, High dose cytarabine 2 g/m^2 over 4 hours starting 4 hours after fludarabine on days 2-6, idarubicin 8 mg/m2 IV days 4-6, and G=CSF SC days 1-7.

Management of CML:

Goal of treatment:
- Primary goal is to eradicate the Ph-positive clones.
- To achieve hematologic complete remission.
- To normalize peripheral blood.

Drugs:
1. Imatinib = 400-800 mg, orally/day.
2. Interferonalfa = IM or subcutaneously, daily.

Algorithm for therapy in newly diagnosed CML patient

- **If patient** is an ideal transplant candidate, then proceed for allogenic stem cell transplant. Observe for molecular remission. If it is not observed then therapy started with Imatinib or IFN or cytarabine.
- If the patient is not an ideal candidate for transplantation, drug therapy is initiated. Imatinib 400mg daily is initiated. After 3 months evaluation for hematologic remission is done. If remission is observed, continue with imatinib for another 9-12 months and then observed and evaluated again. If remission is not observed, imatinib dose is increased to 600-800mg/d for 9 months. If still there is no remission, IFN or cytarabine therapy is initiated.

Management of CLL

Goal of treatment:
- To provide palliation of symptoms.
- To improve overall survival. Reduction in tumor burden.
- Elimination of lymphoblasts in bone marrow.
- Normalisation of peripheral blood count.

Any one of the following criteria should be met to initiate CLL therapy

- Progressive marrow failure, hemoglobin <10 gm/dL or platelet count of <100 × 10^9/L
- Massive (≥6 cm below the left costal margin) or progressive or symptomatic splenomegaly
- Massive (≥10 cm in longest diameter) or progressive or symptomatic lymphadenopathy
- Progressive lymphocytosis with an increase of ≥50% over a 2-month period or lymphocyte doubling time of <6 months
- Autoimmune complications of CLL, that are poorly responsive to corticosteroids
- Symptomatic extranodal involvement (e.g., skin, kidney, lung, spine)
- Disease-related symptoms, including:
  - Unintentional weight loss of ≥10% within the previous 6 months
  - Significant fatigue

o Fever ≥38 °C for 2 or more weeks without evidence of infection
o Night sweats for ≥1 month without evidence of infection

Drugs to be initiated

1. Alemutuzumab = Sc, 3mg/day as 2 hrs infusion and dose increased to 10 mg/day according to response.
2. Chlorambucil = 4-10 mg, orally or iv, daily.
3. Fludarabine = 20 mg/m^2, iv, (daily for 5 days).
4. Rituximab = dose ranges upon patient tolerance.

If no progress then go with HSCT. We can go with single or combination therapy.

Combination therapy

Fludarabine + Cyclophosphamide + Rituximab, improves CR rates compared with fludarabine alone.

Some of the more commonly used treatments include:

- Ibrutinib (Imbruvica), alone or with Rituximab (Rituxan)
- Acalabrutinib (Calquence), alone or with Obinutuzumab (Gazyva)
- Venetoclax (Venclexta) and Obinutuzumab
- Venetoclax alone, or with Rituximab
- Bendamustine and Rituximab (or another monoclonal antibody)
- High-dose Prednisone and Rituximab
- FCR: Fludarabine, Cyclophosphamide, and Rituximab
- PCR: Pentostatin, Cyclophosphamide, and Rituximab
- Chlorambucil and Rituximab (or another monoclonal antibody)
- Obinutuzumab
- Ibrutinib and Obinutuzumab
- Alemtuzumab (Campath), alone or with Rituximab

Treatment of relapsed leukemia

Relapse is the recurrence of leukemic cells at any site after remission has been achieved. Most relapse occurs during treatment or within 2 years of its completion. Bone marrow is the most frequent site of relapse.

- Conventional chemotherapy.
- Allogenic HSCT is the therapy of choice.
- For patients without an HLA- matched sibling, matched unrelated bone marrow or cord blood transplantation may be a reasonable alternative.
- Combination of myeloblative high dose chemotherapy and the graft versus leukemia effect is thought to offer the best chance of survival.

Complications of treatment

- **Tumor lysis syndrome**: It is due to metabolic abnormalities resulting from death of blast cells and release of purines, pyrimidines and intracellular potassium and phosphorous. Uric acid the breakdown product of purines is poorly soluble in plasma and urine. Deposition of uric acid and calcium phosphate crystals in renal tubules lead to acute renal failure.
- **Infection:** it is the cause of death in acute leukemia patients. Fever in a neutropenic patient is a medical urgency. Cefipime is commonly used.
- Secondary malignancies: especially in children. A number of intrinsic and extrinsic factors all contribute to risk of secondary infections. The normal host defense is broken down, damage to mucous membrane mainly in GIT occurs with chemotherapy and radiotherapy .skin infections also occur.

Pathogens commonly causing infections:

Gram negative bacteria	=	Streptococcus, Staphylococcus.
Fungi	=	Candida, Aspergillus.
Protozoa	=	Pneumocytis carinii.
Virus	=	Herpes simplex, Hepatitis.

Prophylactic anti infectives:

Gram negative bacteria	-	Ciproflaxacin.
Candidiasis	-	Nystatin, Fluconazole, Itraconazole.
Herpes simplex	-	Aciclovir.
Pneumocytiscarinii	-	Co-trimoxazole.

Preventive measures:

1. Oral hygiene:
   - Use of mouth washes.
   - Prophylactic anti fungal therapy is given.
   - Attention must be paid to care of dentures.
2. Gut decontamination:
   - Neomycin sulphate, Nystatin, Amphotericin.
   - To reduce burden of potentially pathogenic organisms.
3. Growth factors:
   - G-CSF, given subcutaneously or iv infusion, may reduce the duration of neutropenia upto 7 days.
4. Protective isolation:
   - High efficiency particulate air (HEPA) filtration have been used to reduce infection rates.

References

1. Ries LAG, Eisner MP, Kosary CL, et al. SEER Cancer Statistics Review, 1975–2003. Bethesda, MD: National Cancer Institute. 2006, *http://seer.cancer.gov/csr/1975_2003/*.

2. Macimilian Fleischemarn, et al., (2021). Management of Acute mycloid leukemia: Current Treatment options and future perspectives. Cancers (Basel). Nov. 13(22).

3. Daniel A., Pollyea MD, MS Dale Bixby. 2021, NCCN guidelines insights: Acute Myeloid Leukemia, verion 2021. Vol. 19; Issue 1.

CHAPTER - 39

Surgical Prophylaxis

It is defined as the administration of antibiotics before surgery to prevent surgical site infection.

Surgical Site Infection

- Infections developing at the site of invasive surgical procedure are referred as surgical site infections.
- Surgical site infections occur when pathogenic microorganisms contaminate a surgical wound.
- Surgical site infections are classified as either incisional or involving an organ or space.

Risk Factors for SSIs

- Risk factors for SSIs can be categorized as modifiable (example: *staphylococcus aureus* colonization, weight) and non-modifiable (example: age, sex).
- Risk factors can be divided into host and peri-operative factors which can be further divided into pre-operative, intra-operative and post operative factors.

The following variables were associated with risk of SSI:
- Duration of antibiotic prophylaxis.
- Age
- Elevated ASA score
- Prolonged pre operative hospital stay
- Environment: Moisture and heat
- Malnutrition
- Emergency surgery
- Duration of operation: Prolonged duration increases risk of SSI`S
- Sex

Goals of Antibiotic Prophylaxis

- Reduce the incidence of surgical site infection
- Minimize the effect on the patient`s normal bacterial flora
- Cost effectiveness

Principles of Surgical Prophylaxis

- Prevent SSI – related morbidity and mortality
- Reduce the duration and cost of health care
- Prevent surgical site infection

Table 39.1 ASA Score of patient physical status (American Society of Anesthesiology) [1].

ASA Score	Physical status
1	A normal healthy patient
2	A patient with mild systemic disease.
3	A patient a severe systemic disease that is not incapacitating.
4	Incapacitating systemic disease that is a constant threat to life.
5	Not expected to survive 24 hours with or without operation.

Patient and operative risk factors for SSI'S

➤ **Patient risk factors:** Advanced age, Malnutrition, Obesity, Concurrent infection
➤ Diabetes mellitus, Liver impairment, Renal impairment, Blood transfusion, SmOking
➤ **Operative factors:** Tissue ischaemia, Lack of homeostasis, Tissue damage, Presence of necrotic tissue, Presence of foreign bodies

Surgical site infection risk depends upon a number of patient factors including pre -existing medical conditions, amount and type of resident skin bacteria, perioperative glucose levels, core body temperature fluctuations and preoperative, intra-operative and post operative care. Therefore it is difficult to predict which wounds become infected.

Efficacy of antibiotic prophylaxis: antibiotic prophylaxis was associated with decreased risk of SSI`s, while timing of administration - preoperatively Vs intraoperatively - had no effect on risk.

Surgical Wound Classification

- **Class I/clean:** An infected operative wound in which no inflammation is seen. Clean wounds are primarily closed.
- **Class II/clean contaminated:** Wounds include entry into the oropharyngeal cavity, respiratory, alimentary, urinary tracts under controlled conditions. Major break in a sterile technique is encountered.
- **Class III/contaminated:** Open, fresh, accidental wounds. Acute inflammation is seen.
- **Class IV/Dirty:** Established infection, traumatic wound with retained devitalized tissue.

Table 39.2 Surgical wound classification.

Classification	Infection rate	Pre-operative antibiotics	No pre-operative antibiotics	Antibiotics
Clean	1-3%	5.1	0.8	Not indicated
Clean – contaminated	5-8%	10.1	1.3	Prophylactic antibiotics
Contaminated	20-25%	21.9	10.2	Prophylactic antibiotics
Dirty	30-40%	N/A	N/A	Therapeutic antibiotics

Bacteriology: The micro organisms may present on the patient skin /instruments used in surgery.

Most common organisms in SSI`s

Nose: S.aureus, Pneumococcus, Meningococcus

Skin: S.aureus, S.epidermidis

Mouth/pharynx: Streptococci, Pneumococcus, E.coli

Urinary tract: E.coli, Proteus species

GI tract/colon: E.coli, Klebsiella, Clostridia

Vagina: Streptococci, E.coli, Staphylococcus species

Upper respiratory tract: Pneumococcus, H.influenzea

Common antibiotic selection

- Cefazolin/cefotetan/cefoxitin
- Vancomycin
- Clindamycin+aminoglycoside/aztreonum
- Vancomycin (only G+coverage) can add gentamicin/aztreonum/fluroquinolone to broaden coverage

Antibiotic administration

- Antibiotic prophylaxis for surgery is given within one hour prior to incision.
- Prophylaxis should not exceed beyond 24 hours.
- Postoperative doses of IV antibiotics of upto 24 hours are only required in defined circumstances such as some cardiac and vascular surgeries.

Antimicrobial selection

- First generation cephalosporin antibiotics are the preferred choice.

- Antianerobic cephalosporins are appropriate choices when broad spectrum anerobic and gram negative bacteria are desired.
- Vancomycin may be considered in some cases such as involving implantation of prosthetic device.
- The most commonly used drug is cefazolin.
- Vancomycin is given in the case of documental allergy to cephalosporins.

Table 39.3 Choice of antibiotics based on spectrum.

Antibiotic	Dose	Spectrum
Cefazolin	1-2 g	gram+ve and gram-ve bacteria
Cefoxitin	1-2 g	Broad spectrum
Vancomycin	1 g	G+ve bacteria
Clindamycin+gentamycin	600mg +1.5mg/kg	gram+ve, gram-ve bacteria

Table 39.4 Prophylactic regimens for surgeries: [2, 3].

Type of surgery	Likely pathogens	Recommended regimen
GI Surgery		
Gastroduodenal and oesophageal surgery	Enteric G-ve bacilli, G+ve cocci, oral anaerobes	Cefazolin 1g IV 15 to 30 min before surgery
Appendectomy	Enteric G-ve bacilli, anaerobes, s.aureus	Cefazolin or cefoxitin 1g
Colorectal		Metronidazole 500mg IV + cefazolin 2g IV or
Biliary surgery	Enteric G-ve bacilli, enterococcus anaerobes	Gentamycin 5mg/kg/IV or Cefoxitin 2g IV
	S.aureus, G-ve bacilli	Cefazolin 2g IV
Urogenital		
Transrectal biopsy	S.aureus, G-ve bacilli, anaerobes	Gentamycin + Metronidazole
Uretoscopy,lithotripsy, prostate resection	E.coli	Ciprofloxacin 500mg orally or trimethoprim sulfamethoxazole
Gynecological surgery		Cefazolin 2g
Cesarean section		Cefazolin 2g
Hysterectomy	S.aureus, Streptococci, Enterococci	
	Enteric G-ve bacilli, Streptococci, Enterococcus	

Table 39.5 Prophylactic regimens for surgeries.

Type of surgery	Likely pathogens	Recommended regimen
Head and neck surgery		
Maxillofacial surgery	S. aureus, streptococcus, anaerobes	Cefazolin 2g/ clindamycin 600mg
Head and neck cancer resection	S.aureus, streptococcus, anaerobes	Clindamycin 600 mg
Cardiothoracic surgery	S.aureus, coryne bacterium	
Cardiac surgery		Cefazolin 2g IV every 8 hrs upto 2 doses
Thoracic surgery	S.aureus, S.epidermidis, G-ve bacilli	Cefuroxime 750 mg IV
Vascular surgery		Cefazolin
Abdominal aortal lower extremity vascular surgery	S.aureus, G-ve bacilli, enterococcus	
Neuro surgery		
CSF shunt and craniotomy		Cefazolin 30mg/kg
Spinal surgery	S.aureus, S.epidermidiss	Cefazolin 1g
Orthopedics	S.aureus, S.epidermidis	
Joint replacement surgery		Cefazolin 1g
Closed fracture	primarily staphylococci	Cefazolin
	Staphylococcus aureus	

References

1. Mak PH, Campbell RC et al. The ASA physical status classification: inter-observer consistency. Anaesth Intensive Care 2002;30:633-40
2. American College of Surgeons' proposed guidelines for care of pediatric surgical patients. Journal of the American College of Surgeons, 2014;218:479-48.
3. https://www.asahq.org/standards-and-guidelines/asa-physical-status-classification-system

CHAPTER - 40

Antimicrobial Regimen Selection

Antimicrobials: Antimicrobials are drugs that destroy microbes, prevent their multiplication or growth or prevent their pathogenic action.

Introduction: Choosing an antimicrobial to treat an infection is far more complicated than matching a drug to a known or suspected pathogen.

It is often a systematic approach which takes into account numerous patient and drug related factors.

Antimicrobials are used in three distinct ways:

1. **Empiric therapy:** This is often referred to as Broad spectrum therapy. It covers all the likely pathogens as the infecting organisms have not yet been identified.

2. **Definitive therapy:** Once the infecting organism has been identified, therapy becomes definitive. Antimicrobial is chosen that specifically targets the microorganism identified.

3. **Prophylactic therapy:** Prevent an infection or its re-occurrence.

Consequences of not using the systemic approach: Use of most expensive agents, Potentially more toxic agents, Wide spread resistance, Difficult to treat super- infections, Use for self-limited clinical conditions that are most likely viral in origin.

Systemic approach for selection of Antimicrobials

1. Confirm the presence of infection: Signs and symptoms, Predisposing factor, Careful history and physical exam
2. Identification of the pathogen: Collection of infected material, Stains, Serologies, Culture and sensitivity
3. Selection of presumptive therapy: Host factors, Drug factor
4. Monitor therapeutic response: Clinical assessment, Laboratory/diagnostic tests
5. Assessment of therapeutic failure

Confirm the presence of infection

Infections can be identified by the following: Fever, Elevated WBC count; Swelling, redness, purulent drainage from a visible site

WBC count

Normal: 4000-10000 cells/mm^3

Bacterial infections: Elevated granulocyte count often with immature forms

Neutropenia: low leukocyte counts

Tuberculosis and viral or fungal infections: Lymphocytosis

Identification of the pathogens

- Attempts should be made to microbiologically identify the pathogen.
- Infected body materials (urine, blood) must be sampled, if all possible and practical before the initiation of antimicrobial therapy.
- Gram stain may be helpful for quick detection of potential organisms causing the infection.
- Practitioner related to antimicrobial therapy the organism and its susceptibilities to antimicrobials.
- Once the organism is identified the susceptibility to various antimicrobials is reported as susceptible (S), intermediate (I), resistant (R). This is determined by interpretation of MIC (Minimum Inhibitory Concentration).

Selection of presumptive therapy

Drug factors: Integration of both Pharmacokinetics and pharmacodynamic properties

Aminoglycosides: Concentration dependent effect

Beta lactams: Time dependent bactericidal effects

Hydrophilicity/hydrophobicity: Metronidazole, ampicillin, vancomycin etc

Effective dosing regimens require serum drug concentration to exceed the MIC for at least 40% to 50% of the drug interval.

Host factors

- Drug allergens
- Site of infection
- Age: Renal and hepatic functions varies with age and may affect a patient's ability to eliminate a drug. Aminoglycosides causes renal toxicity. Adults are at a greater risk of meningitis caused by Listeria species.
- Pregnancy: During pregnancy the fetus is at risk for drug teratogenicity and the pharmacokinetic disposition of certain drugs may be altered. Penicillins, cephalosporins and erythromycin appear safe in pregnancy.
- Genetic or metabolic abnormalities: Inherited or acquired metabolic abnormalities may influence

- Antimicrobial therapy: Patients with peripheral vascular disease may have impaired absorption of intramuscularly administered drugs.
- Concomitant drug therapy: It influences the selection of appropriate drug therapy, the dosage and necessary monitoring.
- Underlying disease status: Immunosuppressive diseases; Trauma, burns and surgery; Diabetes mellitus; Chronic lung disease

Combination antimicrobial therapy [1]

Combinations of antimicrobials are generally used to broaden the spectrum of coverage of empiric therapy to achieve synergistic activity against the infection and prevent the emergence of resistance.

Synergism: Penicillins+ Streptomycin /Gentamycin

Disadvantages of combination therapy

- Increased cost, Greater risk of drug toxicity, Super infection with even more resistant bacteria, Result in antagonistic effects
  Ex: Cefoxitin+ Imipenem: They induce   beta lactamases, so more rapid inactivation of penicillins when used together

Monitoring therapeutic response

Patient monitoring should include many of the same parameters used to diagnose the infection.
- The WBC count and temperature should start to normalize
- Radiologic improvement
- Antimicrobials serum concentration should be monitored

Patients not responding to an appropriate treatment in about 2-3 days should be revaluated to ensure that infection is the correct diagnosis, therapeutic drug concentrations are being achieved, and resistance has not developed.

Failure of antimicrobial therapy: Lack of respond over 2-3 days; Drug interaction; Laboratory error; Failure due to drug selection, dosage/route of administration; Mal absorption; Penetration problems; Failure caused by host factors

Conclusion: Optimal use of antimicrobial agents requires consideration of a number of important factors that may influence the choice of an appropriate agent and that determine the most effective dose and route of administration. The goal of therapy is always to maximize efficacy while limiting patients harm.

References

1. Grace C. Lee David S. Burgess Chapter 105: Antimicroial Regimen Selection. Pharmacotherapy A pathophysiologic approach, 10 e.

CHAPTER - 41

Tuberculosis

Introduction to Tuberculosis (TB)

Tuberculosis (TB) is a communicable infectious disease caused by *Mycobacterium tuberculosis*. It can produce silent, latent infection as well as progressive, active disease. Globally, 2 billion people are infected and 2 million to 3 million people die from TB each year.

Tuberculosis is a communicable infectious disease caused by "Mycobacterium tuberculosis". It is a chronic specific inflammatory infectious disease caused by Mycobacterium tuberculosis in humans. The bacteria usually attack the lungs, but TB bacteria can attack any part of the body such as kidney, spine and brain.

There are two conditions of TB- they are latent TB and active TB

Tuberculosis can produce atypical signs and symptoms in infants, the elderly and immunocompromised hosts and it can progress rapidly in these patients--Coinfection with HIV accelerates the progression of both diseases requiring rapid diagnosis and treatment of both diseases.

Epidemiology

Globally, tuberculosis (TB) is the leading cause of death by an infectious disease. In 2018, an estimated 10 million incident TB cases and 1.5 million TB deaths occurred, reductions of 2% and 5%, respectively, from 2017.

Etiology

Causative organism: "Mycobacterium tuberculosis"

M.tuberculosis complex: *M.tuberculosis, M.bovis, M.africanum*

M.Tuberculosis is an aerobic, non spore forming bacillus that resists decolourization.by acid alcohol after staining with basic fuchsin.

- Mycobacterium other than tuberculosis can cause pulmonary disease resembling TB. Strains which effects the humans is 'Hominis'. It thrives in environments where the oxygen tension is relatively high, such as spices of the lungs and the renal parenchyma.

Incubation Period

The incubation period from infection to primary lesions ranges from 2 to10 weeks. Latent infection may persist for life time.

Mode of Transmission

Mycobacterium tuberculosis is transmitted from person by coughing or sneezing, close contacts of TB patients are most to become infected. It is difficult to treat because bacilli divide once in 1-2 days and when the mycobacterium enters into our body it forms caseation sheath. Mycobacterium tuberculae are viable even outside environment for some time. They are not transmitted on inanimate object such as dishes, clothing, bedding; organisms deposited on skin or intact mucosa do not invade tissue.

Factors influencing transmission include –
- Number of organisms in air.
- Concentration of organisms in air.
- Length of time of exposure to contaminated air.
- Immune status of the exposed individual.

Risk Factors

- Patient with latent TB
- Close contact of patients with TB
- Diabetes mellitus: diabetes increases the risk of treatment failure and death combined, death and relapse in patient swith TB. DM has been associated with increased rates of TB, which may be due to blunted T cell mediated immune response.
- Low body weight
- Some medical treatments including corticosteroids or certain medications used for autoimmune diseases
- Alcoholism, Migration from a country with a high number of cases, Diseases that weakens immune system like HIV, crowded living conditions, low socioeconomic status

Pathophysiology

Environmenatal factors like microbial virulence, drug resistance; non-microbial exposure intensity act as risk factors for Mycobacterium Tuberculosis (M.Tb). host factors like genetic, epigenetic, primary immunodeficinecies non genetic like age, immunosuppression also act as risk factors. Because of the exposure to M.Tb the person gets infected. After the treatment, there is clearance of infection or it can proceed to latent TB infection in immunocompromised patients. Based on the primary symptoms the patient is categorized as pulmoanary TB or extrapulmonary TB.

Microorganism enters into our body and Ag-Ab reaction occurs. There is activation of complement system Polymonphonuclear Leukocytes (PMNL) (WBC/PMNL will be activated). Later T-cells and B-cells are activated (CD4, CD8, B-cells). In 2-3 days the microorganism undergoes structural changes as a result of immune mechanism. The modified macrophages resemble epithelial cells called as epithelioid cells. Then epithelioid cells in time aggregate into tight clusters or granulomas. Some constituents of mycobacterial cell wall play a role in formation of granuloma. Some macrophages unable to destroy tubercle bacilli fuse together and form multinucleated giant cells. Around the cluster of epithelioid cells and few giant cells a zone of lymphocytes and plasma cells is formed which is further surrounded by fibroblasts, the lesions at this stage is called hard tubercle. Within 10-14 days caseation sheath is developed which has high lipid content leading to formation of soft tubercle, slowly necrosis will ensue. Caseaous material may undergo liquefaction and extend into surrounding soft tissue. By this stage treatment will be started.

Primary infection

It results from the inhalation of airbrone droplets that contain M.tuberculosis. These particles called droplet nuclei reach the alveolar surface. The organisms are then ingested by macrophages at alveoli. If macrophages inhibit/kill organism, infection is aborted. If not, organisms multiply and macrophages rupture releasing the bacilli which spread to lymph nodes, in hilar mediostinal, retroperitoneal areas. Most commonly, post apical regions of lungs are affected because of high oxygen content. In case of intra vascular dissemination tissues and organs are affected. After 3 weeks of infection by antigen, T-cells are activated and simulate macrophages to become bactericidal that surround the necrotic region in the form of granulomas. At the same time hypersensitivity reactions occur because at activation of T-cells. Over 1-3 months, activated T-cells reach adequate number and shown by a positive skin test, some show radiographic evidence of granulomas.

Re-activation disease

Apices of lungs are most for reactivation due to high oxygen content and 10% patients show reactivation. Organisms within the granulomas emerge and multiply extracellularly, inflammatory responses producing caseating granulomas which will liquify and spread the infection locally and from a hole or cavity in lungs. Some of the necrotic material is coughed out producing droplet nuclei. Bacterial counts are as high as 10^8/ml of cavitary fluid.

Extrapulmonary and Miliary Tuberculosis

Caseating granulomas at extrapulmonary sites can undergo liquefaction, releasing tubercle bacilli and causing symptomatic disease. Extrapulmonary TB without concurrent pulmonary disease is uncommon in normal hosts but more common in HIV-infected patients. Lymphatic and pleural diseases are the most common forms of extrapulmonary TB, followed by bone, joint, genitourinary, meningeal, and other forms. Left untreated, these forms will spread to other organs and may result in death. Occasionally, a massive inoculum of organisms enters the bloodstream, causing a widely disseminated form of the disease known as miliary TB. Miliary TB is a medical emergency requiring immediate treatment.

Clinical Manifestations and Features

Signs and symptoms

Patient presents with weight loss, fatigue, productive cough, fever and night sweats. Frank hemoptysis.

Physical examination:

Dullness, rales, increased vocal fremitus

Diagnosis with algorithm:

Most widely used screening method for tuberculosis infection is the tuberculin skin test. This tuberculin skin test to detect latent TB

Mantoux test:

Mantoux method of PPD (purified protein derivative) administration consists of the Sabcytaneous/Inteadermal S.C/I.D injection of PPD containing five tuberculin units after 48-72 hrs it is checked whether there is hypersensitive reaction occurred or not.

Diagnostic algorithm for TB

After the presumptive TB case-

- ➤ The patient has to be examined for smear test and chest X ray.
- ➤ If it is smear positive and chest X ray suggestive of TB – "programmed management of drug resistant tuberculosis" criteria and Multidrug resistant settings are assessed, based on the results it is confirmed as Mycobacterium TB.
- ➤ If it is smear positive but chest X ray not suggestive of TB – "programmed management of drug resistant tuberculosis" criteria and Multidrug resistant settings are assessed, based on the results it is confirmed as Mycobacterium TB.
- ➤ If smear negative but chest X ray suggestive of TB, then cartridge based nucleic acid amplification test is adviced.
  - (a) The patient is is identified as Mycobacterium TB. positive-
    - ➤ And Rifampicin sensitive: confirmed as Mycobacterium TB patient.
    - ➤ Rifampicin indeterminate- repeat cartridge based nucleic acid amplification test and liquid culture test done to identify the organism.
    - ➤ If rifampicin resistant- "programmed management of drug resistant tuberculosis" guidelines should be followed.
  - (b) If the patient if Mycobacterium TB negative- alternative diagnosis is considered and reffered to a specialist.
    - ➤ If smear negative and chest X ray not suggestive of TB-clinical suspicion if high, then cartridge based nucleic acid amplification test is adviced and same procedure is followed as above.
    - ➤ If the patient is with HIV/AIDS cartridge based nucleic acid amplification test is adviced and the same diagnostic approach is followed.

(Cartridge based nucleic acid amplification test (CB-NAAT, GeneXpert,) is an automated cartridge-based molecular technique which not only detects Mycobacterium Tuberculosis but also rifampicin resistance within two hours and has been endorsed by WHO as an initial diagnostic test in children suspected of having tuberculosis both in pulmonary and specific forms of extra pulmonary tuberculosis)

Criteria for Tuberculin Positivity, by Risk Group

1. Reaction >5mm of induration: HIV + patients; recent TB; fibrotic changes on chest radiograph with prior TB; Patients with organ transplants and other immunosuppressed patients (receiving the equivalent of ≥15 mg/d of prednisone for 1 month or more)
2. Reaction >10mm of induration: Recent immigrants; Injection drug users; Residents and employeesb of the following high-risk congregate settings: prisons and jails, nursing homes and other long-term facilities for the elderly, hospitals and other health care facilities, residential facilities for patients with acquired immunodeficiency syndrome (AIDS), and homeless shelters; Persons with the following clinical conditions that place them at high risk: silicosis, diabetes mellitus, chronic renal failure; Children younger than 4 yr of age or infants, children, and adolescents exposed to adults at high-risk
3. Reaction >15mm of induration: Persons with no risk factors for TB

Radiological Examination

Chest X-ray for pulmonary TB -patchy/nodular infiltrates in the apical area of the upper lobes or the superior segment of the lower lobes

Other tests

Microscopy of the sputum, Sputum culture methods, PCR.

Management

Goals of therapy

1. Rapid identification of a new TB case.
2. Initation of specific anti tubercolosis treatment.
3. Prompt resolution of the signs and the symtoms of disease.
4. Acheivement of a non infectious state in the patient, thus ending isolation.
5. Adherence to the treatment regimen by the patient.
6. Cure of the patient as quickly as possible.
7. Prevent the emergence of Resistance.
8. Eliminate persistant Bacilli From host tissue.
9. Prevent relapse.

Nonpharmacologic Therapy

Debilitated TB patients may require therapy for other medical problems, including substance abuse and HIV infection, and some may need nutritional support.

Surgery may be needed to remove destroyed lung tissue, space occupying infected lesions (tuberculomas), and certain extrapulmonary lesions
Vaccines against TB include BCG and M. vaccae

Treatment Algorithm

Souce: Adapted from American Thoracic Society, Centers for Disease Control and Prevention, Infectious Diseases Society of America. Treatment of tuberculosis [published correction appears in MMWR Recomm Rep 2005;53:1203]. MMWR Recomm Rep 2003;52(RR-11):1–77.

If the patient is identified with abnormal chest radiograph, positive tuberculin test, negative smears and no other diagnosis.

(a) If with high clinical suspicion: treat eith Isoniazid, rifampin, ethambutol, and pyrazinamide for 8 weeeks, obtain cultures. Continue and repeat evaluation at 8 weeks.

    (i)   If initial cultures negative- no change in chest radiographs or symptoms- TB unlikely.

    (ii) Initial cultures negative, radiographic or symptomatic improvement is ssen- diagnose culture negative TB. Treat with isoniazid and rifampin for 8 weeks.

(b) If with low clinical suspicion: No treatments initially; obtain cultures. Repaeat evaluation at 8-12 weeks. Initial cultures negative; no change in chest radiograph- choose of the 3 treatment options

    (i)   Treat with rifampin and/ or isoniazid for 18 weeks.

    (ii) Treat with isoniazid for 9 months

    (iii) Treat with rifampin and pyrazinamide for 8 weeks.

Table 41.1 Classification of Anti-TB Drugs.

Groups	Drugs
Group 1: First-line oral anti-tuberculosis agents	Isoniald (H); Rifampicin (R); Ethambutol (E); Pyrazinamdie (Z)
Group 2: Injectable anti-tuberculosis agensts	Streptomycin (S); Kanamycin (Km); Amikacin (Am); Capreomycin (Cm); Vincomycin (Vi)
Group 3: Fluoroquinolones	Ciprofloxacin (Cfx); Ofloxacin (Ofx); Levofloxacin (Lfx); Moxifloxacin (Mfx); Gatifloxacin (Gfx)
Group 4: Oral second-line anti-tuberculosis agents	Ethionamide (Eto); Prothionamide (Pto); Cycloserine (Cs); Terizidone (Trd); Para-aminosalicyclic acid (PAS); Thioacetazone (Th)
Group 5: Agents with unclear role in treatment of drug-resistnat tuberculosis	Clofazimine (Cfz), Linezolid (Lzd); amoxicillin/clavulanate (Amx/Clv); Thioacetazone (Thz); Imipenem/cilastatin (Ipm/Cin); High dose isoniazid (high dose H); Clarithromycin (Clr)

Pharmacological Treatment

Isoniazid

It is more effective against Mycobacteriam Tuberculosis than both streptomycin and Para-amino Salicyclic Acid (PAS). It is well absorbed from the alimentary tract and is distributed throughout the body water, penetrating easily into the cerebrospinal fluid. It should always be given in cases where there is special risk of meningitis. Isoniazid enters milk in about the same concentration as in the blood. It interferes with pyridoxine metabolism and induces pyridoxine deficiency.

Mechanism of action: INH inhibits the synthesis of mycolic acid and inhibits cell wall synthesis

Indications:

Tuberculosis

Dosage

Adults: 300 mg daily in 1-3 doses. Children: 10-20 mg/kg body wt. in 1-3 doses. Max dose; 300-500mg daily.

Contra-Indications

Drug induced hepatic diseases.

Special Precautions

Chronic alcoholism, Epilepsy, Hepatitis. When Isoniazid is used alone drug resistance develops in all cases within 5 months, hence a combination with other anti-tubercular drugs is advised. **Paediatrics:** Reduced dose necessary. **Pregnancy:** Safety not established. **Lactation:** The drug passes into breast milk. **Elderly:** Increased likelihood of adverse effects.

Side Effects

Peripheral neuropathy and, more rarely, anaemia and pellagra. Mental disturbances convulsions, incoordination, encephalopathy, alcohol intolerance and a variety of allergic effects. Preventable with administrations of Vit. B_6 (Pyridoxine) 50-100 mg orally/day.

Rifampicin

It is highly bacteriocidal to Mycobacterium tuberculosis. Administered orally quick absorption leads to high and well sustained blood levels. Its use in combination with various other anti-tubercular drugs which is considered highlzy effective. Amino salicylic acid may delay absorption of Rifampicin, and if given concurrently, they should be given separately at an interval of 8 to 12 hours.

Mechanism of action: It binds and inhibits bacterial DNA dependent RNA polymerase and prevents RNA synthesis

Indications

Treatment of tuberculosis

Dosage

Adult: (below 50 kg : 450 mg daily as a single dose. **More than 50 kg:** upto 600 mg daily. **Children:**10-15 mg/kg body wt. daily as a single dose.

Contra-Indications

It should not be given to patients who have experienced drug induced liver disease earlier - which may include Jaundice or biliary obstruction.

Special Precautions

Impaired liver functions. Concurrent administration of anticoagulants or oral contraceptives with Rifampicin is to be avoided. Faeces, saliva, sputum, sweat, tears and urine may be discoloured orange red, due to Rifampicin. It is to be used with caution in malnourished or very young patients. **Paediatrics:** Reduced dose necessary. **Pregnancy:** Contraindicated. **Lactation:** Use with caution. **Elderly:** Reduced dose necessary because of adverse effects.

Side Effects

May include nausea, vomiting, skin rash, peripheral neuropathy and liver impairment.

Pyrazinamide

It is the pyrazine analog of nicotinamide. When this drug is used alone the disease is initially controlled but soon relapses because microorganisms rapidly become resistant. When it is administered simultaneously with isoniazid, the bacteria remain sensitive to pyrazinamide. It is well absorbed from the Gastrointestinal tract and distributed throughout the body. Pyrazinamide has been strongly recommended for use in individuals who are to be subjected to pulmonary surgery.

Mechanism of action: Inhibits mycolic acid synthesis and inhibits cell wall synthesis

Indications

Tuberculosis

Dosage

20-35mg/kg body wt in 3-4 divided doses with Maximum of 3gm daily.

Contra-Indications

Hepatic dysfunctions, Gouty arthritis.

Special Precautions

Must be given with other anti-tubercular drugs. Perform liver function and blood uric acid tests regularly. History of diabetes. **Paediatrics:** Use with caution. **Pregnancy:** Contraindicated. **Lactation:** Use with caution. **Elderly:** Use with caution.

Side Effects

Arthralgias, anorexia, nausea and vomiting, dysuria, malaria fever, elevation of plasma uric acid and acute episodes of gout.

Ethambutol

It is well absorbed through Gastro Intestinal Tract and has a long half life. Since it inhibits the growth of M. tuberculosis, use in conjugation with other anti tubercular is considered valuable Mechanism of action: By inhibiting Arabinosyl-transferase enzyme cell wall synthesis is inhibited

Indications

Tuberculosis

Dosage: 15 mg/kg body wt daily as single dose **Retreatment:** 25 mg/kg body weight as single dose for 60 days, then 15 mg/kg body weight to be administered with other anti-tubercular medicines.

Contra-Indications

Hypersensitivity. Optic neuritis, Liver damage. Susceptibility to epilepsy.

Special Precautions

Test visual functions before starting followed by periodic assessment of visual fields treatment. Impaired renal function. **Paediatrics:** Not prescribed under age of 6 years. **Pregnancy:** Safety not established. **Lactation:** Use with caution. **Elderly:** Reduced dose may be necessary.

Side Effects

Dose related adverse effect of retrobulbar neuritis of which the first signs are blurred vision and an inability to distinguish colours.

Second-Line Antituberculosis Drugs

Streptomycin: Streptomycin is one of three aminoglycoside antibiotics (along with Amikacin and Kanamycin) that are active against mycobacteria. Streptomycin is quite active against MAC and several other mycobacteria. can be given safely as intravenous infusions (100 mL of dextrose 5% water or normal saline) over 30 minutes. Streptomycin occasionally causes nephrotoxicity, although it tends to be mild and reversible.

p-Aminosalicylic Acid: Gastrointestinal disturbances are the most common adverse effects.

Cycloserine: Cycloserine is only used to treat MDR-TB. It is well absorbed orally and is best taken on an empty stomach. Most patients reach a maximum dose of 750 mg daily, divided unevenly into two doses. This can be achieved by starting with 250 mg daily for 2 days, followed by 250-mg increments over 2-day intervals.

Table 41.2 Recommended Drug Regimens for Treatment of Latent Tuberculosis (TB) Infection in Adults.

Drug	Duration	Dose	Comments
Isoniazid	Daily 9months	300mg	In HIV infected patient
	BD weekly for 9 months	300mg	DOTS therapy must be used with BD -weekly dosing
	Daily for 6 months	300mg	Used in patient with fibrotic lesions on chest radiographs/children
	BD weekly for 6 months	300mg	DOTS therapy+ BD weekly dosing
Rifampicin	Daily for 4 months	600mg	Patient with isoniazid resistance/who cannot tolerate pyrazinamide

Table 41.3 Drug Regimens for Culture-Positive Pulmonary Tuberculosis Caused by Drug-Susceptible Organisms.

Regimen	Drugs	Initial Phase	Drugs	Continuous Phase
1.	Isoniazid(H), rifampicin(R), Pyrazinamide(Z), Ethambutol(E)	7 days/week for 56 doses or 5days/week for 40 doses	INH/RIF INH/RIF INH/ Rifapentine	7days/week-126 doses or 5days/week for -90 doses BD for 36doses(18 weeks) Once week for 18 doses
2.	H,R,Z,E	7days/week for 14 doses then BD/weekly for 12 doses	H/R	BD/weekly for 36 doses
3.	H,R,Z,E	TID/weekly for 24 doses	H/R	TID/weekly for 54 doses
4.	H, R, E	7days/week for 56 doses	H, R H,R	7days/week for 217 doses BD/weekly for 62 doses

Table 41.4 Therapy for Adults and Children.

First Line Drugs		
First Line Drugs	**Adult dose (max)**	**Children dose (max)**
Isoniazid	5 mg/kg (300 mg)	10-15 mg/kg (300 mg)
Rifampicin	10 mg/kg (600 mg)	10-20 mg/kg (600 mg)
Pyrazinamide	1000 mg (40-55 kg) 1500 mg (56-75 kg) 2000 mg (76-90 kg)	15-30 mg/kg (2 g)
Ethambutol	800 mg (40-55 kg) 1200 mg (56-75 kg) 1600 mg (76-90 kg)	15-20 mg/kg/day (1 g/day)
Rifabutin	5 mg/kg (300 mg)	Unknown

Contd...

Second Line Drugs		
Second Line Drugs	Adult dose (max)	Children dose (max)
Cycloserine	10-15 mg/kg/day (1 g in 2 doses) 500-750 mg/daily in 2 doses	10-15 mg/kg/day (1 g/day)
Ethionamide	15-20 mg/kg/day 500-750 mg/day in a single/two divided doses	15-20mg/kg day (1 g/day)
Streptomycin	1g vials	20-40 mg/kg/day
Amikacin/Kanamycin	1g vials	15-30 mg/kg/day (1 g)
Moxifloxacin	400 mg/day	-

DOTS: (Direct Observation Treatment, Short course)

According to WHO to prevent MDR (multi drug resistant TB)

It is an 8 month therapy

1st, 2nd month- H+R+Z+E+S (streptomycin)

3rd month- H+R+Z+E

4th, 5th, 6th, 7th, 8th months-H+R+E

Doses: H-300mg/day, R-450mg/day, Z-1500mg/day, E-1200mg/day

- Basic and most effective anti- tubercular agents H, R, Z, E
- Newer anti-tuberculars linezolid, clarithromycin, azithromycin (for immunocom-promised patients)
- Corticosteroid should never be used in TB it causes intestinal perforations
- H and R hepatotoxic, H causes vit-B6 deficiency so, Vit. B6 should be given during therapy
- If Hand R are given with Z, E they cause foetal abnormalities

Treatment for meningeal tuberculosis:

DRUGS	DOSE	DURATION
Isoniazid	300mg	9-12 months
Pyrazinamide	1-2g	9-12 months
Ethionamide	15-20mg/kg	9-12 months
Cycloserine	10-15mg/kg	9-12 months

All these drugs penetrate the cerebrospinal fluid readily

Extrapulmonary TB treatment regimen:

DRUGS	DOSE
Isoniazid	300mg
Pyrazinamide	1-2g
Ethambutol	800-1600mg
Rifampicin	600mg

Treatment for bone TB:

Drugs	Dose
Isoniazid	300mg
Pyrazinamide	1-2g
Ethambutol	800-1600mg
Rifampicin	600mg

> It is typically treated for 9 months occasionally with surgical debridement

Treatment regimen for pregnant women:

DRUGS	DOSE
Isoniazid	300mg
Rifampicin	600mg
Ethambutol	800-1600mg

> Duration for 9 months. Isoniazid and ethambutol is relatively safe when used during pregnancy, supplementation with B-vitamins is particularly important. Rifampicin rarely has birth defects and occasionally severe including limb reduction and CNS lesions. Pyrazinamide according to anecdotal information suggests that it may be safe. Ethionamide may be associated with premature delivery, congenital deformation and Down syndrome when used during pregnancy. Streptomycin has been associated with hearing impairment in new born including complete deafness. Cycloserine is not recommended during pregnancy. Fluoroquinolones are avoided during pregnancy

Treatment Regimen for In TB in Renal Failure patients: Isoniazid and rifampicin do not require dose modifications. Pyrazinamide and ethambutol typically require a reduction on dosing frequency

Drug Dose and frequency for Patients with Creatinine Clearance >30ml/min or Patients receiving haemodialysis

Isoniazid	300mg-OD or 900mg-3 times weekly
Rifampicin	600mg-OD or 600mg-3 times weekly
Pyrazinamide	25mg/kg/dose-3 times weekly
Ethambutol	15mg/kg/dose-3 times weekly
Streptomycin	12-15mg/kg/dose 2 or 3 times weekly
Cycloserine	250mg-Odor 500mg/dose-3times weekly

Algorithm for Diagnosis of MDR-TB

Laboratory tests:

(i) Pregnancy test

(ii) HIV test

(iii) Serum creatinine and serum potassium while receiving an injectable drug.

(iv) Thyroid stimulating hormone evry 3 months if receiving ethambutol/ para aminosalicylic acid.

(v) Liver serum enzymes

(vi) Hemoglobin and white blood count monthly.

Clinical assessment:
  (i) Peripheral neuripathy/vibration perception(baseline and monthly) while receiving isoniazid.
  (ii) Audiometry baseline and monthly when receiving an injectable drug.
  (iii) Vision tests baseline and monthly in case of visual toxicity.
  (iv) Electrocardiogram

After the above baseline and routine evaluation:
  1. All patients with rifampicin-resistant TB or MDR-TB
  2. Initiate treatment with second-line regimen. Refer a specimen for SL-LPA (second line anti-TB drugs)
  3. SL-LPA: Resistance to Fluoroquinolone (FQ), second line injectable drug (SLID), or both detected: Initiate individualised MDR-TB treatment based on SL-LPA results and considering use of new drugs and later generation fluoroquinolone. During treatment monitoring, any positive culture suggestive of treatment failure should undergo phenotypic 2nd line drug susceptibility test (DST), if available. Review treatment regimen based on phenotypic DST results
  4. SL-LPA: Resistance NOT detected to both FQ and SLID: • Initiate patient on the shorter MDR-TB treatment regimen if patient meets criteria. If not eligible, initiate an individualised MDR-TB regimen in accordance with national guidelines. In settings with high underlying prevalence of resistance to FQs or SLIDs or for patients considered at high risk of resistance, refer a specimen for culture and phenotypic 2nd line DST. During treatment monitoring, any positive culture suggestive of treatment failure should undergo phenotypic 2nd line DST, if available. Review treatment regimen based on phenotypic DST results.

ATS/CDC/ERS/IDSA, 2019 WHO MDR-TB guideline for Clinical management of patients with multidrug-resistant tuberculosis (MDR-TB).

  1. **Regimens for isoniazid-resistant tuberculosis (Hr-TB):** In patients with confirmed rifampicin-susceptible and isoniazid-resistant tuberculosis, treatment with rifampicin, ethambutol, pyrazinamide and levofloxacin is recommended for a duration of 6 months
  2. **The duration of longer MDR-TB regimens:**
     In MDR/RR-TB patients on longer regimens, a total treatment duration of 18–20 months is suggested for most patients; the duration may be modified according to the patient's response to therapy.
     Group A: fluoroquinolones (levofloxacin and moxifloxacin), bedaquiline and linezolid were considered highly effective and strongly recommended for inclusion in all regimens unless contraindicated.
     Group B: clofazimine and cycloserine or terizidone were conditionally recommended as agents of second choice
     Group C: ethambutol, delamanid, pyrazinamide, imipenem–cilastatin OR meropenem, amikacin (OR streptomycin) ethionamide OR prothionamide, p-aminosalicylic acid

Regimen: group A-include all 3 medicnes + group B –add one or both medicines + group C – add to complete the regimen

3. **Start of antiretroviral therapy in patients on second-line antituberculosis regimens:** Antiretroviral therapy is recommended for all patients with HIV and DR-TB requiring second-line antituberculosis drugs, irrespective of CD4 cell count, as early as possible (within the first 8 weeks) following initiation of antituberculosis treatment.

CHAPTER - 42

Meningitis

Introduction to Meningitis

Meningitis refers to inflammation of sub-arachnoid space by the hematogenous spread in meninges from distal point.

Etiology: It is caused by microorganisms-bacteria, fungi, viruses and parasites

Age Group and Condition	Pathogens
Neonates (<2months)	-Group B-streptococcus, Ecoli,G(-ve)bacilli (ex: Klebsella)
Infants and children (2months-10yr)	-Haemophilus influenza,S.pneumoniae,
Children and adults (>10yr-30yr)	-N.meningitidis,S.pneumo
Adult (30-60yr) and elder (>60yr)	-S.pneumoniae,N.meningitidis
Post neurosurgical	-S.aureus,Gram-ve bacilli(ex:Ecoli,klebsella)
Closed head trauma	-S.pneumoniae,H.influenza
Open head trauma	-S.aureus,Gram-ve bacilli

Risk Factors

- ✓ Alcoholism
- ✓ Bacterial pneumonia
- ✓ Head trauma
- ✓ Sinusitis
- ✓ Immunosuppressants
- ✓ Passive and active exposure to cigarette smoke
- ✓ Presence of cochlear implant

Mode of Spread: Haematogenous/ iatrogenic/ contagious

Pathophysiology

CNS infections are the results of hematogenous spread from primary site or reactivation from latent site or trauma or congenital defects in CNS

The development of bacterial meningitis occurs following the nasopharyngeal colonisation of host by bacterial pathogen with subsequent inflammation of sub-arachnoid space, alterations owing to inflammation and resulting neuronal damage.

Spread from sinus/inner ear/tuberculoma/Naso pharyngeal bacterial colonization/skull fractures/anatomical defects/meningocoele.

Bacteria with the help of their pilli attaches to host epithelial surface receptors. Bacteria release IgA proteases. These deteriorate mucous membrane of nasopharyngeal cavity. These adhered bacteria enter systemic circulation from epithelial cells and overcome host defence mechanism like opsonisation and phagocytosis by formation of resistant polysaccharide capsules. Bacteria invade subarachnoidal space and replicate freely in CSF. They activate host inflammatory pathways. Host immune system causes the bacterial cell death. Bacterial cellwall components like techoic acid, lipotechoicacid, peptidoglycans etc are released out. These components activate capillary endothelial cells and CNS macrophages and stimulate them to release cytokines IL-1, TNF-alfa and other inflammatory mediators like IL-6, IL-8, PAF, PG'S etc. Matrixmetalloprotenases, PAF initiates Coagulation cascade, prostaglandins induce vasodilation. All these events lead to cerebral edema, elevated intracranial pressure, increased blood brain permeability (due to increased endothelial permeability), CSF pleocytosis, reduced cerebral blood flow, cerebral ischemia and finally death. Variability in CSF flow and composition (changes in isotonicity and permeability) leads to meningitis.

Clinical Presentation

Signs and symptoms

- Classic signs and symptoms include fever, chills, vomiting, photophobia, severe headache, and nuchal rigidity associated with Kernig's and Brudzinski's signs. Kernig's and Brudzinski's signs are poorly sensitive and frequently are absent in children.
- Other signs and symptoms include irritability, delirium, drowsiness, lethargy, and coma.
- Clinical signs and symptoms in young children may include bulging fontanelle, apneas, purpuric rash, and convulsions in addition to those just mentioned.
- Seizures occur more commonly in children (20% to 30%) than in adults (0% to 12%)

Diagnosis with Algorithm [1, 2]

Laboratory Tests

- Several tubes of CSF are collected via lumbar puncture for chemistry, microbiology, and hematology tests
- Analysis of CSF chemistries typically includes measurement of glucose and total protein concentrations. An elevated CSF protein of 100 mg/dL or greater and a CSF glucose concentration of less than 50% of the simultaneously obtained peripheral value suggest bacterial meningitis
- The values for CSF glucose, protein, and WBC concentrations found with bacterial meningitis overlap significantly with those for viral, tuberculous, and fungal meningitis.

Therefore, CSF WBC counts and CSF glucose and protein concentrations cannot always distinguish the different etiologies of meningitis.

Other Diagnostic Tests

- Blood and other specimens should be cultured, because meningitis frequently can arise via hematogenous dissemination or can be associated with infections at other sites. A minimum of 20 mL of blood in each of two to three separate cultures per each 24-hour period is necessary for the detection of most bacteremias.
- Gram stain and culture of the CSF is the most important laboratory tests performed for bacterial meningitis.
- Polymerase chain reaction (PCR) techniques can be used to diagnose meningitis caused by N. meningitidis, S. pneumoniae, and Hib (Hemophillus influenzae B).
- Latex fixation, latex coagglutination, and enzyme immunoassay (EIA) tests provide for the rapid identification of several bacterial causes of meningitis, including S. pneumoniae, N. meningitidis, and Hib
- Diagnosis of tuberculosis meningitis employs acid-fast staining, culture, and PCR of the CSF
- The standard diagnostic tests for fungal meningitis include culture, direct microscopic examination of stained and unstained specimens of CSF, antigen detection of cryptococcal or histoplasmal antigens, and antibody assay of serum and/or CSF.

Physical Examination:

- Nuchal rigidity: "neck stiffness"
- Brudzinski sign: severe neck stiffness causes PT's hips and knee to "flex" when neck is flexed.
- Kernig sign: thigh is flexed at hip and knee at 90 angle and subsequent extension in the knee is painful- +ve.
- Altered mental status is measured by "glassgow scale"
  Score: >15: person is intact and normal.
     8 or less comatose condition.
     = 3 unresponsive (or) severe.

Management

Goal

- Amelioration of symptoms
- Prevention of neurological sequalae like coma, deafness
- To prevent morbidity and mortality and to provide supportive care without any delay by vaccination and chemoprophylaxis
- **Cautionary measures:**
  - ✓ Use only anti-metabolites that are bactericidal
  - ✓ Select antimicrobials that have good penetration through blood-brain-barrier (BBB) and achive adequate CSF drug concentrations

✓ Ensure high dose anti-microbials dosage regimens to ensure adequate CSF concentrations that should exceed minimum bacterial concentrations (MBC) of pathogen 8-10 times

Management algorithm for infants and children with suspected bacterial meningitis

1. If there is Suspicion of bacterial meningitis and if immunocompromised, history of CNS disease, papilledema, or delay in performance of diagnostic lumbar puncture- blood cultures are done. Dexamethasone should be initiatewd with empirical antibiotic therapy. CT scan of head shoud be performed and if found negative, perform lumbar puncture and if CSF findings show bacterial meningitis continue the therapy.

2. If patient is not immunocompromised, blood cultures and lumbar puncture can be done. Immediately Dexamethasone should be initiated with empirical antibiotic therapy. CT-scan of head shoud be performed and if found negative, perform lumbar puncture and if CSF findings show bacterial meningitis continue the therapy.

Management algorithm for adults with suspected bacterial meningitis

1. If there is Suspicion of bacterial meningitis and if immunocompromised, history of CNS disease, papilledema, altered consciousness, or focal neurological deficit, or delay in performance of diagnostic lumbar puncture- blood cultures are done. Dexamethasone should be initiatewd with empirical antibiotic therapy. CT scan of head shoud be performed and if found negative, perform lumbar puncture and if CSF findings show bacterial meningitis- perform CSF gram stain. If found positive for gram-ve bacteria- continue the dexamethosaone + targeted anti-microbial therapy.

2. If patient is not immunocompromised, blood cultures and lumbar puncture can be done immediately. Dexamethasone should be initiated with empirical antibiotic therapy. If CSF findings show bacterial meningitis and no positive CSF culture is obtained. Dexamethasone should be continued with empirical antibiotic therapy.

Approach to therapy:

Adjunctive therapy: corticosteroids are given. (Ex: Dexamethasone) and fluids (to maintain electrolyte balance and prevent dehydration).

Empirical therapy:

✓ It is to be instituted as soon as possible to. It is indicated based on patients age, allergy, extent of antibiotic penetration

✓ It should last for 48-72hr, until specific pathogen is identified

✓ Permeability properties like, Molecular size: LMW, HMW antibiotics

✓ Ionic dissociation: Non-ionised at body pH.

✓ Protein bound: Availability of drug in free form for therapeutic effect.

Empirical therapy by age group:

Age	Empirical Therapy
Neonates (<2 months)	Ampicillin+cefotaxime or ceftriaxone
1month -4 yrs	ceftriaxone and vancomycin or cefotaxime
Adults (10-60yrs)	vancomycin+cefotaxime/ceftriaxone
Elders (>60yr)	vancomycin+ampicillin
Open head trauma	vancomycin+cefotamine/ceftriaxone

In addition to this dexamethasone is commonly used in treatment of peadiatric meningitis

- In infants and children with H.influenzae meningitis-dexamethasone-IV-0.15mg/kg-every 6hrs for 2-4days
- After starting of anti-microbial therapy, dexamethasone is stopped
- Monitoring parameters: GI bleeding, hyperglycemia

N.Meningitidis (Meningococcus)

Presence of purpuric and petechial skin lesions may be due to, *H.influenza meningitis/ N.meningitidis* (60% of adults and 90% of pediatric patients). 10-14 days after the onset of the disease the patient develops characteristic immunologic reaction of fever, arthritis and pericarditis. Deafness unilaterally mat develop late in disease course. High dose IV crystalline penicillin G, 50,000 U/kg every 4hrs.

Streptococcus Pneumoniae (Pneumococcus)

- It is the leading cause of meningitis in patients 2 months of age or older
- Neurologic complications are common-coma, seizures
- Empirical therapy is : Vancomycin+ceftriaxone
- Definitive therapy is penicillin-G if MIC is 0.06 µg/ml
- For high resistance S.*pneumoniae*- 3rd generation cephalosporins(ceftriaxone/cefotaxime)
- Even resistance patients are given with MEROPENEM
- For multidrug resistant gram+ve infections: Linezolid+daptomycin-IV
- HCV heptavalent conjugate vaccine for infants between 2 months and 9 yrs of age at 2, 4, 6, 12 to 15 months.
- 13 valent Pneumococcal conjugate vaccine (PCV-13) at 2, 4, 6 and 12-15 months.

H.Inluenzae

- Once up on a time it was the major aetiology for meningitis in children 6 months to 3 yrs of age. Now its severity is declined due to introduction of vaccines.
- Initially Cefotaxime/Ceftriaxone. If bacteria is susceptible-ampicillin may be used
- Alternative therapy: Cefepime and fluroquinolones (Tobramycin)
- Vaccination with HiB conjugate vaccine is given in children at 2 months.

Listeria Monocytogenes

- It is a gram positive organism.

- Penicillin G/ Ampicillin+Aminoglycoside for 3 weeks
- Alternative therapy is Trimethoprim-sulfamethoxazole and Meropenem

G-ve bacillary meningitis

- Elderly patients are at more risk
- For pseudomonas auregenosa- cefotaxime/ceftriaxone+tobramycin.
- Therapy continued for 21 days

Table 42.1 Choice of antibiotics for Gram +ve and gram –ve Meningitis patients.

Organism	First choice antibiotics	Alternative therapy
Gram-Positive Microorganisms		
S.pneumoniae *1. Penicillin susceptible* *2. Penicillin resistant*	*Penicillin-G200,000 units/kg/day/ every 4hIV Vancomycin+cefotaxime/ceftri axone* Cefotaxime or ceftriaxone and vancomycin 30–40 mg/kg/day IV (60 mg/kg/day IV every 6 h)	Cefotaxime 200 mg/kg/day every 4–6 h IV; max: 2g every 4 h Ceftriaxone 100 mg/kg/day every 24 h IVb; max: adults 2g every 12 h Cefepime 50 mg/kg/dose every 12 hb; max: adult 2 g every 8 h IV OR meropenem
S.aureus *Pencillin resistant* *Methicillin resistant*	Nafcillin 200 mg/kg/day every 4 h IV; max: 2 g every 4 h IV *Vancomycin*	*Vancomycin* *Trimethoprim/linezolid*
Listeria monocytogenes	Ampicillin 220–400 mg/kg/day, every 6 h IV or penicillin G max: 2 g every 4 h IV plus gentamicin	Trimethoprim 10 mg/kg/day and sulfamethoxazole 50 mg/kg/day, every 6 h
Gram-negative Microorganisms		
N.meningitidis	Penicillin G 200,000– 300,000 units/kg/day	Cefotaxime 200 mg/kg/day every 4 h; max: 2 g IV every 4 h Ceftriaxone 100 mg/kg/day every 24 h; max: adults 2 g IV every 12 h Chloramphenicole 100 mg/kg/day every 6 h; max: 1.5 g IV every 6 h
Escherichia coli	Cefotaxime or ceftriaxone	Cefepime 50 mg/kg/dose Meropenem 40 mg/kg every 8 h IV; max: adults 1 g every 8 h IV
H.influenza	*Ampicillin* Ampicillin 200–400 mg/kg/day every 6 h *cefotaxime/ceftriaxone*	Ceftriaxone
Pseudomonas auregenosa	Ceftazidime 85 mg/kg/day; +/- *Tobramycin*	Piperacillin 200–300 mg/kg/day + Tobramycine

Prophylactic Therapy for *N.Meningitis*

Drug	Children Dose	Adult Dose
Rifampicin	<1month-5mg/kg >1month-10mg/kg	600mg/kg- BD 2-3 days

Alternative:

Ceftriaxone	125mg	250mg
Oral ciprofloxacin	125mg	500mg

Table 42.2 Choice of antibiotics with dosage for patients with Meningitis based on age.

Antimicrobial agent	Total daily dose (dosing interval in hours)			
	Neonates, age in days		Infants and children	Adults
	0-7[a]	8-28[a]		
Amikacin[b]	15-20 mg/kg (12)	30 mg/kg (8)	20-30 mg/kg (8)	15-20 mg/kg (8)
Ampicilin	150 mg/kg (8)	200 mg/kg (6-8)	300 mg/kg (6)	12 g (4)
Aztreonam	...	...	...	6-8 g (6-8)
Celepime	...	...	150 mg/kg (8)	6 g (8)
Cefotaxime	100-150 mg/kg (8-12)	150-200 mg/kg (6-8)	225-300 mg/kg (6-8)	8-12 g (4-6)
Ceftazidime	100-150 mg/kg (8-12)	150 mg/kg (8)	150 mg/kg (8)	6 g (8)
Ceftriaxone	...	...	80-100 mg/kg (6-8)	4 g (12-24)
Chloramphenicol	25 mg/kg (8-12)	50 mg/kg (12-24)	75-100 mg/kg (6)	4-6 (12-24)
Ciprofioxacin	...	...	...	800-1200 mg (8-12)
Gatifiloxacin	...	...	...	400 mg (24)[d]
Gentamicinb	5 mg/kg (12)	7.5 mg/kg (8)	7.5 mg/kg (8)	5 mg/kg (8)
Meropenem	...	...	...	400 mg (24)[d]
Nafcillin	75 mg/kg (8-12)	100-150 mg/kg (6-8)	200 mg/kg (6)	9-12 g (4)
Oxacillin	75 mg/kg (8-12)	150-200 mg/kg (6-8)	200 mg/kg (6)	9-12 g (4)
Pencillin G	0.15 mU/kg (8-12)	0.2 mU/kg (6-8)	0.3 mU/kg (6)	24 mU (4)
Rifampin	...	10-20 mg/kg (12)	10-20 mg/kg (12-24)[o]	600 mg (24)
Tobramycin[b]	...	...	10-20 mg/kg (6-12)	10-20 mg/kg (6-12)
TMP-SMZ[f]	...	...	10-20 mg/kg (6-12)	10-20 mg/kg (6-12)
Vancomycin[g]	20-30 mg/kg (8-12)	30-45 mg/kg (6-8)	60 mg/kg (6)	30-45 mg/kg (8-12)

Note: TMP-SMZ, trimethoprim-sulfamethoxazole.

[a] Smaller doses and longer intervals of administration may be advisable for very low-birth weight neonates (<2000 g)

[b] Need to monitor peak and trough serum concentrations.

[c] Higher dose recommended for patients with pneumococcal meningitis.

[d] No date on optimal dosage needed in patients with bacterial meningitis.

[e] Maximum daily dose of 600 mg

[f] Dosage based on trimethoprim component

[g] Maintain serum trough concentrations of 15-20 µg/mL

References

1. Tunkel AR, Hartman BJ, Kaplan SL, et al. Practice guidelines for the management of bacterial meningitis. *Clin Infect Dis*. 2004;39(9):1267–1284.
2. Fitch MT, van de Beek D. Emergency diagnosis and treatment of adult meningitis. *Lancet Infect Dis*. 2007;7(3):191–200.

CHAPTER - 43

Respiratory Tract Infections

Introduction to Respiratory Tract Infection

Classification of Respiratory Tract Infection
1. Lower Respiratory Tract Infection: Bronchitis (Acute Bronchitis, Chronic Bronchitis), Bronchiolitis, Pneumonia
2. Upper Respiratory Tract Infection: Otitis Media, Pharyngitis, Acute Bacterial Rhinosinusitis

Lower Respiratory Tract Infection

Bronchitis

Definition: Bronchitis refers to an inflammatory condition of the large elements of the tracheobronchial tree that is usually associated with a generalized respiratory infection. The inflammatory process does not extend to include the alveoli.

Classified as:
1. Acute Bronchitis
2. Chronic bronchitis

Acute Bronchitis

Aetiology

➢ It occurs in all ages.
➢ Occurs during the winter months.
➢ Presence of cold, damp climates and /or the presence of high concentration of irritating substances such as air pollution or cigarette smoke may precipitate attacks.

Infectious agents: [1]

Viral agents – Influenza virus, adeno virus & respiratory syncytial virus.

Bacterial agents – Mycoplasma pneumoniae (most common cause), Chlamydia pneumonia, Bordetella pertussis.

Common cold viruses – Rhinovirus & coronavirus

Pathophysiology

Due to different etiologic factors, there is activation of phagocyte migration, release of proinflammatory mediators (cytokines, enzymes), which are stored in mucous membranes. They act on respiratory tract mucous membranes causing direct impairment of respiratory epilthelium ranging from mild to extensive and may affect bronchial mucociliry function. In addition, the increase in bronchial secretions, which can become thick and tenacious, further impairs mucociliary activity and associated with increased airway hyperreactivity.

Clinical Manifestations and features

> Fever, chills, malaise, headache, coryza, and sore throat.
> Cough is the hall mark of acute bronchitis. Cough is initially non-productive but progresses, yielding mucopurulent sputum.
> Increased sputum, nasopharyngeal secretion.

Diagnosis:

> Chest examination: normal
> Bacterial cultures of expectorated sputum
> Viral antigen detection tests (can be used when specific diagnosis is necessary)
> Cultures, PCR or serologic diagnosis of M.pneumoniae.
> Cultures, Direct fluorescent antibody detection or PCR for B.pertussis.

Management

Goal of therapy

- To provide comfort to the patient
- To treat associated dehydration and respiratory compromise
- To improve quality of life
- Non- pharmacological therapy:
- Patient should be encouraged to drink fluids to prevent dehydration and possibly decrease the viscosity of respiratory secretions
- Bed rest and analgesic-antipyretic therapy are often helpful in relieving the symptoms (fever, malaise and lethargy)

Diagnosis and Management of Acute Bronchitis

The patient is with cough and chest symptoms consistent with acute bronchitis, is the bromchitis uncomplicated

(a) If it is yes – history and physical examination taken to rule out consolidation or other causes of cough.

(b) If it is confirmed as acute bronchitis-patient is treated with protussives, specific and nonspecific antitussives or bronchodilators. Followup after 2 weeks.

If the bronchitis is complicated.

History and physical examination is done. Chest radiography, pulmonary function testing, peak flow measurement, sputum culture tests are done. Then started with appropriate antibiotic therapy.

If symptoms persist after 2 weeks of treatment, consider change in therapy.

Pharmacological therapy

✓ Aspirin or acetaminophen – 650 mg in adults 4 times a day (maximum dose <4g)
  10 – 15 mg /kg per dose in children (maximum dose 60 mg /kg)
✓ Ibuprofen – 200-800mg in adults (maximum dose 3.2g)
  10mg/kg per dose in children (maximum dose-40mg/kg)
✓ Mist therapy and the use of vaporizer may further promote the thinning and loosening of respiratory secretions.
✓ If persistent and mild cough - Dextromethorphan
  Severe cough - Codeine
✓ M.Pneumonia, if suspected or confirmed by culture treated with Azithromycin & Levofloxacin (may be used in adults)

Table 43.1 Selected Nonspecific Antitussive Agents.

Preparation	Dosage	Side effects
Hydromorphone-guaifenesin (e.g., Hycotuss)	5 mg per 100 mg per 5 mL (one teaspoon)	Sedation, nausea, vomiting, respiratory depression
Dextromethorphan (e.g., Delsym)	30 mg every 12 hours	Rarely, gastrointestinal upset or sedation
Hydrocodone (e.g., in Hycodan syrup or tablets)	5 mg every 4 to 6 hours	Gastrointestinal upset, nausea, drowsiness, constipation
Codeine (e.g., in Robitussin A-C)	10 to 20 mg every 4 to 6 hours	Gastrointestinal upset, nausea, drowsiness, constipation
Carbetapentane (e.g., in Rynatuss)	60 to 120 mg every 12 hours	Drowsiness, gastrointestinal upset
Benzonatate (Tessalon)	100 to 200 mg three times daily	Hypersensitivity, gastrointestinal upset, sedation

Chronic Bronchitis

Definition: Chronic bronchitis defined clinically as the presence of chronic cough productive sputum lasting more than 3 consecutive months of the year for the 2 consecutive years without any underlying aetiology of tuberculosis and bronchiectasis.

Aetiology:

- Cigarette smoking, exposure to occupational dusts, fumes and environmental pollution, host factors, and bacterial or viral infections. It primarily affects the adults.

Common bacterial isolates:

- Haemophilus Influenza , Moraxella catarrhalis, Streptococcus pneumonia , E. coli
- Enterobacter species, Klebsiella, Pseudomonas aeruginosa

Pathophysiology

The chronic inhalation of an irritating noxious substance compromises the normal secretory and mucociliary function of bronchial mucosa. In chronic bronchitis, the bronchial wall is thickened, and the number of mucus-secreting goblet cells in the surface epithelium of both larger and smaller bronchi is increased markedly. hypertrophy of the mucous glands and dilation of the mucous gland ducts are also observed. As a result of these changes, chronic bronchitics have substantially more mucus in their peripheral airways, further impairing normal lung defenses. This increased quantity of tenacious secretions within the bronchial tree frequently causes mucous plugging of the smaller airways. Accompanying these changes are squamous cell metaplasia of the surface epithelium, edema and increased vascularity of the basement membrane of larger airways, and variable chronic inflammatory cell infiltration. Continued progression of this pathology can result in residual scarring of small bronchi, augmenting airway obstruction and weakening of bronchial walls.

Clinical manifestation and features

Signs and symptoms:

- Excessive sputum expectoration
- Cyanosis (decreased blood supply – partial death of tissues takes place)

Diagnosis

Physical examination:

- Chest auscultation
- Obesity
- Normal vesicular breathing sounds are diminished
- Clubbing of digits

Chest radiography (increase in anteroposterior diameter of thoracic cage)

Lab tests:

- Erythrocytosis
- Pulmonary function test- decreased vital capacity, prolonged expiratory flow

Management:

Goal of therapy:
- To reduce severity of symptoms
- To achieve prolonged infection free intervals

Non-pharmacological therapy:
- Exposure to bronchial irritants should be reduced
- Patient should reduce or eliminate cigarette smoking.

Management

Clinical algorithm for diagnosis and treatment of chronic bronchitis:
1. If there is suspicion of acute exacerbation of chronic   bronchitis and the symptoms presented are increased dyspnea, increased cough, increased sputum production/ purulence.
2. Assess for risk factors: age, COPD severity 4 exacerbations/year, cardiac disease, antibiotic use in last 3 months, recent corticosteroid use
   (a) Minimal symptoms and no risk factors: Treatment rest, symptomatic treatment observation. If inadequate response, reevlauate sputum culture
   (b) Prominent symptoms and no risk factors: diagnosed as simple chronic bronchitis. Treatemnt: oral antibiotic therapy- with 2nd generation macrolide or $2^{nd}/3^{rd}$ generation cephalosporin; other antibiotics-doxycycline/ amoxicillin also can be used. If inadequate respose in observed, re-evaluate sputum culture.
   (c) Prominent symptoms and risk factors:
       (i) Hospitalization if >/= 2 risk factors FEV1 <50% predicted: Treatemnt: oral antibiotic therapy- with 2nd generation macrolide or $2^{nd}/3^{rd}$ generation cephalosporin; other antibiotics-doxycycline/ amoxicillin also can be used.
       (ii) hospitalization likely if >/=2 risk factors severe symptoms, constant purulent sputum symptom FEV1 <35% predicted. Antibiotic therapy with Fluoroquinolones, beta lactam/beta lactamase inhibitor an be initiated. If hospitalized, empiric IV antibiotic coverage for P. aeruginosa. Adjust antibiotics.

Pharmacological therapy:
- ✓ 1st line option- oral or aerosolised bronchodilators (eg - albuterolaerosol)
- ✓ Beta 2 agonists bronchodilators – salbutamol, salmeterol, formoterol. Chronic inhalation of salmeterol / fluticasone combination improves pulmonary function and quality of life.
- ✓ Second line of drugs-anticholinergics - ipratropium bromide, tiotropium bromide (decreases frequency of cough, severity of cough, and volume of expectorated sputum).
- ✓ Antibiotics are also used.

Table 43.2 Antibiotics of choice for Chronic bronchitis.

Drug	Adult dose/day	Doses schedule
Ampicillin	0.25-0.5 g	4 doses
Amoxicillin	0.5-0.875 g	3-2 doses
Amoxicillinclavulanate	0.5-0.875 g	3-2 doses
Ciprofloxacin	0.5-0.75 g	2 doses
Levofloxacin	0.5-0.75 g	1 dose
Doxycycline	0.1 g	2 doses
Azithromycin	0.25-0.5 g	1 dose

Bronchiolitis

Definition: it is an acute viral infection of lower respiratory tract of infants that affects 50% of children during the first year of life and 100% by 3years.

Etiology: Infectious agents (RSV):
- Respiratory syncytial virus (most common -accounts for about 75% of all cases)
- Parainfluenza virus
- Bacteria (secondary pathogen)

Pathogenesis

- Direct viral inoculation of virus in upper respiratory epithelium leads to inflammation of small airways.
- Immature active immune system in infants fails to clear virus in upper airway. Virus replicates and transfers to lower respiratory tract. The virus continues to infect the epithelial cells of lower airways.
- Clinical features like cough due to inflammatory trigger; tachypnea; lethargy; poor feeding; dehydration is a consequence of these responses.
- RSV infects the superficial layer of airway epithelium, but it triggersn inflammatory response that causes peribronchial edema and mononuclear infiltrate. Sloughing off the epithelium causes varying degrees of obstruction in the distal airways. Complete obstruction of bronchioles stops alveolar ventilation.
- Host cells recognize RSV via toll-like receptors, and secrete inflammatory cytokines (e.g. IFN-γ, IL-1β, IL-4, IL-8). These effectors influence the local tissue environment directly, and also further the inflammatory process by drawing immune cells from the periphery and implicated in sustaining the infection.

Clinical manifestation

Signs and symptoms:
- Mild fever, restlessness, irritability, cough, coryza.
- Vomiting, diarrhoea, noisy breathing, increase in respiratory rate as symptom progress
- Laboured breathing, nasal flaring, grunting.

Diagnosis

Physical examination:

- Tachycardia and respiratory rate of 40-80/min in hospitalised infants
- Wheezing
- Mild conjunctivitis – in 1/3rd patient
- Otitis media in 5-10% of patient

Lab tests:

- peripheral WBC count -normal / slightly elevated
- abnormal arterial blood gases

Treatment:

Goal of therapy:

- to reduce the symptoms
- to improve the quality of life

Management with algorithm

- If the clinical status is - No distress based on the discharge criteria he can be diascharged and home care adviced.

Discharge criteria are: Well appearing/ room air sat >90%; no history of cardiopulmonary disease; low risk for apnea; post conception no witnessed apnea.

Home care: Nasal saline and bilb sunction; small volume frequent feeds; Albuterol Metered dose inhaler with mask and spacer for responders.

- If the patient has severe distress- Then IV, O2, normal saline bolus/ patient has to be intubated.
- Either Albuterol OR racemic Epinephrine OR 3% saline nebulizer OR high flow nasal cannula OR nitric oxide are considered for the treatment options. But id the patient has respiratory failure Intubation is the final option.
- If the patient clinical status shows Poor PO, sat < 90%-- if it is improved, then he can be discharged according to discharge criteria. But if it is still wordened prepare the patient for intubation.
- If the patient does not improve with sunction, then albuterol OR racemic epinephrine has to be initiated. If it is improved, then he can be discharged according to discharge criteria. But if it is still wordened the patient to be treated according to severe distress patient.

Pharmacological therapy:

- ✓ Bronchodilators – salbutamol (aerosol)
- ✓ Antipyretic, analgesic, antiemetic are given to reduce the symptoms.
- ✓ Nebuliser more preferred
- ✓ Ribavirin used for bronchiolitis caused by respiratory syncytial virus.

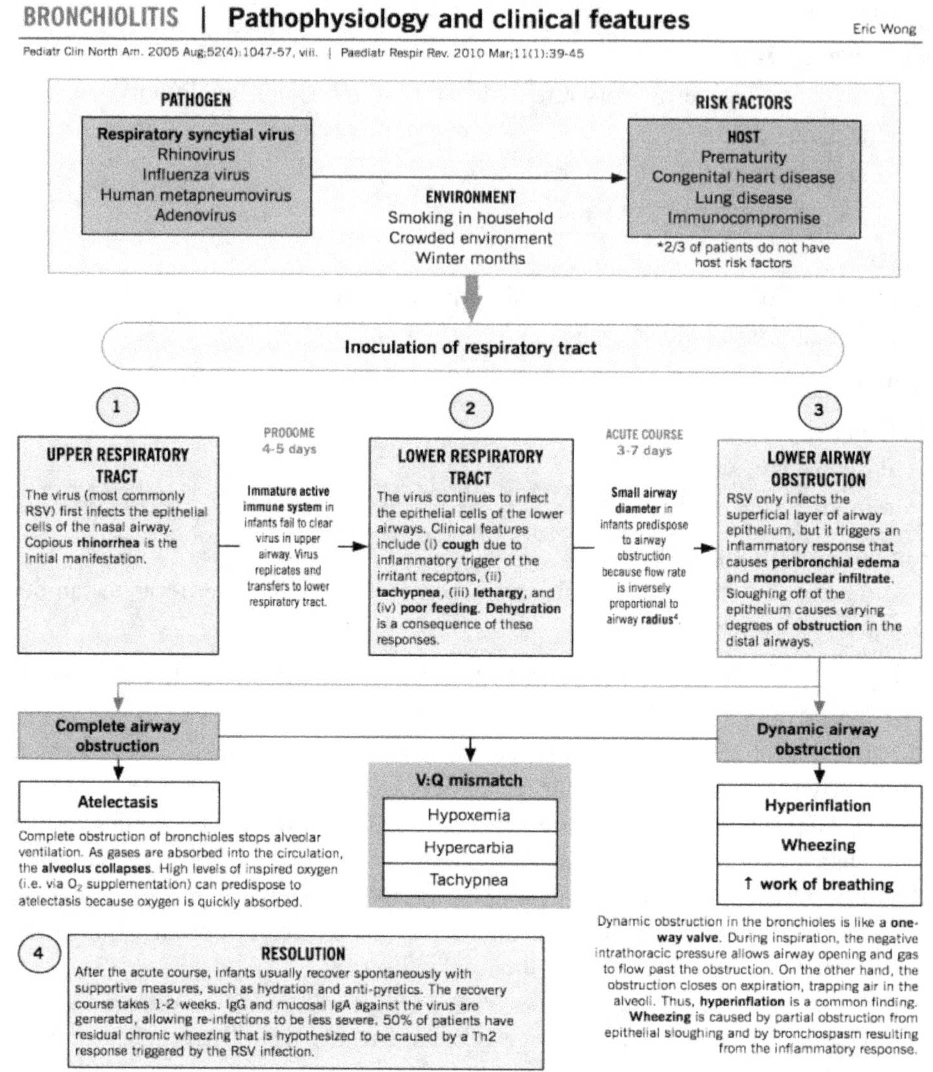

Fig. 43.1 Pathophysiology of Bronchiolitis.

Source: J Matern Fetal Neonatal Med. 2013 Oct;26 Suppl 2:55-9.

Pneumonia

Definition: Pneumonia is an infection that inflames the air sacs in one or both lungs. The air sacs may fill with fluid (purulent material) causing cough with phlegm or pus, fever, chills and difficult breathing.

- It is most common infectious cause of death in united states
- It occurs in persons of all age

Table 43.3 Pneumonia Classification and Risk factors.

Type of pneumonia	Definition	Risk factors
1. Community acquired (CAP)	Pneumonia developing in patients with no contact to a medical facility.	Age >65 years, diabetes mellitus, cardiovascular diseases, pulmonary, renal, and liver diseases, smoking and alcohol disease.
2. Health care associated (HCAP)	Pneumonia developing in patients not in an acute care medical facility but two or more risk factors for MDR pathogens.	Recent hospitalization >or = within past 90 days, recent antibiotic use, chemotherapy, wound care, infusion therapy at either health care facility or home, haemodialysis patients, contact with a family member with infection caused by MDR pathogen.
3. Hospital acquired (HAP)	Pneumonia developing >48 hours after hospital admission.	COPD, ARDS or coma, supine position, age >60years, prior antibiotic exposure, nasogastric tube, enteral nutrition, head trauma, tracheostomy, patient transport.
4. Ventilator associated (VAP)	Pneumonia developing >48 hours after intubation and medical ventilation	Same as hospital acquired.

Pathogenesis

Microorganisms gain access to the lower respiratory tract by three routes. They may be inhaled as aerosolized particles, or they may enter the lung via the bloodstream from an extrapulmonary site of infection; however, aspiration of oropharyngeal contents, a common occurrence in both healthy and ill persons during sleep, is the major mechanism by which pulmonary pathogens gain access to the normally sterile lower airways and alveoli. When pulmonary defense mechanisms are functioning optimally, aspirated microorganisms are cleared from the region before infection can become established; however, aspiration of potential pathogens from the oropharynx can result in pneumonia if lung defenses are impaired. Factors that promote aspiration, such as altered sensorium and neuromuscular disease, may result in an increase in the size of the inoculum delivered to the lower respiratory tract, thereby overwhelming local defense mechanisms.

Causative organisms:

Majority of pneumonia cases acquired in the community: S. pneumoniae (pneumococcus) and M. pneumoniae.

Gram-negative aerobic bacilli and S. aureus are the leading causative agents in hospital-acquired pneumonia

Other causes are – M. pneumoniae, legionella species, C. pneumoniae, H. influenza

In paediatric age group - respiratory syncytial virus, parainfluenza and adenovirus.

Clinical manifestation and features

Signs and symptoms:

- Abrupt onset of fever, chills, dyspnoea, and productive cough
- Pleuritic chest pain
- Rust coloured sputum

- Substantial changes in mental status, hallucination, grand mal seizures, focal neurologic findings with illness

Physical examination:

- Tachypnea and tachycardia
- Inspiratory crackles
- Chest wall retractions and grunting respirations
- Diminished breath sounds over the affected area
- Dullness to percussion

Diagnosis:

- Chest radiograph
- Lab examination - low oxygen saturation on arterial blood gas or pulse oximetry, leukocytes with predominance of polymorphonuclear cells.

Management

Goal of therapy:

- Eradication of offending organism
- Associated morbidity should be minimized
- To improve quality of life

Management algorithm British Thoracic Society (BTS) guidelines for the management of community acquired pneumonia in adults: update 2009)

1. Triage/ initial assessment suggestive of Community Acquired Pneumonia (CAP), and chest X ray reviewed by clinician
2. The patient has to be checked for consolidation, and if the patient meets the criteria for CAP. The patient has to be treated according to clinical judgement and CURB65 severity score (1 point for each feature present: confusion; urea > 7 mmol/l; respiratory rate > 30/min; blood pressure SBP< 90 and DBP< 60mm Hg; age >65 years)
   (a) 0-1 score –low severity and risk of death < 3%; and if no other co-morbid conditions are present in the patient antibiotics have to be started. But of comorbid conditions are present then he has to be hospitalised and course of treatment has to be initiated.
   (b) Score is 2- moderate severity and risk of death is 9%; the patient has to be hospitalised. Immediately supportive care shoud be started. Microbiological investigations to be done and empirical antibiotic therapt to be initiated.
   (c) Id score is 3-5 and risk of death 15-40%; the patient has to be admitted. Supportive care to be started. Microbiological investigations to be done and empirical antibiotic therapt to be initiated. If critical transfer to criticalcare unit especially if CURB score is 4 or 5.

Pharmacological Therapy

Empirical antimicrobial therapy for pneumonia in adults:

1. **Outpatient/community acquired**:
   (a) Previously healthy: If Pathogen-S. pneumoniae, H. influenza, C. pneumoniae, M. pneumoniae

Therapy- macrolide or tetracycilnes

If pathogen viral – oseltamivir or zanamivir

(b) Comorbidities (diabetes, heart/liver/renal disease and alcoholism)-

Therapy – Fluoroquinolone or beta lactam + macrolide

(c) Elderly: Organism- s. pneumoniae, gram negative bacilli

Therapy- penicillin/tazobactam or cephalosporin or carbapenem

fluoroquinolone or beta lactam + macrolide/tetracycline

2. Inpatient/ community acquired:

(a) Non- ICU:

Organism – S. pneumoniae, H. influenzae, M. pneumoniae, S. pneumoniae

Therapy: Fluoroquinolone (or) Beta lactam + Macrolide/Tetracycline.

(b) ICU:

Organism: S. pneumoniae, S. aureus, H. influenzae.

Therapy: beta lactam + macrolide/ fluoroquinolones

If viral – oseltamivir or zanamivir +/- antibiotics for secondary infection.

3. Hospital acquired, ventilator associated, health care associated:

(a) No risk factors for MDR pathogens:

Organism – S. pneumoniae, H. influenzae

Therapy- Ceftriaxone or fluoroquinolone or ampicillin/sulbactam or ertapenem or doripenem

(b) Risk factors for MDR pathogen:

Organism – P. aeruginosa, Acinetobacter species

Therapy- Antipseudomonal cephalosporin or Antipseudomonal carbapenem or beta lactam + Antipseudomonal fluoroquinolone aminoglycoside(amikacin)

(c) Aspiration:

Organism- S. aureus, Enteric gram negative bacilli

Therapy-Penicillin or Clindamycin or Piperacillin/Tazobactam + Aminoglycoside

4. A typical pneumonia:

Organism	Therapy
Legionella pneumophilia	Fluoroquinolone, doxycycline or azithromycin
Mycoplasma pneumonia	Fluoroquinolone, doxycycline or azithromycin
Avian influenza	Oseltamivir
H1N1 influenza	Oseltamivir
Chlamydophila pneumonia	Fluoroquinolone, doxycycline or azithromycin

Criteria for Severe Community-Acquired Pneumonia

Minor Criteria:

RRb ≥30 breaths/minute; $Pao_2/Fio2$ ratiob ≤250; Multilobar infiltrates Confusion/ disorientation; Uremia (BUN level, ≥20 mg/dL); Leukopeniac (WBC count <4000 cells/mm3),

Thrombocytopenia (platelet count, <100,000cells/mm3); Hypotension requiring aggressive fluid resuscitation.

Major Criteria:

Invasive mechanical ventilation Septic shock with the need for vasopressors

Guidelines for the Empirical Treatment of Community-Acquired Pneumonia

1. Outpatients Macrolide/azalide, doxycycline, or fluoroquinolone
2. Inpatients, general medical ward Extended-spectrum cephalosporin + macrolide/azalide or β-lactam/β-lactamase inhibitor + macrolide/azalide or fluoroquinolone
3. Inpatients, intensive care unit Extended-spectrum cephalosporin or β-lactam/β-lactamase inhibitor + fluoroquinolone or macrolide/azalide

Table 43.4 Empirical antimicrobial therapy for pneumonia in paediatric patients: Outpatient/Community acquired.

Clinical setting	Pathogen	Empirical therapy
1 month	*Group B streptococcus, H. influenza, E. coli, S. aureus*	Ampicillin/sulbactam, cephalosporin, carbapenem
1-3 months	*C. pneumoniae, urea plasma, pneumocystis carinii* *S. pneumoniae, S. aureus*	Macrolide/azalide, trimethoprim – sulfamethoxazole Semisynthetic penicillin or cephalosporin
Pre-school aged children	*Viral (rhinovirus, RSV, influenza A & B, adenovirus)*	Antimicrobial therapy not routinely required
Previously healthy, suspected mild-moderate bacterial CAP	*S. pneumoniae, M. pneumoniae* *S. pneumoniae*	Amoxicillin, cephalosporin, macrolide, or fluoroquinolone
Previously healthy, fully immunised school aged and adolescents with mild-moderate CAP	*M. pneumoniae*	Amoxicillin, cephalosporin or fluoroquinolones Macrolide/azalide, fluoroquinolone or tetracycline.
Moderate-severe CAP during influenza virus outbreak	*Influenza A & B, other viruses*	Oseltamivir, Zanamivir
Fully immunised infants and school aged children	*S. Pneumoniae* *M. Pneumoniae*	Ampicillin, Pen G, cephalosporin Beta lactam + macrolide/ fluoroquinolone/doxycycline.
Not fully immunised infants and children, regions with invasive penicillin resistant pneumococcal strains, patients with life threatening infection	*S. pneumoniae, penicillin resistant* *MRSA*	Cephalosporin, Vancomycin/ clindamycin Macrolide/azalide + beta lactam/doxycycline.

Table 43.5 Antibiotic doses for treatment of Bacterial Pneumonia.

Antibiotic class	Antibiotic	Paediatric dose	Adult dose
Penicillin	Ampicillin +/- sulbactam	150-200mg/kg/day	6-12 g/day
	Penicillin/tazobactam	200-300mg/kg/day	12-18g/day
Cephalosporin	Ceftriaxone	50-75mg/kg/day	1-2 g/day
	Cefotaxime	150 mg/kg/day	2-12 g/day
Macrolide	Erythromycin	30-50 mg/kg/day	1-2 g/day
	Azithromycin	10 mg/kg × 1 day and then 5mg/kg/day × 4 days	500mg day 1 and then 250mg/day × 4 days 750mg/day
Fluoroquinolones	Levofloxacin	8-20mg/kg/day	1-2 g/day
	Ciprofloxacin	30 mg/kg/day	
Tetracycline	Doxycycline	2-5mg/kg/day	100-200mg/day
Aminoglycosides	Gentamicin	7.5-10mg/kg/day	7.5mg/kg
Carbapenems	Imipenem	60-100 mg/kg/day	2-4 g/day

Initial Empiric Antibiotic Therapy for Hospital-Acquired Pneumonia

Potential Pathogen

Streptococcus pneumoniae

Haemophilus influenzae

Methicillin-sensitive Staphylococcus aureus

Antibiotic-sensitive enteric Gram-negative bacilli

Escherichia coli

Klebsiella pneumoniae

Enterobacter Sp.

Proteus Sp.

Serratia marcescens

Recommended Antibiotic: Ceftriaxone or Levofloxacin, moxifloxacin, or ciprofloxacin or Ampicillin/sulbactam or Enteropenem

Upper Respiratory Tract Infections

Otitis media:

Definition – Otitis media is an inflammation of the middle ear.

There are three sub types of Otitis media-
- Acute Otitis media
- Otitis media with effusion
- Chronic otitis media

The three are differentiated by –
- Acute signs of infection
- Evidence of middle ear inflammation
- Presence of fluid in the middle ear

Aetiology: More than 709 million cases worldwide each year, half of the cases occur in children under 5 years of age. It is most common in infants and children

Organism involved:

Viral pathogen – Rhinovirus (40-75%)

Bacterial pathogen – S. pneumonia (30-40%) ~ most common cause, H. influenza (30-35%), Moraxella catarrhalis (15-18%)

Risk factors in Acute Otitis media:
- Attendance at a child care centre
- Recent receipt of antibiotic treatment (past 30 days)
- Age younger than 2 years

Pathophysiology:
- Due to Tobacco smoke there is increased nasopharyngeal Streptococcus pneumoniae
- Down syndrome- there is altered defences or structure
- Age 6-16 years – there is immature anatomy physiology and immunity
- Due to Lack of immunisations there is lack of immunity to pathogens
- Day care of children- there is overcrowding and increased infection risk.

All these risk factors are responsible for causing upper respiratory tract infections. Now it leads to inflammation and edema of respiratory mucosa of the nose, nasopharynx and Eustachian tube. It leads to obstruction of the Eustachian tube isthmus.

The obstruction results in accumulation of secretions normally produced in middle ear. Air from middle ear is resorbed into the circulation creating negative pressure. Negative pressure in the middle ear pulls viruses and bacteria into it, infecting and inflaming the middle ear. Most resolve by 72 hours. But if it is not resolved

(a) Systemic release of inflammatory cytokines, which disrupts hypothalamic thermoregulation. It is presented in the patient as fever.

(b) Increased pressure in middle ear stretches tympanic membrane, so there is otalgia in the patient.

(c) Inflammation in middle ear causes vasodilatation of tympanic membrane blood vessels, so there is erythema.

(d) Neutrophillic infiltration, so there is yellow or white pus behind the tympanc membrane

Clinical manifestation and features

Acute otitis media – fever (39°C/102°F), irritability, tugging of ear by children, difficulty sleeping, otalgia (>75% of patients)

Fever is present in less than 25% of patients and, when present, is more often in younger children Examination shows a discolored, thickened, bulging eardrum Pneumatic otoscopy or tympanometry demonstrates an immobile eardrum; 50% of cases are bilateral Draining middle ear fluid occurs (less than 3% of patients) that usually reveals a bacterial etiology.

Middle ear inflammation includes – Erythema of tympanic membrane and otalgia, Fullness or bulging of tympanic membrane, Limited or absent mobility of the tympanic membrane, Otorrhea.

Diagnosis with Algorithm

Diagnosis done based on the three criteria – acute signs of infection, evidence of middle ear inflammation, presence of fluid in middle ear and otoscopic examination.

Laboratory Tests Gram stain, culture, and sensitivities of draining fluid or aspirated fluid if tympanocentesis is performed

Management:

Goal of therapy

- Pain management
- Prudent antibiotic use
- Secondary disease prevention

Nonpharmacologic Therapy

Surgical insertion of tympanostomy tubes (T-tubes) is an effective method for the prevention of recurrent otitis media.

If these children have moderate to severe nasal obstruction in addition to recurrent otitis, adenoidectomy may be of benefit.

Tonsillectomy, however, is not indicated for the treatment of otitis media.

Pharmacological therapy

- ✓ Primary prevention with vaccines should be considered. The "seven valent pneumococcal conjugate vaccine" reduced the occurrence of acute otitis media by 6 – 7 % during infancy.

✓ Symptomatic treatment - To relieve pain – Oral analgesics(Acetaminophen or Ibuprofen)
✓ First line drugs – Amoxicillin (80-90 mg/kg/day)
✓ Second line drugs (if beta lactam producing pathogens are suspected)- Amoxicillin+clavulanate (90 mg/kg/day + 6.4 mg/kg/day in two divided doses)

Table 43.6 Antibiotics for Otitis media: Acute Otitis Media–Excerpts from the AAP 2013 Guidelines with Other Resources.

Antibiotics	Dose
Initial diagnosis Amoxicillin OR	80-90mg/kg/day in 2 divided doses daily
Amoxicillin clavulanate	90 mg/kg/day- amoxicillin 6.4 mg/kg/day-clavulanate in 2 divided doses daily
Alternative treatment if pencillin allergy Cefdinir Cefuroxime Cefpodoxime Ceftriaxone	 14mg/kg/day in 1-2 divided doses 30mg/kg/day in 2 divided doses 10mg/kg/day in 2 divided doses 50mg IM or IV/day for 1-3 days
Failure at 48-72 hours (In children 6 months – 2years of age if symptoms are not severe) Amoxicillin clavulanate	90 mg /kg/day – Amoxicillin 6.4mg/kg/day – clavulanate divided twice daily 30-40mg/kg/day in 3 divided doses
Alternative treatment Ceftriaxone 3 days Clindamycin	

If children 6 years old : 5-7 days course of antibiotic

Surgical insertion of tympanostomy tubes in an effective method for prevention of recurrent otitis media.

Vaccination

- Vaccination against influenza and pneumococcus may decrease the risk of acute otitis media, especially in those with recurrent episodes. Immunization with the influenza vaccine has been associated with up to a 36% reduction in the incidence of acute otitis media infection.

- A conjugate pneumococcal vaccine that is indicated in infants and children has become available and provides a 6% reduction in the frequency of acute otitis media and a 20% reduction in the need for placement of a T-tube

Pharyngitis : [2]

Definition: Pharyngitis is an acute infection of the oropharynx or nasopharynx that results In 1% to 2% of all outpatient visits.

Causative organism:

Bacteria- Group A beta haemolytic streptococcus (GABHS), streptococcus pyogenes

Virus – Rhinovirus, coronavirus, adenovirus

Aetiology: Of all the bacterial causes, GABHS is the most common (15-30% in paediatric, 5-15% in adults)

Pathogenesis:

Asymptomatic pharyngeal carriers of the organism may have an alteration in host immunity (e.g., a breach in the pharyngeal mucosa) and the bacteria of the oropharynx, allowing colonization to become infection.

Clinical manifestation and featues

General signs and symptoms:
- Sore throat of sudden onset (mostly self-limited)
- Fever (resolving in 3 to 5 days)

Signs and symptoms of GABHS pharyngitis:
- Sore throat
- Pain on swallowing
- Fever
- Headache, nausea, vomiting, abdominal pain
- Erythema/Inflammation of the tonsils and pharynx with or without patchy exudates
- Enlarged, tender lymph nodes
- Cough, conjunctivitis and coryza
- Petechiae on the soft palate

Complications of GABHS:
- Acute rheumatic fever/Acute glomerulonephritis/ Reactive arthritis
- Otitis media/rhinosinusitis/peritonsillar abscess

Diagnosis:
- Throat swab and culture
- Rapid antigen detection testing

Treatment:

Goal of therapy
- To improve signs and symptoms
- Prevent transmission to close contacts
- To prevent acute rheumatic fever and other complications

Pharmacological therapy
- ✓ To relieve pain- analgesics (acetaminophen), NSAID'S- Ibuprofen
- ✓ Treatment choice – Penicillin V (250 mg BD/TID orally for 10 days)

  Penicillin G (<27kg – 0.6 million units orally)

  1.2 million units IM orally

  Amoxicillin (50 mg/kg daily for 10 days)

  (25 mg/kg twice daily for 10 days)
- ✓ If penicillin allergy-

  Cephalexin (20 mg/kg/dose orally twice daily for 10 days)

  Azithromycin (12mg/kg orally once daily for 5 days)

  Clindamycin (7mg/kg orally TID for 10 days)

Antibiotics and Dosing for Recurrent Episodes of Pharyngitis

1. Clindamycin:

   Adult dose-600 mg orally divided in 2–4 doses

   Pediatric dose: 20 mg/kg/day in 3 divided doses (max: 1.8 g/day)

2. Amoxicillin-clavulanate:

   Adult dose: 500 mg twice daily

   Pediatric dose: 40 mg/kg/day in 3 divided doses

3. Penicillin benzathine:

   Adult dose: 1.2 million units intramuscularly for one dose

   Pediatric dose: 0.6 million units for under 27 kg (50,000 units/kg)

4. Penicillin benzathine with rifampin:

   Adult dose: 20 mg/kg/day orally in 2 divided doses × last 4 days of treatment with penicillin

   Pediatric dose: As above Rifampin dose same as adults

Acute Bacterial Rhinosinusitis

Definition: Sinusitis is an inflammation and/ or infection of the paranasal sinus mucosa. The term Rhinosinusitis used because it also involves the nasal mucosa.

Causative organism: [3, 4]
- Majority of the cases are viral in origin
- S. pneumoniae and H.influenzae – responsible for 50-70% of bacterial cause in both adults and children.

Clinical presentation:
- "Persistent" signs and symptoms with rhinosinusitis- lasting for ≥ 10 days
- Onset with "severe" signs and symptoms of fever (102°F) and purulent nasal discharge or facial pain lasting for at least 3 – 4days
- Onset with "worsening" signs and symptoms headache, inverse in nasal discharge lasted for 5 to 6 days and initially improving ("double sickening")

Signs and symptoms:
- Anterior nasal discharge/ Nasal congestion and obstruction/ Facial congestion and fullness/ Facial pain or pressure/ Fever/ Headache/ Ear pain/pressure/fullness
- Dental pain/ Fatigue/ Halitosis

Treatment:

Goal of therapy-
- To reduce signs and symptoms
- Eradicating bacterial infection with antimicrobial therapy
- Preventing complications
- Preventing progression from acute to chronic
- Minimizing duration of illness

Pharmacological therapy:
- ✓ Nasal decongestants sprays – phenylephrine, oxymetazoline (reduces the inflammation by vasoconstriction)
- ✓ Mucolytics -guaifenesin (to decrease the viscosity of nasal secretions)
- ✓ Antimicrobial therapy to reduce symptoms
- ✓ First line treatment – amoxicillin

Table 43.7 Antibiotic choice for Rhinosinusitis.

Therapies	Children dose	Adult dose
Empirical therapy Amoxicillin-clavulanate	45mg/kg/day p/o twice daily	500 mg/125 mg p/o TID or 875 mg/125 mg p/o BD
Doxycycline	-	100 mg p/o BD
Beta lactam allergy Levofloxacin	10-20 mg/kg/day p/o every 12-24 hours	500mg p/o OD
Risk for antibiotic resistance Amoxicillin clavulanate	90 mg/kg/day p/o twice daily	2,000mg/125mg p/o twice daily
Levofloxacin	10-20mg/kg/day p/o every 12-24 hrs	500 mg p/o once daily
Severe infection requiring hospitalization Ampicillin-sulbactam	200-400mg/kg/day IV every 6 hours	1.5-3 g IV every 6 hours
Ceftriaxone	50mg/kg/day IV every 12 hours	1-2 g IV every 12-24 hours
Cefotaxime	100-200mg/kg/day IV every 6 hours	2g IV every 4-6 hours

Duration of antibiotics course -10 to 14 days

Recommended duration for adults – 5 to 7 days

Case Study of Viral Pneumonia

Subjective data:

A male patient of age 65 years was admitted in the hospital with the complaints of fever with chills and rigors along with SOB and cough with expectoration since 5 days. Symptoms like burning micturation, vomiting, loose stools, abdominal pain, chest pain, bleeding were not found.

He has a past medical history of Diabetes mellitus since 12 years. Hypertension since 25 years, Hypothyroidism since 15 years, No medication history was specified. His surgical history states that he underwent a thyroid cyst surgery. Physical examination specifies that he was conscious, coherent and cooperative. And his vitals were normal.

- CBC: It indicates low levels of hemoglobin and RBC
- Biochemical investigations: Serum creatinine (4mg/dL) and blood urea (94mg/dL) levels were high.
- Serum electrolytes: Low levels of serum sodium (128.7mmol/lit) and serum chlorides (87.9mmol/lit) were found.
- Liver function tests: Serum bilirubin levels were high (1.8mg/dL)
- Urine analysis: Presence of pus cells (3-4/hpf), albumin and glucose were reported.

Other investigations:

Fungal culture and sensitivity (bronchial wash) - Aspergillus flavus was grown on culture

ADA test: 30 U/L (normal range 0-20 U/L)

Procalcitonin: 0.628ng/ml (normal range 0.05-0.25ng/ml)

Glycatedhemoglobin: 9.2 (normal range – <6 percent)

Disc diffusion test (sputum): Acinetobacter baumanii was isolated.

Radiological report:

Grade I- LV diastolic dysfunction

Diagnosis:

From the above subjective and objective data the patient was diagnosed to be suffering with the following: Viral Pneumonia, Influenza A, ARF, Type II DM, HTN, Hypothyroidism.

Treatment given:

Drugs	Generic Name
Inj. Meropenam	Meropenam
Inj. Solumedrol	Methyl prednisolone
Inj. Pantop	Pantoprazole
T. Udiliv	Urso deoxy cholic acid
T. Heptral	8- adenosine methionine
Inj. Lasix	Furosemide
Syp. Potklor	Potassium chloride

Drugs	**Generic Name**
T. Claribid	Clarithromycin
T. Doxy	Doxycycline
T.Fluvir	Oseltamivir
T. Nerosave	N-acetyl cycstine + taurive
T. Thyronorm	Levothyroxine
T. Atorvas	Atorvastatin
Inj. Forcan	Fluconazole
Caps. Amantrel	Amantidine
Inj. Moxiflox	Moxifloxacin
Inj. Clexave	Enoxaparin sodium
T. Duphalac	Lactulose
T.Ecospirin	Aspirin
Inj. Colistin	Cholystimethate
Neb. Duolin	Ipratropium bromide
Neb. Budecort	Budesonide
Neb. Mesna	Mesna
Inj. Voriconazole	Voriconazole
Inj. Metoclopramide	Metoclopramide
Inj. Nova rapid	Insulin aspartate
Inj. Lantus	Insulin glargine
Targocid	Teicoplanin
Inj. Muccinac	Acetyl cystine
T. Tonact	Atorvastatin+ Fenofibrate
T.Unicontine	Theophylline
Inj. Albumin	Albumin

Pharmacist interventions:

- Propranolol should be avoided as it interacts with diuretics and increases serum potential so other anti-hypertensive like ACE inhibitors or ARB are recommended.
- Gradual tampering of propranolol or use of alternative drug like nadolol can be used for treating portal hypertension.
- Sclerotherapy to close off blood vessels and stop bleeding, coagulation therapy to seal off torn vessels can be given in case of Mallory Weiss.
- As the patient is having diabetes, there is a high risk of developing fatty liver and liver cirrhosis and most of the oral anti diabetic agents are metabolized in liver in such case biguanides IIor III generation, sulphonyl ureas can be recommended.
- The use of statins is currently contraindicated in the presence of active liver disease or persistent unexplained increase in liver amino transferees.
- Cessation of alcohol intake is advised.

- Lose weight if he /she tries to maintain a healthy life.
- Take steps to reduce high B.P.
- Keep your LDL and triglyceride levels within recommended limits.
- Vaccines to protect the liver against Hepatitis A &B
- Avoid NSAIDS(Ibuprofen, naproxen, and other herbal medications)
- Decrease salt intake as it is useful in both HTN and ascites.

Assignment

1. **What are the signs and symptoms of viral pneumonia?**

   The signs and symptoms of viral pneumonia may change in severity
   - Fever
   - Cough that is likely to be initially but may produce yellow or green mucus after 1-2 days
   - SOB, shaking, chills, muscle ache, fatigue.
   - Malaise, weakness, loss of appetite, blue tint of lips.
   - Some people may also experience sore throat or headache depending on the underline cause of the viral infection.
   - A child with viral pneumonia may develop noticeable wheezing and their skin and lips often take blue tint from lack of oxygen. They are also likely to lose their appetite.
   - Adults over 65 yrs of age may experience abnormally low body temp, confusion and dizziness.

2. **What are the clinical manifestations and risk factors?**
   - The primary target cells are those of respiratory epithelium. The typical influenza syndrome includes fever, cough, and general aches for 3-7 days but lassitude, cough and evidence of small airways disease may persist for weeks. Laryngotracheal bronchitis, pneumonia and unexplained fever are prominent manifestations.
   - Less frequent complications include myositis, various neurologic disorders and Reyes syndrome.
   - Adults are more likely to have complications of bacterial pneumonia and worsening of COPD or CHF.

   Risk factors:
   - h/o smoking, alcoholism
   - Longer pre-operative stays and longer operative procedures.
   - Thoracic or upper abdominal sites of surgery
   - Massive obesity, old age, males were also associated with increased incidences of pneumonia
   - Chronic obstructive lung disease
   - Heart diseases (contracting pneumonia almost 2 fold)

- Viruses spread easily when effected people sneeze or cough. Coming with a contaminated surface also transmit the virus.

3. **What are the common causative types of virus?**

They include the following:

- Influenza virus A and B
- Para influenza
- Herpes Simplex Virus (HSV)
- Adeno virus which cause bronchitis and the common cold
- The varicella zoster virus that causes chicken pox and shingles
- Respiratory syncytial virus which is most serious in young children but can cause cold like symptoms in all ages

4. **How is viral culture tests performed?**

Testing method	Specimen types
Bacterial culture	Blood, sputum, pleural fluid, lung aspirates, bronchoscope specimens.
Myco bacterial culture	Blood, sputum, pleural fluid, lung aspirates, bronchoscope specimens, gastric aspirates.
Viral culture	Nasopharyngeal specimens, oropharyngeal specimens, lung aspirates, bronchospasmic specimens, sputum.
Antigen detection	Nasopharyngeal specimens, oropharyngeal specimens, urine, pleural fluid.
Antibody detection	Serum.
Nucleic acid detection (PCR)	Nasopharyngeal specimens, oropharyngeal specimens, lung aspirates, bronchospasmic specimens, sputum, blood, pleural fluid.

❖ Microscopy and culture

Microscopy and culture of sputum or other lower respiratory tract specimens and blood cultures are the main Diagnostic tools for identifying the microbial etiology of pneumonia provides good evidence of likely causative microorganisms

Direct immunofluorescence microscopy and isolation in cell cultures have been the standard diagnostic approach for the detection of viral pathogens in respiratory specimens.

❖ Haemagglutination inhibition assay of Influenza virus with monoclonal antibodies- antigen detection

Haemagglutination is inhibited when antibodies are present because antibodies to the influenza virus will prevent attachment of the virus to RBC.The high dilution of antibody that prevents haemagglutination is called the H1 titer. Human monoclonal antibodies generated from single human B cells were tested to characterize their ability to inhibit haemagglutination against viruses.

❖ Nucleic acid detection

Nucleic acid detection tests, such as PCR, have many features that make them attractive tools for diagnosing the etiology of respiratory tract infections. These test can detect very low levels of nucleic acid from potentially all respiratory pathogens, do not depend on the viability of the target microbe, can provide results within a clinically relevant time frame, probably less affected by prior antibiotic administration than culture based methods and have the potential to provide supplementary information such as the presence of antibiotic resistance genes.Nucleic acid detection assays have been particularly useful for diagnosing infections that are difficult or impossible to rapidly diagnose by other methods.

5. **What is the role of viruses in etiology of viral pneumonia?**

A. Influenza virus:

When influenza virus is introduced into the respiratory tract by aerosol or by contact with saliva or other respiratory secretions from an infected individual it attaches to and replicates in epithelial cells. The virus replicates in cells of both the upper and lower respiratory tract .viral replication combined with the immune response to infection lead to destruction and loss of cells lining the respiratory tract. As infection subsides the epithelium isregenerated, a process that can take up to a mouth, cough and weakness may persists for up to 2 weeks after infection.

B. Para influenza virus:

HPLV infection of the airway epithelium causes extensive change in cellular gene expression and stimulates increased production of numerous cytokines and chemokines that either have antiviral functions themselves or attract and activate cells infected with HPIV1 has indicated tht the NF-KB,IRF3 and type 1 IFN pathways play a major role in regulating the cellular antiviral and inflammatory response to HPIV1 infection, and the HPIV1C proteins normally suppress the activation of these pathways correlating with the microarray data, elevated nasal wash concentrations of inflammatory cytokines, including IL-8/CXCL8, Macrophage Inflammatory Protein-1 Alpha (MIP-1 alpha/CCL3), RANTES/CCL5 and CXCL9, have been described in case series of children with HPIV disease. Patients with primary HPIV infections also developed detectable IFN responses during acute infection. CXCR3 ligands such has IP-10 and I-TAC, which attract activated TH1 cells to the infected epithelium are the dominant side chemokines known to be produced during HPIV infection and are secreted by the airway epithelium as well as by monocytes and neutrophils. High concentrations of IL- 8 and IP-10, inparticular, have been correlated with more severe HPIV disease. It is under weather the association between the magnitude of inflammatory responses and disease severity reflects a specific pathogenic feature of viruses or the magnitude of virus replication resulting in increased immune responses or both.

6. How is viral pneumonia differentiated from bacterial pneumonia?

Viral pneumonia	Bacterial pneumonia
• Most likely to affect healthy people with strong immune system. • Antibiotics do not work. • Can be severe and fatal. • Viral pneumonia spreads from person to person.	• Most likely to affect someone with lowered immune system or someone who is recovering from a respiratory infection. • Antibiotics are prescribed. • May be more aggressive and difficult to treat. • Bacterial pneumonia does not spread.

In the bacterial pneumonia there will likely be a much more visible presence of fluid in the lungs than viral pneumonia .Bacterial pneumonia is also more likely to enter the blood stream and infect other parts of the body. In some cases, viral pneumonia can lead to a secondary bacterial pneumonia.

7. What diagnostic techniques are used for diagnosis?

- Physical examination: Decreased air flow, crackling in the lungs, wheezing when breathing and rapid heart rate.
- Chest X-ray.
- Sputum culture to test secretions from the lungs.
- Nasal swab test to check for viruses such as flu.
- Complete blood count with differential to look for inflammatory changes.
- Arterial blood gas.
- Computed tomography scan of the chest area.
- Blood culture.
- Bronchoscopy, which is rarely needed for diagnosing viral pneumonia.

8. What is included in supportive care for viral pneumonia?

- Oxygen is the patient is dyspneicor hypoxemic.
- Beta agonist, if bronchospasm is present.
- Fluids, if dehydration is present.
- Acyclovir if varicella or herpes pneumonia is suspected.
- Respiratory isolation.
- Isotonic sodium chloride solution should be administered to patients who are in shock.
- Antibiotics if infiltrate is seen on the chest radiograph.
- Mechanical ventilation if respiratory failure is present or impending.

9. What are the medications used for viral pneumonia?

Table 43.8 Medications used for viral pneumonia.

Virus	Treatment	Prevention andior Infection Control Measures
Influenza virus	Oseltamivir; 75 mg PO BID times 5-10 days Zanamivir: 2 inhalations (2 times 5 mg) bid times 5-10 days	Contact and respiratory droplet isolatin (gloves, gown, and mask); vaccination
Parainfluenza virus	No treatment available	Contact and respiratory droplet isolation (gloves, gown and mask)
Respiratory syncitial virus	Ribavirin: 6 g inhaled delivered over 18 hours each day or 2 g inhaled for 3 hours every 8 hours with palvizumab (15 mg/kg IV or IVIG 500 mg/kg every other day	Palivizumab: 15 mg/kg IV q month or IVIG 500 mg/kg every other day for 5 to 7 doses; contact and respiratory droplet isolation (gloves, gown, and mask)
Adenovirus	Cidofovir: 5 mg/kg IV q week times 2, then q 2 weeks	Contact and respiratory droplet isolation (gloves, gown, and mask)
Cytomegalovirus	Ganiclovir: 5 mg/kg IV q 12 hours (induction); 5 mg/kg IV q 24 hours (maintenance); or Forscarnet 90 mg/kg IV q 12 hours (induction); 90 mg/kg IV q 24 hours (maintenance)	Ganiclovir: 5 mg/kg IV q 24 hours or Faoscarnet 90 mg/kg IV q 24 hours or Valacyclovir 2 g 4 times daily; Valgancyclovir 900 mg PO daily; standard infection control measures
Herpes simplex virus and varicella virus	Acyclovir; 10mg/kg IV q 8 hours	Valgancyclovir 500 mg bid; famiciclovir 250 mg bid; contact and respiratory droplet isolation (gloves, gown and mask) for varicella virus infections

Case Study of LRTI- Pneumonia with Uncontrolled Diabetes mellitus

Summary

A female patient of age 58 years was admitted in hospital with chief complaints of high grade fever associated with chills, infective cough, SOB since 1 week. She is having a past medical history of type II diabetes and coronary artery disease and is on medications- Clopilet (75mg), Angizem (120mg), Aztor (20mg), Repace (25mg) and on insulin. She has undergone stenting in 2011 and sling operation was performed in 2009. Her vitals were checked and temperature was 100F, BP 130/70 mm/Hg and pulse rate was found to be 94 beats/min. Other examinations include- decreased haemoglobin and leukocytosis.

*CBP revealed – decreased haemoglobin and leukocytosis. Urine examination indicated presence of pus cells, epithelial cells, glucose and few bacteria in urine. LFT results were normal. Serum electrolytes revealed hyperkalemia. GRBs found to be 391mg/dL.

Treatment

Trade name	Generic name	Category	Route	Dose	Frequency
Inj. Pan	Pantoprazole	Antacid	IV	40mg	OD
Inj. Zofer	Ondansetron	Anti-emetic	IV	4mg	TID
Inj. PCM	Paracetemol	Anti-pyretic	IV	1g	Stat
Inj. Magnex fort	Cefoperazone+ sulbactum	Anti biotic	IV	1.5mg	BD
HAI	Human actrapid insulin	Anti-diabetic	According to GRBS		
Syp. Ascoril	Ambroxol+mucolytic	Mucolytic	p/o	15ml	TID
Inj. Clarbid	Clarithromycin	Antibiotic	IV	500 mg	BD
Neb. Duolin	Salbutamol+ Ipratropium	Bronchodilator	P/N	1 resp	TID
Neb. Budecart	Budesonide	Corticosteroid	P/N	1 resp	BD
Neb. Mesna	Mesna	Uro protective+ bronchodilation	P/N	1 amp	BD
T. Clopitab	Clopidogrel	Anti- platelet	P/O	75 mg	OD
T. Aztor	Atorvastatin	Hypo- lipidemic	P/O	20mg	OD
T. Repace	Losartan	Anti- hypertensive	P/O	25mg	OD
T. Dilizem SR	Dilitiazem	Anti- angina	P/O	90 mg	OD
Syp. Potklor	Potassium chloride	Potassium supplement	P/O	15ml	TID
T. Istamet	Sitagliptin+ Metformin	Hypoglycemic	P/O	50/ 500mg	OD
T. Bispec	Solifenacin	Anti- muscurnic	P/O	5mg	OD
T. Clarbid	Clarithromycin	Antibiotic	P/O	500mg	BD
Neb. Formonide	Formotrol+Budesonide	Bronchodilator+Corticos teroid	P/N		
T. Mucinoc forte	Acetyl cysteine	Mucolytic	p/o	600mg	TID
IVF. NS	Normal saline	Electrolyte replenisher	IV	30ml/hr	
HAI 50 units with NS 50ml	Insulin+NS	Anti-diabetic	IV		
Syp. Duphalac	Lactulose	Laxative	p/o	20ml	Stat

Progress chart: On this day of admission patient was conscious and stable. Upon diagnosis, medications were prescribed. No fresh complaints were observed. Cardiac medications were also used along with prescribed medications. GRBs was checked regularly

Pharmacist interventions: Based on the patient's condition many drugs were prescribed and most of them have interactions. Most of the interactions result in prolongation of QT- interval, risks for arrhythmias and electrolyte loss. It is important to monitor cardiac functions and electrolyte levels. Use of steroids may increase the chances for hyperglycemia. GRBs should be monitored regularly.

Patient counselling:

- Patient is advised to stay hygiene
- To have plenty of water and healthy diet
- Take medications regularly
- Avoid dust
- Avoid stressful conditions

Assignment

1. **What are the risk factors for LRTI- Pneumonia?**

   Pneumonia is an infection of lung parenchyma.

   Risk factors include the following-

   - Age- infants to 2 years and above 65 years
   - Bed ridden patients
   - Patients with history of stroke, swallowing problems
   - Weak immune patients
   - Smoking & alcohol consumption
   - Misuse of drugs
   - History of certain chronic conditions like asthma, heart failure, diabetes, cystic fibrosis
   - Hospitalised patients
   - Other conditions like HIV, organ transplant
   - Malnutrition

2. **What clinical signs, symptoms and lab tests are consistent with pneumonia in this patient?**

   Clinical signs & symptoms in this patient are-

   High grade fever since 7days associated with chills

   Productive cough since 7days

   Shortness of breath SOB

   Dyspnoea + Temperature 100°C

   Tachycardia

   Lab tests:

   Blood test — - WBC-21,700cells/cumm leukocytosis

   Urine tests — - appearance-turbid with few bacteria

   - pus cells-8 to10/HPF

   - epithelial cells-7 to8/HPF

   - Glucose-+++

   Chest X-ray: multiple patch opacities underlying consolidation moderate pleural effusion.

3. How can the etiologic organism be determined? What are the causative organisms?

A sample of sputum or blood test or urine test is taken and inspected in laboratory for presence of bacteria/virus.

Generally- gram staining is done to identify bacteria.

Culture test and culture sensitivity tests are also done.

Viral detection- PCR tests, antibody or antigen detection, Rapid molecular assays, Rapid influence detection test.

-causative organisms for pneumonia:

- Bacteria- Streptococcus pneumoniae, Haemophilus influenzae, Mycobacterium tuberculosis, gram negative bacilli like Klebsiella pneumoniae, E.coli, Enterobacter, Proteus
- Atypical bacteria- Mycoplasma pneumoniae, Chlamydia pneumoniae, Legionella pneumophilia
- Viruses- Influenza viruses, Human para influenza viruses, Adenoviruses, Rhinoviruses, Human meta pneumovirus

Fungal- Pneumocystis pneumonia, coccidioidomycosis, Histoplasma capsulatum, Crystococcus

4. How should pneumonia be treated?

Table 43.9 Treatment Options for Community-Acquired Pneumonia.

Class	Generic name	Brane Name	Adult Dosing
Macrolides	Azithromycin	Zithoromax	500 mg po for 1 day, followed by 250 mg po once daily for 4 days
	Clarithromycin	Biaxin Blaxin XL	IR: 250 mg po q 12h for 7 days ER: 1,000 mg po every day for 7 days
	Erythromycin	Ery-Tab	250 mg po qid
Tetracyclines	Doxycycline	Vibramycin	100 mg po q12h for 5-7 days
Respiratory floroquinolones	Levofloxacin	Levaquin	750 mg po once daily for 5 days
	Moxifloxacin	Avelox	400 mg po once daiyly for 7-14 days
Beta-Lactams			
Pencillin	Amoxicillin	Amoxil	1,000 mg po qid (plus a macrolide or doxycycline)for a minimum of 5 days
	Amoxicillin-clavulanate	Augmentin	2,000 mg po bid (plus a macrolide or doxycycline) for a minimum of 5 days
Cephalosporins	Cefuroxime	Ceftin	500 mg po bid (plus a macrolide or doxycycline) for a minimu of 5 days
	Ceftriaxone	Rocephin	1-2 g IM daily for a minimum of 5 days
	Cefpodoxime	Vantin	200 mg q12h for 14 days

ER: extended-release; IR: immediate-release.

5. What are the criteria for assessing the severity of CAP?

The two best studied tools that are endorsed by infectious diseases society of America / ATS guidelines are-

- Pneumonia severity index (PSI)- developed to define mortality risk
- Categorizes patient into 5 classes
- CURB-65-developed by British thoracic society and the score obtained is associated with a rising mortality risk
- PSI- uses demographic characteristics, historical findings, physical examination findings, laboratory data. All these are assigned a score and when cumulated, patient is categorized.
- CURB-65 - involves confusion, uremia, respiratory rate of atleast 30 breaths/min, BP of <90mm/Hg systolic <60 mm/hg diastolic & age of atleast 65years

Table 43.10 Predicted mortality and recommended site of care.

System & score	Predicted 30-day Mortality %	Recommended site of care
PSI strata 1-2	0.1 to 0.7	Out patient
PSI strata 3	0.9 to 2.8	Admit to ward
PSI strata 4-5	9.3 to 27	Admit, consider ICU
CURB-65 score 0 to1	0.7 to 2.1	Out patient
CURB-65 score 2	9.2	Admit to ward
CURB- 65 score>3	14.5 to 57.0	Admit to ICU

6. What is the impact of drug resistant *Streptococcus pneumoniae* in the management of CAP?

The impact of drug resistant *Streptococcus pneumoniae* in CAP is mainly on anti-microbial selection

- DSRP are distributed world wide and these are mainly resistant to Penicillins and also few other anti-pneumococcal agents
- In these cases, it causes a great deal of confusion in choosing empirical treatment for pneumonia
- Generally for penicillin sensitive strains, penicillin or amino penicillin in standard dose is effective
- for High level penicillin resistance- third generation cephalosporins – cefixime new anti-pneumococcal fluroquinolones like gatifloxacin, moxifloxacin
- for high prevalence of high level macrolide resistance - fluroquinolones

7. What treatment options are available for influenza virus infection for pneumonia?

Treatment options available for influenza virus infection for pneumonia –

Antiviral agents- Oseltamivir- 75mg-BD for 5 days

    150mg-BD for 10 days

    Zanamivir- 10mg-BD

Acyclovir- 200mg to 800mg

Ganciclovir- 500mg

Ribavirin- 200 to 600 mg

Cidofovir- 75mg/ml-IV

8. What agents are available for immunoprophylaxis against Respiratory tract infections?

Agents available for immunoprophylaxis against RTI are as follows-

- PCV 13 (Prevnar 13), prevents 13 of most severe types of **S.pneumoniae**
- PPSV23 (pneumovax 23), protects against additional 23 streptococcus

Pneumoniae serotypes

Given either by IM or SC route

- PCV 10- new vaccine for pneumoniae
- Influenza vaccination for flu infections

References

1. L Collins, Alexander C Schmidt. (2012). Pathogenesis of acute respiratory illness caused by human parainfluenza viruses. *Current Opinion in Virology,* 2(3), 294-299.
2. Martin-Loeches I, Lisboa T, Rhodes A, Moreno RP, Silva E, Sprung C, et al. Use of early corticosteroid therapy on ICU admission in patients affected by severe pandemic (H1N1)v influenza A infection. *Intensive Care Med.* 2011 Feb. 37(2):272-83
3. Adenovirus. *Am J Transplant.* 2004 Nov. 4 Suppl 10:101-4.
   Chu CM, Cheng VC, Hung IF, Wong MM, Chan KH, Chan KS, et al. Role of lopinavir/ritonavir in the treatment of SARS: initial virological and clinical findings. *Thorax.* 2004 Mar. 59(3):252-6.
4. G. Blair Sarbacker et al., Preventing and Treating Community-Acquired Pneumonia: A Focus on Men. *US Pharm.* 2018;43(8):21-25.

CHAPTER - 44

Gastroenteritis

An infection or inflammation of the digestive tract particularly the stomach and intestines. It is frequently referred to as stomach or intestinal flu.

Epidemiology

In US 179M episodes of acute gastroenteritis each year leading to 6, 00,000 hospitalizations and over 5000 deaths.

In underdeveloped and developing countries acute gastroenteritis involving diarrhoea is leading cause of mortality in infants and children younger than 5yrs of age.

Etiology

Most are caused by viruses and some are caused by bacteria or other organisms.

Viruses- Calciviruses, rotaviruses, astroviruses and adenoviruses.

Bacteria- Campylobacter bacterium, E.coli.

Parasites- Entamoeba histolytica, Giardia lamblia and Cryptosporidium.

Bacterial Toxins- Poisonous by-products caused by bacteria and contaminated food.

Some strains of staphylococcal bacteria produce toxins that can cause gastroenteritis.

Chemicals- Lead poisoning

Drugs- Certain drugs such as antibiotics can cause gastroenteritis in susceptible people and can irritate the digestive tract.

Infectious Gastroenteritis

E. Coli infection - Common problem for travellers to countries with poor sanitation. Infection caused by drinking contaminated water or eating contaminated raw fruits and vegetables.

Campylobacter infection - The bacteria are found in animal faeces. Infection is caused by consuming contaminated poor or water eating undercooked meat and not washing your hands after handling infected animals.

Shigellosis - Bacteria are found in faeces. An infected person may spread the bacteria to food or surfaces if they don't wash their hands after going to toilet.

Viral gastroenteritis - Viruses are found in human faeces. Infection is caused by person to person contact such as touching contaminated hands faeces or vomit, by drinking contaminated water and food.

Pathophysiology

Virus 70% (rotavirus, norovirus, adenovirus, enterovirus)

Bacteria 10-20% (Campylobacter jejuni, Salmoneela spp, E.coli, Shigella, Yersinia)

Others < 10%- (Giardia lamblia, Entamoeba histolytica)

Due to these there is pathogenic infiltration of GIT. Because of this there is noxious stimuli and GIT inflammation, so stimulation of visceral nerve afferents occurs causing abdominal pain. Pathogen toxins stimulate enteric chloride secretion and interaction with enteric nervous system. Hence there is increased GI fluid secretion resulting in dairrhoea. Alteration of brush border activity, so impaired absorption of substances in small intestine. Capacity for water reabsorption inlarge intestine is overwhelmed resulting in dairrhoea.There is release of 5HT form enterochromaffin cells, so activation of CTZ in area prostema, hence stimulation of vomiting centre which results in nausea and vomiting.

Clinical Manifestation and Features

Signs and Symptoms

> - Diarrhoea/ Nausea and vomiting/ Headache muscle aches/joint aches
> - Fever or chills/ Sweating or clammy skin/ Abdominal cramps and pain
> - Loss of appetite/ Bloody stools/ Dry lips / Dizziness.

Emergency medical treatment- If diarrhoea is lasted for 3 days or more.

Risk factors

> - Age-Infants and young children are at increased risk due to their immature immune system
> - Elderly at increased risk due to weakened immune system/ Living in crowded areas
> - Travelling-especially to areas where water and food can be contaminated.
> - people residing in hospital clinics/ Not taking proper food.

Diagnosis

The symptoms of gastroenteritis are usually enough to identify the illness.

But it is important to identify the cause as different types of gastroenteritis respond to different to treatment.

Diagnostic method includes.

- ➢ Medical history
- ➢ Physical examination-It helps in assessing the presence and degree of dehydration. Mucous membranes and skin should be examined carefully.
- ➢ Signs of dehydration- Dry mouth, dry skin, skin tightening.
- ➢ Blood test- It is used to identify the presence of shigella, campylobacter or salmonella or determination of specific antibodies.
- ➢ Stool test-verifies the presence of WBC, Bacteria, Virus, Parasites.

Management

Goals

- ➢ To treat the symptoms
- ➢ Prevent the spread of infections
- ➢ To identify complications
- ➢ To improve the quality of life

Non pharmacological

- Take plenty of fluids
- Consume foods or drinks rich with Potassium
- Avoid eating high dairy, fruit or high fiber foods
- Oral rehydration drinks to keep electrolytes balanced.
- Admission to hospital and IV fluid replacement in severe cases.

Acute Gastroenteritis: Evidence-Based Management of Pediatric Patients

Antiemetic- Reduce vomiting and nausea

- Ondansetron   4-8mg BD
- Domperidone   10mg before meals
- Metoclopramide   5-10mg P/O   0.25mg IV

Table 44.1 Treatment for Watery diarrhoea.

Ecoli	Children	Adults
	Azithromycin 10mg/kg OD 3days	Ciprofloxacin 750mg OD
	Ceftriaxone 50mg/kg OD IV 3 days	Rifaximin 200mg p/o 3times OD
	Azithromycin 1000mg p/o 1 day	500mg P/O 3 days.
Vibrio cholerae	Erythromycin 30mg/kg/day 8hrs	Doxycycline 300mg p/o
	P/O 3 days	1 day
	Azithromycin10mg/kg OD 3days	Tetracycline500mgP/O QD 3days.
Dysentric diarrhoea		
Campylobacter	Azithromycin 10mg/kg/day	Azithromycin 500mg P/O species
	P/O 3-5 days	OD
	Erythromycin 500mg p/o	
	every 6hrs 3days	
Shigella species	Azithromycin 10mg/kg OD	Ciprofloxacin 750mg p/o 3days OD
	Ceftriaxone 50mg/kg/day	Levofloxacin 500mg OD
	IV 3 days	3 days
	Azithromycin 500mg OD	3days.

Pharmacological treatment

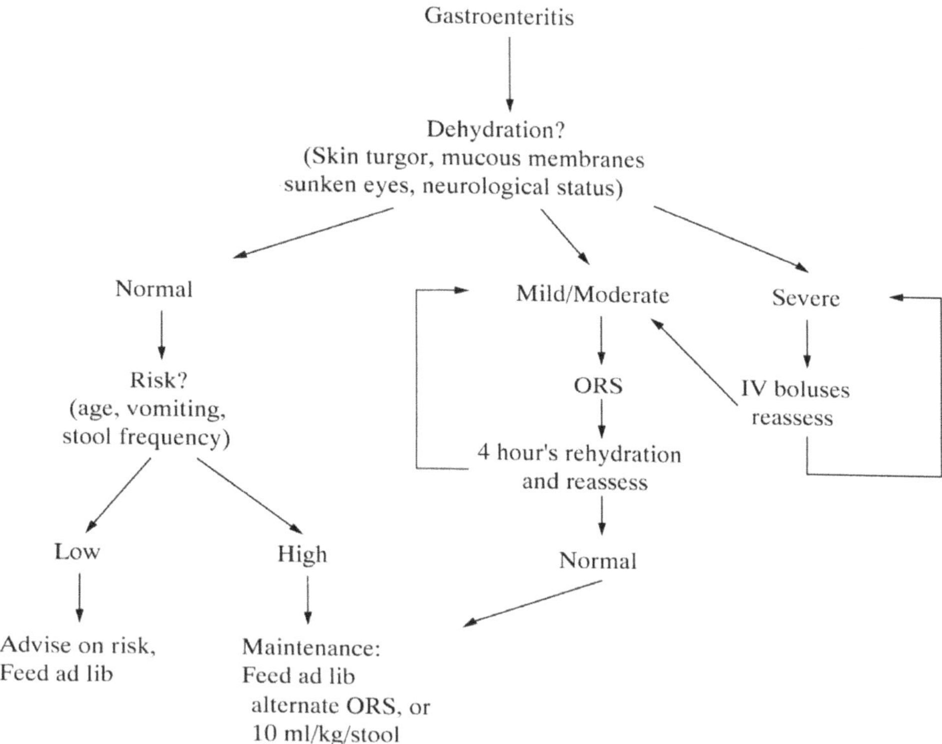

Fig. 44.1 Algorithm for management of Acute gastroenteritis.

Traveller's diarrhoea

Prophylaxis:

Norfloxacin400mg (or) Ciprofloxacin750mg p/o
Rifamixin200mg1-3times upto 2weeks

Treatment: Ciprofloxacin750mg p/o 1day (or) 500mg-12hrs- 3days

Levofloxacin1000mg p/o (or) 500mg p/o 3days

Azithromycin1000mg p/o 1 day (or) 500mg p/o 3days.

References

1. Guerrant RL. Van Gilder T, Steriner TS et al., Infactious Disease society of America Practice diarhoea. Clin Dis 2001; 32(3): 331-351.
2. Theilman NM, Gurerant RL. Clinical Practice Acute, infectious diarrhea. N. Engl J Med. 2004; 350(1): 38-47.

CHAPTER - 45

Endocarditis

Introduction to Endocarditis

Endocarditis is an inflammation of the inner layer of the heart, the endocardium. It usually involves the heart valves. When the endocardium becomes damaged, bacteria from the blood stream can become lodged on the heart valves or heart lining. The resulting infection is known as Endocarditis.

Epidemology

The incidence of infective endocarditis in a general population has been estimated at between 2-6 cases per 1 lakh persons per year.

It occurs in 1-3% of patients after valvular heart surgery.

Etiology

The cause is typically a bacterial infection and less commonly a fungal infection.

Bacterial

Staphylococcus aureus followed by streptococci of the viridians group and coagulase negative staphylococci are the most common organisms responsible for infective endocarditis.

Fungal:

Candida albicaus -24-26%; Histoplasma capsulatum; Aspergillus – 25%

Risk Factors

A predisposing factor, however, may be absent in up to 25% of cases. Some of the more important risk factors include
- Presence of a prosthetic valve (400-fold increased risk)
- Previous endocarditis (400-fold increased risk)
- Complex cyanotic congenital heart disease (e.g., single-ventricle states)
- Surgically constructed systemic pulmonary shunts or conduits
- Acquired valvular dysfunction (e.g., rheumatic heart disease)
- Hypertrophic cardiomyopathy

- Mitral valve prolapse with regurgitation
- Intravenous drug abuse

Pathophysiology [1]

Infective endocarditis (IE) is an uncommon infection, occurring as a complication in varying percentages of bacteremic episodes. The ability of an organism to cause endocarditis is the result of interplay between the predisposing structural abnormalities of the cardiac valve for bacterial adherence, the adhesion of circulating bacteria to the valvular surface, and the ability of the adherent bacteria to survive on the surface and propagate as vegetation or systemic emboli. Certain bacteria, if present in the bloodstream, may colonize the initially sterile vegetation composed of fibrin and platelets; bacterial growth enlarges the vegetation, further impeding blood flow and inciting inflammation that involves the vegetation and adjacent endothelium. There is formation of immune complexes secondary to infection. Part of vegetation embolize systemically, obstructing arteries. Infection destroys infected valve. Complications which develop are- Mitral regurgitation, Aortic stenosis, Aortic insufficiency. Immune complex deposit in the kidney produce damage to glomeruli causing glomerulonephritis. Immune complex deposit subcutaneously and cause Osler's nodes (tender, raised, red lesions found on hands and feet). There is decreased blood flow to organs perfused by obstruction of arteries so organ infarction is seen. Because of infected valve, valve is unable to fulfil normal functions and so there is cardiac valve insufficiency and regurgitation. The true incidence of endocarditis complicating each of the bacterial species causing IE is difficult to estimate. About 20%-30% of individuals with community-acquired staphylococcal bacteremia develop IE.

Clinical Manifestations and Features

Signs and Symptoms

Fever, malaise, fatigue, weight loss, coughing, septic embolism, stroke or gangrene of fingers, heat murmur, low red blood cells, night sweats, rigors, anaemia, spleen enlargement etc.,

Peripheral manifestations ("stigmata") of endocarditis

- **Osler nodes:** Purplish or erythematous subcutaneous papules or nodules on the pads of the fingers and toes. These lesions are 2 to 15 mm in size and are painful and tender. These nodes are not specific for IE and may be the result of embolism, immunologic phenomena, or both.
- **Janeway lesions:** Hemorrhagic, painless plaques on the palms of the hands or soles of the feet. These lesions are believed to be embolic in origin.
- **Splinter hemorrhages:** Thin, linear hemorrhages found under the nailbeds of the fingers or toes. These lesions are not specific for IE and more commonly are the result of traumatic injuries.

Table 45.1 The Duke criteria for the clinical diagnosis of infectious endocarditis.

Major criteria

Positive blood culture

Two separate blood cultures positive for microorganism consistent with infectious endocarditis (viridians streptococcus, streptococcus bovis, gram-negative Hacek bacilli, staphylococcus aureus, or community-acquried enterococci in the absence of a primary focus)

or

recovery of a microorganism consistent with infectious endocarditis from blood cultures drawn more than 12 hours apart

or

recovery of a microorganism consistent with infectious endocarditis from all of three or most of four or more blood cultures. With first and last drawn more than one hour apart

or

single positive blood culture for Coxiella burnetii or phase 1 immunoglobulin G antibody titer greater tha 1:800

Evidence of endocaridal involvement

Positive echocardiography (oscillating intrcardiac mass on valve or supporting structures, or in the path of regurgitant jets, or on implanted material in the absence of an alternative anatomic explanation; intracardiac abscess; new partial dehiscence of prosthetic valve)

New valvular regurgitation (increase or change in preexisting murmur not sufficient)

Minor criteria

Fever of at leat 38.0°C (100/4°F)

Immunologic phenomena: glomerulonephritis, Osler nodes, Roth spots, rheumatoid factor

Microbiologic evidence: positive blood culture that does not meet major criteria, serologic evidence of active infection with organism consisten with infectous endocarditis

Predisposing heart condition or history of injection drug use

Vascular phenomena: major arterial emboli, septic pulmonary infarctions, mycotic aneurysm, intracranial hemorrhage, conjunctival hermorrhages, Janeways lesions

Note: A definitive diagnosis of endocarditis can be made in patients with two major critiera, one major and three minor criteria, or five minor criteria.

HACEK = Haemophilus species. Aggregatibacter actinomycetemcomitans, Cardiobacterium hominis, Elkenella corrodens, and Kingella kingae.

Adapted with permission from Durack DT. Lukes AS. Bright DK; Duke Endocarditis service. New criteria for diagnosis of infective endocarditis: utilization of specific echocardiographic findings. Am J Med. 1994;96(3): 203.

Durack DT, Lukes AS, Bright DK; Duke Endocarditis Service. New criteria for diagnosis of infective endocarditis: utilization of specific echocardiographic findings. *Am J Med*. 1994;96(3):200–209.

- Distal lesions are more likely the result of trauma, whereas proximal lesions tend to be associated with IE.

- **Petechiae:** Small (usually 1 to 2 mm in diameter), erythematous, painless, hemorrhagic lesions. These lesions appear anywhere on the skin but more frequently on the anterior trunk, buccal mucosa and palate, and conjunctivae. Petechiae are nonblanching and resolve after a few days.

- **Clubbing of the fingers:** Proliferative change in the soft tissues about the terminal phalanges observed in long-standing endocarditis. Roth spots. Retinal infarct with central pallor and surrounding hemorrhage.
- **Emboli:** Embolic phenomena occur in up to one-third of cases and may result in significant complication

Diagnosis

1. Blood Culture Test: Three sets of blood cultures should be collected over 24hours. WBC count may be normal or slightly elevated. Non specific findings include anaemia, thrombocytopenia.
2. Transthoracic Echocardiogram TTE: It's a non radiating imaging test used to view and its valves. It is used to find the damage or abnormal movements of heart.
3. Transesophageal Echocardiogram TEE: It is done when a transthoracic echocardiogram doesn't provide enough information. It is used to view heart by way of oesophagus.
4. Electrocardiogram: It may be done to get a better view of hearts electrical activity.
5. Chest X-Ray: It is used to view lungs and see if they have collapsed or if fluid has built in them.

Management

Goals of treatment

- Relieve the signs and symptoms of disease.
- Decrease morbidity and mortality associated with infection.
- Eradicate the causative organism with minimal drug exposure.
- Prevent IE in high risk patients with appropriate prophylactic antimicrobials.

Non pharmacological treatment

- Surgery: It is an important adjunct to management of endocarditis in certain patients.
- Valve Replacement:
- Surgical replacement of diseased or damaged heart valve.
- The new valve may be mechanical or biological tissue from an animal or human donor.
- Indications of surgery include heart failure, persistent bacteria.

Treatment algorithm [2]

If there is clinical suspicion of Infective endocarditis (IE), classify according to duke's criteria

(a) Definite IE
(b) Possible/rejected IE but high suspicion :
Assess if it is due to native valve. If yes repeat echo, microbiology, imaging for embolic events, cardiac CT.
OR assess if it is due to prosthetic valve- repeat echo/ microbiology/ cardiac CT, imaging for embolic events. Then according to the criteria categorise as definite/ possible/ rejected IE.
(c) Rejected IE and low suspicion

Pharmacological Management

Streptococcal endocarditis

Streptococci are a common cause of endocarditis.

Most viridian *streptococci* are sensitive to penicillin G with MIC of 0.12 mcg/ml or less.

Recommended therapy in the uncomplicated case caused by fully susceptible strains in native valves is

➢ 4 weeks of either high dose of penicillin G or ceftriaxone.

➢ 2 weeks of combined or penicillin G or ceftriaxone therapy plus gentamicin.

➢ Vancomycin is effective and dug of choice for patient with a history of immediate type of hypersensitivity reaction to penicillin.

➢ For patients with complicated infection (extracardiac foci), combination therapy with aminoglycoside and pencillin or ceftraixone for 2 weeks followed by pencillin or ceftraxone for another 2 weeks.

➢ For patients with endocarditis of prosthetic valves treatment is extended for 6 weeks.

Suggested Regimens for Therapy of Native-Valve Endocarditis Due to Penicillin-Susceptible Viridans Streptococci and Streptococcus bovis (Minimum Inhibitory Concentration ≤0.1 mcg/mL)

1. Aqueous crystalline penicillin G sodium 12–18 million units/24 h IV either continuously or in six equally divided doses for 4weeks or Ceftriaxone sodium 2 g once daily IV or IM for 4weeks

2. Aqueous crystalline penicillin G sodium 12–18 million units/24 h IV either continuously or in six equally divided doses for 2weeks With gentamicin sulfatec 1 mg/kg IM or IV every 8 h for 2weeks

3. Vancomycin hydrochloride 30 mg/kg per 24 h IV in two equally divided doses, not to exceed 2 g/24 h unless serum levels are monitored for 4 weeks

Therapy of NVE Caused by Strains of VGS and Streptococcus gallolyticus (bovis) Relatively Resistant to Penicillin

1. Aqueous crystalline penicillin G sodium 24 million U/24 h IV either continuously or in 4–6 equally divided doses for 4weeks + Gentamicin sulfate† 3 mg/kg per 24 h IV or IM in 1 dose for 2weeks

2. Vancomycin hydrochloride‡ 30 mg/kg per 24 h IV in 2 equally divided doses for 4weeks

Staphylococcal Endocarditis

Staphylococcus aureus has become more prevalent as a cause of endocarditis because of increased IV drug abuse, central venous replacement therapy, catheters, valve coagulase-negative staphylococci are causes of PVE.

- For patients with left sided IE 6 weeks of nafcillin or oxacillin with gentamicin.

- If patient has allergy to pencillin, first generation cephalosporins are effective.
- Daptomycin 6mg/kg/day fore the treatment S.aureus bacteremiaassociated with right sided native valve endocarditis.
- Vancomycin is preferred for methicillin resistant staphylococci.

Treatment of Staphylococcus Endocarditis in IV Drug Abusers

➢ IE in IV drug abusers is most frequently caused by *S.aureus*.

➢ 2 week course of nafcillin or oxacillin plus an aminoglycoside may be effective.

Therapy for Endocarditis Due to Staphylococcus in the Absence of Prosthetic Material

1. Methicillin-Susceptible Staphylococci Regimens for non-β-lactam-allergic patients Nafcillin sodium or oxacillin sodium 2 g IV every 4 h for 4–6weeks with optional gentamicin
2. Regimens for β-lactam-allergic patients Cefazolin (or other first-generation cephalosporins in equivalent dosages) with optional addition of gentamicinb 2g IV every 8 h for 4–6 weeks
3. Methicillin-Resistant Staphylococci Vancomycin hydrochloridec 30 mg/kg per 24 h IV in two equally divided doses, not to exceed 2 g/ 24 h unless serum levels are monitored for 4–6weeks

Treatment of Staphylococcal Endocarditis in the Presence of a Prosthetic Valve or Other Prosthetic Material

1. Regimen for Methicillin-Resistant Staphylococci

   Vancomycin hydrochloride 30 mg/kg per 24 h IV in 2 or 4 equally divided doses, not to exceed 2 g/24 h unless serum levels are monitored for ≥6weeks duration

   With rifampin 300 mg orally every 8 h for ≥6weeks

   And with gentamicin sulfate 1 mg/kg IM or IV every 8 h for 2weeks

2. Regimen for Methicillin-Susceptible Staphylococci

   Nafcillin sodium or oxacillin sodium 2gIV every 4 h for ≥6weeks

   With rifampin 300 mg orally every 8 h for ≥6weeks

   And with gentamicin sulfate 1 mg/kg IM or IV every 8 h for 2weeks

Enterococcal Endocarditis [3]

Enterococci cause 5% to 18% of endocarditis cases and are not worthy for following reasons

1. No single antibiotic is bactericidal; MIC's to penicillin are relatively high, Resistance to all available drugs.
2. Treatment requires 4-6 weeks of high dose penicillin G or ampicillin plus gentamicin for cure.

Standard Therapy for Endocarditis Due to Enterococci

Antibiotic Dosage and Route Duration (wks) Comments

1. Aqueous crystalline penicillin G sodium: 18–30 million units/24 h IV either continuously or in six equally divided doses; 4–6 weeks **duration** ; Four-week therapy recommended for patients with symptoms 3 months in duration

   With gentamicin sulphate: 1 mg/kg IM or IV every 8 h; **duration of therapy**: 4–6

2. Ampicillin sodium: 12 g/24 h IV either continuously or in six equally divided doses ; duration of therapy: 4–6weeks

   With gentamicin sulfate 1 mg/kg IM or IV every 8 h 4–6

3. Vancomycin hydrochloride: 30 mg/kg per 24 h IV in two equally divided doses, not to exceed 2 g/24 h unless serum levels are monitored; duration of therapy: 4–6weeks; Vancomycin therapy is recommended for patients allergic to β-lactams; cephalosporins are not acceptable alternatives for patients allergic to penicillin.

Therapy for Endocarditis Involving a Native or Prosthetic Valve or Other Prosthetic Material Resulting From Enterococcus Species Caused by Strains Resistant to Penicillin, Aminoglycosides, and Vancomycin

1. Linezolid 600 mg IV or orally every 12 h for >6weeks

   or

   Daptomycin 10–12 mg/kg per dose for >6 weeks

Therapy for Endocarditis Due to HACEK Microorganisms (Haemophilus parainfluenzae, Haemophilus aphrophilus, Actinobacillus actinomycetemocomitans, Cardiobacterium hominis, Eikenella corrodens, and Kingella kingae)

1. Ceftriaxone sodium: 2 g once daily IV or IM for 4weeks OR
2. Ampicillin sodium: 12 g/24 h IV either continuously or in six equally divided doses for 4weeks
3. With gentamicin sulfated 1 mg/kg IM or IV every 8 h for 4weeks

Antifungal Agents used for the Treatment

1. Fluconazole 400mg daily only reduced in severe renal falilure patients
2. Voriconalzole –IV thrapy preferred initially
3. Amphoterecin B- 3mg/kg/24 H
4. Micofungin -200mg daily
5. Capsofungin 70mg loading, 50-100mg dily
6. Flucytosine- 100mg /kd/day in 3 divided doses reduced with renal dysfunction

Prevention

➢ If you are at increased risk of developing endocarditis, its important that you practise good oral and dental hygiene. Regularly washing your skin with an antibacterial soap will help to lower your skin of developing a skin infection. It is also very important to wash any cut or grazer carefully as soon as you notice them to prevent them being infected.

Prophylactic Regimens for Dental, Oral, Respiratory Tract, or Esophageal Procedures

1. Standard general prophylaxis: Amoxicillin Adults: 2 g; children: 50 mg/kg orally1h before procedure
2. Unable to take oral medications: Ampicillin Adults: 2 g intramuscularly (IM) or intravenously (IV); children: 50 mg/kg IM or IV within 30 min before procedure
3. Allergic to penicillin:
   Clindamycin - Adults: 600 mg; children: 20 mg/kg orally1h before procedure
   OR
   Cephalexin or cefadroxil - Adults: 2 g; children: 50 mg/kg orally1h before procedure
   OR
   Azithromycin or chlarithromycin - Adults: 500 mg; children: 15 mg/kg orally1h before procedure
4. Allergic to penicillin and unable to take oral medications:
   Clidamycin - Adults: 600 mg; children: 20 mg/kg IV within 30 min before procedure
   OR
   Cefazolin Adults 1 g; children: 25 mg/kg IM or IV within 30 min before procedure

Prophylactic Regimens for Genitourinary Gastrointestinal (Excluding Esophageal) Procedures

1. High-risk patients: Ampicillin plus gentamicin-
   (a) Adults: Ampicillin 2g intramuscularly (IM) or intravenously (IV) plus gentamicin 1.5 mg/kg (not to exceed 120 mg) within 30 min of starting the procedure; 6 h later, ampicillin1g IM/IV or amoxicillin 1 g orally.
   (b) Children: Ampicillin 50 mg/kg IM or IV (not to exceed 2 g) plus gentamicin 1.5 mg/kg within 30 min of starting the procedure; 6 h later, ampicillin 25 mg/kg IM/IV or amoxicillin 25 mg/kg orally.
2. High-risk patients allergic to ampicillin/amoxicillin: Vancomycin plus gentamicin
   (a) Adults: Vancomycin 1 g IV over 1–2 h plus gentamicin 1.5 mg/kg IV/IM (not to exceed 120 mg); complete injection/infusion within 30 min of starting the procedure.
   (b) Children: Vancomycin 20 mg/kg IV over 1–2 h plus gentamicin 1.5 mg/kg IV/IM; complete injection/infusion within 30 min of starting the procedure.
3. Moderate-risk patients: Amoxicillin or ampicillin
   (a) Adults: Amoxicillin 2g orally1h before procedure, or ampicillin 2 g IM/IV within 30 min of starting the procedure.
   (b) Children: Amoxicillin 50 mg/kg orally1h before procedure, or ampicillin 50 mg/kg IM/IV within 30 min of starting the procedure.

4. Moderate-risk patients allergic to ampicillin/amoxicillin: Vancomycin
   (a) Adults: Vancomycin 1 g IV over 1–2 h; complete infusion within 30 min of starting the procedure.
   (b) Children: Vancomycin 20 mg/kg IV over 1–2 h; complete infusion within 30 min of starting the procedure.

References

1. Que YA, Moreillon P. Infective endocarditis. Nat Rev Cardiol. 2011;8:322–36.
2. Gilbert Habib, Patrizio Lancellotti, Bernard lung. 2015 ESC Guidelines on the management of infective endocarditis: a big step forward for an old disease. BMJ journals-Heart; 2016;102 (13).
3. Ricahrd watkin et al., British Society of Antimicrobial Chemotherapy (BSAC) guidelines for the diagnosis and treatment of endocarditis: What the cardiologist needs to know., Heart (British Cardiac Society), 2012; 98(10):757-9.

CHAPTER - 46

Urinary Tract Infections

Introduction to UTI

A urinary tract infection is an infection that can occur in any area of the urinary tract, which includes the ureters, bladder, kidneys, or urethra.

Classification

- Lower UTIs: Infections of the bladder (cystitis) ,infections of the urethra (urethritis) and prostate (prostatitis)
- Upper UTIs: Infections of the kidneys (pyelonephritis)

Both upper and lower UTI are further divided into complicated and uncomplicated

Urethritis: Infection of anterior urethral tract dysuria, urgency and frequency of urination.

Cystitis: Infection to urinary bladder dysuria, frequency and urgency, pyuria and hematuria.

Acute pyelonephritis: Infection of one/both kidneys; sometimes lower tract also. pyuria, fever, painful micturition

Chronic pyelonephritis: Particular type of pathology of kidney; may/may not be due to infection.

Epidemiology

- 150 million people per year become infected
- 20% of women between ages 20-65 suffer one attack per year
- Approximately 50% of women develop a UTI at least once.
- 1%-6% of general practitioner visits are for UTIs.

Epidemiology of UTI worldwide-150 million cases year- 90 cystitis, 10% pyelonephritis, 75 sporadic, 25 recurrent, 2% complicated

Risk factors for urinary tract infection

- Developing a UTI is approximately 30 times higher in women than in men. The incidence of bacteriuria in pregnant women is 2% to 10%, which is approximately twice that of similarly aged nonpregnant women. The incidence of acute symptomatic pyelonephritis in pregnant women with untreated bacteriuria also is high. Many factors contribute to the increased susceptibility of the pregnant female to infection; these include hormonal changes, anatomic changes, progressive urinary stasis, and glucose in the urine.

- Patients with spinal cord injuries, stroke, atherosclerosis, or diabetes may have neurologic dysfunction that can cause UTI. The neurologic dysfunction can cause urinary retention, which may lead to catheterization. Furthermore, prolonged immobilization facilitates hypercalciuria and stone formation in some of these patients.
- Previous antimicrobial use (within the previous 15–28 days) has been shown to increase the relative risk for UTI in women by approximately three- to sixfold. mechanism for increased risk is alteration of normal flora of the urogenital tract and predisposition to colonization with pathogenic bacterial strains.
- Diabetes mellitus has often been associated with an increased risk for UTI because of glucose in the urine, which both promotes bacterial growth and impairs leukocyte function.
- **Females:** Shorter urethra, sexual intercourse, contraceptives, incomplete bladder emptying with age. Mechanism may be related to alterations in vaginal flora that allow for bacterial overgrowth and subsequent infection.
- **Males:** Prostatic hypertrophy, bacterial prostatitis, age

Etiology

Complicated/ Nosocomial UTI:

E.coli (gram-ve), Klebsiella pneumoniae (gram negative enteric bacteria), Proteus spp (gram negative enteric bacteria), Pseudomonas aeruginosa (gram-ve), Enterococcus spp(gram+ve)

Enterobacter spp (gram-ve), Staphylococcus saprophyticus (gram+ve)

Uncomplicated UTI:

E.coli (most common gram negative bacteria), Staphylococcus saprophyticus (gram+ve)

Klebsiella pneumoniae (gram-ve), Proteus spp (gram-ve), Pseudomonas aeruginosa(gram-ve)

Enterococcus spp (gram+ve)

Most are caused by single organisms except in patients with stones, indwelling urinary catheters or chronic renal abscesses

Pathogenesis

4 routes of bacterial entry to urinary tract.

1. **Ascending infection:** Most common route/ Organisms ascend through urethra into bladder.
2. **Hematogenous spread:** Blood borne spread to kidneys/ Occurs in bacteraemia/ Mostly spread by Streptococcus aureus
3. **Lymphatogenous spread:** Men- through rectal and colonic lymphatic vessels to prostrate and bladder/ Women- through peri-uterine lymphatics to urinary tract.
4. **Direct extension from other organs:** Pelvic inflammatory diseases/ Genito-urinary tract fistulas

Predisposing factors like immunocompromised, diabetes, elderly, stagnant urine, urine reflux, indwelling urinary catheter, stent, nephrostomy tube. So there is impairment of body's usual defense system, stagnant urine allow bacterial accumulation. Later bacterial proliferation and finally leading to Upper UTI or pyelonephritis.

In persons with Lower UTI infections, bacteri's unique pilli allow them to adhere to renal parenchyma and proceed to bacterial proliferation. Bacteria present irritate urinary epithelium and stimulates urinary reflux. Symptoms observed are urinary urgency, increased frequency. Pathogens use enzymes to reduce nitrate to nitrite and there is increased colony count, bacterial culture, and turbid urine. Inflammatory response is initiated and there is inflammation of renal parenchyma and capsule, cytokines are released systemically. As a result of this persons have flank pain, fever, malaise, nausea, vomiting,

Clinical manifestations and clinical features

Signs and symptoms

- pain or burning when urinating (dysuria);
- frequent urination;
- sudden urge to urinate (bladder spasm);
- pain during sexual intercourse;
- fatigue;
- general feeling of being unwell (malaise);
- vaginal irritation; and
- In elderly patients, subtle symptoms such as altered mental status (confusion) or decreased activity may be signs of a UTI.
- frequent or persistent urge to urinate without much urine passing when you go;
- sense of incomplete emptying of the bladder;
- loss of bladder control (urinary incontinence);
- a feeling of pressure or pain in the lower abdomen or pelvis;
- foul odor to the urine;
- urine that is milky, cloudy, reddish, or dark in color;
- blood in the urine;
- back pain, flank (side) pain, or groin pain; fever or chills;

Vaginal itching is not a typical symptom of a UTI. It may be a sign of bacterial vaginosis or a vaginal yeast infection.

Clinical manifestations depending on site of infection [1, 2]

Urethritis: Discomfort in voiding, Dysuria, Urgency, frequency

Cystitis: dysuria, urgency and frequent urination, Pelvic discomfort, abdominal pain, Pyuria

Haemorrhagic cystitis: Visible blood in urine, irritating, voiding symptoms

Pyelonephritis: Invasive nature, Suprapubic tenderness, Fever and chills, White blood cell casts in urine, Back pain, Nausea and vomiting

Complications include sepsis, septic shock and death

Diagnosis with Algorithm

Observe the symptoms of the patient- Dysuria/ frequency/ suprapubic tenderness/ urgency/ polyuria/ haematuria.

(a) If severe i.e. > 3 symptoms of UTI and no vaginal discharge or irritation; 90% culture positive is present. Then initiate empirical treatment.

(b) If urine cloudy-Send the urine for dipstick test with nitrite test.

    (i) Positive nitrite and leucocytes and blood 92% Positivie Predictive Value (PPV) or positive nitrite alone-treatment with first line agent on local management of infection guidelines.

    (ii) If negative nitrite and positive leucocyte then it is UTI or other diagnosis likely. Review time of specimen. Treat if severe symptoms or consider delayed antibiotic prescription and send the urine for culture test.

    (iii) If negative nitrite, leucocytes and blood 76% Negative Predictive Value (NPV) OR negative nitrite and leucocyte positive blood or protein. UTI is unlikely and consider other diagnosis. Reassure and give advice on management of symptoms.

(c) If symptoms are mild i.e. if symptoms are < 2 symptoms of UTI. Obtain the urine specimen. If urine not cloudy 97% NPV, consider other diagnosis.

- **Urinalysis** is done to examine the urine for red blood cells, white blood cells and bacteria.
- **Urine culture** to determine the type of bacteria in the urine.
- **Intravenous pyelogram (IVP)**, a series of X-rays of the bladder, kidneys and ureters after a special dye is injected
- **Ultrasound**, a test that uses sound waves to form images of internal organs
- **Cystoscopy**, a test that uses a special instrument fitted with a lens and a light source (cystoscope) to see inside the bladder from the urethra
- **CT scan**, a type of X-ray that takes cross sections of the body

Laboratory examination

Uncontaminated, midstream urine sample used.

Methods for urine collection:

1. Stick on bags
2. Catheterization
3. Suprapubic aspiration (SPA) – gold standard for urine collection

Laboratory findings

Normal Findings
- pH - 4.6 – 8.0
- Appearance- clear
- Colour – pale to amber yellow
- Odour – aromatic
- Blood – none
- Leukocyte esterase – none
- WBC- absent
- Bacteria- absent

Abnormal findings
- pH – Alkaline (increases)
- Appearance – cloudy
- Colour - deep amber
- Odour – foul smelling
- Blood – maybe present
- Leukocyte esterase – present
- WBC- present (Pyuria)-WBC $> 10 \times 10^6$/L
- Bacteria- present

Diagnostic Criteria for Significant Bacteriuria
1. ≥102 CFU coliforms/mL or ≥105 CFU noncoliforms/mL in a symptomatic female
2. ≥103 CFU bacteria/mL in a symptomatic male
3. ≥105 CFU bacteria/mL in asymptomatic individuals on two consecutive specimens
4. Any growth of bacteria on suprapubic catheterization in a symptomatic patient
5. ≥102 CFU bacteria/mL in a catheterized patient

Treatment with algorithm:

Goals of antimicrobial therapy:
- ➢ Elimination of infection
- ➢ Relief of acute symptoms
- ➢ Prevention of recurrence and long term complications

Pathogen Specific Treatment: [3]

Pathogen	Treatment options
➢ *Escherichia coli*	ceftriaxone 50mg/kg i.v./I.M. OD
➢ *Pseudomonas aeroginosa*	gentamycin 6-7.5mg/kg i.v. q 8h/qday
➢ Klebsiella sps	
➢ Enterobacter sps/Proteus sps	ceftadizine 100-150mg/kg/day i.v. q 8hr
➢ Enterococcus sps	ampicillin 100-200mg/kg/day 6 hr

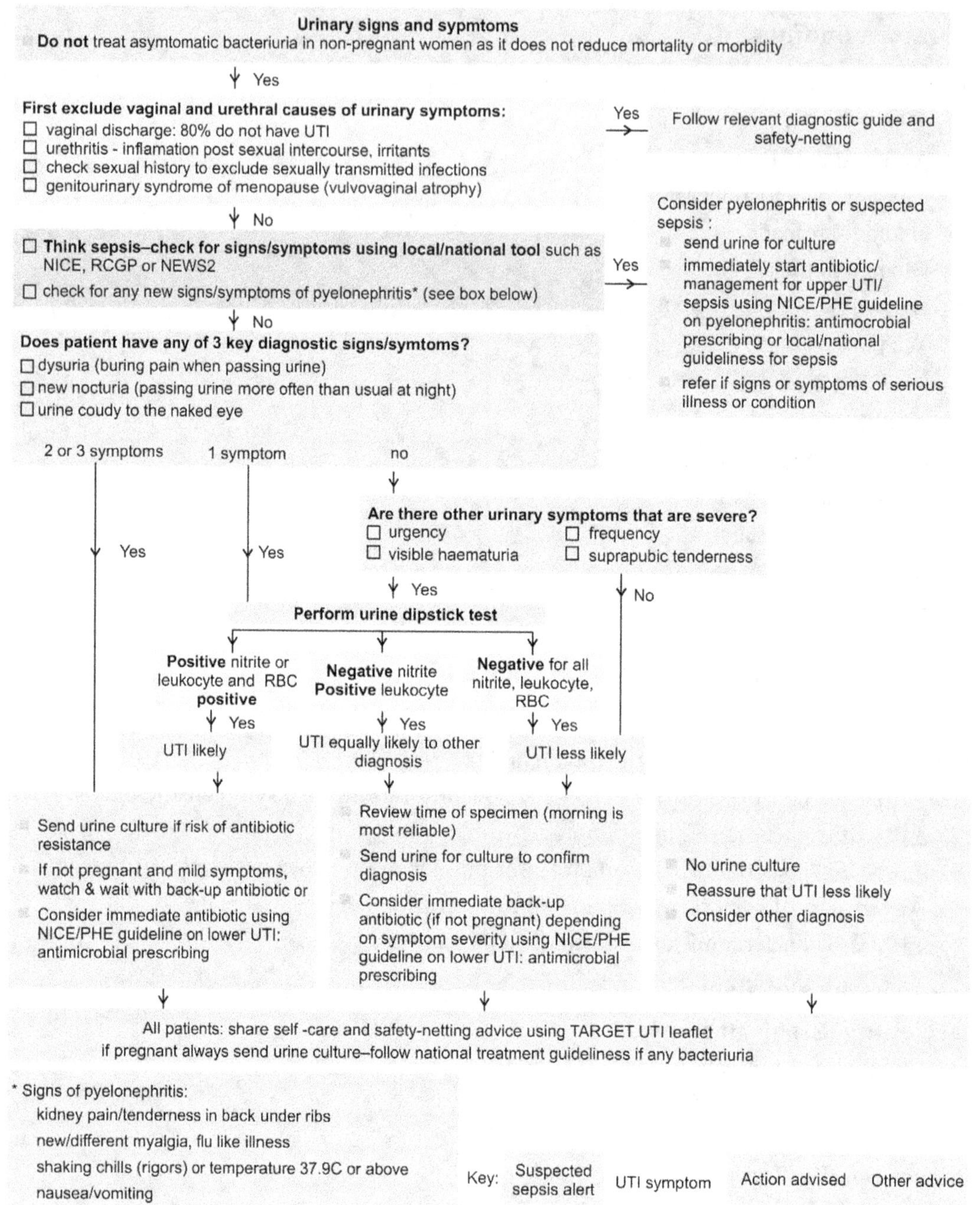

Fig. 46.1 Flowchart for women aged under 65 years with suspected UTI.

Source: Clinical-Pathways.org.UK/Sites/default/files/referral-support/Urology/Pheutiflow chart-under 65 women.pdf.

Flowchart for infants/children under 16 years with suspected UTI

Check temperature and symptoms in all infants/children- unexplained fever 38°C or more OR loin pain/ tenderness suggesting pyelonephritis:

- If yes- Consider referral to a paediatric specialist Test urine within 24 hours If urine test positive, treat with antibiotic.
- If no- Management depends on age and symptoms:
    - (i) Infants younger than 3 months: Most common symptoms: fever, vomiting, lethargy, irritability, poor feeding, failure to thrive Less common: abdominal pain, jaundice, haematuria, offensive urine, then Refer urgently to paediatric specialist care AND send a urine sample for urgent microscopy and culture.
    - (ii) Infant or child over 3 months with suspected UTI: Most common symptoms: fever, frequency, dysuria, abdominal pain, loin tenderness, vomiting, poor feeding, dysfunctional voiding, changes to continence Less common: lethargy, irritability, haematuria, offensive urine, failure to thrive, malaise, cloudy urine, then Perform a urine dipstick test.
    - (a) Positive nitrite and positive leucocyte: Treat as UTI AND start antibiotic Send urine for culture if: • under 3 years • suspected pyelonephritis • risk of serious illness • past UTI • no response to treatment and urine sample not already sent
    - (b) Positive Nitrite Negative leucocyte: Treat as UTI AND start antibiotic if dipstick on fresh urine sample Send urine for culture to confirm diagnosis and reassess with result Repeat urine if not fresh (as old samples can give false positives)
    - (c) Negative nitrite Positive leucocyte: Send urine for culture Under 3 years: start antibiotic and reassess with culture result Over 3 years: only start antibiotics if good clinical evidence of UTI; leucocytes may indicate infection outside urinary tract
    - (d) Negative nitrite and Negative leucocyte: UTI unlikely Do not start antibiotics Exclude other causes Send urine for culture if: • suspected pyelonephritis • risk of serious illness • under 3 months • recurrent UTI • no response to treatment within 24-48 hours and urine sample not sent • symptoms and dipsticks results do not correlate.

Commonly used antibiotics in UTI

Oral therapy

1. **Sulfonamides:** Trimethoprim-sulfamethoxazole (TMP-SMX): These agents generally have been replaced by more agents due to resistance. This combination is highly effective against most aerobic enteric bacteria except Pseudomonas aeruginosa. High urinary tract tissue levels and urine levels are achieved, which may be important in complicated infection treatment. Also effective as prophylaxis for recurrent infections
2. **Penicillins:** Ampicillin Amoxicillin–clavulanic acid Carbenicillin indanyl: Ampicillin is the standard penicillin that has broad-spectrum activity. Increasing Escherichia coli resistance has limited amoxicillin use in acute cystitis. Drug of choice for enterococci

sensitive to penicillin. Amoxicillin-clavulanate is preferred for resistance problems. Carbenicillin indanyl is only indicated for the treatment of urinary tract infections.

3. **Cephalosporins:** Cephalexin Cephradine Cefaclor Cefadroxil Cefuroxime Cefixime Cefzil Cefpodoxime: They may be useful in cases of resistance to amoxicillin and trimethoprim-sulfamethoxazole.

4. **Tetracyclines:** Tetracycline Doxycycline Minocycline: These agents have been effective for initial episodes of urinary tract infections.

5. **Nitrofurantoin:** This agent is effective as both a therapeutic and prophylactic agent in patients with recurrent UTIs

Parenteral therapy:

1. **Aminoglycosides:** Amikacin, Tobramycin: Gentamicin and Tobramycin are equally effective; Gentamicin is less expensive. Tobramycin has better pseudomonal activity

2. **Pencillin:** Amphicillin+sulbactum, Ticarcillin-clavulanate, Pepericilliin+tazobactum: These agents generally are equally effective for susceptible bacteria. The extended-spectrum penicillins are more active against P. aeruginosa and enterococci and often are preferred over cephalosporins.

3. **Cephalosporin:** Ceftriaxone, Ceftazidime: Second- and third-generation cephalosporins have a broad spectrum of activity against gram-negative bacteria

4. **Carbapenams/Monobactams:** Imipenam+Cilistiatin, Meropenam: These agents have broad spectrum of activity, including Gram-positive, gram-negative, and anaerobic bacteria

5. **Fluroquinalones:** Ciprofloxacin, Levofloxacin, Gatifloxacin: These agents have broad-spectrum activity against both gram-negative and gram-positive bacteria. They provide urine and high-tissue concentrations and are actively secreted in reduced renal function.

Treatment regimen for lower UTI in adults:

1. **Acute Uncomplicated cystitis:** Trimethoprim+ Sulfamethoxazole 160/800mg BID 3days

Nitrofurantoin [100mg]	BID 5days
Ciprofloxacin [250-500mg]	BID 3days
Levofloxacin 250mg	OD 3days
Augmentin 500/125mg	BID for 7 days

2. **Acute uncomplicated pyelonephritis :**

   Outpatient management-Ciprofloxacin 500 mg PO BID 7 days

   Levofloxacin 750 mg PO daily 5 days

   Alternatives or Definitive Therapy after susceptibility is confirmed

   Trimethoprim/sulfamethoxazolec 160/800 mg PO BID 14 days

   Cefpodoxime proxetil 200 mg PO BID 10–14 days

   Inpatient management or in those unable to take oral medications

   Ciprofloxacin 400 mg IV q12hr 7 days

   Levofloxacin 500 mg IV q24hr 7 day

   May add aminoglycoside pending culture results. Complete the course with PO antibiotics after afebrile for 48 hr

3. **Complicated UTI:** Trimethoprim+Sulfamethoxazole   1tab BID 7 -10days
    Ciprofloxacin [250-500mg] BID 7 -10days
    Amoxicillin + Clavulanate [500mg+125mg] 8hrly 7-10days
4. **Recurrent infections:** Nitrofurantoin [50mg] OD 6 months
    Trimethoprim + sulphamethoxazole OD 6 months
5. **Acute bacterial prostatitis:** Ceftriaxone 1–2 g IV q24hr
   Ciprofloxacin 400 mg IV q12hr
   Levofloxacin 500 mg IV q24hr
6. **Chronic Bacterial Prostatitis:** Ciprofloxacin 500 mg PO BID 4–6 wk
   Levofloxacin 500 mg PO daily 4–6 wk
   Trimethoprim 100 mg PO BID 4–12 wk
   Doxycycline 100 mg PO BID 4 wk

Empirical Treatment of Urinary Tract Infections

1. **Acute uncomplicated cystitis:** E. Coli, S. Saprophyticus:
    1. Trimethoprim-sulfamethoxazole × 3 days
    2. Quinolone × 3 days
2. **Pregnancy:** E. Coli, S. Saprophyticus- 1. Amoxicillin-clavulanate × 7 days
    2. Cephalosporin × 7 days
3. **Trimethoprim-sulfamethoxazole** × 7 days
4. **Acute pyelonephritis**
    (a) Uncomplicated: E. coli-
        1. Trimethoprim-sulfamethoxazole × 14 days
        2. Quinolone × 14 days
    (b) Complicated: E. coli, Proteus mirabilis, K. pneumoniae, Pseudomonas aeruginosa, E. fecalis –
        1. Quinolone × 14 days
        2. Extended-spectrum penicillin Plus aminoglycoside

Treatment for certain conditions:
1. **Bacteriruria in pregnancy:** To prevent risk of pyelonephritis
   A 7 day course with following antibiotics-cephalexin, nitrofurantoin, Amoxicillin is given. Tetracyclines, sulphonamides and fluoroquinolones should be avoided.
   Regimen: 1. Amoxicillin-clavulanate × 7 days
        2. Cephalosporin × 7 days
        3. Trimethoprim-sulfamethoxazole × 7 days
2. **For relapsing UTI**: 7-10 day course is required. If the patient is not responding a 2 week course is required. Structural abnormalities are corrected by surgery. A 6 week course is required for chidren, adults with continuous symptoms and those who have high risk of renal damage.
3. **UTI in men**: men require prolonged therapy. A urine culture should be obtained before treatment. If G-ve bacteria are presumed, trimethoprim-sulfamethoxazole or a

fluoroquinolone is preferred for 10-14 days initially. If recurrent then a 6 week regimen is followed.

4. **Catheterized patients**: systemic antibiotic therapy should be avoided. Catheter removed as soon as possible. Treatment as described for complicated infections should be started.

Antimicrobial Agents Commonly Used for Chronic Prophylaxis against Recurrent UTIs
1. Nitrofurantoin 50–100 mg nightly
2. Trimethoprim 100 mg nightly
3. Trimethoprim 80 mg + Sulfamethoxazole 400 mg 0.5–1 tablet nightly or 3/week
4. Norfloxacin 200 mg/day
5. Cephalexin 125–250 mg/day
6. Cefaclor 250 mg/day
7. Cephradine 250 mg/day
8. Sulfamethoxazole 500 mg/day

References

1. Clinical pharmacy and therapeutics by Roger Walker, Clive Edwards; 3rd edition; page 503 – 511.
2. Applied therapeutics the clinical use of drugs by Mary Anne konda- kimble; 8th edition; page 456 – 465 [Guideline] Gupta K, Hooton TM, Naber KG, et al. International clinical practice guidelines for the treatment of acute uncomplicated cystitis and pyelonephritis in women: A 2010 update by the Infectious Diseases Society of America and the European Society for Microbiology and Infectious Diseases. *Clin Infect Dis.* 2011 Mar. 52(5):e103-20.
3. Hooton TM, Stamm WE. Diagnosis and treatment of uncomplicated urinary tract infection. *Infect Dis Clin North Am* 1997;11:551-581.
4. Warren JW, Abrutyn E, Hebel JR, et al. Guidelines for antimicrobial treatment of uncomplicated acute bacterial cystitis and acute pyelonephritis in women. Infectious Diseases Society of America (IDSA). *Clin Infect Dis* 1999;29:745-758.
5. NICE 2018. Urinary tract infection (lower): Antimicrobial prescribing.

CHAPTER - 47

Malaria

Introduction to Malaria

- Malaria is a vector borne infection caused by protozoan parasites of plasmodium species.
- It is wide spread in tropical and subtropical regions.

Different species of causative organisms:

- Plasmodium falciparum: most common deadly type of malarial infection.
- Plasmodium vivax: most common and causes relapse if treatment was not completed.
- Plasmodium ovale
- Plasmodium malariae
- Plasmodium knowlesi

Mode of transmission: Malaria is transmitted through the bite of an infected female anopheles mosquito. Other transmission include from mother to unborn child through blood transfusion.

Epidemiology:

- Malaria remains the world`s most devastating human parasite infection.
- Malaria effects over 40% of the world`s population.
- WHO estimates that there are 350-500 million cases of malaria worldwide.
- In India 2 million cases and 1000 deaths occur annually.
- 75% of cases are caused by plasmodium falciparum and 20% by plasmodium vivax.

Vectors:

- Anopheles culicifacies- rural, peri urban
- An.fluviatilis- forest, hilly areas
- An. Stepensi- urban, industrial
- An. Minimus- foot hills
- An. Philippinensis and an. Sundaicus

Life span: 10-12 days

Choice of host: Anthrophilic species

Breeding habits: Moving water, wells, fountain, garden pools,

Time of biting: Night time

Pathophysiology

The erythrocytic phase causes extensive hemolysis, which results in anemia and splenomegaly. The most serious complications usually are associated with P. falciparum infections. Infants and children younger than 5 years of age and nonimmune pregnant women are at high risk for severe complications from falciparum malaria. The complications associated with falciparum malaria are primarily a result of the high parasitemia and the ability of the parasites to sequester in capillaries and postcapillary vessels of organs such as the brain and the kidney.

Incubation period:
- It is usually 7-30 days
- Increased in *P. malariae* and reduced in p. falciparum.

Clinical presentation:

Usual symptoms include fever, headache, muscle pain, anorexia, nausea, hepatomegaly, splenomegaly, anemia, jaundice, dehydration.

P. falciparum infection:
- This is the most dangerous type of malarias and patients are either killed or cured.
- The onset is insidious with malaise, headache and vomiting.
- Jaundice due to hemolysis and hepatic dysfunction.
- Hepatomegaly, splenomegaly, anaemia, thrombocytopenia, parasitaemia(blood).

Other symptoms:

Neurological: coma, hypoglycaemia, seizures, cerebral malaria.

Respiratory: pulmonary edema, secondary bacterial pneumonia.

Cardiovascular: shock, cardiac failure

Renal: acute renal failure, haemoglobinuria (black water fever)

Severe manifestations/complications of *P. falciparum* malaria and their immediate management:
Coma:
- Maintain airway
- Nurse on side
- Exclude other treatable causes of coma (ex: hypoglycaemia, meningitis)
- Avoid harmful axillary treatments such as corticosteroids, heparin and adrenaline

Hyperpyrexia: Tepid sponging, fanning, cooling blanket, antipyretic drug (paracetamol)

Convulsions: Maintain airway/ Treat with diazepam or paraldehyde injection

Severe anaemia: Transfer fresh whole blood or packed cells

Acute pulmonary edema: Give oxygen, 250ml of blood, give diuretic, and stop intravenous fluids. Harmofilter and intubate and add PEEP (Positive end expiratory pressure) or CPAP (Continuous positive airway pressure) in life threatening hypoxemia.

Acute renal failure: Exclude prerenal causes/ Fluid resuscitation/ Peritoneal dialysis

Shock: Suspect G-ve septicaemia/ Take blood cultures/ Give parenteral anti-microbials/ Correct hemodynamic disturbances

Aspiration pneumonia: Give parenteral antimicrobial drugs/ Physiotherapy/ Give oxygen

Specific therapy:
- Intravenous artesunate
- Mefloquine should be avoided due to increased risk of post-malaria neurologic syndrome.
- Absorption and intrauterine growth retardation from parasitisation of the maternal side of the placenta are frequent.
- Previous splenectomy increases the risk of severe malaria.

P. vivax and *P. ovale* **infection:**
- Illness starts with days of continued fever before development of classical bouts of fever on alternate days
- Fever with rigors and temperature rises to about 40° C
- Cold
- Flush phase leading to profuse perspiration (repeat 48 hours later)
- Splenomegaly, hepatomegaly, tenderness, anaemia
- Relapses are frequent in first 2 years after leaving malarious area.

P. malariae **infection:**
- Mild symptoms and bouts of fever every third day.
- Parasitaemia may persist for many years with occasional recudescence of fever or without producing any symptoms
- Chronic condition causes glomerulonephritis and long term nephrotic syndrome in children

Diagnosis with algorithm
- ➤ Malaria suspected based on clinical findings and exposure history.
- ➤ Perform one or more of the following below malaria tests immediately
  - (a) Rapid diagnostic test done using lateral flow immunochromatography assay and preliminaty result to be provided.
  - (b) Microscopic examination of blood films-if it is ngative repeat testing as indictaed. If it is positive, identification of species to be done. Calculate the % of paracitemia. Subsequent monitoring of parasite density is indicated for monitoring response to therapy.
  - (c) Nucleic acid amplification test to be done. If it is negative, testing to be repeated as indicated. If it is positive Calculate the % of paracitemia. Subsequent monitoring of parasite density is indicated for monitoring response to therapy.

Diagnosis:

Blood examination: thin and thick blood film

Dipstick test: not as effective when parasite levels are below 100 parasites/ml of blood.

PCR: to determine the species of plasmodium

Chest X-ray: helpful if respiratory symptoms are seen

CT-Scan: to evaluate evidence of cerebral edema or haemorrhage

CBP (increased ESR)

Quantitative buff coal technique

Urine analysis

Immunochromatographic tests for malaria antigens (detects plasmodium lactate dehydrogenase of several species)

Management

Nonpharmacological:
- Use of nets and repellent containing 30-50% DEET (N, N-diethyl-3-methylbenzamide) should be applied to exposed areas of skin to avoid mosquito bites.

Table 47.1 Pharmacological management.

Drug	Mechanism of Action	Mechanism of resistance
Artemisinin and Derivatives	Production of toxic heme-adducts	Not known at this time
Atovaquone	Inhibits mitochondrial electron transport in the cytochrome bc, complex	Nucleotide polymorphisms in the cytochrome b gene
Proguanil	Inhibits dihydrofolate reductase-thymidylate synthase	Mutations in the amino acid sequence near the dihydrofotate-reductase binding site
Pyrimethamine	Inhibits *Plasmodium* dihydrofolate-reductase	Mutations in dihydrofolate-reductase binding site
Sulfadoxine	Inhibition of *Plasmodium* dihydropteroate synthase	Mutations in dihydropteroate synthase gene
Chloroquine/Hydroxychloroquine	Production of toxic heme adducts	Production of a chloroquine efflux transporter
Quinine/Quinidine	Production of of toxic heme adducts	Production of an efflux transporter; amplification of *pfmdr 1* gene
Mefloquine	Production of toxic heme adducts There is also a *cytosolic* mode of action	Amplification of *pfmdr 1* gene that accumulates drug in digestive vacuole away from cytosolic site of action
Primaquine	Production of reactive oxygen species	Not known at this time

Mild *P. falciparum* malaria

- *P. falciparum* is resistant to chloroquine and sulfadoxine-pyrethamine (fansidar) almost worldwide, an artemicinin based treatment is recommended.

- Co-artemeter contains artemeter and lumefantrine and is given as 4 tables at 0, 8, 24, 36, 48 and 60 hours.
- Alternatives are quinine by mouth (600mg of quinine salt every 8 hours for 5-7 days), together with or followed by either doxycycline (200mg OD for 7days) or clindamycin (450mg every 8 hrs for 7 days) or atovaquone-proguanil (4 tablets OD for 3 days).
- Doxycycline and artemether should be avoided in pregnancy.
- Artesunate (200 mg orally OD for 3 days) followed by mefloquine (1g orally on day 2 and 500 mg orally on day 3) may be used.

Complicated *P. falciparum* malaria

- Severe malaria should be considered in any nonimmune patient with a parasite count greater than 2%
- Management includes antimalarial chemotherapy, active treatment of complications, fluid and electrolyte and acid-base balance and avoidance of harmful ancillary treatment.
- **Treatment of choice:** IV artesunate – 24 mg/kg at 0, 12, 24 hrs and then once a day for 7 days. If patient gets recovered then oral artesunate 2mg/kg OD is preferred.
- **Quinine salt:** loading dose infusion of 20mg/kg over 4 hrs (max 1.4 g) followed by maintenance doses of 10 mg/kg as 4 hr infusions 2-3 times daily upto max. of 100mg per dose
- Patients should be monitored by ECG (QRS duration and QT interval)
- Mefloquinone should not be used for severe malaria since no parenteral form is available
- Exchange transfusion may be beneficial for nan-immune patients with persisting high parasitaemias (>10 % circulating erythrocytes)

Management of non-falciparum malaria

- *P. vivax, P. ovale, P. malariae* infections should be treated with Oral chloroquine: 600mg chloroquine base followed by 300 mg base in6 hrs, then 150mg base 12 hourly for 2 more days
- Radical care is achieved by using a course of primaquine (15mg daily for 14 days) while destroys hypnozoite phase in liver
- Late relapses can be treated by prescribing antimalarial drugs in suppressive doses

Prevention

- Clinical attacks of malaria may be preventable with chemoprophylaxis using chloroquine, atovaquone plus proguanil (malaria) doxycycline or mefloquine
- Using permethrin impregnated mosquito or insecticide treated bed nets, electronic mosquito repellants, intermittent preventive treatment in pregnant women.

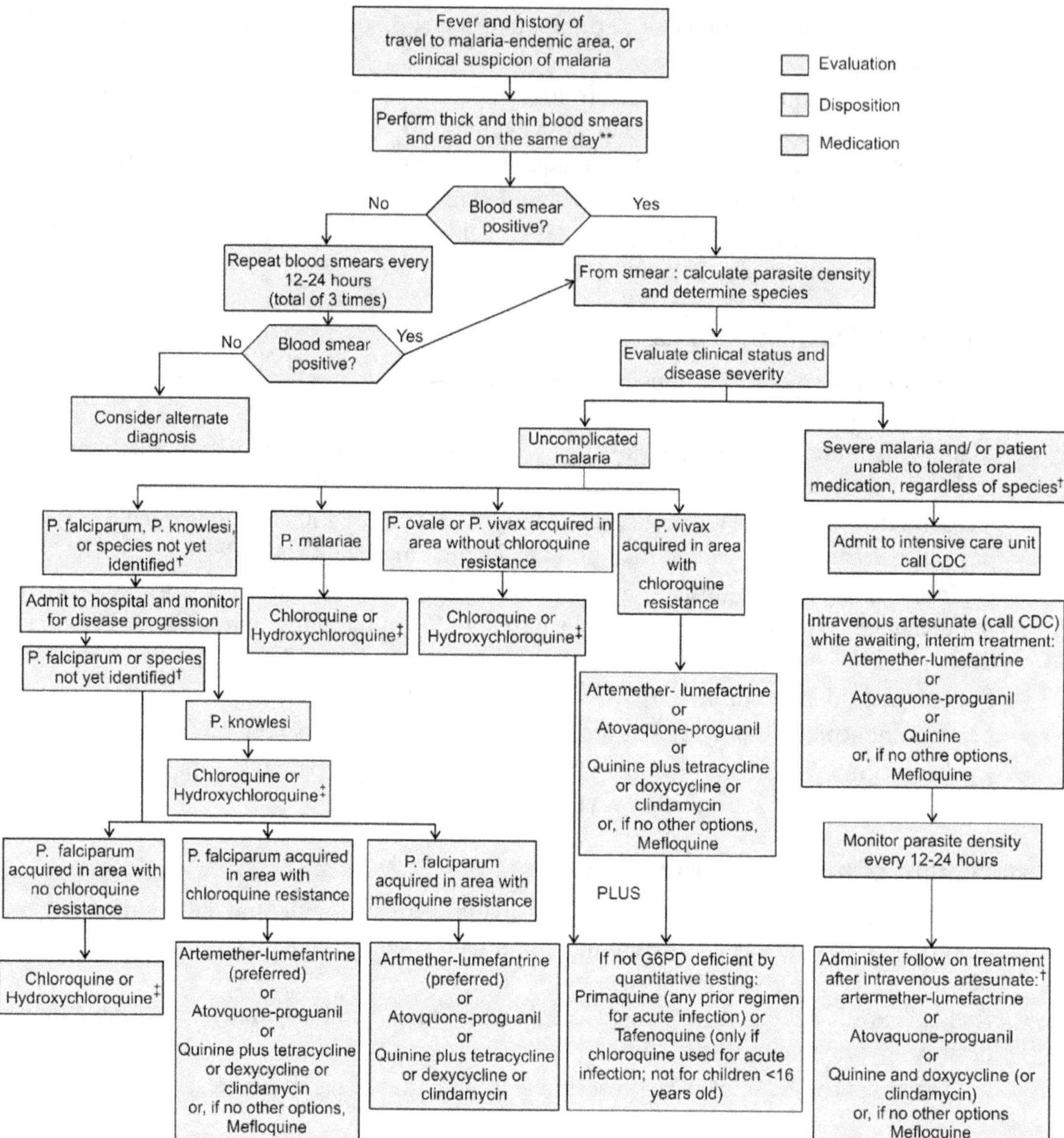

Fig. 47.1 Algorithm for diagnosis and management of malaria.

Source: cdc.gov/malaria/resources/pdf/algorithm.pdf.

CDC Algorithm for the management of malaria

Table 47.2 Chemoprophylaxis of malaria: in non-immune.

Antimalarial tablets	Adult prophylactic dose	Regimen
Chloroquine resistance high • Mefloquine	250mg weekly	2-3 weeks before travel and continued till 4 wks after
• Doxycycline	100mg daily	Started 1 wk before and continued until 4 wks after travel
• Malarone	1 tablet daily	From 1-2 days before travel until 1wk after return
Chloroquine resistant absent • Chloroquine • Proguanil	300mg base weekly 100-200 mg daily	Started 1 wk before and continued until 4 wks after return

Case Study of Malaria

Summary

A 38 years old woman got admitted in the hospital with these symptoms. She had fever with chills and rigors associated with generalized body weakness and pain, she doesn't had a past medical history. She underwent CBP which revealed abnormal haemoglobin levels and platelet count was very low and also low RBC levels. Peripheral smear has shown microcytic hypochromic RBC. Which indicate abnormal HB levels and also serum iron level was low (39 micro gm/dl) ultra sound abdomen revealed Hepatomegaly – Grade II. The smear for malarial parasite revealed presence of schizonts of plasmodium vivax. ESR levels were noted, vitals were abnormal with temperature 100.1 degree F and pulse: 132 bpm, liver function tests revealed low levels of SGPT and SGOT.

Diagnosis: Based on the CBP and Hematology reports, she was finally diagnosed with Malaria with Thrombocytopenia. She also has microcytic hypochromic anemia which was not noticed properly.

Trade name	Generic name	Dose	Route	Frequency
T.Dolo	Paracetamol	650 mg	P/O	TID
T.Rantac	Ranitidine	150mg	P/O	BD
T.Zincovit	Vitamins	1tab	P/O	BD
T.Doxy	Doxycycline	100mg	P/O	BD
T.Malarid	Primaquine	15mg	P/O	OD
T.Montek-LC	Montelukast and levocetrizine	5/10mg	P/O	SOS
	Artemether			BD
T.Lumerax	Iron +Folic acid	480mg	P/O	
T.Orofer-XT	Vitamin C	1tab	P/O	OD
T.Limcee	Normal saline	1tab	P/O	OD
N.S	Ringerlactose			
RLDNS	Dextrose normal saline	100ml/hr	I.V	

Daily Progress

Day 3- c/o fever at night with episodes of vomitings and complaint of head ache. Day 4 – c/o swelling of B/L parotid area. Day 6- c/o headache, no other complaints. Day 7- Patient was discharged and she was conscious stable at time of discharge.

Discharge Medications

T.Doxy 100mg BD 1day

T.Dolo 650mg BD 3days

T.Rantac 150mg BD 2days

T.Zincovit 1tab OD 30days

T.Malaraid 15mg OD 9days

T.Orofer-XT OD 9days

T.Limcee OD 30 days

T.Montek LC OD 15days

T.Lumerox 80mg BD 1day

Pharmacist Interventions

Patient has a problem of microcytic hypochromic anemia which was not mentioned clearly in case sheet. Care must be taken in order to normalize iron content and haemoglobin content. Primaquine and lumefantrine has a chance of getting interacted resulting in risk of irregular heart rhythm. Hence time of administration of the above 2 drugs must differ by atleast 3-6 hrs

Patient Counselling

- Proper hygiene conditions maintained.
- Apply mosquito repellentgels to avoid mosquitobite.
- Iron rich diet like cereals, ricebreads, cooked beans, lentils, Nut are to be taken.
- Garlic increases blood count.
- Broccoli-excellent source of Vit K it regenerates blood platelets.
- Proper diet maintenance.

Assignment

1. **What are the signs and symptoms of malaria in this patient?**
   Fever with chills and rigors, associated with generalized body weakness and pain, headache, fever at nights with episodes of vomitings.
2. **Which blood studies are to be performed in diagnosis of malaria?**
   - Thick and thin blood smears to identify the presence and the type of parasite.

- Rapid diagnostic test: It detects presence of parasite.
- PCR /Molecular test: to determine the species of plasmodium.
- Antibody test: To determine the patients past malaria.
- Drug resistance test: To test if the parasite is resistance to the drug.
- Blood test: To determine the count of RBC, WBC, Platelets, how serious the condition is and if it causes any further problems like anemia or kidney failure.

3. **What complications are associated with plasmodium falciparum malaria?**

   Coma, Hyperpyrexia, Convulsions, Severe anemia

   Acute pulmonary edema, Acute renal failure, Shock

   Aspiration pneumonia

4. **What is the incubation period of malaria infection?**

   Each plasmodium species has typical incubation period

   P.Falciparum -14days

   P.Vivax -12-18 days

   P.Ovale – 18-40 days

5. **How is malaria treated during pregnancy?**
   - Uncomplicated malaria:

     First trimester: Quinine + clindamycin – given for 7 days if this fail then Artesunate + Clindamycin - 7 days if Clindamycin in unavailable then Quinine monotherapy is given.

     Second and third trimester: Artesunate + Clindamycin – 7days

     Quinine +Clindamycin – 7 days

     Doses: Quinine – 10mg/kg TID

     Clindamycin – 10 mg/kg BD

     Chloroquine -300mg weekly

     Artesunate – 2.4 mg /kg
   - **Complicated malaria** : Parenteral therapy should be given in pregnant with severe anemia without any delay

   First trimester: Artesunate and quinine are given

   Second and third trimester: Artesunate is given in parenteral route because quinine is associated with recurrent hypoglycemia.

6. **How is malaria treated in children?**
   - ➢ Treatment for Chloroquine resistant patient:

     Species: P.vivax and Chloroquine resistant P. falciparum
     - Treatment: Chloroquine 10mg /kg stat followed by 5 mg /kg at 6hrs, 24 hrs ,48 hrs
     - Chloroquine 10mg/kg followed by 10mg/kg at 24 hrs , 5mg at 48 hrs
     - In case of vivax to prevent relapse: Primaquine – 0.25 mg /kg day -14days

- In case of falciparum malaria a single dose of Primaquine is given for gametocytidal action
- Primaquine – 0.75 mg/kg

➢ Treatment for Chloroquine resistant P. falciparum:

Species:

Chloroquine resistant P.falciparum

Artesunate – 4mg/kg - 7day OD

Mefloquine – 25 mg/kg divided into 2 doses at 4-6 hours

A single dose of Primaquine for gametocydal action

Primaquine – 0.75 mg/kg

➢ Treatment of multidrug resistant P.falciparum:

Quinine – 10 mg/kg TID for 7-10 days

In case of chinconism Quinine 10 mg salt /kg/dose TID for 3-5 days + tetracycline's 4mg/kg /dose QID for 7-10 days

Doxycycline 3mg/kg/day BD for 7-10 days

Clindamycin 20mg /kg /day divided 3 times daily

For gametocyte action: Primaquine 0.75 mg/kg

➢ For severe and complicated malaria:

Initially IV therapy later replaced with oral administration.

Quinine salt 20 mg salt/kg diluted in 10ml glucose by infusion over 4 hrs.

Then 12 hrs after the salt, given maintenance dose of over 2 hrs.

This maintenance dose should be repeated every 8 hrs from beginning of previous infusing until the patient can swallow, then quinine tablet 10mg/kg 8hrly to complete 7 days course.

If IV therapy cannot be done IM is done in anterior thigh.

 Half the dose in each anterior thigh.

If possible IM quinine should be diluted in normal saline Quinine 300mg salt /ml saline.

➢ Alternative drug other than quinine in severe malaria

Artesunate 24mg /kg IV followed by 1.2 mg /kg at 12, 24hrs

Artemether 3.2 mg/kg IM followed by 1.6 mg /kg for 6 days .if able to swallow daily dose given orally .

Artesunate 60mg per ampoule dissolved in 0.6 ml of 5% NaoH dilute with 3-5 ml with 5% dextrose and given immediately by bolus.

7. **What are the possible adverse effects of anti malarials?**

- **Chloroquine:** Nausea, vomiting, anorexia, itching, headache, epigastricpain, uneasiness

- **Prolonged high dose:** Loss of hearing, rashes, photoallergy, myopathy, mental disturbances, graying of hair

- **Mefloquine:** Dizziness, Nausea, vomit, diarrhea, abdominal pain, sinus

- **Quinine:** Highly toxic, Chinconism, Ringing ears, Nausea, Vomit, GI irritation, Headache, Visual defects, Diarrhea
- **Pyrimethamine:** Nausea, Rashes, Folate deficiency
- **Proguanil:** Vomit, Rash, Hematuria

8. Pharmacotherapeutic regimen of malaria?

Mild falciparum malaria: Coartemether 0, 8, 24, 36 hrs

Alternative: quinine 600mg every 8 hrs 5-7 day Doxycycline 200mg, Clindamycin 450 mg, artesunate – 200mg

- Complicated falciparum: Artesunate: IV 24mg/kg at 0, 12, 24 then OD

  Quinine salt – 20mg/kg 4 hrs, 10mg/kg 4 hrs
- Non falciparum malaria : -

  Chloroquine : 600mg Followed by 300 mg in 6 hrs

  Followed by 150 mg in 12 hourly for 2 months

  Primaquine :15mg daily for 14 days which destroy hypozoites.

References

1. Karolina – Anthoula Akinosoglou. The management of malaria in a adults. Clin Med (Lond).2011. Octs;11(5):497-501.
2. Treatment of Malaria: Guidelines for Clinicians. Cdc-giv. Available at https://www.cdc.gov/malaria/diagnosis-treatment/clinicianl.html.

CHAPTER - 48

HIV (Human Immuno Deficiency Virus)

Introduction to HIV

HIV stands for "human immunodefiency virus" which is the cause of AIDS (Aquired immunodefiency syndrome).

Epidemiology and Transmission [1]

- Infection with human immunodeficiency virus (HIV) occurs through three primary modes: sexual, parenteral, and perinatal.
- Sexual intercourse, primarily receptive anal and vaginal intercourse, is the most common vehicle for transmission.
- The probability of HIV transmission from receptive anorectal intercourse is 0.1% to 3% per sexual contact and 0.1% to 0.2% per sexual contact for receptive vaginal intercourse. Condom use reduces the risk of transmission by approximately 20-fold.
- Individuals with genital ulcers or sexually transmitted diseases, such as syphilis, chancroid, herpes, gonorrhea, *Chlamydia,* and trichomoniasis, are at great risk for contracting HIV.
- The use of contaminated needles or other injection-related paraphernalia by drug abusers has been the main cause of parenteral transmissions of HIV.
- Healthcare workers have a small risk of occupationally acquiring HIV, mostly through accidental injury, most often, percutaneous needle stick injury.
- Perinatal infection, or vertical transmission, is the most common cause of pediatric HIV infection. The risk of mother-to-child transmission is approximately 25% in the absence of breast-feeding or antiretroviral therapy. Breast-feeding can also transmit HIV.

Etiology

HIV is a member of the genus *Lentivirus,* part of the family *Retroviridae.* Lentiviruses have many morphologies and biological properties in common. Many species are infected by lentiviruses, which are characteristically responsible for long-duration illnesses with a long incubation period. Lentiviruses are transmitted as single-stranded, positive-sense, enveloped RNA viruses. [2]

Types: Two types of HIV have been characterized: HIV-1 and HIV-2. HIV-1 is the virus that was initially discovered and termed both LAV (Lymphadenopathy Associated Virus) and HTLV-III (Human T cell Lymphotropic Virus III). HIV-1 is more virulent and more infective than HIV-2.

Structure and Genome: HIV is different in structure from other retroviruses. It is roughly spherical with a diameter of about 120 nm, around 60 times smaller than a red blood cell. It is composed of two copies of positive-sense single-stranded RNA that codes for the virus's nine genes enclosed by a conical capsid composed of 2,000 copies of the viral protein p24. The single-stranded RNA is tightly bound to nucleocapsid proteins, p7, and enzymes needed for the development of the virion such as reverse transcriptase, proteases, ribonuclease and integrase. A matrix composed of the viral protein p17 surrounds the capsid ensuring the integrity of the virion particle.

This is, in turn, surrounded by the viral envelope, that is composed of the lipid bilayer taken from the membrane of a human host cell when the newly formed virus particle buds from the cell. The viral envelope contains proteins from the host cell and relatively few copies of the HIV Envelope protein, which consists of a cap made of three molecules known as glycoprotein (gp) 120, and a stem consisting of three gp41 molecules that anchor the structure into the viral envelope. The Envelope protein, encoded by the HIV *env* gene, allows the virus to attach to target cells and fuse the viral envelope with the target cell's membrane releasing the viral contents into the cell and initiating the infectious cycle. HIV can infect a variety of immune cells such as CD4$^+$ T cells, macrophages, and microglial cells. HIV-1 entry to macrophages and CD4$^+$ T cells is mediated through interaction of the virion envelope glycoproteins (gp120) with the CD4 molecule on the target cells membrane and also with chemokine co-receptors.

Pathogenesis [3, 4, 5]

HIV virus entry into the human body and gp160 (gp120+gp41) mediated binding of virus to CD4+ receptors and proteins present on macrophages, monocytes, dendritic cells takes place. Gp 120 binds virus to CD4+ receptors with high affinity. Chemokine recptors enhance further association of CCR5 and CXCR5 (R5 viruses use CCR5 and X4 viruses use CXCR4 as coreceptors). Clinical picture may show coexistence of R5 & X4 or DUAL TYPE (R5X4). INSIDE the host cell: Uncoating in preparation for replication is started. Reverse transcription for propogation in host using reverse transcriptase takes pace. Single strand RNA is converted into DNA, which is then translated into RNA. Integration of ds DNA into host cell chromosome by INTEGRASE. Replication of virus (proviral DNA →mRNA→viral peotiens). Regulatory proteins Tat, Nef, Rev are synthesized. Assembly of virion particles beneath hostcell lipid bilayer is seen. Nucleocapsid synthesis by viral ss RNA is initiated. The next step i.e. packing & budding through host lipid layer takes place. Maturation of virion by functional proteins formation and progression of infection proceeds by causing cell lysis. T lymphocyte induced killing and apoptosis. CD4+ cell destruction & compromising of immune function is started. Gradually the person becomes immunocompramised dut to CD4+ cells invasion and apotosis and leads to AIDS.

Clinical Manifestation and Features

Primary HIV infection:

Asymptomatic, Acute retroviral syndrome

Clinical stage 1:

Persistent generalised lymphadenopathy.

Clinical stage 2:

Moderate unexplained weight loss, Herpes zoster, Angular cheilitis,

Recurrent oral ulceration, Papular pruritic eruptions, Seborrheic dermatitis, fungal nails infections.

Clinical stage 3:

Unexplained severe weight loss (>10% of presumed or measured body weight), Unexplained chronic diarrhea for >1 month, Unexplained persistent fever for >1 month (>37.6°C, intermittent or constant), Persistent oral candidiasis (thrush), Oral hairy leukoplakia, Pulmonary tuberculosis (current), Severe presumed bacterial infections (e.g., pneumonia, empyema, pyomyositis, bone or joint infection, meningitis, bacteremia) , Acute necrotizing ulcerative stomatitis, gingivitis, or periodontitis ,Unexplained anemia .

Clinical stage 4:

Pneumocystis pneumonia , Recurrent severe bacterial pneumonia , Chronic herpes simplex infection (orolabial, genital, or anorectal site for >1 month or visceral herpes at any site), Esophageal candidiasis (or candidiasis of trachea, bronchi, or lungs), Extrapulmonary tuberculosis, Kaposi sarcoma , Cytomegalovirus infection (retinitis or infection of other organs), Central nervous system toxoplasmosis , HIV encephalopathy, Cryptococcosis, extrapulmonary (including meningitis), Disseminated nontuberculosis mycobacteria infection, Progressive multifocal leukoencephalopathy.

Diagnosis with algirithm of HIV

> HIV-1/HIV-2 antigen/antibody combination immunoassay to be done
> If test is positive-HIV-1/HIV-2 antibody differentiation immunoassay to be done. The result can be categorized as
> (a) HIV-1 +ve   HIV-2 -ve   HIV-1 antibodies detected
> (b) HIV-1 -ve   HIV-2 +ve   HIV-2 antibodies detected
> (c) HIV-1 +ve   HIV-2 +ve   HIV antibodies detected
> (d) HIV-1 –ve or indeterminate   HIV-2 -ve. Then nucleic acid test NAT to be done.
> HIV-1 NAT +ve –it is confirmed as Acute HIV-1 infection
> HIV-1 NAT –ve it is confirmed as negative for HIV-1
> If the result is negative for HIV-1 and HIV-2 antibodies and p24 antigen, then no HIV disease in the patient.

ELISA, which detects antibodies against HIV-1. The ELISA test is both highly sensitive (>99%) and highly specific (>99%)

False Positive: Occur in multiparous women; recent recipients of hepatitis B, HIV, influenza, or rabies vaccine; patients with multiple blood transfusion, liver disease, and renal failure; or those on chronic hemodialysis.

False Negative: Occur if the patient is newly infected and the test is performed before antibody production is adequate. The minimum time to develop antibodies is 3 to 4 weeks from initial exposure, with greater than 95% of individuals developing antibodies after 6 months.

Surrogate Markers:
- Occur if the patient is newly infected and the test is performed before antibody production is adequate. The minimum time to develop antibodies is 3 to 4 weeks from initial exposure, with greater than 95% of individuals developing antibodies after 6 months. Viral load is reported as the number of viral RNA copies per millilitre.
- Because HIV attacks and destroys cells bearing the CD4 receptor, the number of CD4 lymphocytes in the blood is a surrogate marker of disease progression.
- The normal adult CD4 lymphocyte count ranges from 500 to 1600 cells/mcL, or 40% to 70% of all lymphocytes.
- CD4 counts in children are age-dependent, with younger children having higher CD4 counts. Depletion of CD4 cells has been associated with the development of opportunistic infections and other AIDS malignancies.

Management

Goals of therapy:
1. To decrease morbidity and mortality
2. Improve quality of life
3. Achieve maximum suppression of HIV infection.
4. Achieve plasma viral load less than lower level of quantitation.

Pharmacological treatment:

General Approach to Treatment of Human Immunodeficiency Virus Infection
- Regular, periodic measurement of plasma HIVRNA levels and CD4 cell counts is necessary to determine the risk of disease progression in an HIV infected individual and to determine when to initiate or modify antiretroviral treatment regimens.
- Treatment decisions should be individualized by level of risk indicated by plasma HIV RNA levels and CD4 counts.
- The use of potent combination antiretroviral therapy to suppress HIV replication to below the levels of detection of sensitive plasma HIV RNA assays limits the potential for selection of antiretroviral-resistant HIV variants, the major factor limiting the ability of antiretroviral drugs to inhibit virus replication and delay disease progression.
- The most effective means to accomplish durable suppression of HIV replication is the simultaneous initiation of combinations of effective anti-HIV drugs Persons with acute

primary HIV infections should be treated with combination antiretroviral therapy to suppress virus replication to levels below the limit of detection of sensitive plasma HIV RNA assays.

- HIV-infected persons, even those with viral loads below detectable limits, should be considered infectious and should be counseled to avoid sexual and drug-use behaviors that are associated with transmission or acquisition of HIV and other infectious pathogens.

The two established targets for anti-HIV attack are: (a) HIV reverse transcriptase: Which transcripts HIV-RNA into proviral DNA. (b) HIV protease: Which cleaves the large virus directed polyprotein into functional viral proteins. Some newer targets are:

1. Fusion of viral envelope with plasma membrane of CD4 cells through which HIVRNA enters the cell.
2. Chemokine coreceptor (CCR5) on host cells which provide anchorage for the surface proteins of the virus.
3. HIV-integrase: Viral enzyme which integrates the proviral DNA into host DNA. [6]

Classification of Anti-Hiv Drugs

1. **Anti-Retrovirus**
   (a) Nucleoside reverse transcriptase inhibitors (NRTIs): Zidovudine (AZT), Didanosine, Stavudine, Lamivudine, Abacavir, Emtricitabine, Tenofovir (Nt RTI); **MOA:** Nucleic acid analogues mimic the normal buiding blocks of DNA, preventing transcription of viral RNA to DNA.
   (b) Nonnucleoside reverse transcriptase inhibitors (NNRTIs): Nevirapine, Efavirenz, Delavirdine; **MOA:** alter the confirmation of the catalytic site of reverse transcriptase and directly inhibit its action.
   (c) Protease inhibitors: Ritonavir, Atazanavir, Indinavir, Nelfinavir, Saquinavir, Amprenavir, Lopinavir; **MOA:** inhibit the final stages of HIV replication, reslting in the formation of non-infective viral particles.
   (d) Entry (Fusion) inhibitor: Enfuvirtide ; **MOA: B**ind to viral gp41 or gp 120 or host cell CD4+ or chemokine receptors
   (e) CCR5 receptor inhibitor: Maraviroc
   (f) Integrase inhibitor: Raltegravir; **MOA:** prevent the transfer of proviral DNA strands into the host chromosomal DNA

Treatment of HIV Infection: Antiretroviral Regimens Recommended in Antiretroviral-Naive Persons

1. **Nonnucleoside Reverse Transcriptase Inhibitor (NNRTI)–Based Regimens:**
   (a) Preferred: Efavirenz + lamivudine + zidovudine (or tenofovir DF or stavudine) except for pregnant women or women with pregnancy potential
   (b) Alternatives: Efavirenz + emtricitabine + zidovudine (or tenofovir DF or stavudine) except for pregnant women or women with pregnancy potential
      or

Efavirenz + (lamivudine or emtricitabine) + didanosine except for pregnant women or women with pregnancy potential **or**

Nevirapine plus (lamivudine or emtricitabine) + zidovudine (or stavudine or didanosine)

2. **Protease Inhibitor (PI)–Based Regimens**

   (a) Preferred: Lopinavir/ritonavir + lamivudine + zidovudine (or stavudine)

   (b) Alternatives:
   - Amprenavir/ritonavir + lamivudine (or emtricitabine) + zidovudine (or stavudine)
   - Atazanavir + lamivudine (or emtricitabine) + zidovudine (or stavudine)
   - Indinavir-ritonavir + lamivudine (or emtricitabine) + zidovudine (or stavudine)
   - Lopinavir-ritonavir + emtricitabine + zidovudine (or stavudine)
   - Nelfinavir + lamivudine (or emtricitabine) plus zidovudine (or stavudine)
   - Saquinavir-ritonavir + lamivudine (or emtricitabine) + zidovudine (or stavudine)

3. **Triple Nucleoside Reverse Transcriptase Inhibitor–Based Regimen**

   (Only as an alternative to NNRTI- or PI-based regimens when these cannot be used as preferred therapy)

   Abacavir + lamivudine + zidovudine

   Abacavir +lamivudine + stavudine

Therapeutic regimens: Whenever treatment is instituted, it should be aggressive (HAART) with at least 3 anti-HIV drugs. The optimum response to any regimen is reduction of plasma HIV-RNA to undetectable levels (less than 50copies/μl) within 6 months.

- All regimens should have 2 NRTI+1NNRTI.
- Lamivudine is to be included in all regimens.
- NRTI can be zidovudine or stavudine.
- NNRTI can be nevirapine or efavirenz.
- Efavirenz is preferred in patients with hepatic dysfunction and in those concurrently receiving rifampin. Efavirenz is not to be used in pregnant women.

Antiretroviral drug combinations to be avoided:

1. Zidovudine + stavudine: Pharmacodynamic antagonism
2. Stavudine + didanosine: Increased toxicity (neuropathy, lactic acidosis)
3. Lamivudine + didanosine: Clinically not additive

Post-exposure prophylaxis of HIV Basic (2 drug) regimen (for low risk) :

Zidovudine 300 mg + Twice daily

Lamivudine 150 mg for 4 weeks

Expanded (3 drug) regimen (for high risk) patients: Zidovudine 300 mg + Twice daily

Lamivudine 150 mg + Indinavir 800 mg Thrice daily (or another PI) All for 4 weeks

Characteristics of Antiretroviral Agents for the Treatment of Adult Human Immunodeficiency Virus (HIV) Infection

1. Nucleoside reverse transcriptase inhibitors:

Drug	Dose	Frequency	t ½
Abacavir	300mg	BD	1.5 hr
Didanosine	200mg	BD	1.4hr
Emtricitabine	400mg	OD	10hr
Lamivudine	150mg	BD	5hr
Stavudine	40mg	BD	1.4hr
Tenofovir	300mg	OD	1.7hr
Zidovudine	200mg	TID	1.1hr

Non nucleoside reverse transcriptase inhibitors:

Drug	Dose	Frequency	t ½
Delavirdine	400mg	TID	5.8hr
Efavirenz	600mg	OD	48hr
Nevirapine	200mg	OD	25hr

Protease inhibitors:

Drug	Dose	t ½
Indinavir	800mg	43 hr
Lopinavir	400mg	6.5hr
Ritonavir	600mg	8.8hr
Saquinavir	1200mg	80hr

Treatment during pregnancy:

- Pregnant women should be treated as like non pregnant adults.
- Abacavir, emtricitabine, lamivudine or zidovudine should be avoided.
- IV zidovudine is given intrapartum depending on mothers viral load.

Prevention and Control:

1. Safe sex / Sex education
2. Prevention of blood borne HIV transmission
3. Antiretroviral therapy/ Combination therapy
4. Post exposure prophylaxis
5. Refraining i/v drug use
6. Monogamous relationships

WHO updates HIV treatment guidance for pregnant women and preventing HIV infection in babies

Table 48.1 Three options for PMTCT programmes.

	Woman receives:		Infant receives:
	Treatment (for CD4 count $\leq$350 cells/mm^3)	**Prophylaxis (for CD4 count > 350 cells/mm^3)**	
Option A*	Triple ARVs starting as sppm as diagnosed, *continued for life*	*Antepartum*: AZT starting as early as 14 weeks gestation *Intrapartum*: at onset of labour, sdNVP and first dose of AZT/3TC *Postpartum*: daily AZT/3TC through 7 days postpartum	Daily NVP from birth through 1 week beyond complete cessation of breastfeeding; or, of not breastfeeding or if mother is on treatment, through age 4-6 weeks
Option B*	*Same initial ARVs for both*		Daily NVP of AZT from birth through age 4-6 weeks regardless of infant feeding method
	Triple ARVs starting as soon as diagnosed, *continued for life*	Triple ARVs starting as early as 14 weeks gestation and continued intrapartum and through childbirth if not breastfeeding or until 1 week after cessation of all breastfeeding	
	Same for treatment and prophylaxis		
Option B+	Regardless of CD4 count, triple ARVs starting as soon as diagnosed,^{c} *continued for life*		Daily NVP of AZT from birth through age 4-6 weeks regardless of infant feeding method

Recommended Antiretroviral Agents for Initial Treatment of Established Human Immunodeficiency Virus (HIV) Infection

1. **Dual NRTIs Options**: preferred: Tenofovir + Emtricitabine

    Abacavir + lamivudine

    Alternatives: Zidovudine + Lamivudine

    Didanosine + (Lamivudine or Emtricitabine)

2. **NNRTIs (one NNRTIs + two NRTIs)**: preferred : Efavirenz

    Alternatives: Nevirapine

3. **PIs (one or two PIs + two NRTIs)**: preferred : Atazanavir + ritonavir

    Fosamprenavir + Ritonavir twice daily

    Lopinavir/Ritonavir (coformulated) twice daily

    Alternatives: Atazanavird

    Fosamprenavir

    Fosamprenavir + ritonavir once daily

    Lopinavir/ritonavir (coformulated) once daily Saquinaivr + ritonavir

Therapies for Common Opportunistic Pathogens in HIV-Infected Individuals

Fungi

1. Candidiasis oral- Fluconazole 200 mg orally single dose or 100 mg orally for 5 days **or** Nystatin 500,000 units oral swish 4–6 times daily for 7–10 days **or** Clotrimazole 10 mg (1 troche) orally 5 times daily for 7–10 days
2. Cryptococcal meningitis: Amphotericin B 0.5–1.0 mg/kg/day intravenously for a minimum of 2 weeks with or without flucytosine 100–150 mg/kg/day orally in 4 divided doses followed by Fluconazole 100 to 200 mg/day, orally
3. Histoplasmosis: Amphotericin B 0.5–1 mg/kg/day intravenously for 6–8 weeks or Itraconazole 200–400 mg/day orally for 3 months
4. Coccidioidomycosis: Amphotericin B 0.5–1 mg/kg/day intravenously for $\geq$6–8 weeks

Protozoa

1. Toxoplasmic encephalitis: Pyrimethamine 200 mg orally once then 50–100 mg/day plus Sulfadiazine 1–1.5 g orally four times daily and Folinic acid 10–20 mg orally daily for a minimum of 28 days

Bacteria

1. Salmonella enterocolitis or bacteremia: Ciprofloxacin 500–750 mg orally twice daily for 14 days or Trimethoprim (160 mg)–sulfamethoxazole
2. Shigella enterocolitis Ciprofloxacin 500 mg orally twice daily for 5 days

Viruses

1. Mucocutaneous herpes simplex Acyclovir 1–2 g/day orally in 3–5 divided doses for 7–10 days

   or Valacyclovir 500 mg orally every 12 hours for 7–10 days

   or Famciclovir 500 mg orally every 12 hours for 7–10 days
2. Varicella-zoster Acyclovir 30 mg/kg/day intravenously in 3 divided doses or 4 g/day orally for 7–10 days

   Or Valacyclovir,1g orally every 8 hours for 7–10 days
3. Cytomegalovirus Ganciclovir 7.5–10 mg/kg/day in 2–3 divided doses intravenously for 14 days

   Or Foscarnet 180 mg/kg/day in 2 or 3 divided doses intravenously for 14 days

References

1. Barbara G. Wells. Pharmacotherapy Handbook, Seventh Edition, Copyright © 2009 by The McGraw-Hill Companies, Inc.
2. International Committee on Taxonomy of Viruses *(2002)*. "61.0.6. Lentivirus". National Institutes of Health. Retrieved February 28, 2006.
3. Levy JA (1993). "HIV pathogenesis and long-term survival". AIDS. 7(11): 1401–10
4. Reeves JD, Doms RW (2002). "Human Immunodeficiency Virus Type 2" (PDF). Journal of General Virology. 83 (Pt 6): 1253–65.
5. Chan DC, Fass D, Berger JM, Kim PS (1997). "Core structure of gp41 from the HIV envelope glycoprotein" (PDF). Cell. 89 (2): 263–73.

6. National Institute of Health (June 17, 1998). "Crystal structure of key HIV protein reveals new prevention, treatment targets" (Press release). Archived from the original on February 19, 2006. Retrieved September 14, 2006.

7. Fletcher C. Human immunodeficiency virus infection. In: DiPiro JT, Talbert RL, Yee G, et al, eds. *Pharmacotherapy: A Pathophysiologic Approach.* 9th ed. New York, NY: McGraw-Hill Education; 2014:2034.

CHAPTER - 49

AIDS and Opportunistic Infections

When a person with HIV gets certain infections (called opportunistic infections, or OIs) or specific cancers, they will get diagnosed with AIDS (also known as HIV Stage 3), the most serious stage of HIV infection. AIDS is also diagnosed if a person's CD4 cells falls below a certain level.

What are opportunistic infections?

Opportunistic infections (OIs) are infections that occur more frequently and are more severe in people with weakened immune systems, including people with HIV. OIs are less common now than they were in the early days of HIV because better treatments reduce the amount of HIV in a person's body and keep a person's immune system stronger. [1]

Table 49.1 Common Opportunistic Infections [2,3].

Candidiasis of bronchi, trachea, esophagus, or lungs	This illness is caused by infection with a common (and usually harmless) type of fungus called *Candida*. Candidiasis, or infection with *Candida*, can affect the skin, nails, and mucous membranes throughout the body. Persons with HIV infection often have trouble with *Candida*, especially in the mouth and vagina.
Invasive cervical cancer	This is a cancer that starts within the cervix, which is the lower part of the uterus at the top of the vagina, and then spreads (becomes invasive) to other parts of the body. This cancer can be prevented by having care provider perform regular examinations of the cervix
Coccidioidomycosis	This illness is caused by the fungus *Coccidioides immitis*. It most commonly acquired by inhaling fungal spores, which can lead to a pneumonia that is sometimes called desert fever, San Joaquin Valley fever, or valley fever. The disease is especially common in hot, dry regions of the southwestern United States, Central America, and South America.
Cryptococcosis	This illness is caused by infection with the fungus *Cryptococcus neoformans*. The fungus typically enters the body through the lungs and can cause pneumonia. It can also spread to the brain, causing swelling of the brain. It can infect any part of the body, but (after the brain and lungs) infections of skin, bones, or urinary tract are most common.
Cryptosporidiosis, chronic intestinal (greater than one month's duration)	This diarrheal disease is caused by the protozoan parasite *Cryptosporidium*. Symptoms include abdominal cramps and severe, chronic, watery diarrhea.

Contd...

Cytomegalovirus diseases (particularly retinitis) (CMV)	This virus can infect multiple parts of the body and cause pneumonia, gastroenteritis (especially abdominal pain caused by infection of the colon), encephalitis (infection) of the brain, and sight-threatening retinitis (infection of the retina at the back of eye).
Encephalopathy, HIV-related	This brain disorder is a result of HIV infection. It can occur as part of acute HIV infection or can result from chronic HIV infection. Its exact cause is unknown but it is thought to be related to infection of the brain with HIV and the resulting inflammation.
Herpes simplex (HSV): chronic ulcer(s) (greater than one month's duration); or bronchitis, pneumonitis, or esophagitis	Herpes simplex virus (HSV) is a very common virus that for most people never causes any major problems. HSV is usually acquired sexually or from an infected mother during birth. In most people with healthy immune systems, HSV is usually latent (inactive). However, stress, trauma, other infections, or suppression of the immune system, (such as by HIV), can reactivate the latent virus and symptoms can return. HSV can cause painful cold sores (sometime called fever blisters) in or around the mouth, or painful ulcers on or around the genitals or anus. In people with severely damaged immune systems, HSV can also cause infection of the bronchus (breathing tube), pneumonia (infection of the lungs), and esophagitis (infection of the esophagus, or swallowing tube).
Histoplasmosis	This illness is caused by the fungus *Histoplasma capsulatum*. *Histoplasma* most often infects the lungs and produces symptoms that are similar to those of influenza or pneumonia. People with severely damaged immune systems can get a very serious form of the disease called progressive disseminated histoplasmosis. This form of histoplasmosis can last a long time and involves organs other than the lungs.
Isosporiasis, chronic intestinal (greater than one month's duration)	This infection is caused by the parasite *Isospora belli*, which can enter the body through contaminated food or water. Symptoms include diarrhea, fever, headache, abdominal pain, vomiting, and weight loss.
Kaposi's sarcoma (KS)	This cancer, also known as KS, is caused by a virus called Kaposi's sarcoma herpesvirus (KSHV) or human herpesvirus 8 (HHV-8). KS causes small blood vessels, called capillaries, to grow abnormally. Because capillaries are located throughout the body, KS can occur anywhere. KS appears as firm pink or purple spots on the skin that can be raised or flat. KS can be life-threatening when it affects organs inside the body, such the lung, lymph nodes, or intestines.
Lymphoma, multiple forms	Lymphoma refers to cancer of the lymph nodes and other lymphoid tissues in the body. There are many different kinds of lymphomas. Some types, such as non-Hodgkin lymphoma and Hodgkin lymphoma, are associated with HIV infection.
Tuberculosis (TB)	Tuberculosis (TB) infection is caused by the bacteria *Mycobacterium tuberculosis*. TB can be spread through the air when a person with active TB coughs, sneezes, or speaks. Breathing in the bacteria can lead to infection in the lungs. Symptoms of TB in the lungs include cough, tiredness, weight loss, fever, and night sweats. Although the disease usually occurs in the lungs, it may also affect other parts of the body, most often the larynx, lymph nodes, brain, kidneys, or bones.
Mycobacterium aviumcomplex (MAC) or Mycobacterium	MAC is caused by infection with different types of mycobacterium: *Mycobacterium avium*, *Mycobacterium intracellulare*, or *Mycobacterium kansasii*. These mycobacteria live in our environment,

Contd...

kansasii, disseminated or extrapulmonary. Other Mycobacterium, disseminated or extrapulmonary.	including in soil and dust particles. They rarely cause problems for persons with healthy immune systems. In people with severely damaged immune systems, infections with these bacteria spread throughout the body and can be life-threatening.
Pneumocystis cariniipneumonia (PCP)	This lung infection, also called PCP, is caused by a fungus, which used to be called *Pneumocystis carinii*, but now is named *Pneumocystis jirovecii*. PCP occurs in people with weakened immune systems, including people with HIV. The first signs of infection are difficulty breathing, high fever, and dry cough.
Pneumonia, recurrent	Pneumonia is an infection in one or both of the lungs. Many germs, including bacteria, viruses, and fungi can cause pneumonia, with symptoms such as a cough (with mucous), fever, chills, and trouble breathing. In people with immune systems severely damaged by HIV, one of the most common and life-threatening causes of pneumonia is infection with the bacteria *Streptococcus pneumoniae*, also called *Pneumococcus*. There are now effective vaccines that can prevent infection with *Streptococcus pneumoniae* and all persons with HIV infection should be vaccinated.
Salmonellasepticemia, recurrent	*Salmonella* are a kind of bacteria that typically enter the body through ingestion of contaminated food or water. Infection with salmonella (called salmonellosis) can affect anyone and usually causes a self-limited illness with nausea, vomiting, and diarrhea. *Salmonella* septicemia is a severe form of infection in which the bacteria circulate through the whole body and exceeds the immune system's ability to control it.
Toxoplasmosis of brain	This infection, often called toxo, is caused by the parasite *Toxoplasma gondii*. The parasite is carried by warm-blooded animals including cats, rodents, and birds and is excreted by these animals in their feces. Humans can become infected with it by inhaling dust or eating food contaminated with the parasite. *Toxoplasma* can also occur in commercial meats, especially red meats and pork, but rarely poultry. Infection with toxo can occur in the lungs, retina of the eye, heart, pancreas, liver, colon, testes, and brain. Although cats can transmit toxoplasmosis, litter boxes can be changed safely by wearing gloves and washing hands thoroughly with soap and water afterwards. All raw red meats that have not been frozen for at least 24 hours should be cooked through to an internal temperature of at least 150°F. *Contd...*
Wasting syndrome due to HIV	Wasting is defined as the involuntary loss of more than 10% of one's body weight while having experienced diarrhea or weakness and fever for more than 30 days. Wasting refers to the loss of muscle mass, although part of the weight loss may also be due to loss of fat.

Prevention of opportunistic infections

The best ways to prevent getting an OI are to get into care and to take HIV medications as prescribed.

- Prevent exposure to other sexually transmitted infections.

- Don't share drug injection equipment. Blood with hepatitis C in it can remain in syringes and needles after use and the infection can be transmitted to the next user.
- Getting vaccinated
- Understand what germs you are exposed to (such as tuberculosis or germs found in the stools, saliva, or on the skin of animals) and limit exposure to them.
- Don't consume certain foods, including undercooked eggs, unpasteurized (raw) milk and cheeses, unpasteurized fruit juices, or raw seed sprouts.
- Don't drink untreated water such as water directly from lakes or rivers.

References

1. Koehler JE, Sanchez MA, Garrido CS, et al. Molecular epidemiology of bartonella infections in patients with bacillary angiomatosis-peliosis. N Engl J Med. Dec 25 1997;337(26):1876-1883
2. Houpikian P, Raoult D. Blood culture-negative endocarditis in a reference center: etiologic diagnosis of 348 cases. Medicine (Baltimore). May 2005;84(3):162-173.
3. Kikendall JW, Friedman AC, Oyewole MA, Fleischer D, Johnson LF. Pill-induced esophageal injury. Case reports and review of the medical literature. Digestive diseases and sciences. Feb 1983;28(2):174-182.

CHAPTER - 50

Superficial Fungal Infections

Introduction to Fungal Infections

Fungi are the extremely common organisms which are wide spread in nature. Fungi are broadly divided into yeasts or moulds.

Yeasts are oval or round shaped, reproduce by budding. Moulds are a mass of hyphae that grown by branching and tubular extensions.

Morphological classification

A:-Moulds – They are hyphae in the form.

Ex: - ringworm (or) dermatophytosis.

B:-Yeast –   Single cell that bud to reproduce.

Ex:-Cryptococcus neoformans.

C:-Yeast like form pseudo hyphae

Ex: - candida albicans.

D:-Dimorphic Fungi –Fungi having yeast form in tissue &mould in culture

Ex:-blastomyces dermatitis.

Human fungal infections fall into two categories.

1. Superficial infections of skin or mucosa.
2. Deep seated or systemic infection.

Diseases are classified into 4 groups

According to pathogenicity

1. Superficial mycoses
2. Mucocutaneous mycoses
3. Subcutaneous mycoses
4. Deep mycoses

Pathogenesis

Compared with bacterial, viral, and parasitic disease, less is known about the pathogenic mechanisms and virulence factors involved in fungal infections. Analogies to bacterial diseases come the closest because of the apparent importance of adherence to mucosal surfaces, invasiveness, extracellular products, and interaction with phagocytes. In general, the principles applied to fungal infections. Most fungi are opportunists, causing serious disease only in individuals with impaired host defence systems. Only a few fungi are able to cause disease in previously healthy persons.

Immunity to fungal infections.

  A. Pathogenic fungi are able to survive and multiply slowly in no activated macrophages.
  B. When macrophages are activated by cytokines from T-cells the growth is restricted and the fungi digested.

Superficial Infection

This type of infections affects the outermost skin and hair. These include candida infections and dermatophytosis.

  1. **Candida Infections**

  It occurs in three forms;

  1. Vulvovaginal.
  2. Oropharyngeal.
  3. Oesophageal.

  Vulvovaginal:

  Causative Agent: Candida albicans, candida galbrata.

  Risk Factors: Oral genital contact, contraceptive use, intrauterine devices, antibiotics.

  Clinical Presentation of Vulvovaginal Candidiasis

  General: Often involves both the vulva and the vagina

  Symptoms: Intense vulvar itching, soreness, irritation, burning on urination, and dyspareunia **Signs**: Erythema, fissuring, curdy "cheese"-like discharge, satellite lesions, edema

  Laboratory tests: Vaginal pH—normal, saline and 10% KOH microscopy—blastospores or pseudohyphae

  Other diagnostic tests: Candida cultures not recommended unless classic signs and symptoms with normal vaginal pH and microscopy is inconclusive or recurrence is suspected

  Treatment:

  Goals of Therapy: Complete resolution of symptoms in patients who have symptomatic vaginal candidiasis

Treatment for Uncomplicated Vulvovaginal Candidiasis

1. Over the Counter/Topical Vaginal Products

   Clotrimazole 1% cream 1 applicator or 100-mg tablet 1 100 mg tablet × 7 days

   Miconazolea 2% cream 1 applicator or 100-mg suppository 1 100 mg suppository × 7 days

   Ticonazole 6.5% cream 1 applicator or 300-mg ovule 1 ovule × 1 day

2. Prescription/Topical

   Econazole 150-mg tablet 1 tablet × 3 days

   Nystatin 100,000-unit tablet 1 tablet × 14 days

   Terconazole 0.4% cream 1 applicator × 7 days

3. Oral Products

   Ketoconazole 200 mg 1 tablet twice daily × 5 days

   Itraconazole 200 mg 1 tablet twice daily × 1 day

   Fluconazole 150 mg 1 tablet × 1 day

Treatment for complicated Vulvovaginal Candidiasis

1. Complicated **Vulvovaginal Candidiasis** occurs in patients who are immunocompromised or have uncontrolled diabetes mellitus.

2. The main approach to the treatment of these individuals is to increase the length of therapy. Current recommendations are to lengthen therapy to 10 to 14 days regardless of the route of administration

3. Treatment options are same as above for uncomplicated vulvovaginal candidiais

Oropharyngeal & Oesopharyngeal

Causaive Agent: Candida tropicalis, candida krusei.

Risk Factors for Development of Oropharyngeal and/or Esophageal Candidiasis

1. **Use of steroids and antibiotics:** Suppression of cellular immunity and inhibition of phagocytosis by steroids, including chronic use of inhaled and topical steroids

2. Dentures Enhanced adherence of Candida to acrylic material of dentures, reduced saliva flow under surfaces of denture fittings, improperly fitted dentures, or poor oral hygiene; these provide a milieu conducive to survival of microorganisms

3. Disruption of oral mucosa due to chemotherapy and radiotherapy, ulcers, endotracheal intubation trauma, and burns- Oral mucositis induced by radiation and breaks in physical barrier of oral epithelium, which is protective against invasion by microorganisms; altered rate of mucosa regeneration by cancer chemotherapy, which increases vulnerability to infection.

4. **Drugs:** Reduced immunity due to drug-induced neutropenia or cell-mediated immunit

5. **Neonates or elderly:** Immature immune system of neonates who usually acquire infection during birth to a mother with vaginal candidiasis or from exposure to infected bottle nipples or to skin of adult care giver. Elderly—Unclear if this is the direct effect of age per se or contribution from dentures or underlying comorbidity

6. **Diabetes:** Higher than normal numbers of C. albicans cultured from saliva of daibetic patients. May be related to the elevated glucose levels and reduced chemotactic factor in saliva, altered neutrophil function, and reduced saliva volume and flow

7. **Malignancies:** Chemotherapy disrupt oral mucosa and also cause xerostomi

8. **Nutritional defiencies:** May be related to dietary restriction or GI absorption problem

Pathogenesis:

The presence of Candida usually stimulates antibody formation and cell-mediated immunity in most healthy adults without causing any signs or symptoms of infection. Effective antifungal host-defense mechanisms in the oral cavity play an important role in maintaining the colonizing organisms in low numbers for years in the absence of inflammation. The changeover of the role of Candida from commensal to pathogenic in the human host usually occurs when host defenses are impaired.

Clinical Presentation

Oropharyngeal Candidiasis

Symptoms:

Symptoms are diverse and range from none to sore, painful mouth, burning tongue, metallic taste, and dysphagia and odynophagia with involvement of hypopharynx

Signs:

Signs are variable and may include diffuse erythema and white patches on the surfaces of buccal mucosa, throat, tongue, or gums. Constitutional signs are absent

Laboratory Tests:

Scraping of an active lesion for microscopic examination can help confirm the diagnosis (presence of psuedohyphae and budding yeast) but is usually not necessary. Cultures are also not necessary since isolation of Candida does not distinguish between colonization and true infection. Cultures may be taken in patients responding poorly to therapy to determine the infecting species and to predict likely drug resistance

Esophageal Candidiasis

Symptoms:

Typically the symptoms are dysphagia, odynophagia, and retrosternal chest pain but may be asymptomatic in some patients. Although rare, epigastric pain may be the dominant symptom

Signs:

Constitutional signs, including fever, occasionally occur. Physical findings may range from a few to numerous white or beige plaques of variable size. Plaques may be hyperemic or edematous, with ulceration in more severe cases. Most advanced cases may occur with increased mucosal friability and narrowing of lumen. Uncommon complications include perforation and aortic–esophageal fistula formation.

Laboratory Tests:

The best test is upper GI endoscopy (more useful than barium swallow); helps exclude other causes of esophagitis (e.g., viral, aphthous ulcers). Diagnosis is confirmed by the histologic presence of Candida in biopsy lesions taken during endoscopy. Cultures to look for drug-resistant Candida are warranted in patients who require endoscopy.

Laboratory Diagnosis of Fungal Infections

- CSF- Microscopic observation under India ink preparation
- Direct microscopy – gram staining
- Cultures on sabouraud dextrose agar
- Serological tests for detection of capsular antigen
- CSF finding mimic like tuberculosis
- In CSF- latex test for detection of antigen
- Blood cultures
- ELISA

Laboratory Diagnosis of Fungal Diseases:-

- Specimen collection –skin crapping; - nail clipping/scrapping; - Hair; -exudates
- Biopsy materials; -respiratory -body fluids, CSF

Laboratory Diagnosis of Mycoses

1. A. Direct examination
   *10-30% KOH
   *Histological stains H&E
   B. PAS
   *Indian ink
   *Wet mount
2. **Isolation & Culture** SDA Media with/Without Antibiotics: Macroscopic examination of culture; Microscopic examination
3. **Biochemical Tests:** Rapid kits for yeast; urea test
4. **Special Test:** In Vitro hair perforation test; Germ tube test; chlamydoconidia formation test
5. **Serological Tests:** Latex agglutination; CFT; precipitation.

Treatment & Prevention

*Topical therapy

*application of topical azoles, compound terbinafin, oral grisofulvin

Table 50.1 Treatment of fungal infections.

1. **Amphotericin-B**
   Spectrum of activity: Candida spp., Aspergillus spp. and other filamentous fungi, life-threatening infections with the endemic fungi Coccidioides immitis, Histoplasma capsulatum and Blastomyces dermatitidis Reports of resistance in non-albicans Candida spp.
   Properties: Delivered topically or systemically, most frequently used in IV form for treatment of systemic fungal infections; oral tablets used mainly to treat thrush and gastrointestinal candidiasis; conventional formulations are nephrotoxic; lipid-associated formulations have reduced nephrotoxicity

2. **Nystatin**
   Spectrum of activity: Candida spp. and Aspergillus spp.
   Properties: Oral formulation used for topical treatment of oropharyngeal candidiasis

3. **Terbinafine**
   Spectrum of activity Candida spp., Aspergillus spp., dermatophytes and dimorphic fungi
   Properties: Topical and oral formulations used in treatment of cutaneous and nail dermatophyte infections; lipophilic and accumulates in skin, hair, sebum and nail plate

4. **Ketoconazole**
   Spectrum of activity: Candida spp., all dermatophytes, Malassezia furfur, B. dermatitidis, C. immitis, H. capsulatum, Paracoccidioides brasiliensis and Phialophora spp. NOT Aspergillus spp.
   Properties: Oral formulations previously used in treatment of systemic infections; largely supplanted by other azole antifungals

5. **Fluconazole**
   Spectrum of activity: Cryptococcus spp., and many Candida spp., including C. albicans NOT Aspergillus spp. or some non-albicans Candida spp., e.g. C. glabrata and C. krusei Reports of resistance
   Properties: Water-soluble oral capsules (or tablets), suspension or IV formulation used extensively in prophylaxis; treatment of choice for mucocutaneous candidiasis in neutropenic patients and one of the preferred treatments for oral candidiasis in patients with HIV infection

*Pityriasis responds to topical therapy

*1% Selenium sulphide

*Azoles-ketoconazole

*Oral azoles

*Skin- azoles, inhibits cytochrome 450 dependent enzyme systems at the demethylation step from lanosterol to ergo sterol.

*Hair- griseofulvin, oral, affects micro tubular system.

2. Dermatophytosis

Dermatophytosis (or) tineas are the superficial mycotic infection of the skin. They are caused by 3 genera (or) dermatophytes fungi.

-Trichophyton, Epidermophyton, Microsporum

Risk Factors Include: Moist conditions, Prolonged exposure to sweaty clothes, Failure to bath regularly, Many skin folds, Sedentary, Confinement to bed

The Most Commonly Occuring Infections Include

Tinea Pedi's (athlete's foot), Tinea mannum (palms), Tinea cruris (jock itch)

Tinea corporis (smooth skin), Tinea capitis (scalp), Tinea barbae (beard),

Tinea unguium (nail plate), Pityriasis versicolor

Tinea Pedis: It is also called as athlete'sfoot. It is most common type of fungal infection. Sharing of wash places (i.e., in shower rooms) & of swimming pools predisposes to infection. Most cases are caused by one of three organisms -1. Trichophyton rubrum (most common and most stubborn); 2. Trichophyton mentagrophytes var. interdigitale; 3. Epidermophyton floccosum

Common three clinical patterns: Soggy interdigital scaling, particularly in the fourth and fifth interspace (all 3 organisms); A diffuse dry scaling of the soles (usually T. rubrum); Recurrent episodes of vesication (usually T. mentographytes var.interdigitale)

Tinea of the Nails: Toe nail infection is usually associated with tinea pedis. The initial changes occur at the free edge of the nail, which becomes yellow crumbly. Finger nail lesions are similar, but less common, and are sudden seen without a chronic T. rubrum infection of the skin of the same hand.

Tinea of the Scalp: Mostly seen in the children. Fungi coming from the human sources caused bald and scaly areas, with minimal inflammation and hairs broken off 3-4 mm from the scalp. Hair loss associated may be permanent. Favus, caused by trichophyton schoenleini, is foul smelling yellowish crusts surrounding many scalp hairs, and sometimes leading to the scarring alopecia

Complications: Fierce animal ringworm of the scalp can lead to the permanent scarring alopecia. Epidemics of ringworm occur in schools, Usual appearance of a fungal infection can be masked by mistreatment with topical steroids (tinea incognito)

Table 50.2 Differential Diagnosis.

S.No.	Area	Differential Dignosis
01	Scalp	Alopecia areta , seborrheic eczema, carbuncle, abscess, trichotillomania
02	Feet	Erythema , interdigital intertrigo , eczema
03	Trunk	Discoid eczema, psoriasis, candiddiasis
04	Groin	Candidiasis, erythrasma, intertrigo, irritant and allergic contact and dermatitis neurodermatitis
05	Nails	Paronychia, trauma, ageing changes.
06	Hands	Chronic eczema, granuloma annular xerosis, dyshidrotic eczema.

Table 50.3 Treatment for Dermatophytosis.

S no	Clinical form	Areas involved	Treatment
01	Tinea pedis	Foot & between toes	Butenafine topical for 2-4 weeks Fluconazole 150mg (1 per week)for about 1-4 weeks
02	Tinea mannum	Palmar surface of hands	Emollients with lactic acid Ketoconazole 200mg daily for 4 weeks
03	Tinea cruris	Proximal thighs and buttocks	Clotrimazole BD, itraconazole 200-400 mg /day for 1 week
04	Tinea corporis	Globous skin of trunk	Econazole or miconazole (BD) Terbinafine250mg/day for 2 weeks.
05	Tinea capitis	Scalp, hair follicles	Ketoconazole or povidone Iodine shampoo
06	Tinea barbae	Hair and follicles of beard and moustaches	Removal of beard,mustache Ketoconazole (twice a week)
07	Tinea unguinum	Toe nails	Terbinafine 250mg/day for 6 weeks(fingers) 12 weeks(toe)

References

1. Ameen M. Epidemiology of Superficial fungal infections Clin. Dermatol 2010; 28:197.

2. Weinstein A, Berman B. Topical treatment of common superficial tinea infections. Am Fam Physician, 2002, May 15,65(10);2095-102.

CHAPTER - 51

Invasic Fungal Infections

Introduction to Invasive Fungal Infections

In humans, fungal infections occur when a invading fungus takes over an area of the body and is too much for the immune system to handle

Types of Fungi

- Some of the common types of fungalinfections are athletes foot, yeast infection, jock itch, ring worm

Epidemiology: 4th most common skin disease in 2010. Major cause of morbidity and mortality in the immunocompromised patient. 20% to 30% of fatal infections in patients acute Leukaemia. 10% to 15% with lymphoma. 5% solid tumours

Etiology:

- Systemic mycoses such as, *cryptococcosis, blastomycosis, paracoccidiodmycosis, sporotrichosis histoplasmosis, coccidiodomycosis* are caused by primary or pathogenic fungi that can disease in both health and immunocompromised individuals
- In contrast, mycoses caused by opportunistic fungi such as *c.albicans ,aspergillosis spp, trichosporon,torulopsis(candida) glabrata, fusorium, alternaria* and *mucor* generally are found only in the immunocompromised host

Pathogenesis:

Most fungal infections are acquired as a result of accidental inhalation of airborne conidia Ex: H.capsulatum found in contaminated by bat, chicken. C.neoformans— associated with pigeon droppings. Bacterial flora of the skin and mucous membranes compete with fungi for growth. Alterations in the balance of normal flora caused by the use of antibiotics or alterations in nutritional status can allow the proliferation of fungi such as Candida, increasing the likelihood of systemic invasion and infection.

Symptoms:

Skin changes such as: Reddish, Itching, and Cracking

Diagnosis:

Generally accomplished by:
- Careful examination of clinical symptoms
- Serological tests
- Histopathologic examination
- Culture of clinical specimen

Specific Fungal Infections

HISTOPLASMOSIS: Member of the "Phylum-ascomycota". It is caused by inhalation of dust borne microconidia of the dimorphic fungus Histoplasma Capsulatom.

Epidemiology: Although it is found world wide, certain areas of North and Latin America are recognized as endemic areas. In the US, most disease is localized along the Ohio and mississippi river valleys.

Types: 2 major forms of histoplasmosis are of Pulmonary and Disseminated

Pulmonary: It occurs when microconidia are inhaled. Form lesions in the hilar and mediastinal nodes

Types of pulmonary histoplasmosis:
- Asymptomatic pulmonary histoplasmosis
- Acute
- Mediastinal granuloma
- Fibrosing mediastinitis
- Chronic cavitary

Disseminated: Occurs primarily in immunocompromised individuals. In healthy individuals "H capsulatom" is similar to TB. In immunocompromised individuals, H capsulatom is able to spread from the lungs into other organs. Patient's display fever, malaise or skin lesions.

Risk Factors: Chemotherapy, Smoking, Antibiotics, HIV & AIDS, Steroids

Symptoms: Fever, Headache, Chills, Muscle aches, Dry cough, Chest discomfort

Diagnosis: Lung secretions, Blood or urine, Biopsied lung tissue, Bone marrow

Treatment:
- Non-HIV: oral ketoconazole or iv amphotericin B
- HIV: 12 -week primary anti fungal therapy.
- Life long suppressive therapy with itraconazole.
- Hospitalization: amphotericin B
- Non hospitalization: itraconazole 200mg -12weeks
- Once course is done:- life long suppressive therapy with Oralazoles or amphotericin B (1-1.5mg/kg-weekly)

- Fluconazole 800 mg/day orally as induction, followed by 400 mg/day, was effective in 88% of patients, but relapses occurred in approximately one-third of patients, and in vitro resistance developed in approximately 50% of patients who relapsed.

Blastomycosis

- Also known as "North American Blastomycosis".
  Blastomycetic dermatitis and Gilchrist's disease.

Causative Agent: Caused by Blastomyces dermatitidis

Signs and Symptoms:

- Fever, Night sweats, Cough, Muscle aches or Joint pains
- Weight loss, Chest pain, Fatigue

Risk Factors:

- Occupational exposures
- Residence in an area of endemicity
- Immuno compromise

Diagnosis:

Tests:

- **Chest X-ray:** Lobarpneumonia, mass like or cavitary lesions, diffuse interstitial infiltrates, or signs of adult respiratory distress syndrome.
- **Sputum, smear and culture:** Large, oval, broad based budding yeast.
- **Fungal blood culture:** Positive
- **B.dermatitidis PCR:**Presence of B. Dermatitidis
- **Anthrocentesis:** Large, oval, broad- based budding in yeasts field.

Treatment:

- **Non HIV Patients:**
  Some may recommend Ketoconazole therapy for the treatment of self limited pulmonary disease

Type of disease	Treatment
➢ **Pulmonary:**	
Life threatening	AmphotericinB IV 0.7-1mg/kg/day(total dose-1.5-2.5g)
Mild to moderate	Itraconazole-200mg-orally-BD > 6M
➢ **Disseminated**	
CNS	AmphotericinB 0.7-1mg/kg-OD IV(total dose 1.5-2.5g)
Non-CNS:	
Life threatening	AmphotericinB 0.7-1mg/kg-OD IV (total dose-1.5-2.5g)
Mild to moderate	AmphotericinB 200-400mg-orally-daily> 6 M
➢ **Immunocompromised**	
Acute disease	AmphotericinB 0.7-1mg/kg-OD-IV(total dose- 1.5-2.5g)
Suppressive therapy	Itraconazole 200-400mg-orally-daily

> **HIV Patients**
  Should receive chronic suppressive therapy with Oral azole antifungal
  Itraconazole has become the drug of choice for non life threatening histoplasmosis in HIV infected patients

Coccidioidomycosis

- It is commonly known as coccidioidomycosis, valley fever.
- It is a mammalian fungal disease.

Epidemiology: It is found in South Western and Western United States, as well as in parts of Mexico and South America.

Causative Agent: Caused by infection with coccidiodes immites.it is a dimorphic fungus.

Signs and Symptoms: Asymptomatic (60% of patients), Fever, Headache, Cough, Sore throat, Myalgia, Fatigue

Risk Factors:

- Pregnancy, Aids patient, Males gender
- Neonates, Patients with B or AB blood type, Corticosteroids
- Immuno – suppressive agents, Chemotherapy

Pathophysiology: When individuals come in contact with contaminated soil during ranching, dust storms, or proximity to construction sites or archaeologic excavations, arthroconidia are inhaled into the respiratory tree, where they transform into spherules, which reproduce by cleavage of the cytoplasm to produce endospores. The endospores are released when the spherules reach maturity. Similar to histoplasmosis, an acute inflammatory response in the tissue leads to infiltration of mononuclear cells, ultimately resulting in granuloma formation

Diagnosis:

- **Sputum smear or culture:**check a sample of the matter that is discharged while coughing (sputum) for the presence of coccidioides organisms
- **Blood test:** check for antibodies against the fungus that cause valley fever
- **Chest X Ray :** check for characteristic abnormalities

Treatment:

- **Antifungals**

  AmphotericinB IV (0.5-1.5mg/kg/OD)
  Ketoconazole (400mg-Italy-daily)IV / oral
  Fluconazole (400-800mg-daily)
  Itraconazole (200-300mg-orally-BD either capsules or Solution form

- **Primary respiratory disease** — 3-6 months course of therapy
- **Patients with disease outside the lung** — 400mg/day (oral azole)
- **Meningeal disease** — Fluconazole 400mg/day-orally (Some May initiate 800mg or 1000mg) **Itraconazole** (400-600mg/day)

Cryptococcosis

- It is a non contagious, systemic mycotic infection. Also known as cryptococcal disease is a potentially fatal fungal disease

Causative Agent: It is caused by ubiquitous encapsulated soil yeast Cryptococcus neoformans

Signs and Symptoms: Fever, Pleuritic chest pain, Hemoptysis, Vision changes, Vomiting, Malaise, Cough, Headache, Nausea, shortness of breath (SOB).

Risk Factors: DM, Chronic failure, AIDS

Diagnosis:

- **Microscopic examination ; Blood test ; Antigen test**
- **CSF-** Reveals elevates opening pressure, CSF Pleocytosis, leukocytosis, a decreased CSF glucose, an elevated CSF protein and a positive cryptococcal antigen
- **Latex agglutination:** C.neoformans can be detected in 60% by India ink smear of CSF and cultured in more than 90%

Treatment:

- ➢ **Non immunocompromised:**
  - Isolated pulmonary disease Fluconazole-200mg-400mg-orally-daily* 3-6M
  - Acute CNS disease Amphotericin B IV(0.7-1mg/kg/orally/day)*6-10W

    (Or)

    Fluconazole 400-800mg orally- daily * 10-12 W

    (Or) Itraconazole 400-800mg Italy – daily * 10-12 W
  - CNS disease: Amphotericin B-IV0.7-1mg/kg/day+5-flucytosine 100mg/kg/day – orally * 6-10W

    (or)

    Amphotericin B IV 0.1-1 mg/kg/day * 10W
- ➢ **Immunocompromised:**
  - Non CNS and extra pulmonary disease same as non immunocompromised
  - CNS   AmphotericinB IV 0.7-1mg/kg/day*2W

    Followed by Fluconazole 400-800mg-8-10W

    Fluconazole 20mg- 6-12M
- ➢ **HIV infected :**
  - Maintenance therapy Fluconazole 200-400mg- lifelong-orally
- ➢ **Cryptoccocal meningitis** AmphotericinB with flucytosine – 6W

Candida Infections

Eight species of candida are regarded as clinically important pathogens in human.

- Those are of C.albicons, C.tropicalis, C.parapsilosis C.kruvesis C.skillatoidoa C.guilliermondi C.lusitaniae & C.Globrata
- Skin infections includes athletes foot, oral thrush, nail fungus etc

Risk Factors:
- Diabetes, Hypothyroidism, Over weight, Infants, Inflammatory disorders: weaken immune system
- Pregnant women : working in wet conditions

Pathogenesis: After Candida invades the dermis or enters the bloodstream, polymorphonuclear leukocytes (PMNs) play a major role in the defense of the patient because PMNs are capable of damaging pseudohyphae and can phagocytize and kill blastoconidia.8 In addition to neutrophils, lymphocytes, monocytes, macrophages, complement, and eosinophils play a role in the prevention of infection. Adherence of C.albicans is important in the pathogenesis of oral candidiasis and subsequent colonization of the GI tract. Because evidence suggests that the GI tract is often the portal of entry for Candida in disseminated disease, factors that alter the adherence of Candida are crucial in the development of local and systemic infection

Signs and Symptoms:
- Rashes, Red or purple patches, Scaling, Cracks, Soreness

Hematogenous Candidiasis

Describer the clinical circumstances in C hematogenous seeding to deep organs such as eye, brain, heart and kidney occurs.

Causative Agent: Candida spp

Signs and symptoms:
- Itching, Fever, White patches, Hypotension, Redness, Swelling, Soleness

Risk Factors: Diabetes, Renal failure, Immuno deficiency disease, Mechanical ventilation
- Immuno suppressants, Haematologic malignancies, Corticosteroids. Prior fungal colonization

Diagnosis: Blood culture – helps to identify the specific bacteria as fungi causing the infection.

Treatment

1. **Prophylaxis of candidemia**
   (a) Non neutropenic patients: High risk patients –Fluconazole IV/PO – 400mg daily
   (b) Neutropenic patients : Fluconazole IV/PO – 400mg daily
   (c) Solid organ transplantation (Liver): Amphotericin B IV, 10-20mg / daily or lipoosmal amphotericin B. or fluconazole 400 mg orally daily

2. **Treatment of candidemia & Acute hematagenously disseminated candidiasis :**
   (a) Nonimmunocompromised host: 2Weeks after last positive blood culture

   C.albicans, C.tropicalis, C.parapsilosis: Amphotericin B IV 0.6mg / kg / day

   Loading dose then 50mg IV daily

       Patients intolerant or refractory to therapy:

       Amphotericin B lipid complex IV 5mg/kg/day

   Liposomal amphotericin B IV 3-5mg/kg/day

      C.krusei: Amphotericin B IV > 1mg/kg/day

      C.lusitaniae: Fluconazole IV/PO 6mg/kg/day

      C.glabrata: Amphotericin B IV > 0.7 mg/kg/day

3. **Hepatosplentic candiadisis:** Fluconazole IV/PO 6mg/kg/day
4. **Urinary candiadisis:** High risk: Removal of urinary Tract instruments, Stents by foley, catheters and 7-14 days; Fluconazole 200mg orally – daily

Candiduria: Presence of candida organism in the urine is called as candidura. Most common lesions are either candida cystitis or hematogenously disseminated renal abscesses.

Treatment: Initial therapy of candida cystitis – should focus on removal of urinary catheters. Changing catheters will eliminate candidura in 20% people. Discontinuation will eradicate – 40% people.

- Asymptomatic à rarely requires therapy.
- Fluconazole – 200mg /day - 14days - negative urine culture.
- Bladders irrigation – amphotericin B (50 mg in 500 ml sterile water instilled – BD into Bladders)
- Neutropenic Micafugin 100mg/ day IV

Aspergillosis:

- Caused by infection by fungi of the genus aspergillus.
- Aspergillus has been characterized into these specific A.fumigatus, A.flavus A.niger

Causes: Allergic reactions, Stored grain, Marijuana leaves, Compost piles, Decaying vegetation

Signs And Symptoms: Fever, Headache, Chills, Eye symptoms, Cough, Skin lesions

Risk Factors: Acute leukaemia, Immuno suppressive therapy, Diabetes mellitus (DM)
- Cystic fibroses, Chronic granulomatous disease, Pre – existing cavity

Diagnosis:

- Biopsy -test lung tissue, Blood test, Check for anti bodies, allergens & fungus
- Chest X-ray, CT –scan, sputum stain & culture à to examine bronchial mucus
- Imaging test – reveals a fungal mass

Treatment:

Oral corticosteroids :-Treating allergic bronchopulmonary

Anti -fungal medications:-Itraconazole, Voriconazole , Amphotericin B (1–1.5mg /kg/day)

Surgery : Surgery to remove the fungal mass is the First choice of the treatment.

Embolization: Stops lungs bleeding caused by an aspergilloma.

Aspergilloma: Also known as mycetoma or fungus ball. It's a clump of mold which exists in a body cavity such as a paranasal sinus or an organ – Lung. Caused by genes- aspergillus

Causes: chronic lung conditions, TB, Advanced sarcoidosis, Cystic fibrosis, Lung cancer, Histoplasmosis

Symptoms: Chest pain, Cough, Fatigue, Fever, Weight loss, Coughing up blood

Invasive Aspergillosis

- Patient often   present and classic sign and symptoms of acute pulmonary embolus ; pleuritic chest pain, fever, hemoptysis a friction rub and a wedge – shaped infiltrate on chest radiograph.
- Demonstration of aspergillus by repeated culture and microscopic examination tissue provides the most firm diagnosis.

Treatment: Antifungal therapy should be initiated in

1. Persistent fever
2. Esher over nose, sinuses or palate.
3. Nodular densities , new cavity lesions, wedge shaped inface&
   - Primary therapy voriconazole
   - Patients who cannot tolerate voriconazole->amphotericin B can be used(1 to 1.5mg/kg/day)
   - Capsofugin->invasive aspergillus & who are intolerant to amphotericin B.

References

1. Sobel TD. Vulvovaginal candidiasis. Lancet 2007 Jun 9. 369(9577):1961-71.
2. Knox KS. Perspective on coccidiomyosis and histoplasmosis. AMJ Raspir Crit Care Med. 2014 March 15, 189(6): 752-3.

CHAPTER - 52

Viral Diseases

There are different types of viral diseases, they are
1. Herpes simplex
2. Varcille (chicken pox)
3. Herpes zoster (shingles)
4. Rubella (measles)
5. Epedemic parotitis (mumps)
6. Herpangina
7. Intecteous mononucleoses
8. Eyetomegatic inclusion desease

1. Herpes simplex virus:

It is of two types
1. Herpes simplex 1
2. Herpes simplex 2

Herpes simplex 1:

It is also known as cold sore

➤ According to WHO, 67%of population under age 50yr have HSV-1

Signs and symptoms:

Symptoms include

Watery blisters in skin/mucous membrane of mouth, lips, nose or genitals

➤ Pharynx, intraoral sites, lips, eyes and skin above waist are more frequently involved

➤ $1°$ infection typically occurs at younger age and it is often asymptomatic

➤ It does not cause significant morbidity

➤ All $1°$ infections occurs from contact with an infected person who is releasing the virus

➤ Incubation period is 3-9 days

➤ It is acquired from contact with contaminated saliva, active perioral lesions, crowing and poor oral hygienes

➤ Most common pattern of sympotomatic $1°$ HSV infection arises between ages of 6months to 5 years

➢ Acute herpetic gingivostomatitis (primary herpes) is accompanied by
  ❖ Anterior cervical lymphadenopathy
  ❖ Chills, fever (103-105F)
  ❖ Nausea
  ❖ Anorexia
  ❖ Irritability
  ❖ Sore mouth lesions

Herpes simplex 2:

It is adapted best to the genital zones, predominately through sexual contact

➢ Typically involves genitalia, skin below waist

➢ HSV-2 increases due to
  ❖ Partly to lack of prior exposure to HSV-1
  ❖ Sexual activity
  ❖ Lack of barrier conception

Treatment:

If infection is diagnosed early, antiviral medications can have significant influence

Table 52.1 Therapy for Herpes simplex virus.

Therapy/prophylaxis	Drug	Therapeutic regimen
Acute therapy (duration: 7-10 days), dialy doses		
First choice	Acyclovir	(3–5) 5 × 400 mg p.o.
Severe cases		3 × 5 – 10 mg/kg i.v.
Alternatives	Valacyclovir	2 – 3 × 1,000 mg or 3 × 500 – 1,000 mg (expert opinion
Therapy for recurrent	Acyclovir	3 × 400 mg p.o. for 5-10 days
Herpes simplex infectio virus	Valacyclovir	2 × 1,000 mg for 5-10 days
episodes	Famciclovir	2 × 500 mg for 5-10 days
Long-term	Acyclovir	2-3 × 400-800 mg
Prophylaxis (duration: at least 90 days)	Valacyclovir	2 × 500 mg
	Famciclovir	2 × 500 mg

2. **Varicella (chicken pox):**
   ➢ It is similar to herpes simplex virus (HSV)
   ➢ Chicken pox represents 1° infection with VZV

Etiology:
- Presumed to be spread through air droplets
- Direct contact with active lesions
- Arise between ages 5-9

Clinical features:
- Symptomatic phase usually begins with
    - Malaise/ Pharyngitis/ Rhinitis
      Additional symptoms include
    - Headache/ Myalgia/ Nausea/ Anorexia/ Vomiting
- Rash begins on face, trunk followed by involvement of extremities
- Each lesion rapidly progresses through stages of
    - Erythema/ Vesicle/ Pustule/ Hardened crust
- Lesions typically continue to erupt for 4 days
- Affected individuals are contagious from 2 days before exanthema until all lesions crust
- Vermillion border of lips and palate are most common sites of involvement followed by buccal mucosa
- Lesions are painless, prevalence and number of oral lesions correlate with severity of extra oral infection
- Mild cases, often only ½ oral ulcerations upto 30 lesions and persists for 5-10days

Treatment
- Warm bath soap/baking soda
- Application of calamine lotion
- Systematic diphenhydramine
    - to relieve pruritis
- Antipyretics should be given to reduce fever
- Antiviral medications such as
    - Acyclovir
    - Valcyclovir
    - Famciclovir
      (These drugs are shown to reduce duration and severity if administrated with in first 24 hrs of rash)

Medications used for the treatment of Varicella ZosterVirous (VZV) infection

1. **Acyclovir:**

   MOA: stops the replication of viral DNA by competitive inhibition of viral DNA polymerase, incorporation into and termination of the growing viral DNA chain and inactivation of viral DNA polymerase.

   CI: Hypersensitivity to acyclovir

   Dose: Pediatric- 20mg/kg per dose orally 4 times daily for 5 days

         Adult: 800mg orally 4 times daily for 5 days

   AE: Diarrhoea

2. **Varicella zoster immunoglobulin:**
   MOA: Antibodies obtained from pooled human plasma of individuals with high titres of varicella zoster provides immunity
   CI: Severe reaction
   Dose: Adult and pediatric- 125 IU/10kg given within 96 h of exposure
   AE: Headache, local injection pain, dizziness
   Varicella vaccines available
   1. Varicella virus vaccine live 0.5 ml SC – at 12-15 months, 2nd dose at 4-6 years
   2. MMRV virus vaccine live – 0.5 ml SC- at 12-15 months, 2nd dose at 4-6 years

3. **Herpes zoster (Shingles):**
   After initial infection with chicken pox, virus is transported up the sensory news presumably establishes latency in dorsal spinal ganglia, occurs ofter reactivation of virus
   Prediposing factors for re activation are
   - immunosupression/HIV-infection/ Treatment with cytoxic/immunosupressive drugs
   - Radiation/ Presence of malignancies/ Old age
   - Alcohol abuse / Stress

Clinical features:
Clinical features are grouped into 3 phases
1. Prodome
2. Acute
3. Chronic

Prodome:
During initial viral replication active ganglionitis develops with resultant neuronal necroses and severe neuralgia
Inflammatory reactions's are responsible for prodromal symptoms of intense pain that precedes rash in more than 90% cases
- Prodome is accompanied by
  - Fever
  - Malaise
  - Headache
- All these symptoms normally present 1-4 days before development of cutaneous/mucosal lesions
- As pain intensifies, it causes
  - Burning
  - Tingling
  - Itching
  - Boring and prickly sensation

Acute:
Begins as involved skin develop clusters of vesicles set on erythematous base

- With in 3-4 days, vesicles becomes pustular, ulcerate crusts developing after 7-10 days
- Oral lesions occurs trigeminal nerve involvement
- Lesion often extend to midline
- In most common cases significant bone necroses lose of teeth in areas involved herpes zoster

Chronic:

Approximately 15% of affected patients progress to chronic phase of herpes zoster

- It is characterized by pain and persists longer than 3 months after initial presentation of acute rash
- Pain is described as
  - ❖ Burning
  - ❖ Throbbing
  - ❖ Itching
  - ❖ Stabbing often with flares caused by light stroking of area

Treatment

Antipyretics

Antipruritics such as diphenhydramine

Antiviral medications-acyclovir, valaciclovir and famciclovir accelerate healing of cutaneous and mucosal lesions

Antibiotics to treat secondary infections

1. Acyclovir: 8 mg five times daily for 7-10 days
2. Famcyclovir : 500 mg 3 times daily for 7 days
3. Valcyclovir: 1000mg 3 tmes daily for 7 days

4. **Rubella (measles):**
   - Infection produced by a virus in family paramyxovirus belonging to genus morbillivirus
   - In most cases it arises in winter and spread through respiratory droplets
   - Incubation period is 10-12days
   - The effected individuals are infectious form 2 days before becoming symptomatic until 4 days often appearance of associated rash
   - Virus is associated significant lymphoid hyperplasia often involves sites such as
     - ❖ Lymph nodes
     - ❖ Tonsils
     - ❖ Adenoids
     - ❖ Peyer'spatch
   - There are 3 stages infection and each stage lasts 3 days justifying designation is nine-day measles
   - First 3 days are dominated by 3 C's
     - ❖ Coryza (running nose)

- ❖ Cough (brassy and uncomfortable)
- ❖ Conjunctivitis (red, watery, photophobic eyes)
- ➢ Fever typically accompanies these symptoms
- ➢ During initial stage, most distinctive oral manifestation
  - ❖ Less often on soft palate
  - ❖ With in these areas are numerous small, blue white maculous
- ➢ As second stage begins, fever continuous, maculopapular and erythomatous rash begins
- ➢ In third stage, fever ends, rash begins to fade

Treatment and prognoses:
- ➢ Good vaccination
- ➢ Fluids, non asprin antipyretics

5. Epidemic parotitis (Mumps):

Infection caused by virus in family paramyxovirus
- ➢ It involves exocrine glands
  - ❖ Pancreas
  - ❖ Choroid plexus
  - ❖ Mature ovaries
  - ❖ Testes
- ➢ Salivary glands are the major sites

Clinical features:
- ❖ Prodromal symptoms-Low grade fever
- ❖ Headeche
- ❖ Malaise
- ❖ Anorexia
- ❖ Myalgia
  - ➢ Parotid gland is involved most frequently but sublingual & submandibular glands also affected
  - ➢ Discomfort and swelling develop in tissues surrounding lower half of external ear
  - ➢ Enlargement typically peaks with in 2-3 days
  - ➢ Pain is most intense during this period of maximal enlargement
  - ➢ Chewing movement if jaw increases pain
  - ➢ Enlargement of glands usually begins on one side
  - ➢ Unilateral involvement is most common
  - ➢ Most oral manifestation is redness of enlargement of Wharton's and Stensen's glands

Progress and prognosis:
- ➢ Non aspirin analgesics
- ➢ Antipyretics
- ➢ Avoid sour foods and drinks

6. Herpengina:

Herpengina begins with acute onset of significant

- ❖ Sore throat
- ❖ Dysphasia, Fever
- ❖ Occasionally accompanied by cough
- ❖ Rhino rhea, Anorexia
    - ➢ It begins with acute onset of significant

        Vomiting, diarrhea, Myalgia, headache
    - ➢ Small number of oral lesions usually 2-6 develop in posterior areas of mouth, usually soft palate, tonsils pillars

        Affected areas begins as red macules

        Form fragile vesicles that rapidly ulcerate
    - ➢ Systemic symptoms resolve within few days
    - ➢ Ulcerations usually take 7-10days to heal

7. Infectious mononucleosis:

It is a symptomatic disease resulting from exposure to Epstein-bass virus (EBV, HHV-4)

- ➢ Infection usually occurs by intimate contact
- ➢ Interfamilial spread is common
- ➢ Children usually becomes infected through contaminated salvia on fingers and other objects

Clinical features:

- ➢ Most EBV infection children are asymptomatic
- ➢ Children younger than 4 years of age with symptoms
    - ❖ Fever, Lymphadenopathy, Pharyngitis, Rhinitis
    - ❖ In adults Prodomal fatigue, Malaise anorexia
- ➢ Body temperature may reach 104F, It lasts from 2-14 days
- ➢ Lingual tonsils can become hyperplastic
- ➢ Lymphoid enlargement

Treatment: In most cases resolves within 4-6 weeks. Non aspirin containing antipyretics

1. Acyclovir : 600-800 mg po 5 times /day for 7-10 days
2. Valcyclovir: 3g/day for 14 days
3. Prednisone : 60mg PO daily followed by 10 day taper
4. Prednisolone: 0.7 mg/kg for 4 days followed by tapered dose
5. Dexamethasone: 0.3mg/kg for 1 dose

Nonpharmacologic Treatment

Nonpharmacologic treatment is an essential part of managing IM.

The mainstay of therapy includes restriction of activity. Adequate rest is important, but bed rest is not required.[2] It is also important to stay hydrated and maintain adequate nutrition because IM may lead to a decrease in appetite. Maintaining adequate hydration is even more important in individuals taking NSAIDs for symptomatic relief to avoid renal insufficiency.

Case Study of Dengue with Thrombocytopenia

Summary

A 25 years old woman got admitted into the hospital with complaints of fever and chills, nausea. She doesn't have any medical history and medication history. Her vitals were normal but have slight fever. She underwent CBP and her platelet levels were completely low. Day 1 0.76 lakhs/cumm, Day 2 0.81 lakhs/cumm. Dengue serology was also performed and the reports were revealed. NS 1(non-specific antigen):- positive.

Diagnosis: Initially the condition of patient was assumed to be enteric fever with thrombocytopenia based on symptoms. But based on dengue serological test and also based on platelet levels it finally proved that she was diagnosed with dengue fever with thrombocytopenia.

Her inpatient therapy included:
1. Inj: Monocef – Ceftriaxone - 1gm, BD.
2. Inj: Pan - Pantoprazole - 40mg, OD.
3. Inj: Zofer - Ondansetron - 4mg, BD.
4. Inj: Infupar - Paracetamol -1gm, SOS.
5. Tab: Dolo - Paracetamol - 650mg, TID.
6. Tab: Supradyn - Multivitamin, OD.

Daily progress:

For 3 days patient is stable and conscious on normal diet.

Pharmacist interventions:

No interaction of drugs and adverse effects were noted. Regular check of platelet count must be done; decreased platelet count may lead to dangerous situation.

Patient counseling:
1. Patient should take rest, drink plenty of fluids to prevent dehydration, avoid mosquito bites while febrile.
2. Juice or pulp made from papaya, effective not only in fighting symptoms but also curing it.
3. Diet with beans which contain vitamin B_9 or folate greatly boost blood platelet count.
4. Garlic acts a blood purifier and also increases blood platelet count.

5. Fruits like oranges and vegetables like spinach are rich in vitamin B_9.
6. Broccoli excellent source of vitamin K regenerate blood platelets.
7. Proper diet maintained.
8. Regular medication intake.

Assignment

1. **What is dengue hemorrhagic fever?**

   Dengue hemorrhagic fever is caused by dengue virus and is characterized by increase vascular permeability, hypovolemia, abnormal blood clotting mechanism. The fever usually continues for 2-7 days and can be as high as 105° F possibly with convulsions and other complications and other symptoms like frequent vomiting, abdominal pain and bleeding under the skin.People with compromised immune system, older adult, infants, small children, and pregnants are at high risk.

2. **Which dietary and activity modifications are beneficial during treatment of dengue?**

   Dietary modifications:

   * Drink plenty of oral fluids (orange water, coconut water, ginger water) or oral rehydration solution to prevent dehydration.
   * Eat fruits like papaya inorder to increase platelet count and overcome thrombocytopenia.
   * A high protein diet in accordance with the patient is recommended as it helps to battle the virus fast.
   * Hot soup intake increase the strength and helps to fight the joint pain also help in increasing apetite and improve taste of mouth.

   Activity modifications:

   * Avoid outdoor activities.
   * Bed rest is recommended in patients with symptomatic dengue fever
   * Permit the patients to graduaaly resume their previous activities, specially during the long period recovery.

3. **What physical findings are characteristic of severe dengue?**

   * Signs of peritoneal effusion, pleural effusion or both.
   * More hemorrhagic findings
   * Conjuctivital infection.
   * Optic neuropathy.
   * Pharyngeal infection.
   * Generalized lymphadenopathy.
   * Tachycardia, bradycardia, conduction defects.

4. **What are the causes of thrombocytopenia in dengue?**

   Thrombocytopenia is common in patients with dengue virus infections. With a possible focus, about the mechanism. There is a direct correlation between activation and depletion of platelets in patients. A kinetic description of platelet count shows significant decrease on fourth day of illness.

A high number of dengue virus genome copies have been found in activated platelets and thus is a high binding of C_3 and I_gG on surface of their platelets .Dengue infection has been found to activate the intrinsic pathway of apoptosis.

5. **What is the most common electrolyte abnormality in patients with severe dengue?**

Hyponatremia-The levels of sodium play a significant role in the prognosis of dengue fever and associated complications.

6. **What is the immunopathology of severe dengue?**

Most patients who develop severe dengue were notably infected priorly with one or more dengue serotype. When an individual is infected with another serotype secondary infection. Then it produces low levels of non neutralizing antibodies which are directed surface protiens when bounded by macrophages, monocytes F_c receptor there by fail to neutralize virus from Ag-Ab complex increases viral into macrophages (bear infection) death of virus.

7. **When is the transfusion of fresh frozen plasma indicated in the treatment dengue?**

Patients with internal or GI bleeding mass require transfusion and the patient with coagulopathy i.e (bleeding disorder) may require fresh frozen plasma.

8. **What are the difference between serotype 1 and serotype 2 dengue?**

Dengue (serotype 1) patients comprised – 469 patients (76%) out of which

DENV 1pts - 103(22.0%)

DENV 2pts - 268(57.1%)   others rests serotype

In all, DENV 1-41.6%pts, DENV-2pts-46.3% required hospital admission.

Univariet analysis showed significant difference between patients for the predominant serotypes,

In terms of gender, $DENV_1$-68.5%

$DENV_2$-highest   proportion in malesis 74.3% comparatively.

Patients required for 1^0 care- DENV 1 – 83%

DENV 2- 45.9%

2^0 care –DENV 1- 53%

DENV2-more common-60.8%

DENV 1 symptoms – redeyes

DENV 2-more likely present joint pains.

Platelets count, DENV - cases – lowest platelets count

Viral RNA level, DENV 1- two time higher than 2

DENV 2- lower.

9. **When is the oral rehydration indicated for management of dengue?**

Oral rehydration therapy is recommended for patients with moderate dehydration caused by high fever and vomiting, patients with suspected or known dengue fever should have their platelet count and haematocrit measured daily from 3rd day of lines until 1-2 days after defervescence.

References

1. A'varez DM, Castilo E, Duarte LF, Arrigada J et al, Current antivirals and Nvel Botanical Molecules Interfering with Herpes Simplex Virus Infection. Front Microbiol. 2020. 11:139.

CHAPTER - 53

Influenza

Introduction to Influenza Infection

- Influenza is also referred as Flu
- It is a viral infection that affects mainly the nose, throat, bronchi and occasionally tongue.
- It's caused by RNA virus family orthomyxoviridae which affects birds and mammals
- It is associated with high mortality and high hospitalization rates among the persons younger than age 6 years.

Structure of virion:

- The major reservoir of influenza virus exists in birds and animals
- Many influenza viruses have been isolated from wide range of birds and animals
- Animal reservoir provides new strains of influenza virus by recombination between influenza viruses of man, animal and birds

Period of infectivity:

The virus is present in nasopharynx a couple of days before and couple of days after the onset of symptoms.

The incubation period is about 18-72 Hrs

Host factors:

It affects all ages and people of both sexes children constitutes an important link in the transmission chain.

Highest mortality rate during epidemic occurs among people more than 65 yrs of age, infants under 18 months and persons with DM, CHD, and respiratory ailments.

Ab appear in about 7 days of attack and search maximum level about 2 weeks about 2 weeks and often 8-12 months Abs level drops to pre infection levels.

'H' Ab neutralize the virus while 'N' Ab modifies the infection.

2 Ab develop in respiratory tract after infection.

Pathogenesis:

The virus enters the respiratory tract and causes inflammation and necrosis of superficial epithelium of francheat and proncheal mucosa followed by secondary bacterial invasion.

Initially there is virus attachment to the cell membrane followed by virus replication, production of cytokines, granzymes and cytotoxic factors. This results in airway inflammation and alveolitis. Because of airway inflammation there is damage of airway epithelial cells and endothelial cells. Airway hyperactivity and narrowing takes place. So there is exacerbation of bronchial asthma and COPD. Due to alveolitis there is damage of alveolar epithelial cells and endothelial cells which causes pneumonia.

Clinical Manifestation and features:

Common symptoms:

Chills, fever, sore throat, muscle pain, severe headache, coughing, non productive cough rhinitis, fatigue, diarrhea, dizziness

Complications may include exacerbation of underlying co morbidities primary viral phenomena or other respiratory issues like sinusitis, bronchitis and otitis, encephalopathy and rye syndrome.

Signs and symptoms typically resolve in 3-7 days. Cough & malaise may persists for more than 2 weeks

There are different viral subtypes of influenza which are classified as type A type B type C. All the three subtypes are antigenically distinct

Both influenza A and B viruses have two distinct surface antigens Hemoglutinin (H) and Nuraminidase (N)

'H' antigen initiates infection fallowing attachment of virus to susceptible cell 'N' antigen is responsible for release of virus from infected cell.

Influenza A virus is unique because it is frequently subject virus to antigenic variation

Antigenic changes occurs to lesser degree in type B and Influenza 'C' appears to be antigenically stable

When antigenic changes are sudden, complete or major changes it is called Shift, and it appears as a result of genetic recombination of human with animal or avian virus

When antigenic changes are gradual it is called drift & it involves point mutations in the gene owing to selection pressure by immunity in host population

Diagnosis with algorithm:
 - ➢ Gold standard for diagnosis of influenza is viral culture
 - ➢ Chest radiograph should be obtained if pneumonia is suspected
 - ➢ Rapid antigen and point of care tests, direct fluorescence antibody test
 - ➢ PCR assay may be used for rapid detection of virus

 Rapid influenza test:
 - ➢ These test are 70%accurate for determining of patient has been infected with influenza virus &90% accurate for determining the type of influenza pathogen
 Eg: Direct antigen flu A, Direct antigen Flu A+B

Prevention:
> ➢ The best means to decrease the morbidity and mortality associated with influenza is to prevent infection through vaccination.
> ➢ Annual vaccination is recommended for all persons age 6 months or older and caregivers of children less than or equal to 6 months of age
> ➢ The yearly vaccination should start approximately 2 weeks before the flu season begins
> ➢ Since influenza virus is subjected to genetic mutation with HA and NA proteins, new Vaccines consists of different influenza strains needed develop each year

Influenza vaccines

Killed vaccines:

Killed vaccines are inactivated vaccines
> ➢ Subcutaneous route, A single inoculation (0.5ml) is usually given, in persons with no previous immunological experience 2 doses of vaccine, separated by an interval of 3-4 weeks are considered necessary to induce satisfactory antibody levels
> ➢ The protective value of vaccine varies between 70-90% and immunity lasts for only 3-6 months revaccination on an annual basis is recommended
> ➢ Killed vaccine can produce fever, local inflammation at site of infection and rarely Gillian-bare syndrome (an ascending paralysis)
> ➢ Since vaccine strains are grown in eggs, persons allergic to eggs may develop & hyper sensitivity symptoms

Live Attenuated Influenza Vaccine (LAIV)

LAIV is made with live attenuated viruses and is approved for intranasal administration in healthy people between 2 and 49 yrs of age

The advantage of LAIV include its ease of administration, intranasal rather than intramuscular administration and the potential induction of broad mucosal and systemic immune response
> ➢ It is approved for children over age of 2 yrs in part because it causes increase in asthma over reactive airway disease in those younger than 5 years
> ➢ The adverse effect associated with LAIV is running nose/ Congestion/ Sore throat/ Headache
> ➢ It should not be given to immunosuppressed patients

New Vaccines:

Split virus vaccines:

Also known as sub virion vaccine
> ➢ It is highly purified vaccine, due its lower antigenicity it requires several doses than single dose.
> ➢ It is recommended for children

Neuraminidase specific vaccine:

It is sub unit vaccine containing only N antigen which induces antibodies only to the neuraminidase antigen of the prevailing influenza virus.

> Antibody to neuraminidase reduces both the amount of virus replication in the respiratory tract and the ability to transmit virus to contacts

Recombinant vaccine:

By using recombinant technique the desired antigen properties of a virulent strain can be transferred to another strain known to be low virulence

Anti viral Drug:

All antiviral drugs inhibit viral replication but they act in different ways to achieve this. The drugs that are effective against influenza A virus & B viruses

Eg : Amantadine, rimantadine, oseltamivir and zanamivir

Amantadine: For the treatment of influenza A, oral Dose: 200mg

Rimantadine: For the treatment of influenza A; Dose-200mg/day in 1 to 2 doses for 7 days

Zanamivir: For the treatment of influenza A and B; oral inhalation- 2 inhalations twice daily for 5 days

Oseltamivir: Influenza A and **Influenza** B; 200mg capsules twice daily for 5 days

Symptomatic drugs: Analgesics Decongestants, Antihistamines, Anesthetics.

References

1. R. World Health Organisation Bell D, Nicoll A et al, Nonpharmacological Interventions for Pandemic Influenza, international measures. Emerg. Infect. Dis. 2006, Jan. 12(1): 81-7.

CHAPTER - 54

Sexually Transmitted Diseases

The spectrum of sexually transmitted diseases (STDs) has broadened from the classic venereal diseases gonorrhea, syphilis, chancroid, lymphogranuloma venereum, and granuloma inguinale — to include a variety of pathogens known to be spread by sexual contact.

Table 54.1 Type of STD disease with associated pathogen.

Disease	Associated pathogen
Bacterial	
Gonorrhea	Neisseria gonorrheae
Syphilis	Treponema pallidum
Chancroid	Haemophilus ducreyi
Granuloma inguinale	Calymatobacterium granulomatis
Campylobacter infection	Campylobacter jejuni
Group B streptococcus infections	Group B streptococci
Chlamydial	
Non gonococcal urethritis	Chlamydia trachomatis
Lymphogranuloma venereum	C. trachomatis type L
Viral	
AIDS	HIV
Herpes genitalis	Herpes simplex virus
Viral hepatits	Hepatitis A,B,C,D viruses
Condylomata acuminate	Human papilloma virus
Mycoplasmal	
Non gonococcal urethritis	Ureaplasma urealyticum
Protozoal	
Trichomoniasis	Trichomonas vaginalis
Amoebiasis	Entamoeba histolytica
Giardiasis	Giardia lamblia
Fungal	
Vaginal candidiasis	Candida albicans
Parasitic	
Scabies	Sarcoptes scabiei
Pediculosis pubis	Phthirus pubis

Because of the large number of infected individuals, the diversity of clinical manifestations, the changing drug-susceptibility patterns of some pathogens, and the high frequency of multiple STDs occurring simultaneously in infected individuals, the diagnosis and management of patients with STDs are much more complex today than they were a decade ago.

The varied spectrum of clinical syndromes produced by common STD's is determined not only by the etiologic pathogens but also by differences in male and female anatomy and reproductive physiology.

Table 54.2 Clinical presentation of various syndromes.

Syndrome	Commonly implicated pathogens	Common clinical manifestations
1. Urethritis	Chlamydia trachomatis, herpes simplex virus, Neisseria gonorrhea, Trichomonas vaginalis, Ureaplasma urealyticum	Urethral discharge , dysuria
2. Epididymitis	C. trachomatis, N.gonorrhea	Scrotal pain, inguinal pain, flank pain
3.Cervicitis/ Vulvovaginitis	C.tracomatis, Gardnella vaginalis, HSV, HPV, N.gonorrhea	Abnormal vaginal discharge, vulvular itching, dysuria.
4.Genital ulcers (painful)	H.ducreyi, HSV	Pustular lesions
5.Genital ulcers (painless)	T.pallidum	Single papular lesion
6. Genital warts	HPV	Multiple lesions
7.Pharyngitis	C.trachomatis, HSV, N.gonorrhea	Acute pharyngitis, cervical lymphadenopathy
8.Proctitis	C.trachomatis, HSV, N.gonorrhea, T.pallidum	Constipation, anorectal discomfort, mucopurulent renal discharge
9.Salpingitis	C.trachomatis, N.gonorrhea	Lower abdominal pain, purulent cervical/ vaginal discharge, swelling, fever

Gonorrhea

It is an infection caused by gram negative diplococcus bacteria Neisseria gonorrheae. Humans are the only known natural host of this intracellular parasite. It can reside in the uterus, cervix, rectum, throat. Because of its rapid incubation period and the large number of infected individuals with asymptomatic disease, gonorrhea is difficult to control.

Pathophysiology

On contact with a mucosal surface lined by columnar, cuboidal, or noncornified squamous epithelial cells, the gonococci attach to cell membranes by means of surface pili and are then pinocytosed. The virulence of the organism is mediated primarily by the presence of pili and other outer membrane proteins. Bacterial porins and proteins form pores in host cell membranes, inducing endocytosis by host epithelial cells. Bacterial invade and replicate within columnar epithelail cells. Damage to host immune response occurs. Bacterial phagocytosis by circulating monocytes. Due to Unsuccessful eradication of pathogen, bacterial proteins block Phagolysosomal fusion and PMN oxidative burst takes place. Due to various mechanisms host immunity is avoided. After mucosal damage is established, polymorphonuclear leukocytes (PMNs) invade the tissue, sub mucosal abscesses form, and purulent exudates are secreted.

Clinical Manifestation and Features

Individuals infected with gonorrhea can be symptomatic or asymptomatic, have complicated or uncomplicated infections, and have infections involving several anatomic sites. Interestingly, most of the symptomatic patients who are not treated become asymptomatic within 6 months, with only a few becoming asymptomatic carriers of the disease.

Signs and Symptoms

Men

Incubation period: 1-14 days

Symptoms onset: 2-8 days

Signs: Purulent urethral or rectal discharge, anorectal pruritus, mucopurulent discharge, bleeding

Complications: Disseminated gonorrhea

Women

Incubation period: 1 -14 days

Symptoms onset: 10 days

Signs: Abdominal vaginal discharge, uterine bleeding, purulent urethral or rectal discharge

Complications: Pelvic inflammatory disease, infertility, disseminated gonorrhea.

Diagnosis

Diagnosis of gonococcal infections can be made by Gram stained smears, culture methods based on the detection of cellular components of the gonococcus (e.g., enzymes, antigens, DNA, or lipopolysaccharide) in clinical specimens. Various stains have been used to identify gonococci microscopically, with the Gram stain the most widely used in clinical practice.

Alternative methods of diagnosis have been developed, including enzyme immunoassay, DNA probe techniques and nucleic acid amplification techniques employing polymerase chain reaction (PCR) and ligase chain reaction (LCR).

Treatment

N. gonorrhoeae are susceptible to a variety of antibiotics.

1. All gonorrhea treatment regimens recommended by the CDC consist of various oral or parenteral cephalosporins and fluoroquinolones given as a single dose. These regimens have documented efficacy in the treatment of urethral, cervical, rectal, and pharyngeal infections.

   As a result, concomitant treatment with doxycycline or azithromycin is recommended in all patients treated for gonorrhea. While none of the single-dose regimens recommended for gonorrhea in the CDC guidelines is effective against chlamydia, azithromycin (2 g) as a single dose is highly effective in eradicating both gonorrhea and chlamydia.

   Ceftriaxone, the only parenteral agent included in CDC recommended first-line agents for the treatment of gonorrhea, is administered intramuscularly (IM) as a single 125-mg dose. Ofloxacin is useful in eradicating both N.gonorrhoeae and C.trachomatis.

   Spectinomycin is still the preferred alternative for patients unable to tolerate the recommended cephalosporin or fluoroquinolone regimens.

   Treatment of gonorrhea during pregnancy is essential to pre-vent ophthalmia neonatorum. Ophthalmia neonatorum is the most common ophthalmic infection in newborns (1.6% to 12%), although membranes of the vagina, pharynx, or rectum also can be colonized. Conjunctival involvement usually develops within 7 days of delivery and is characterized by intense, bilateral conjunctival inflammation with chemosis.If not treated promptly, corneal ulceration and blindness can develop. Because the law in most states requires neonatal prophylaxis with topical ocular antimicrobials, gonococcalo phthalmia neonatorum is rare in the United States.

   The American Academy of Pediatrics recommends that either silver nitrate (1%), tetracycline (1%), erythromycin (0.5%) be instilled in each conjunctival sac immediately postpartum. Infants born to infected mothers should receive an IM or intravenous (IV) injection of ceftriaxone 25–50 mg/kg (not to exceed 125 mg).

Table 54.3 Pharmacotherapy for types of Gonorrhoal infections.

Type of infection	Recommended dose	Alternative dose
1. Uncomplicated infections of the cervix, urethra and rectum in adults	Ceftriaxone 250mg IM OD + Azithromycin 1g p/o OD (OR) Doxycycline 100mg p/o BD Daily for 7days	Cefixime 400mg p/o OD + Azithromycin 1g p/o OD (OR) Doxycyclin 100mg p/o BD Daily for 7 days
2. Uncomplicated infections of the pharynx	Ceftriaxone 250mg IM OD + Azithromycin 1g p/o OD (OR) Doxycyclin 100mg p/o BD for 7 days	
3. Disseminated gonococcal infection in adults	Ceftriaxone 1g IM/ IV every 24 hours	Cefotaxime 1g IV every 8hrs (OR) Ceftizoxime 1g IV every 8hrs
4. Uncomplicated infections of cervix, urethra, rectum in children	Ceftriaxone 125mg IM OD Ceftriaxone 1g IM OD	
5. Gonococcal conjunctivitis in adults 6. Infants born to mother with gonococcal infection	Erythromycin(0.5%) ointment (opthalmic) in a single application	Ceftriaxone 25-50mg/kg IM or IV once

Syphilis

Syphilis usually is acquired by sexual contact with infected mucous membranes or cutaneous lesions; although on rare occasions it can be acquired by nonsexual personal contact, accidental inoculation, or blood transfusion. The causative organism of syphilis is Treponema pallidum, a spirochete.

After sexual contact, the organism penetrates the intact mucous membrane or a break in the cornified epithelium, and spirochetemia occurs. The clinical presentation of syphilis is varied with progression through multiple stages possible in untreated or inadequately treated patients.

Pathogenesis

Inoculation with trepanaoma palladium from direct contact with infected lesion. There is penetration intomucous membranes and microscopic abrasions in skin. It is now primary syphilis (10-90 days of incubation) if primary syphilis left untreated or unresponsive to therapy, it develops into 2^0 syphillis (weeks-months after 1^0syphillis). The primary syphilis gradulally invade dermal leucocytes, macrophages and lymphocytes infiltrate site of infection and cause endarteritis, periarteritis. In this course of time spirochetes multiply and spread throughout body with varying dermal and systemic manifestations. If 2^0 syphillis left untreated or unresponsive to therapy, it develops into latent syphilis or tertiary syphilis (months-years after primary infection). In 2^0 syphillis infiltration causes epidermal hyperkeratosis, capillary proliferation and endothelial swelling which is presented as alopecia, macule lesions, fever, sore throat, headache.

Clinical Manifestation and Features

Primary Syphilis

The primary stage, characterized by the appearance of a chancre on cutaneous or mucocutaneous tissue exposed to the organism, is highly infectious. Even without treatment, chancres persist only for 1 to8 weeks before healing spontaneously.

Secondary Syphilis

The secondary stage of syphilis is characterized by a variety of mucocutaneous eruptions resulting from widespread hematogenous and lymphatic spread of T. pallidum.

Skin lesions can be either generalized or localized to a small portion of the body and with the exception of follicular lesions, are nonpruritic. Generalized lymphadenopathy also is seen in the majority of patients, as are nonspecific symptom such as mild and transitory malaise, fever, pharyngitis, headache, anorexia, and arthralgia. If untreated, secondary syphilis disappears in 4 to 10 weeks; however, lesions may recur at any time within 4 yrs.

Latent Syphilis

By definition, persons with a positive serologic test for syphilis but with no other evidence of disease have latent syphilis. Latent syphilisis further divided into early and late latency. During early latency, the patient is considered potentially infectious because of the 25% risk of spontaneous mucocutaneous relapse. The U.S. Public Health Service defines early latency as 1 year from the onset of infection, late latency is considered noninfectious, although the patient remains a host.

Tertiary Syphilis and Neurosyphilis

If left untreated, syphilis can slowly produce an inflammatory reaction in virtually any organ in the body. Manifestations of this disease progression were referred as tertiary syphilis.

These clinical manifestations now are differentiated into two sub groups based on the presence or absence of central nervous system (CNS) involvement: neurosyphilis or tertiary syphilis.

Congenital Syphilis

In pregnant women with syphilis, T. pallidum can cross the placenta at any time during pregnancy. The risk of fetal infection is greatest in pregnant women with primary and secondary syphilis and declines in pregnant women with late disease. Symptoms can be seen during the first months of life (early congenital syphilis) or later in childhood or adolescence (late congenital syphilis).

Diagnosis

Because T.pallidum is difficult to culture invitro, diagnosis is based primarily on dark field or direct fluorescent antibody microscopic examination of serous material from a syphilitic lesion.

Serologic tests are the mainstay in the diagnosis of syphilis and are categorised as nontreponemal or treponemal.

Common nontreponemal tests include
- The Venereal Disease Research Laboratory (VDRL) slide test
- Rapid Plasma Reading (RPR) card test
- Unheated Serum Reagent (USR) Test
- The Toluidine Red Unheated Serum Test (TRUST).

Treponemal tests include - The fluorescent Treponemal antibody absorption test.

Treponemal tests are more sensitive than nontreponemal test and are used to confirm the diagnosis.

Treatment

Parentral penicillin G is the drug of choice for all stages of syphilis. Because T. pallidum multiplies slowly, single doses of short- or intermediate-acting penicillins do not provide the prolonged, low-level exposure to penicillin required for eradication of the treponeme. As a result, benzathine penicillin G is the only penicillin effective for single-dose therapy.

The recommended treatment for syphilis of less than 1 year's duration is benzathine penicillin G 2.4 million units as a single dose. In patients with syphilis of greater than 1 year's duration and normal CSF examination, benzathine penicillin G is administered weekly for three successive doses.

Patients with abnormal CSF findings should be treated as having neurosyphilis. Preferred regimens for neurosyphilis provide treatment over 10 to 14 days with parenteral penicillin G administered every4 hours.

Because T.pallidum resistance to penicillin has not emerged, the primary need for alternative drugs in treating syphilis is for penicillin-allergic patients.

Alternative regimens recommended for penicillin-allergic patients are doxycycline 100 mg orally twice daily or tetracycline 500 mg orally four times daily for 2 to 4 weeks depending on the duration of syphilis infection.

Alternative treatment regimens should be used only in cases of documented penicillin allergy, and given concerns regarding patient compliance with these regimens.

Other antibiotics used successfully in treating syphilis include various

β-lactam antibiotics; however, none offers significant ad-vantages over benzathine penicillin G. ceftriaxone isconsidered effective in eradicating incubating syphilis whwn given as single 125mg dose.

For pregnant patients, penicillin is the treatment of choice at the dosage recommended for that particular stage of syphilis. To ensure treatment success and prevent transmission to the fetus, some experts advocate an additional IM dose of Benzathine penicillin G 2.4 million units 1 week after completion of the recommended regimen.

Table 54.4 Drug Therapy and Follow up for Syphilis.

Stage of syphilis	Recommended regimens	Follow up serology
Non Penicillin Allergic Patients		
1. Primary, secondary or latent syphilis (<1yr duration)	Benzathine penicillin G 2.4 million units in a single dose	Quantitative non treponemal tests at 6 and 12 months
2. Late latent syphilis (> 1yr duration)	Benzathine penicillin G 2.4 million units IM once a week for 3 weeks	Quantitative non treponemal tests at 6, 12, 24 months
3. Neurosyphilis	Aq-crystalline pen G 18-24 million units IV for 10-14 days (or) Aq-crystalline pen G 2.4 million units IM daily plus probenecid 500mg orally 4 times daily both for 10-14 days	CSF examination every 6 months until the cell count is normal
4. Congenital syphilis	Aq-crystalline pen G 50,000 units/kg IV every 12hrs during the first 7 days of life and every 8 hrs for total of 10days (or) Procaine pen G 50,000 units/kg IM daily for 10 days	Serologic follow up only recommended if antimicrobials other than pen are used
Penicillin Allergic Patients 1. Primary , secondary or early latent syphilis	Doxycycline 100mg orally 2times daily for 14 days (or) Tetracycline 500mg orally 4times daily for 14 days, Ceftriaxone 1g IM/IV daily for 8-10 days	Same as for non pen allergic patients

Most patients treated for primary and secondary syphilis experience the Jarisch-Herxheimer reaction after treatment. This benign, self-limiting reaction is characterized by flulike symptoms, such as transient headache, fever, chills, malaise, arthralgia, myalgia, tachypnea, peripheral vasodilation, and aggravation of syphilitic lesions. The Jarisch-Herxheimer reaction is independent of the drug and dose used and should not be confused with penicillin allergy. It usually begins within 2 to 4 hours of initiating therapy, peaks at 8 hours, and is complete within 12 to 24 hours. Most reactions can be managed symptomatically with analgesics, antipyretics, and rest. Steroids and antihistamines have been administered prior to initiation of syphilitic therapy.

References

1. Workowski KA, Berman S, Centres for Disease Control and Prevention. Sexually transmitted diseases treatment guidelines 2010. MMWR. Recomm. Rep. 2010; 59:1-110.

CHAPTER - 55

Alcoholic Liver Disease

Introduction to Alcoholic Liver Disease

Alcoholic liver disease is a term that encompasses the liver manifestations of alcohol over consumption which includes Fatty liver, Alcoholic hepatitis, chronic hepatitis with liver cirrhosis.

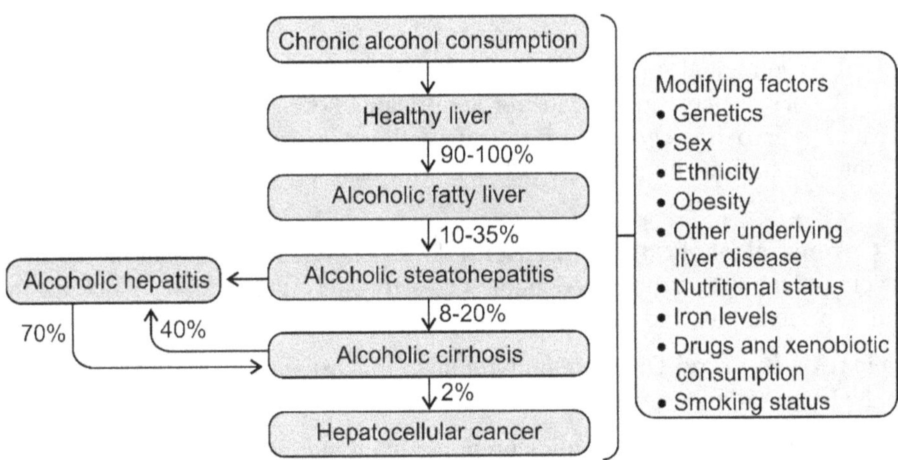

Fig. 55.1 Risk factors and causes of Alcoholic Liver disease.

Alcoholic fatty liver (steatosis): It refers to accumulation of fatty **acids** in the liver cells and fatty globules are present in hepatocytes throughout the liver. Steatosis is invariable if alcohol intake exceeds 80 g of alcohol/day. A large portion of cytoplasm of affected hepatocytes is occupied by a single large triglyceride occlusion but liver function is often normal. It is reversible with abstinence but may progress to cirrhosis if alcohol intake persists. Death due to direct fatty liver is rare and usually caused by acute liver failure or fat embolism.

Acute Alcoholic Hepatitis (Steatohepatitis): It refers to an inflammation of hepatocytes and 10-35% of heavy drinkers develop hepatitis. There is fatty changes, liver inflammation and necrosis. Alcohol consumption increases the permeability of GIT and results in increase in absorption of endotoxins released from gut bacteria.as a reslut liver macrophages release inflammatory cytokines TNF-alpha, IL-6 to induce liver inflammation. This further continues to either hepatitis or hepatocyte damage.

Alcoholic cirrhosis: Cirrhosis is the most common type of alcoholic liver injury and is usually of nodular type. It is characterized by extensive fibrosis that damages the liver architecture. 10-20% of heavy drinkers develop cirrhosis.

Liver Cirrhosis

Introduction

Fibrosis is defined as excessive accumulation of proteins, such as collagen in liver, extra cellular matrix. If fibrotic disease progresses the collagen bands progress to bridging fibrosis and eventually cirrhosis.

Cirrhosis is defined as a diffuse process characterized by fibrosis and a conversion of the normal hepatic architecture into structurally abnormal nodules. The end result is destruction of hepatocytes and their replacement by fibrous tissue.

Epidemiology

Acute variceal bleeding and spontaneous bacterial peritonitis are life-threatening complications of cirrhosis. Associated conditions causing significant morbidity include ascites and hepatic encephalopathy. Approximately 50% of patients with cirrhosis develop ascites during 10 years of observation and half of the cirrhotic patients who develop ascites will die within 2years of diagnosis.

Etiology: Chronic alcoholic liver disease: 15% of individuals who drink for more than a decade develop alcoholic cirrhosis. Alcohol seems to injure the liver by blocking the normal metabolism of protein, fats, and carbohydrates.

Chronic hepatitis B, C and D: Infection with this virus causes inflammation of and low grade damage to the liver that over several decades can lead to cirrhosis.

Non-alcoholic steatohepatitis: Fat builds up in the liver and eventually causes scar tissue. This type of hepatitis appears to be associated with diabetes, protein malnutrition, obesity, coronary artery disease, and treatment with corticosteroid medications. This disorder is similar to that of alcoholic liver disease but patient does not have an alcohol history.

Primary biliary cirrhosis: May be asymptomatic or complain of fatigue, pruritus, and non-jaundice skin hyperpigmentation with hepatomegaly. There is prominent alkaline phosphatase elevation as well as elevations in cholesterol and bilirubin.

Primary sclerosing cholangitis: It is a progressive cholestatic disorder presenting with pruritus, steatorrhea, fat soluble vitamin deficiencies, and metabolic bone disease. There is a strong association with inflammatory bowel disease (IBD).

Autoimmune hepatitis: This disease is caused by the immunologic damage to the liver causing inflammation and eventually scarring and cirrhosis.

Hereditary hemochromatosis: Usually presents with family history of cirrhosis, skin hyperpigmentation, diabetes mellitus, pseudogout, and/or cardiomyopathy, all due to signs of iron overload.

Wilson's disease: Autosomal recessive disorder characterized by low serum ceruloplasmin and increased hepatic copper content on liver biopsy.

Alpha 1-antitrypsin deficiency (AAT): Autosomal recessive disorder. Patients may also have COPD, especially if they have a history of tobacco smoking. Serum AAT levels are low.

Cardiac cirrhosis: Due to chronic right sided heart failure which leads to liver congestion.

Galactosemia, Cystic fibrosis, Drugs or toxins, Certain parasitic infections (such as schistosomiasis)

Pathogenesis

Mechanisms of alcoholic liver disease: Alcohol contributes to liver injury through a multitude of ways. Alcohol is metabolized to acetaldehyde; both alcohol and acetaldehyde have toxic effects on hepatocytes via formation of free radicals like $H2O2$, $O2-$. Damaged hepatocytes in turn release mediators that recruit innate and adaptive immune cells that perpetuate further liver injury. Earlier alcohol lesion of steatosis is mediated by effects of alcohol or lipogenesis and fatty acid oxidation. Alcohol also has direct effects on intestinal microbiome and gut permeability that allows bacterial products to reach liver, and further stimulate immune response and liver injury. Finally, despite immune stimulation, the immune response is ineffective in combating the injury/infection. Chronic ethanol consumption, leads to formation of gut derived endotoxins. These now act on kupfer cells to release cytokines like IL-1α, IL-1β, IL-6 and TNF. These activate the inflammatory process, recruit T cells, neutrophils. Now there is activation of HSC, which causes the formation of collagen in extracellular matrix. Over the time collagen deposits in the intracellular spaces and forms nodules and then to fibrosis.

Complications of Cirrhosis

Portal hypertension and varices: Portal hypertension is defined by an elevation in blood pressure in the portal system. Different causes are known and include a pre-, intra-, or posthepatic block. Portal hypertension is also classified according to the sinusoidal system. Portal pressure becomes elevated by either an increase in blood flow (Q), an increase in resistance (R), or both. Regulation of the vascular tone in the splanchnic system includes intrinsic and extrinsic aspects. A variety of metabolic end-products (e.g. adenosine), endothelium-derived substances (e.g. nitric oxide), and certain neurotransmitters (e.g. acetylcholine) are known to relax the tone and thus produce vasodilation. Important vasoconstrictor influences on splanchnic arterioles include circulating agents (e.g. angiotensin), endothelium-derived substances (e.g. endothelin), and again neurotransmitters (norepinephrine). Besides vascular tone, structural changes (thrombosis, fibrosis, shear stress, and cell regeneration) add to overall hepatic resistance. Further consequences of portal hypertension include an increase in blood flow which leads to a hyperdynamic state with fluid retention, leading to secondary involvement of other organs, such as cirrhotic cardiomyopathy, hepatopulmonary syndrome and hepatorenal syndrome. Finally, portal hypertension will end up in the formation of collateral vessels. Varices can involve the whole gastrointestinal tract and are a frequent source of bleeding.

Ascites

As cirrhosis of the liver becomes severe, there is severe portal hypertension and hepatic insufficiency lead to splanchnic arterial vasodilatation and decreased peripheral resistance. The resulting systemic hypotension causes increased activity of the sympathetic nervous system and renin–angiotensin–aldosterone system, which causes increased sodium and water retention and vasoconstrictor production. Signals are sent to the kidneys to retain salt and water in the body. The excess salt and water first accumulates in the tissue beneath the skin of the ankles and legs because of the effect of gravity when standing or sitting. This accumulation of fluid is called edema or pitting edema. As cirrhosis worsens and more salt and water are retained, fluid also may accumulate in the abdominal cavity between the abdominal wall and the abdominal organs. This accumulation of fluid (called ascites) causes swelling of the abdomen, abdominal discomfort, and increased weight.

Spontaneous bacterial peritonitis: Fluid in the abdominal cavity (ascites) is the perfect place for bacteria to grow. Normally, the abdominal cavity contains a very small amount of fluid that is able to resist infection well, and bacteria that enter the abdomen (usually from the intestine) are killed or find their way into the portal vein and to the liver where they are killed. In cirrhosis, the fluid that collects in the abdomen is unable to resist infection normally. In addition, more bacteria find their way from the intestine into the ascites. Therefore, infection within the abdomen and the ascites, referred to as spontaneous bacterial peritonitis occurs. It is a life- threatening complication. Some patients have no symptoms, while others have fever, chills, abdominal pain and tenderness, diarrhea, and worsening ascites.

Hepatic Encephalopathy

Hepatic encephalopathy (HE) can be defined as a central nervous system disturbance with a wide range of neuropsychiatric symptoms, and which is associated with hepatic insufficiency and liver failure. Symptoms of HE are thought to result from an accumulation of gutderived nitrogenous substances in the systemic circulation as a consequence of decreased hepatic functioning and shunting through portosystemic collaterals bypassing the liver. Once these substances enter the central nervous system, they cause alterations of neurotransmission that affect consciousness and behavior. Ammonia is the most commonly cited culprit in the pathogenesis of HE.

Stages of Encephalopathy

Stage I prodrome: The patient is alert, slow mentation, euphoria, occasional depression, confusion, restless, irritable, disoriented speech, tremor.

Stage II impending coma: Stage I signs amplified, lethargic, sleepy, loss of sphincter control, yawning, grimacing, blinking, hyperactive.

Stage III stupor: Arousable, but generally asleep, significant confusion, confusion, incoherent speech, severe tremor, hyperactive.

Stage IV coma: Unarousable, or responds only to pain, hyperactive

Stage V coma: Unarousable

Hepatorenal Syndrome

Patients with worsening cirrhosis can develop the hepatorenal syndrome. This syndrome is a serious complication in which the function of the kidneys is reduced. It is a functional problem in the kidneys, that is, there is no physical damage to the kidneys. Instead, the reduced function is due to changes in the way the blood flows through the kidneys themselves. The hepatorenal syndrome is defined as progressive failure of the kidneys to clear substances from the blood and produce adequate amounts of urine even though some other important functions of the kidney, such as retention of salt, are maintained. If liver function improves or a healthy liver is transplanted into a patient with hepatorenal syndrome, the kidneys usually begin to work normally. Elevated levels of splanchnic nitric oxide production and central hypovolemia lead to decrease in cardiac preload, cardiac output; splanchnic arterial vasodilationand decreased vascular resistance. Final outcome id decreased effective arterial blood volume. As a result there is stimulation of systemic vasoconstrcitors-RAAS, Arginine Vasopresin (AVP). Angiotensin, aldosterone cause potent vasoconstriction. In the late stage of cirrhosis, there is decreased production of local vasodilators and increased production of local vasoconstrictors. This leads to hepatorenal syndrome.

Coagulation Defects

- Complex coagulation derangements can occur in cirrhosis. These derangements include the reduction in the synthesis of coagulation factors, excessive fibrinolysis, disseminated intravascular coagulation, thrombocytopenia, and platelet dysfunction.
- Vitamin K–dependent clotting factor, including factor VII, is affected early.
- The net effect of these events is the development of bleeding diathesis.

Clinical Manifestations and Features

Signs and symptoms

- Asymptomatic, hepatomegaly, pruritis, splenomegaly
- Jaundice, palmar erythema, spider angiomata, hyperpigmentation
- Gynecomastia, reduced libido, ascites, edema, pleural effusion
- Respiratory difficulties, malaise, anorexia, weight loss, encephalopathy

Diagnosis with Algorithm

Laboratory investigations:

The following findings are typical in cirrhosis:
- Thrombocytopenia
- AST and ALT are moderately elevated, with AST > ALT.
- Alkaline phosphatase - slightly elevated but less than 2-3 times the upper limit of normal
- Gamma-glutamyl transferase – correlates with AP levels. Typically much higher in chronic liver disease from alcohol.
- Bilirubin - Levels elevate as cirrhosis progresses.
- Albumin - levels fall as the synthetic function of the liver declines with worsening cirrhosis since albumin is exclusively synthesized in the liver
- Prothrombin time - increases since the liver synthesizes clotting factors.
- Leukopenia and neutropenia - due to splenomegaly with splenic margination.
- Coagulation defects - the liver produces most of the coagulation factors
- Imaging: liver will be highly ecogenic and will be irregular in shape

Table 55.1 CHILD PUGH classification & end stage disease score.

Score	1	2	3
Bilirubin (mg/dl)	1-2	2-3	>3
Albumin (IU)	>3.5	2.8-3.5	<2.8
Ascites	None	Mild	Moderate
Encephalopathy	None	Mild-moderate	Severe to coma
PT (sec)	1-4	4-6	>6

Class A = total score of 5-6

Class B = total score of 7-9

Class C = total score of 10 and more

Treatment of Cirrhosis

General Approaches to Treatment

The clinical manifestations of cirrhosis are protean and it is difficult to provide overall management guidelines. General approaches to therapy should include:

1. Identifying and eliminating, where possible, the causes of cirrhosis (e.g., alcohol abuse).
2. Assessing the risk for variceal bleeding and beginning pharmacologic prophylaxis when indicated. Reserve prophylactic endoscopic therapy for patients with contraindications or intolerance to β-adrenergic blockers. Endoscopic therapy is also appropriate for patients suffering acute bleeding episodes. Variceal obliteration with endoscopic techniques is the recommended treatment of choice in patients with acute bleeding.

3. Evaluating the patient for clinical signs of ascites and managing with pharmacologic therapy (e.g., diuretics and paracentesis). Careful monitoring for spontaneous bacterial peritonitis should be used in patients with ascites who undergo acute deterioration.
4. Monitoring for hepatic encephalopathy, which is a common complication of cirrhosis that requires clinical vigilance and treatment with dietary restriction, elimination of central nervous system depressants, and therapy to lower ammonia levels.
5. Monitoring frequently for signs of hepatorenal syndrome, pulmonary insufficiency, and endocrine dysfunction is necessary.

Treatment with Algorithm

1. Once the cirrhosis is diagnosed, the patient is to be checked if he is stable. If yes, check for model end stage liver disease score. If ≥15 consider referral to a transplant centre.
2. If score is < 15, then monitor for complications
   (a) Surveillance for varices
   (i) If there is acute bleeding-shift the person to intensive care unit
      Large –bore IV line to be established. Complete blood count, serum electrolyte levels to be estimated. Immediately somatostatin or somatostatin analogue is to be given and antibiotic has to be started.
   (ii) Medium or large varices are observed- beta blockers have to be initiated and /or endoscopic variceal ligation has to be done.
   (iii) Small varices are observed- periodic endoscopy has to be initiated.
   (b) If the person is identified with ascites- salt restriction is implemented. Diuretics have to be started. If the edema is not controlled paracentesis has to be initiated.
   (c) If the person is identified with hepatic encephalopathy- disaccharides or rifamixin is to be initiated. Paracentesis can be started to control edema.
   (d) Screening for hepatocellular carcinoma every 6-12 months using imaging.

Management

Portal Hypertension & Variceal Bleeding

It involves 3 strategies-
   (a) Primary prophylaxis
   (b) Treatment of acute variceal hemorrhage
   (c) Secondary prophylaxis
   (a) **Primary prophylaxis:** Nonselective β-blockers primary prophylaxis for patients with cirrhosis and small, medium or large varices and no history of bleeding
      MOA: block β1 reduces cardiac output, block β2 splanchnic constriction leads to reductions in portal pressure. Therapy should aim for a heart rate of 55–60 beats/minute or a 25% reduction from baseline
      Propranalol-10mg-OD
      Nodolol-20mg-OD

(b) Acute Variceal Hemorrhage: Symptoms include hematemesis, melena.

Goals of treatment:

1. Adequate fluid resuscitation with packed RBC, frozen plasma, platelets
2. Correction of coagulopathy & thrombocytopenia.
3. Control bleeding & prevent rebleeding.
4. Preserving liver function.
5. Airway management.

Somatostatin: It is a naturally occurring 14-aminoacid peptide with $t_{1/2}$ -1 min, given i/v. Mechanism of action is to decrease the splanchnic blood flow. So there will be decrease in portal inflow through inhibition of vasodilatory GI peptides including glucagon, vasoactive intestinal peptide, and calcitonin gene.

Vasopressin: It is a Non-selective vasoconstrictor. It causes Splanchnic vasoconstriction-so decrease in splanchnic blood flow. ADRS: HTN, headache, coronary ischemia, MI, arrhythmia

Octreotide: It is a synthetic peptide. It is a selective potent vasoconstrictor that reduces portal and collateral blood flow by constricting splanchnic blood vessles. t1/2: 10-22 min; IV-50-100mcg/hr for 3-5 days. Monitoring parameters: hyperglycemia, cardiac conduction abnormalities.

(c) Secondary Prophylaxis:

1. For preventing rebleeding- Combination of endoscopic variceal ligation + nonselective β blockers as the initial approach is recommended.

   Propranolol-20mg or Nadolol-20-40mg.

   Endoscopic band ligation (EBL) or endoscopic variceal ligation (EVL) An elastic band is placed around the mucosa and submucosa of the esophageal area containing the varix, leading to strangulation, fibrosis, and ideally obliteration of the varix. Side effects are Moderate bleeding, hypotension, gastrointestinal discomfort, esophageal ulceration, and perforation.

2. Transjugular Intraheaptic Portosystemic Shunt (TIPS) is very effective. A conduit between the hepatic vein and intrahepatic segment of the portal vein with an expandable metal stent is placed during an angiographic procedure. This channel allows blood to return to the systemic circulation and reduces portal pressure.

3. Balloon tamponade bleeding is controlled by direct compression of the varices at the gastroesophageal junction or at the bleeding site by a Sengstaken-Blakemore tube or Lintern tube (gastric varices only). The tube is passed through the mouth and into the stomach. A balloon is then inflated, which applies direct compression to the varices.

4. Sclerotherapy Injection of 0.5 to 5 mL of a sclerosing agent (e.g., concentrated saline: 11.5% NaCl or ethanolamine oleate [Ethamolin]) into each varix at points about 2 cm apart to induce immediate hemostasis (cessation of bleeding within 2 to 5 min)

Pharmacological Management of Hepatic Encephalopathy

Factors that Precipitate Hepatic Encephalopathy

(a) Excess nitrogen load: Bleeding from gastric and esophageal varices, paptic ulcers, constipation, excess dietary protein, azotemia, infection

(b) Fluid and electrolyte abnormalities: hypokalemia, alkalosis, hypovolemia, excessive vomiting

Initial management:

- After identifying and removing precipitating causes of hepatic coma, therapeutic management is aimed primarily at reducing the amount of ammonia or nitrogenous products in the circulatory system.

- In general, the **2006 European Society for Clinical Nutrition and Metabolism (ESPEN)** recommends an energy intake of 35 to 40 kcal/kg of body weight/day and a protein intake of 1.2 to 1.5 g/kg of body weight/day is recommended for cirrhotic patients and those awaiting liver transplantation surgeries.

1. **Thiamine:** Reverses mental confusion

   Dose: 100-200mg/day

   Monitoring parameters: Mental status, ↓nystagmus

2. **Vit-K:** Prevent bleeding secondary to decreased production of factors II, VII, IX, X.

   Dose: 10-15 mg/day not exceeding 3 doses.

   Monitoring parameters: Hypersensitivity, fever, chills

3. **Spironolactone:** Diuresis in ascites, specific for antagonising pre-existing hyperaldosteronism

   Dose: 200-400mg/day

   Monitoring parameters: Weight, mental status, serum K, urine Na+K+, BUN, B.P

4. **Sodium tetradecyl sulphate:** Sclerosing agent for esophageal bleeding

   Dose: 05-2ml of 1.5% solutions about 2 cm apart

   Monotoring parameters: Signs of GI bleeding, fever, chest pain, local irritation.

5. **Lactulose:** Lactulaose is broken down in GI lumen to form lactic, acetic and formic acids. Acidification of colonic contents converts ammonia into the less readily absorbed ammonium ion. Back diffusion of ammonia from the plasma into the GI tract may also occur. The net result is a lower plasma ammonia concentration. The absorption of other protein breakdown products (e.g., aromatic amino acids) may also be reduced. Lactulose-induced osmotic diarrhea may also decrease the intestinal transit time available for ammonia production and absorption, and may help clear the GI tract of blood.

   Dose: 15-45 ml dose 2-3 times daily or an enema (300ml +700ml water retained for 1 hr, may be continued over the long term to prevent recurrent encephalopathy.

   Adverse effects: Flatulence, diarrhoea, and abdominal cramping

6. **Neomycin:** Sterilises gut to prevent bacterial breakdown of protein and thus decrease serum NH_3 levels.

Dose: 2-6g/day p/o or rectal.

Monitoring parameters: mental status, diarrhea, bacterial over growth, renal function, ototoxicity.

➤ **The ACG guidelines state that combination therapy of lactulose** and neomycin may be reasonable in patients who do not respond to monotherapy.

➤ **Rifamixin:** Rifaximin is a synthetic antibiotic structurally related to rifamycin. It displays a wide spectrum of antibacterial activity against gram-negative and gram-positive bacteria, both aerobic and anaerobic. It is an available option as potential treatment if patient is nor responding to neomycin therapy.

Management of Ascites [1]

Grading of ascites

1. **Grade 1 ascites:** mild ascites only detectable by ultrasound.
2. **Grade 2 ascites:** moderate ascites evident by moderate symmetrical distension of abdomen.
3. **Grade 3 ascites:** large or gross ascites with marked abdominal distension.

Goals of treatment: To mobilize ascitic fluid; to diminish abdominal discomfort, back pain, and difficulty in ambulation; as well as to prevent complications (e.g., bacterial peritonitis, hernias, pleural effusions, hepatorenal syndrome, and respiratory distress). The goal is a weight loss of 0.5 to 1 kg/day, which corresponds to a net fluid volume loss of about 0.5 to 1 L/day

Grade 1 or mild ascites- no treatment

Grade 2 or moderate ascites:

➤ Patients with moderate ascites can be treated as outpatients and do not require hospitalization unless they have other complications of cirrhosis. Renal sodium excretion is not severely impaired in most of these patients, but sodium excretion is low relative to sodium intake.

➤ Initial management is Dietary sodium restriction (< than 2g/day)

➤ Fluid restriction to <1.5 L/day if serum sodium is < 120–125 mmol/L

➤ Diuretics: Patients with the first episode of grade 2 (moderate) ascites should receive an aldosterone antagonist such as spironolactone alone, starting at 100 mg/day and increasing stepwise every 7 days (in 100 mg steps) to a maximum of 400 mg/day if there is no response (Level A1). In patients who do not respond to aldosterone antagonists, as defined by a reduction of body weight of less than 2 kg/ week, or in patients who develop hyperkalemia, furosemide should be added at an increasing stepwise dose from 40 mg/day to a maximum of 160 mg/day (in 40 mg steps) (Level A1).

➤ Furosemide + spironolactone (a ratio of 40 mg of furosemide to every 100mg of spironolactone is an appropriate starting regimen).

➤ The doses of both oral diuretics can be increased simultaneously every 3 to 5 days (maintaining the ratio) to achieve adequate response. Usual maximal doses are 400 mg/day of spironolactone and 160 mg/day of furosemide. Hyponatremia,

hyperkalemia, metabolic alkalosis, and uncommonly hypokalemia occur as side effects of diuretic therapy in patients with ascites.
- Amiloride 10–40 mg/day may be substituted for spironolactone in patients who develop tender gynecomastia

Grade 3 ascites or large ascites:
- If refractory ascites is present, may consider midodrine 7.5 mg three times daily as add-on therapy to diuretics
- **Refractory ascites**: If tense ascites is present, may use large-volume paracentesis. Paracentesis involves the removal of ascitic fluid from the abdominal cavity with a needle or a catheter. Although paracentesis can remove large amounts of ascitic fluid (e.g., 10 L), removal of as little as 1 L of fluid may provide considerable relief from the painful stretching of skin and the respiratory distress that occurs with massive ascites. The ascitic fluid often reaccumulates rapidly after paracentesis owing to transudation of fluid from the interstitial and plasma compartments into the peritoneal cavity. The major complications of overly aggressive, large-volume paracentesis include hypotension, shock, oliguria, encephalopathy, and renal insufficiency. Other potential complications of paracentesis are hemorrhage, perforation of the abdominal viscera, infection, and protein depletion.
- Large volume paracentesis alone is associated, however, with paracentesis-induced circulatory dysfunction (PICD). 4 Intravenous (IV) albumin infusions are commonly administered to prevent PICD following large volume paracentesis.
- Administer albumin at a dose of 6–8 g/L of ascitic fluid removed (if more than 5 L is removed at one time)
- No upper limit of weight loss if massive edema is present, 0.5 kg/day in patients without edema
- Drugs as NSAIDs, ACE Inhibitors and ARBs should be avoided also to prevent renal failure.
- **Alternative treatments are available for management of refractory ascites**: Transjugular intrahepatic portosystemic shunt (TIPS) is another option for patients who are refractory to the pharmacologic interventions described above.

Management of Spontaneous Bacterial Peritonitis [2]
- The presence of more than 250 polymorphonuclear cells/mm3 (PMN) is diagnostic for SBP, antibiotic therapy should be intiated.
- Since the most common causative organisms of SBP are Gram-negative aerobic bacteria, such as E. coli, the first line antibiotic treatment are third-generation cephalosporins (Level A1). Alternative options include amoxycillin/clavulanic acid and quinolones such as ciprofloxacin or ofloxacin. However, the use of quinolones should not be considered in patients who are taking these drugs for prophylaxis against SBP
- 3rd generation cephalosporins:
  Cefotaxime (2 g every 8–12 hours) or
  Ceftriaxone (2 g/day IV) for 5–10 days.

- If PMNL counts are less than 250 cells/cumm, but signs of infection are there, empiric therapy should be given.
- Ofloxacin 400 mg orally twice daily
- If ascetic fluid PMN counts are greater than 250 cells/cumm and clinical suspicion of SBP is present ,
  Albumin: 1.5 mg/kg on admission; 1 mg/kg on hospital day 3
  Guidelines suggest using this albumin regimen with antibiotics
  If SCr is >1 mg/dL, BUN > 30 mg/dL, or total bilirubin more than 4 mg/dL
- Prophylaxis against SBP:

  Twice daily norfloxacin or trimethoprim –sulfamethoxazole should be used for 7 days.

Recommendations:
- In patients with gastrointestinal bleeding and severe liver disease ceftriaxone is the prophylactic antibiotic of choice, whilst patients with less severe liver disease may be given oral norfloxacin or an alternative oral quinolone to prevent the development of SBP (Level A1).
- Patients who recover from an episode of SBP have a high risk of developing recurrent SBP. In these patients, the administration of prophylactic antibiotics reduces the risk of recurrent SBP. Norfloxacin (400 mg/day, orally) is the treatment of choice (Level A1). Alternative antibiotics include ciprofloxacin (750 mg once weekly, orally) or co-trimoxazole (800 mg sulfamethoxazole and 160 mg trimethoprim daily, orally), but evidence is not as strong as that with norfloxacin (Level A2).

Management of Hepatorenal Syndrome

Diagnostic Criteria for Hepatorenal Syndrome in Cirrhosis

1. Cirrhotic patients with ascites
2. Serum creatinine >133 µmol/L (1.5 mg/dL)
3. No improvement of serum creatinine ($\downarrow$ to a level of ≤133 µmol/L) after at least two days along with a. Diuretic withdrawal and b. Volume expansion with albumin (1 g/kg of body weight per day up to a maximum of 100 g/day)
4. The absence of shock
5. No current or recent treatment with nephrotoxic drugs
6. The absence of parenchymal kidney disease as indicated by
   (a) Proteinuria >500 mg/day,
   (b) Microhematuria (>50 red blood cells per high power field),
   (c) And/or abnormal renal ultrasonography
- Development of Renal failure secondary to liver cirrhosis.
- Primary mechanism responsible for deterioration of renal functions is renal hypo perfusion.
- Criteria in patients with cirrhosis and ascites: SCr greater than 1.5mg/dL.

Subtypes of HRS:

➤ HRS is classified into two types: type 1 HRS, characterized by a rapid and progressive impairment in renal function (increase in serum creatinine of equal to or greater than 100% compared to baseline to a level higher than 2.5 mg/dL in less than 2 weeks), and type 2 HRS characterized by a stable or less progressive impairment in renal function (Level A1).

➤ Type 1: Doubling of SCr to greater than 2.5 mg/dL or a 50% reduction in CrCl to less than 20 mL/minute/1.73 m^2 in less than 2 weeks.

➤ Type 2: Non rapid progression of worsening of renal function. Associated with high mortality

Treatment:

➤ HRS is associated with a high mortality rate (within 2 weeks of diagnosis of type-1 HRS and within 6 months of type-2 HRS). The definitive treatment for type-1 and type 2 HRS is liver transplantation, which is the only treatment that assures long-term survival.

Management of type 1 hepatorenal syndrome:

➤ Drug therapy of type 1 hepatorenal syndrome Terlipressin (1 mg/4–6 h intravenous bolus) in combination with albumin should be considered the first line therapeutic agent for type 1 HRS. The aim of therapy is to improve renal function sufficiently to decrease serum creatinine to less than 133 lmol/L (1.5 mg/dl) (complete response). If serum creatinine does not decrease at least 25% after 3 days, the dose of terlipressin should be increased in a stepwise manner up to a maximum of 2 mg/4 h. For patients with partial response (serum creatinine does not decrease < 133micromoles /L, or in those patients without reduction of serum creatinine treatment should be discontinued within 14 days (Level A1).

➤ Potential alternative therapies to terlipressin include norepinephrine or midodrine plus octreotide, both in association with albumin.

➤ Renal replacement therapy may be useful in patients who do not respond to vasoconstrictor therapy, and who fulfill criteria for renal support.

Management of type 2 hepatorenal syndrome

➤ Type-2 HRS manifests itself as a progressive disease and, therefore, patients do not present acutely with deterioration in kidney function. No particular treatment exists for type-2 HRS. The main clinical problem in type-2 HRS is refractory ascites, which can be controlled by large volume paracentesis along with IV albumin or TIPS.

➤ Terlipressin plus albumin is effective in 60–70% of patients with type 2 HRS.

➤ Liver transplantation for appropriate candidates may be the best option for end-stage liver disease and its complications. Transplantation is generally considered in patients with refractory ascites, severe hepatic encephalopathy, esophageal or gastric varices and hepatorenal syndrome. Because of the shortage of organs available and significant complications associated with transplantation, therapeutic alternatives should be considered to avoid the necessity for transplantation.

Case Study of Liver Abscess

Summary

A male patient of age 40 years was admitted to the male medical ward with complaints of right upper abdominal pain since 7 days, no H/O fever, vomiting. No H/O constipation, no H/O burning micturition, Patient is anaemic, leucocytic and had an elevated ESR (40mm/hr). RBS was elevated (86mg/dL). Prothrombin time was found to be increased (16.9 sec). Direct bilirubin (0.3mg/dL), SGPT, SGOT also elevated, alkaline phosphatase enzyme (263IU/L) were also abnormally high. Serum Cr- 3.3mg/dL; BUN- 161mg/dL. US abdomen – hepatomegaly with liver abscess. Right pleural effusion diagnosis: Chest X-ray-elevated dome of hemidiaphragm

Diagnosis: The patient was diagnosed with liver abscess

The inpatient therapy was:

Trade name	Generic name	Route	Dose	Frequency
Inj. Futaz	Piperacillin+tazobactum	IV	4.5g	BD
Inj Metrogyl	Metronidazole	IV	100ml	TID
Inj Pan	Pantoprazole	IV	40mg	OD
Tab Ultracet	Tramadol	Oral	50mg	BD
Tab Becosules	Vit B complex	Oral		OD

Assignment

1. How common is bacterial abscess of the liver and types of liver abscess?

Liver abscess is a pus-filled mass inside the liver common cause are abdominal conditions such as appendicitis diverticulitis due to hametogenous spread through the portal vein.

The Three major forms of liver abscess, classified by cause:

- Amoebic liver abcess due to entamoeba histolyica accounts for 10% cases. the incidence is much higher in developing countries

- Pyogenic liver abcess, which is most often polymicrobial, accounts for 80% of hepatic abscess cases in U.S.

- Fungal abscess, most often due to candida species accounts for less than 10% of cases

A Pyogenic liver abscess, infection is caused by bacteria and is usually polymicrobial. The majority of cases are caused by ascending infection from bilary tract pathology (bilary strictures) due to the liver dual blood supply from the portal vein and the hepatic artery, an infectious focus in the gastrointestinal tract or bacteremia exposes the liver to high bacterial loads. Complications include sepsis, pneumonia and abscess rupture into the peritoneum / thorax

2. **Which organism is associated with fungal abscess of liver?**

   Most candida species are involved:-

   ➢ Candida albcians; Candida auris ; Candida glabrata

   ➢ Candida rugosa; Candida tropicalis

   ➢ Candida dubliniensis and Histoplasma capsulatum

   Bacterial causes of the liver abcess :-

   ➢ Streptococcus species (including Enterococcus); Escheria species

   ➢ Staphylococcus species; Klebsiella species

   ➢ Anaerobes; Pseudomonas species

   ➢ Proteus species; Entamoeba Histolytica

3. **What are the signs and symptoms in this patient?**

   • Fever; Malaise; Right upper quadrant pain

   • Anorexia; Weight loss; Nausea

   • Vomitings; Symptoms of diaphragmatic irritation

   The signs and symptom observed in this patient are

   • Upper abdominal pain, Fever, Vomitings

4. **What are the risk factors?**

   ➢ Diabetis mellitus,

   ➢ Hepatobiliary diseases (Cholithiasis, Transplant recipients, Hepatic tumors)

   ➢ Pancreatitis, Gastrointestinal Malignary (colorectal carcinoma)

   ➢ Crohns Diseases, Smoking and alcohol

5. **What is the recommended long term monitoring of liver abscess treatment?**

   ➢ Aggressively seek an underlying source of abdominal pathology

   ➢ Perform weekly serial CT (or) Ultrasound examination to document progress of therapy after discharge of the abscess cavity

   ➢ Continue radiological evaluation to document progress of therapy after discharge

   ➢ Drain care may be required. Maintain drains until the out put is less than 10 ml /day

   ➢ Monitor fever curves. Persistent fever after 2 weeks of therapy may indicate the need for more aggressive damage

   ➢ Patients will require prolonged parenteral antimicrobial therapy that may continue after discharge. Monitoring of medication levels, renal functions and blood counts may be needed. Enteral nutrition is preferred route unless it is CI.

6. **What are the indications and contraindiactions for the surgical treatment of liver abscess?**

   Open surgery can be performed by either of following two approaches;

   • A Transpirental approach allows for abscess drainage and abdominal exploration to identify previously undetected abscess and the location of an etiologic source

   • For higher posterior lesions, a posterior transpleural approach can be used

   • Laproscopic (or) Percutaneously

Indications:

- Signs of peritonitis
- Existence of a known abdominal surgical pathology (diverticuar abscess)
- Failure of previous drainage attempts
- Presence of complicated, Multiloculated, thick walled abscess with various with viscous pus
- Shock with multisystem organ failure is a contraindication for surgery

7. **Which antimicrobial agents/regimen used in treatment of liver abscess?**

- Antibiotics should be wide spectrum. The antibiotic therahy should consists of a combination of an aminoglycoside with either Metronidazole (or) Clindamycin (or) Beta lactam antibiotic with anaerobic coverage
- Incase of Staphylococci (or) Streptococcal infection a Penicillinase resistant penicillin or first generation cephalosporins can be used
- The antibiotic treatment in liver abscess secondary to biliary disease should consists of Ampicillin or Uriedopenicillin combined with an aminoglycoside
- The length of an antibiotic therapy should individualized on the basis of the number of abscess and the clinical resaponse. Patients with multiple abscesses should receive antibiotics for 4 – 6 weeks.

First choice:

1. Monotherapy with a Beta-lactam inhibitor
   Piperacillin + Tazobactum   3.375-4.5g IV every 6 hrs
   Ticarcillin + Clavulanate   3.1 g IV every 4 hrs
2. Combination therapy
   Ceftriaxone +   1g IV every 24hrs
   Metronidazole   500mg IV every 8 hrs
3. Combination therapy
   Ciprofloxacin +   400 mg IV every 12 hrs
   Metronidazole   500mg IV every 8 hrs

8. **How are systemic Antifungal agents used for treatment?**

- Amphotericin B (ambisome) – 500mg

- Fluconazole (Diflucan) – 250 – 500 mg

9. **What are the causes of liver abscess?**

- Appendicitis
- Diverticulitis
- Pyogenic abscess- bacteria one (or) more species
- Amoebic Abscess – amoebs which are single celled parasites (protozoa) most common isentamoeba hiistolytica
- Fungal abscess- candida species
- Parasitic abscess – rare, assosciated with helminths

References

1. EASL clinical practice guidelines on the management of ascites, spontaneous bacterial peritonitis, and hepatorenal syndrome in cirrhosis. Clinical Practice Guidelines. Journal of Hepatology.
2. Fernández J, Ruiz del Arbol L, Gómez C, Durandez R, Serradilla R, Guarner C, et al. Norfloxacin vs ceftriaxone in the prophylaxis of infections in patients with advanced cirrhosis and hemorrhage. Gastroenterology 2006;131:1049–1056.

CHAPTER - 56

Drug Induced Liver Disorders

Introduction to Liver Disorders

Drug induced liver disease is a rare but potentially fatal, often debilitating and largely unpredictable outcome of drug treatment.

Drugs can cause liver disease in several ways, some drugs are directly injurious to the liver, and others are transformed by the liver into chemicals that can cause injury to liver directly or indirectly.

Drug-induced liver disease can have many different clinical presentations: idiosyncratic reactions, allergic hepatitis, toxic hepatitis, chronic active toxic hepatitis, toxic cirrhosis, and liver vascular disorders.

The liver function affects almost every other organ system in the body, but there are no specific diagnostic tests for drug induced liver disease.

Patterns of Drug Induced Liver Disease [1]

A. Hepatocellular injury
- Centrolobular necrosis
- Steatohepatitis
- Phospholipidosis
- Generalized hepatocellular necrosis

B. Toxic cirrhosis

C. Cholestatic injury

D. Liver vascular disorders

E. Mixed hepatocellular and cholestatic injury

A. Hepatocellular injury: Hepatocellular injury is characterized by significant elevations in the serum aminotransferases, which usually precede elevations in total bilirubin levels and alkaline phosphatase levels. Hepatocellular injury can lead to fulminant hepatitis.

- **Centrolobular Necrosis:** Centrolobular necrosis is often a dose-related, predictable reaction. It also can be associated with idiosyncratic reactions. Also called direct or metabolite-related hepatotoxicity, centrolobular necrosis is usually the result of the production of a toxic metabolite.

- **Steatohepatitis:** Also known as steatonecrosis. It results from the accumulation of fatty acids in the hepatocyte. Drugs or their metabolites that cause steatonecrosis by affecting fatty-acid esterification and oxidation rates within the mitochondria of the hepatocyte. This eventually disrupts the homeostasis of the hepatocyte. The liver biopsy is marked by a massive infiltration by polymorphonuclear leukocytes, degeneration of the hepatocytes, and the presence of Mallory bodies.
- **Phospholipidosis [2]:** Phospholipidosis is the accumulation of phospholipids instead of fatty acids. The phospholipids usually engorge the lysosomal bodies of the hepatocyte.
- **Generalized Hepatocellular Necrosis:** It mimics the changes associated with the more common viral hepatitis. Many drugs that are associated with toxic hepatitis produce metabolites that are not inherently toxic to the liver. Instead, they act as haptens, binding to specific cell proteins and inducing an autoimmune reaction.

B. Toxic Cirrhosis [3]: The scarring effect of hepatitis in the liver leads to the development of cirrhosis. Methotrexate causes periportal fibrosis in most patients who experience hepatotoxicity. The lesion results from the action of a bioactivated metabolite produced by CYP450.

C. Cholestatic Injury: It primarily involves the bile canalicular system. The inability of the liver to remove bile causes intrahepatic accumulation of toxic bile acids and excretion products, this leads to cholestatic injury. In some cases, progressive destruction of the cholangiocytes leads to the vanishing bile duct syndrome. Drug induced cholestasis can occur as an acute disorder or as a chronic disorder.

D. Liver Vascular Disorders: Focal lesions in hepatic venules, sinusoids, and portal veins occur with various drugs. Peliosis hepatitis is a rare type of hepatic vascular lesion that can be seen as both an acute and a chronic disease. [4]

Table 56.1 Types of liver injury patterns induced by drugs.

Liver disorders	Drugs inducing liver disorders
Hepatocellular injury	Acarbose, allopurinol, losartan
Centrolobular necrosis	Acetaminophen
Steatohepatitis	Alcohol, sodium valproate
Phospholipidosis	Amiodarone
Generalized hepatocellular necrosis	Isoniazid, ketoconazole
Toxic cirrhosis	Methotrexate
Cholestatic injury	Erythromycin, tetracycline,
Liver vascular disorders	Androgens, estrogens, tamoxifen

Mechanisms of Drug Induced Liver Disease

1. **Acetaminophen:** The main pathway of acetaminophen metabolism at low doses is formation of sulaftes and glutathione conjugates with the help of enzymes sulfotransferase, uridine diphosphate and glucoronosyl transferase. It also undergoes oxidation by CYP-450 at high doses to form reactive electrophile N-Acetyl –p-benzoquinone imine NAPQI, allowing the elecrophile to exert damaging effects within the cell via covalent bonding. It leads to cell necrosis.

2. **Isoniazid:** The primary means for INH metabolism is through acetylation by N-acetyltransferase (NAT-2) in the liver generating acetyl isoniazid. Acetyl isoniazid can undergo hydrolysis to form acetylhydrazine and non toxic Isonicotinic acid. Polymorphisms of NAT-2 have been identified in the population that relegates humans to be either 'rapid' or 'slow' acetylators. Slow acetylators shunt some INH to a secondary metabolic pathway of oxidation via cytochrome P450 producing hydrazine and non toxic isonicotinic acid. It appears that both acetylhydrazine and hydrazine, generated by rapid and slow acetylators respectively are capable of participating in reactions that generate oxidative stress e.g. free radicals. Hydrazine may induce Cytochrome P450 (specifically CYP2E1), increasing production of additional toxic metabolite. Thus, hepatotoxicity may occur in both rapid and slow acetylators.

3. **Alcohol Induced Liver Damage:** Mechanisms of alcohol induced liver damage. Alcohol consumption alone, or with its metabolites, disrupts the gut integrity by various mechanisms, including increased reactive oxygen species (ROS), inducible nitric oxide synthase (iNOS), alteration of microRNAs, proliferation of Gram-negative bacteria, and changes in bacterial species. These factors alone, or in combination, mediate increased gut permeability and subsequent bacterial or microbial translocation into intestinal lumen and thus an increase in lipopolysaccharide (LPS) in the portal circulation. The excess of LPS in the liver affects immune, parenchymal, and non-immune cells and in response there is release of various inflammatory cytokines, and recruitment of neutrophils and other inflammatory cells. Persistence of the above mentioned factors are hallmark of alcoholic liver disease (ALD).

4. **Sodium Valproate:** Parent drug or its metabolites can trigger outer mitochondrial rupture These drugs disrupt beta oxidation of lipids and oxidative energy production within the hepatocyte.

   In acute cases, interruption of beta oxidation leads to micro vesicular steatosis

   In chronic disease, micro vascular disease is present

   Interruption of beta oxidation leads to depletion of ATP which can cause liver cell necrosis & further leads to hepatic failure and death.

References

1. Murray KF. Drug-related hepatotoxicity and acute liver failure. J Pediatr Gastroenterol Nutr 2008;47:395–405.

2. Lullman H, Lullman R, Wasserman O. Drug-induced phospholipidosis, II. Tissue distribution of the amphiphilic drug chlorphentermine. CRC Crit Drug Rev Toxicol 1975;4:185–218.

3. Gunawan B, Kaplowitz N. Mechanisms of drug-induced liver disease. Clin Liver Dis 2007;11:459–475

4. https://accesspharmacy.mhmedical.com/content.aspx?bookid=689§ionid=48811442#57523512

CHAPTER - 57

Gastroesophageal Reflux Disease (GERD)

Introduction

GERD refers to symptoms or mucosal damage that results from abnormal reflux of the stomach contents into the esophagus.

When the esophagus is repeatedly exposed to refluxed material for prolonged periods of time, inflammation of the esophagus (esophagitis) occurs. It can progress to erosion of the squamous epithelium (erosive esophagitis).

GERD progresses in organs other than the esophagus such as the lungs or larynx is referred as atypical or extraesophageal GERD.

Epidemiology

Occur in people of all ages but it is more common in those older than age 40 years. Mortality is rare but has a significant impact on quality of life.

Etiopathogenesis

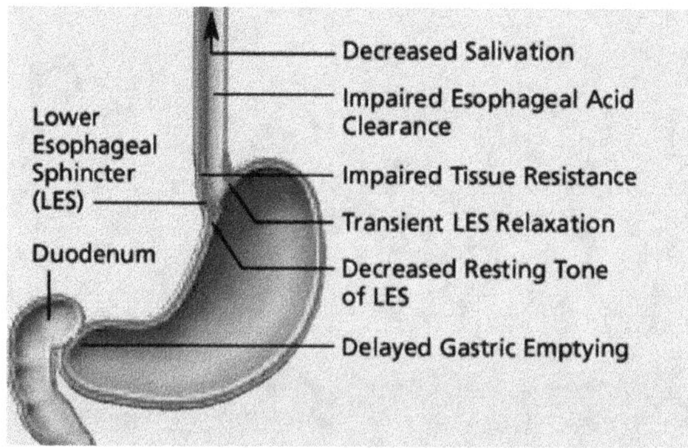

Fig. 57.1 Pathogenesis of GERD[1].

Source: Peter J K. GERD pathogenesis, pathophysiology, and clinical manifestations. Cleve Clin J Med, 2003 Nov;70 Suppl 5:S4-19.

The key factor is the abnormal reflux of gastric contents from the stomach into the esophagus.

Gastroesophageal reflux is associated with

1. Defective Lower Esophageal Sphincter (LES) pressure or function.

   Decreased LES pressure related to

   (a) Spontaneous transient LES relaxations

   (b) Transient increase in intraabdominal pressure

   (c) Atonic LES

2. Problems with other normal mucosal defence mechanisms like

   (a) Anatomic factors

   (b) Esophageal clearence

   (c) Mucosal resistance

   (d) Gastric emptying

   (e) Epidermal growth factor

   (f) Salivary buffering

1. **Lower Esophageal Sphincter Pressure:** The lower oesophageal sphincter is a defined zone at the distal oesophagus with an elevated basal resting pressure. The sphincter is normally in a tonic contracted state, preventing the reflux of gastric material from the stomach, but relaxes on swallowing to permit the free passage of food into the stomach.

   Decreased LES pressure related to: Mechanisms

   (a) Spontaneous transient LES relaxations that are not associated with swallowing, exact mechanism is not known, but oesophageal distension, vomiting, belching and retching have all been shown to cause relaxation of LES. It also depends on the degree of sphincter relaxation, efficacy of oesophageal clearance, gastric volume, intragastric pressure and patient position.

   (b) Transient increase in intra-abdominal pressure: An increase in intraabdominal pressure that occurring during straining, bending over, coughing, eating may overcome weak LES and thus lead to reflux.

   (c) LES may be atonic, thus permitting free reflux.

   Other factors which decrease the LES pressure are: foods and medications

   Foods and medications that worsen GERD symptoms

   1. **Decrease LES pressure**

      Foods: Fatty meals, garlic, carminatives, onions, choclate, coffee, tea, cola, chilli

      Medications: Anticholinergics, ethanol, barbiturates, caffeine, nicotine, nitrates, tetracycline, dopamine, estrogen, dihydropyridine calcium channel blockers

   2. **Direct Irritants to the Esophageal Mucosa**

      Foods: Spicy foods, tomato juice, orange juice, coffee

      Medications: Alendronate, aspirin, iron, quinidine, NSAIDs, KCl

2. **Problems with Mucosal Defence Mechanisms**

   (a) **Anatomic factors:** The most important factor related to the presence or absence of symptoms in patients with hiatal hernia is the LES pressure. The size of the hiatal hernia is proportional to the frequency of transient LES relaxations. Patients with low LES pressure and large hiatal hernia are more likely to experience gastro esophageal reflux following increase in intraabdominal pressure.

(b) Oesophageal clearance: The problem is that the acid produced remains too much time in contact with the esophageal mucosa. This contact time is in turn dependent on the rate at which the esophagus clears the noxious material,as well as frequency of reflux.

(c) Mucosal resistance: The mucus secreted by the glands within the mucosa and submucosa contribute to the protection of the esophagus. Bicarbonates moving from the blood to the lumen can neutralize acidic refluxate in the esophagus. When the mucosa is repeatedly exposed to the refluxate in GERD or if there is a defect in the normal mucosal defence, hydrogen ions diffuse into the mucosa, leading to the cellular acidification and necrosis that ultimately cause esophagitis.

(d) Gastric emptying: Delayed gastric emptying can contribute to gastroesophageal reflux. Factors that increase gastric emptying / gastric volume such as smoking and high fat meals are often associated with gastroesophageal reflux.

Composition of Refluxate

Refluxed contents include gastric acid, pepsin, bile acid and pancreatic enzymes. The composition, pH and volume of the refluxate are important aggressive factors in determining the consequences of reflux.

Clinical Manifestation and Features

Typical symptoms: heart burn, water brash (hyper salivation), belching, regurgitation.

These symptoms may be aggravated by activities that worsen gastroesophageal reflux such as recumbent position, bending over, eating meals containing high amount of fat.

Atypical symptoms: Non allergic asthma, chronic cough, hoarseness, pharyngitis, chest pain, dental erosions, recurrent sore throat, recurrent laryngitis.

Alarm symptoms: These are indicative of complications of GERD.

The symptoms are continual pain, dysphagia (difficulty swallowing), odynophagia (pain with swallowing), unexplained weight loss, choking.

Complications of GERD

Esophagitis or inflammation of the oesophagus is one of the complications of GERD. If it is left untreated, esophagitis may cause bleeding, ulcers and chronic scarring.

Other major complication include Barretts esophagus in people with chronic or longstanding GERD. Barrett's oesophagus results when normal cells of the esophagus are replaced with the cells similar to those of the intestine. This increases the risk of esophageal cancer.

Classification Systems for Endoscopically Determined Esophagitis

The Savary-Miller Classification System of Esophagitis

Grade 0 Normal esophageal mucosa

Grade 1 Erythema or diffusely red mucosa, edema causing accentuated folds

Grade 2 Isolated round or linear erosions extending from the gastroesophageal junction upward, not involving entire circumference

Grade 3 Confluent erosions extending around entire circumference or superficial ulceration without erosions

Grade 4 Complicated cases; erosions as in grade 3 plus deep ulcerations, strictures, or columnar epithelium-lined esophagus

Grade 5 Presence of Barrett's metaplasia

Diagnosis with Algorithm

- ➢ **History:** If classic symptoms of heartburn and acid regurgitation dominate a patient's history, then they can help establish the diagnosis of GERD with sufficiently high specificity, although sensitivity remains low compared to 24-hour pH monitoring. The presence of atypical symptoms, although common, cannot sufficiently support the clinical diagnosis of GERD.
- ➢ **Testing:** No gold standard exists for the diagnosis of GERD. Although 24-hour pH monitoring is accepted as the standard with a sensitivity of 85% and specificity of 95%, false positives and false negatives still exist. Endoscopy lacks sensitivity in determining pathologic reflux but can identify complications (eg, strictures, erosive esophagitis, and Barrett's esophagus). Barium radiography has limited usefulness in the diagnosis of GERD and is not recommended.
- ➢ **Therapeutic trial:** An empiric trial of anti-secretory therapy can identify patients with GERD who lack alarm or warning symptoms and may be helpful in the evaluation of those with atypical manifestations of GERD, specifically non-cardiac chest pain

Useful tool in the diagnosis is the clinical history, including both presenting symptoms and associated risk factors.

For mild and typical symptoms no need of invasive esophageal evaluation.

Diagnostic Tests include

- • **Endoscopy:** It is the preferred technique for assessing the mucosa for esophagitis, barretts esophagus and diagnosing complications.
- • **Ambulatory pH monitoring:** Identifies patients with excessive esophageal acid exposure and helps determine if symptoms both typical and atypical are acid related.
- • **Esophageal manometry:** Used to ensure the proper placement of esophageal pH probes and to evaluate esophageal peristalsis and motility prior to antireflux surgery.
- • Combined impedence pH monitoring
- • High Resolution Esophageal Pressure Topography (HREPT)

Treatment with Algorithm

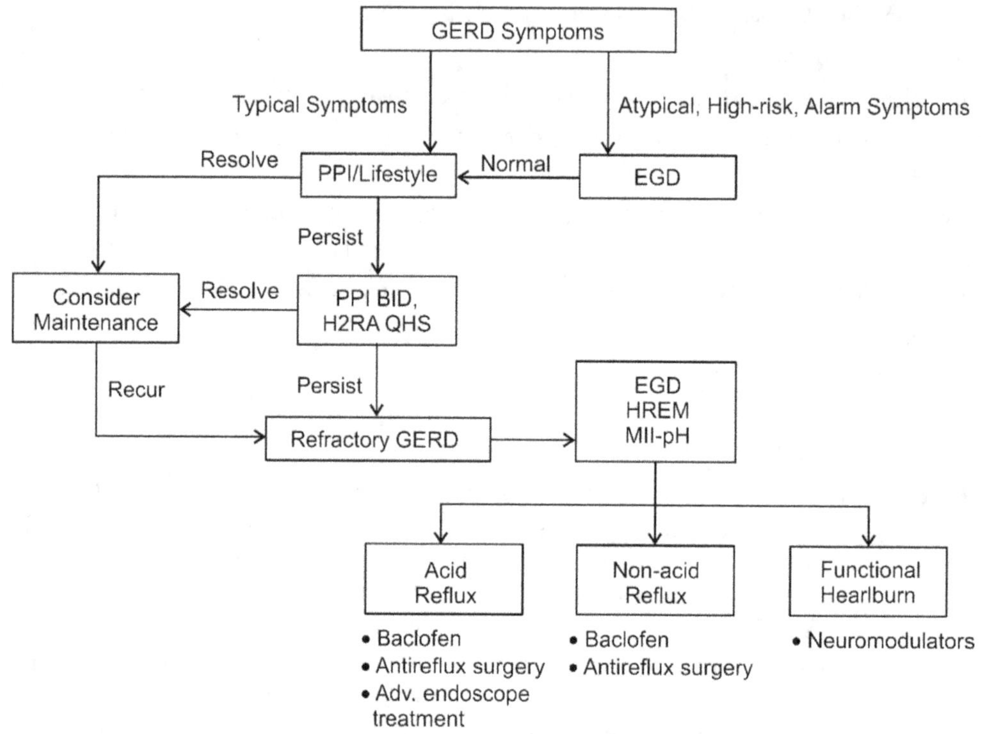

Fig. 57.2 Algorithm for Diagnosis and Management of GERD.

Source: Wai-Kit Lo et al., Medical management of GERD: Algorithms and Outcomes. Failed Anti-reflux therapy. Chapter. pp 19-23.

Management

Goal:

1. Reduce / eliminate the patients' symptoms
2. Decrease frequency, recurrence and duration of reflux
3. Promote healing of injured mucosa
4. Prevent long term complications

Therapy

To augment defense mechanisms that prevent reflux or decrease the aggressive factors that worsen reflux or mucosal damage.

The therapy is directed at

(a) Decreasing the acidity of the refluxate:
   - Antacids

- H2 receptor antagonits
- Proton pump inhibitors
(b) Decreasing the gastric volume
(c) Improving gastric emptying:
- Metoclopramide
- Cisapride
(d) Increasing LES pressure:
- Bethanechol
- Metoclopramide
(e) Enhancing esophageal acid clearence:
- Bethanechol
(f) Protecting the esophageal mucosa:
- Alginic acid
- Sucralfate

The treatment for GERD is categorised into one of the following modalities
1. Life style modifications and patient directed therapy with antacids, non-prescription H2 receptor antagonists and/ or non-prescription proton pump inhibitors.
2. Pharmacologic intervention with prescription strength acid suppression therapy.
3. Interventional therapies (antireflux surgery and endoscopic therapies)

Life style modifications
- Elevate the head of the bed (increases esophageal clearance), sleep on a foam edge
- Dietary changes
  - avoid foods that decrease LES pressure (fats, choclate, alcohol, peppermint)
  - avoid foods that have direct irritant effect on esophageal mucosa (spicy foods,
- Orange juice, tomato juice, coffee)
  - include protein rich meals in diet
- Eat small meals and avoid eating immediately prior to sleeping
- Weight reduction
- Stop smoking
- Avoid alcohol
- Avoid tight fitting clothes

- Discontinue the drugs which promote reflux (Ca channel blockers, beta blockers, nitrates, theophylline)
- Take drugs with plenty of fluids / water

Antacids and Antacid Alginic Acid Products

Antacids provide immediate symptomatic relief for mild GERD and often used concurrently with acid suppression therapies, but for frequent use in case of chronic symptoms.

MOA: An antacid with alginic acid is not a potent acid neutralizing agent and does not enhance LES pressure, but it forms a viscous solution that floats on the surface of gastric contents. This serves as a protective barrier for the esophagus against reflux of gastric contents and reduces frequency of reflux episodes.

Antacids have a short duration of action and needs frequent administration through out the day to provide continuous acid neutralization.

Ex: Gaviscon

ADR's: Diarrhoea or constipation, alterations in mineral metabolism

Proton Pump Inhibitors [1] [3]

Ex: Dexlansoprazole, Esomeprazole, Lansoprazole, Omeprazole

MOA: They block gastric acid secretion by inhibiting H+K+ATPase pump in gastric parietal cells, results in profound and long lasting antisecretory effects.

Twice daily use is indicated in patients not responding to standard once daily therapy.

ADR's: Headache, dizziness, somnolence, diarrhoea, constipation, nausea, enteric infections, vit b12 deficiency, hypomagnesia, bone fractures.

These are available in different formulations like capsules, tablets, intravenous etc

Patients should take oral PPIs in the morning 15-30mins before breakfast.

Omeprazole

It is a gastric proton pump inhibitor. Omeprazole is a substituted benzimidazole derivative acts on the final step of acid production &therefore controls intragastric acidity irrespective of stimulus. It markedly inhibits basal & stimulated gastric acid secretion. Thus it is antisecretory drug which is very effective for rapidly healing peptic ulcers & erosive oesophagitis,& for reducing gastric acid hyper-secretion in patients with Zollinger-Ellison syndrome.

Indications: Duodenal and gastric ulcers, reflux or ulcerative oesophagitis. Zollinger-Ellison syndrome. NSAID-induced ulcers.

Dosage: Gastric ulcer; 20 mg once daily for 8 wks, in severe cases increase to 40 mg once daily. Reflux oesophagitis; 20 mg once daily for 4wks, Refractory cases 40 mg once daily. Duodenal ulcer; 20 mg once daily for 4 wks. Zollinger Ellison syndrome; 60 mg once daily. Maintenance therapy 20-120 mg adjusted to response, doses over 80 mg daily should be divided in 2 doses.

Contra-Indications

Hypersensitivity, neonates.

Special Precautions: Exclude the presence of gastric malignancy. Impaired renal & hepatic functions. Paediatrics: Not recommended. Pregnancy: Safety not established. Lactatio: Safety not established. Elderly: No special problem.

Side Effects: Skin rash, nausea, headache, diarrhoea, constipation and flatulence. Increased risk of enteric infections due to reduced acid secretion.

Histamine 2 Receptor Antagonists [2] [4]

Ex: Cimetidine, ranitidine, famotidine, nizatidine

MOA: Competetive antagonist at H2 receptor.

Blocks H2 receptors in parietal cells which suppresses basal and meal stimulated acid secretion.

H2 receptor antagonists in divided doses are effective for treating mild to moderate GERD. Standard doses given twice daily are beneficial for symptomatic relief of mild GERD. Patients not responding to standard doses require higher doses. Prolonged courses are frequently required.

ADR's: Headache, somnolence, fatigue, dizziness, constipation or diarrhoea.

Cimetidine: It competitively inhibits histamine induced gastric secretion. All phases (basal, psychic, neurogenic, gastric) of secretion are suppresse whereas it has no effect on gastric and esophageal motility.

Indications: Duodenal, gastric, recurrent & stomal ulceration. Oesophageal reflux diseases &other conditions where a reduction of gastric acid is beneficial including persistent dyspeptic symptoms. Zollinger-Ellison syndrome. Stress ulcers and gastritis.

Dosage: Benign gastric ulcer: 400 mg twice at breakfast & bedtime. Acute duodenal ulcer: 800 mg at bed time. Prophylaxis of recurrent duodenal ulcer maint dose of 400 mg at bed time. Peptic oeophagitis: 0.8-1.6 gm daily. Persistent dyspeptic symptoms: 200 mg 4 times daily. Max. period of treatment should be 4 wks. 800-1600 mg/day depending on severity of symptom, has to be given in 4 divided doses. Maintenance 400 mg at bedtime. Injection: Children: 20-25 mg/kg body wt. Neonates: 10-15mg/kg BID.

Contra-Indications- Hypersensitivity.

Special Precautions: Exclude presence of gastric malignancy. Impaired renal function, i.v. injecton by slow infusion. Pregnancy: Safety not established. Lactation: Present in breast milk. No known effect on the baby. Elderly: Dosage may have to be reduced.

Side Effects: Headache, dizziness, bowel upset, rash, diarrhoea, confusion, hallucinations, delirium, convulsions. Gynaecomastia. Sodium & water retention. Impotence.

Promotility Agents

Useful as an adjunct to acid suppression therapy in patients with a known motility defect.

Ex: Cisapride - has the efficacy with H2 receptor antagonists in treating patients with mild esophagitis.

Metoclopramide - a dopamine antagonist increases LES pressure and accelerates gastric emptying in reflux patients.

It has got central anti-dopaminergic effect and thereby raises threshold for vomiting at chemoreceptor trigger zone. Its effects on the G.I. tract are thought to result from blocking of dopaminergic receptors; potentiation of cholinergic effects and/or a direct action on smooth muscle. Metoclopramide, stimulates the release of prolactin.

Indications: Nausea and vomiting, gastritis, gastro-oesophageal reflux, heart burn. Hiccups. Pre/post-operative nausea, vomiting. Radiological examinations. Diagnotic procedures in gastroenterology. Lactation failure.

Dosage: 10 mg thrice daily children 0.5 mg/kg body wt per day in 3-4 divided doses.

Contra-Indications: Hypersensitivity, gastro-intestinal haemorrhage, obstruction or perforation. Epilepsy or extra-pyramidal syndrome. Phaeochrom- ocytoma. Breast carcinoma.

Special Precautions: Injectable should not be diluted as this will upset the isotonicity and stability. I.V. injection should be given slowly as it may cause fling of anxiety and restlessness. Renal or hepatic insufficiency. Paediatrics: Reduced dose necessary. Pregnancy: Safety not established. Lactation: Drug passes into breast milk. Elderly: Reduced dose may be necessary.

Side Effects: Restlessness, drowsiness, fatigue, lassitude, extra-pyramidal effects, tardive dyskinesia, motor restlessness, galactorrhoea & gynae comastia.

Mucosal Protectants

Ex: Sucralfate: Non absorbable aluminium salt of sucrose octasulfate.

Useful for management of radiation esophagitis and bile or non-acid reflux GERD. It is a basic aluminium salt of sulfated sucrose, inherently viscous in acidic medium, polymerizing into a sticky gel like consistency. It precipiates surface proteins at ulcer base & acts as acid resistant physical barrier preventing acid, pepsin & bile from coming in contact with the ulcer base.

Indications: Duodenal & gastric ulcer, chronic gastritis, post-prandial reflux oesophagitis, bile reflux.

Dosage: 1 gm four times daily before meals for 4 wks.

Contra-Indications: Severe renal dysfunction, hypophosphataemia.

Special Precautions: Hypophosphatemia, renal dysfunction, Interferes with absorption of tetracyclines, H2 block, phenytoin, digoxin quinolones. Paediatrics: Use with caution. Pregnancy: Safety not established. Lactation: Use with caution. Elderly: No special problem.

Side Effects: Dry mouth, nausea, constipation.

Combination Therapy

Acid suppressing agent and a promotility agent or mucosal protectant is a useful combination therapy.

Using the omeprazole sodium bicarbonate immediate release product in addition to once daily PPI therapy offers an alternative for noctural GERD symptoms.

Maintenance Therapy

- Consider long term therapy to prevent complications and worsening of esophageal function who have symptomatic relapse after discontinuation of therapy.
- Most patients require standard doses to prevent relapses.
- H2RAs - effective maintenance therapy in patients with mild disease.
- PPI - for treatment of moderate to severe esophagitis.
- Once daily dose of esomeprazole 20mg, omeprazole 20mg, lansoprazole 30mg, rabeprazole 20mg. Low doses or alternate day regimen is effective with milder symptoms.
- Maintenance therapy by which patients take their PPI only when they have symptoms may be effective for patients with endoscopy negative GERD.

Interventional Approaches

- **Antireflux Surgery:** The goal of antireflux surgery is to reestablish the antireflux barrier, to position the lower esphageal sphincter within the abdomen where it is under positive pressure and to close any associated hiatal defect.

  It should be considered in patients

  (a)   Who fail to respond to pharmacologic treatment

  (b)   Who opt for surgery because of life style considerations like age, prolonged treatment duration

  (c)   Who have complications of GERD

Complications with surgery include gas bloat syndrome (inability to belch or vomit), dysphagia, vagal denervation, splenic trauma and very rarely death.

Endoscopic Therapies

Include endoscopic sewing devices and endoluminal application of radiofrequency heat energy (Stretta procedure).

An endoscopic sewing device and full thickness plication devices reduces symptoms of heart burn and regurgitation and improve the quality of life scores.

The stretta device delivers radiofrequency energy through specialized needles placed into the submucosal tissue of the esophagus while monitroing esophageal mucosal surface temperatures, resulting in an increase in the LES reflux barrier.

Therapeutic Approach to GERD in Adults

Patient presentation   **Recommended treatment regimen**

1. Intermittent, mild heart burn

Life style modifications + patient directed therapy
Antacids:
- Maolox or Mylanta 30ml as needed or after meals and at bed time
- Gaviscon 2tabs after meals and at bed time
- Calcium carbonate 500mg, 2-4tabs as needed
        (and/or)
Non prescription H2RA (twice daily)
- Cimetidine 200mg /   - Nizatidine 75mg
- Famotidine 10mg/   - Ranitidine 75mg
        (or)
Non prescription PPI (once daily)
- Omeprazole 20mg

2. Symptomatic relief of GERD

Life style modifications + prescription strength acid suppression therapy
H2RA (6-12 weeks)
- Cimetidine 400mg twice daily /   - Famotidine 20mg twice daily
- Nizatidine 150mg twice daily/   - Ranitidine 150mg twice daily
        (Or)
PPI (4-8 weeks) once daily
- Esomeprazole 20mg/   - Lansoprazole 15mg
- Omeprazole 20mg/   - Pantoprazole 40mg
- Rabeprazole 20mg

3. Healing of erosive esophagitis or patients with mod to severe symptoms or complications

Life style modifications +
PPI (4-16 weeks) twice daily
- Esomeprazole 20-40mg /day
- Lansoprazole 30mg /day
- Omeprazole 20mg /day
- Rabeprazole 20mg /day
- Pantoprazole 40mg /day
(or)
H2RA (8-12 weeks)
- Cimetidine 400mg four times a day / 800mg twice daily
- Famotidine 40mg twice daily/   - Nizatidine 150mg four times a day
- Ranitidine 150mg four times a day

4. Interventional Therapies

Antireflux surgery and endoscopic therapies

Case Study of Gastroesophageal Reflux Disease

Summary

A 65-year-old female patient was admitted in the hospital with the symptoms of throat pain and vomiting since 2 days after taking food and liquids, difficulty in talking since one week. He has past medical history of type 2 diabetes mellitus. He has hypothyroidism and dyslipidemia, recurrent ischemic stroke and hypertension. He uses the medication: metformin, Telma, thyronorm, tonact. He has slight weakness in left hand, On examination: temperature is afebrile, blood pressure: 90/60mm Hg. Pulse rate: 98bpm, respiratory rate: 22 cycles/min. Urine analysis included hazy appearance and increase in pus cells, complete blood picture shown abnormal values in WBC: 19,100 cells/cumm; RBC: 3.09 milli cells/cumm. Sensitivity: sensitive to magnexforte. Endoscopy has revealed hiatal hernia. And also abnormal random blood sugar values.

Diagnosis: Based on the evidence from urine analysis, complete blood picture, urine culture and sensitivity testing and endoscopy, finally, she has diagnosed with **severe GERD with urinary tract infection**.

Inpatient therapy included

S.no	Drug name	Drug	Dose	Frequency	ROA
1	Magnexforte	Multivitamin	1.5gm	BD	IV
2	Deplatt-a	Aspirin+clopidogrel	75MG	OD	PO
3	Tonact	Atorvastatain	40mg	HS	PO
4	Eltroxin	Thyroxine	50mcg	OD	PO
5	Novomix	Insulin	8units	BD	SC
6	Zofer	Ondansetron	4mg	BD	IV
7	Limcee	Viamin c	500mg	BD	IV
8	Pan	Pantaprazole	40mg	BD	IV
9	Pulmoclear	Acebrophylline+acetyl cysteine	1tab	BD	PO
10	Syp. Sucralfate	Sucralfate	10ml	TID	PO
11	Syp. Vroncorex	Terbutaline+bromhexine	5ml	TID	PO
12	Neb Duolin	Levosalbutamol+ipratropium		TID	P/N
13	Neb Formonid	Formeterol+budesonide	0.5mg	BD	P/N
14	Lesuride	Levosulpiride	25mg	BD	IV
15	Rene guard	Cefixime+K.Clavulanate	200mg	BD	IV
16	Niftas	Nitrofurantoin	50mg	OD	PO
17	Forcan	Fluconazole	150mg	OD	PO
18	Zosyn	Piperacillin+tazobactum	4,5mg	TID	IV
19	Claribid	Clarithromycin	500mg	BD	PO

Day to day progress: Day 1: he was conscious and coherent, vomiting, throat pain. Day 2: hypoglycemia was noticed, dysphagia was present. Hence usage of RT feed: 200ml/ 2nd hourly. Day 3: cough while swallowing, dysphagia, no vomits. Day 4: dysphagia decreased. Day 5: complaints of throat irritation. Day 6: cough present, mild relief of dysphagia. Day 8: dysphagia continued for next 6 days. Day 18: 2 episodes of vomiting, cough decreased, complaint of coffee coloured vomiting. Day 19: cough decreased. Day 20: patient was symptomatically better and discharge d in a stable condition.

Discharge Medications:

S.No	Drug name	Drug	Dose	Frequency
1	T.Clopilet	Clopidogrel	75mg	OD
2	T.Tonact	Atorvastatin	40mg	HS
3	T.Eltroxin	Thyroxine	50mcg	
4	Syp. Sucralfate	Sucralfate	10ml	TID
5	Neb duolin	Levosalbutamol+ipratropium	3 ml	TID
6	T.Niftas	Nitrofurantoin	50mg	OD
7	T.Forcan	Fluconazole	150mg	OD
8	Neb Formonide	Formeterol+budesonide	0.5mg	BD
9	T.Claribid	Clarithromycin	500mg	BD
10	T.Sompraz.O	Esmoprazole	40mg	OD
11	T.Pan	Pantaprazole	40mg	OD
12	Inj.Novorapid	Insulin	100UNITS	SC
13	T.Galvus met	Vildagliptin + metformin	50/500	OD

Pharmacist interventions: Initially hypoglycemia: was seen in the patient, this may be due to usage of metformin.

Replacement with combination drug like galvus+metformins (galvus met) decreases the risk of development of hypoglycemia.

Patient Counselling

- Avoid tomato products, caffeine, citrus fruits, chocolates, spicy food, garlic and onion.
- Avoid eating before bedtime: it takes 4-5 hrs to food empty a meal to stomach, so wait at least 3 hrs after eating to go to bed.
- Avoid clothing that is tight in abdominal area.
- Reduce fat rich diet/ meal.
- Maintain healthy weight.
- Eat small, frequent meals.
- Maintain an upright posture while eating and for 45-60minutes afterward. Avoid bending over or below your waist after meals.

Assignment

1. What causes gastroesophageal reflux disease (GERD)?

Gastroesophageal reflux disease occurs when the amount of gastric juice that refluxes into the esophagus exceeds the normal limit, causing symptoms with or without associated esophageal mucosal injury (ie, esophagitis).

2. What are the typical symptoms of gastroesophageal reflux disease (GERD)?

Typical esophageal symptoms include the following:
- Heartburn/ Regurgitation/ Dysphagia/
- Abnormal reflux can cause atypical (extraesophageal) symptoms, such as the following:
- Coughing and/or wheezing/ Hoarseness, sore throat/ Otitis media
- Noncardiac chest pain/ Enamel erosion or other dental manifestations

3. What are some complications associated with gastroesophageal reflux disease (GERD)?

Patients with GERD may also experience significant complications associated with the disease, such as esophagitis, stricture, and Barrett esophagus. Approximately 50% of patients with gastric reflux develop esophagitis.

4. What are the first-line medications for the treatment of mild to moderate gastroesophageal reflux disease (GERD)?

H2 receptor antagonists are the first-line agents for patients with mild to moderate symptoms and grades I-II esophagitis. Options include ranitidine (Zantac), cimetidine, famotidine and nizatidine.

7. What is the efficacy of proton pump inhibitors (PPIs) for the treatment of gastroesophageal reflux disease (GERD)?

A research review by the Agency for Healthcare Research and Quality (AHRQ) concluded, on the basis of grade A evidence, that PPIs were superior to H2 receptor antagonists for the resolution of GERD symptoms at 4 weeks and healing of esophagitis at 8 weeks. In addition, the Agency for Heathcare Research and Quaity (AHRQ) found no difference between individual PPIs (omeprazole, lansoprazole, pantoprazole, and rabeprazole) for relief of symptoms at 8 weeks. For symptom relief at 4 weeks, esomeprazole 20 mg was equivalent, but esomeprazole 40 mg superior, to omeprazole 20 mg.

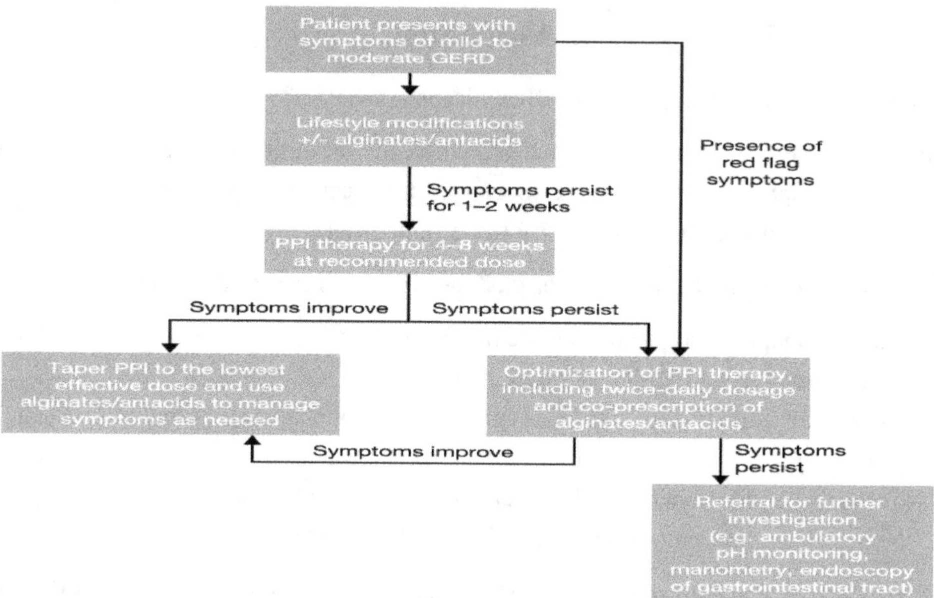

Fig. 57.3 Algorithmic approach to management of gastro-esophageal reflux disease (GERD).

8. Which medications in the drug class Prokinetics are used in the treatment of Gastroesophageal Reflux Disease?[5]

Prokinetics: Prokinetic agents, such as metoclopramide, improve the motility of the esophagus and stomach and increase the lower esophageal sphincter (LES) pressure to help reduce reflux of gastric contents. They also accelerate gastric emptying.

Prokinetic agents are somewhat effective but only in patients with mild symptoms; most patients usually require acid-suppressing medications, such as PPIs. Long-term use of prokinetic agents may have serious, even potentially fatal, complications and should be discouraged.

Metoclopramide: Metoclopramide is a GI prokinetic agent that increases GI motility, increases resting esophageal sphincter tone, and relaxes the pyloric sphincter.

Table 57.1 Pharmacological management of GERD by Prokinteic agents.

Drug Classification/ Mechanism	Sites of Activity	Indications	Dose	Other Properties
Dopaminergic D$_2$-Antagonist Drugs				
Metaclopramide	GES, stomach, intestine, CRTZ	Vomiting disorders. Gastroesophageal reflux, delayed gastrc emptying, ileus/pseudoobstruction	0.2 to 0.5 mg/kg PO, IV TID: 0.01 to 0.02 mg/kg/h infusion	α_2-adrengeric antagonist β_2-adrengeric antagonist 5-HT$_4$-serotonergic antagonist 5-HT$_3$- serotonergic antagonist

Contd...

Drug Classification/ Mechanism	Sites of Activity	Indications	Dose	Other Properties
Dopaminergic D$_2$-Antagonist Drugs				
Domperidone	GES, CRTZ	Vomiting disorders, gastroesophagel reflux	0.05 to 0.1 mg/kg PO BID	β$_2$-adrengeric antagonist α$_2$-adrengeric antagonist
Cisapride	GES, stomach. Intestine. CRTZ	Gastroespphageal reflux, delayed gastric emptying, ileus/pseudoobstruction, constipation, chemotherapy-induced vomiting	0.1 to 0.5 mg/kg PO TID (doses as high as 0.5 to 1 mg/kg have veen used in some dogs)	5-HT$_3$-serotonergic antagonist 5-HT$_1$-serotonergic antagonist 5-HT$_2$-serotonergic antagonist
Mosapride	Stomach	Delayed gastric emptying	0.25 to 1 mg/kg PO BID	None
Prucalopride	Stomach, colon	Delyaed gastric emptying, constipation	0.14 to 0.2 mg/kg PO BID	None
Tegaserod	Intestine, colon	Constipation, ileuspseudobstruction	0.05 to 0.1 mg/kg PO or IV, BID	5-HT$_1$-Serotonergic antagonist
Motillin-like Drugs				
Erthyromycin	GES, stomach intestine, colon	Gastroespphageal reflux, delayed gastric emptying, constipation (dogs)	0.5 to 1 mg/kg PO IV TID	5-HT$_3$-serotonergic antagonist
Acetylcholinesterase Inhibitors and Cholinomimetic Agents				
Ranitidine	Stomach, colon	Delayed gastric emptying, constipation	1 to 2 mg/kg PO BID-TID	H$_2$-histaminergic antagonist
Nizatidine	Stomach, colon	Delayed gastric emptying, constipation	2.5 to 5.0 mg/kg PO SID	H$_2$-histaminergic antagonist
Bethanechol	Esophagus	Canine idiopathic megaesophagus	Dog: 5 to 15 mg/dog PO TID	
Nitric Oxide Donors				
AMU-301		Stomach	Diabetic gastroparesis	Not yet established
Prostanolds				
Misoprostol		Colon	Constipation	Dog: 2 to 5 μg/kg PO TID-OID

CRTZ, chemoreceptor trigger zone; GES, gastroesophageal sphincter; SID, standardized ileal digestible.

Robert J . Washabau. Prokinetic agents. https://veteriankey.com/prokinetic-agents/

References

1. Peter JK. GERD pathogeneisis, pathophysiology and Clinical Manifestations. Cleve Clin J Med, 2003 Nov to Suuply 5:54-19.

2. Wai-Kit Lo et al., Medical management of GERD: Algorithms and Outcomes. Failed Anti-reflux therapy chapter PP.19-23.

3. Anvari M, Allen C, Marshall J, et al. A randomized controlled trial of laparoscopic Nissen fundoplication versus proton pump inhibitors for treatment of patients with chronic gastroesophageal reflux disease: One-year follow-up. *Surg Innov*. 2006 Dec. 13(4):238-49.

4. Katz PO. Medical therapy for gastroesophageal reflux disease in 2007. *Rev Gastroenterol Disord*. 2007 Fall. 7(4):193-203.

5. Pohle T, Domschke W. Results of short-and long-term medical treatment of gastroesophageal reflux disease (GERD). Langenbacks Arch Surg. 2000;385:317–23.

CHAPTER - 58

Inflammatory Bowel Disease

Introduction to IBD

Inflammatory bowel disease is a group of inflammatory conditions of the colon and small intestine. There are two types of IBD:

1. **Ulcerative Colitis (UC): A** mucosal inflammatory condition, confined to rectum and colon.
2. **Crohn Disease (CD): A** transmural inflammation of gastrointestinal (GI) of mucosa, that may occur in any part of the GI tract

Etiology

Idiopathic that is, spontaneous in origin.

The etiology of both the conditions is unknown.

Risk Factors [1]

1. Infectious agents: The microflora of GI tract triggers the development of IBD. Micro-organism like Mycobacterium, Measles species, E.coli, Clostridium official etc. causes the relapse.
2. Genetic Factors: Markers for CD: CARD 15; CARD 23 R (Caspaise Recruitment Domain)
3. Markers for UC: HLA DR 2, HLA DR 3 (Human Leykocyte Antigen)
4. Immunological factors: Leucocytes, plasma cells, neutrophils, macrophages are infiltrated into bowel wall in Crohn disease and infiltrated into mucosal layers in Ulcerative colitis.
5. Adhesion molecules – Alpha Intigrins at the site of inflammation helps in infiltration of leucocytes, macrophages, mast cells etc.
6. Diet: Refine sugar, chemical additives etc.
7. Non Steroidal Anti- Inflammatory Drugs: This is mainly in the case of UC.
8. Smoking

Pathophysiology [2]

The microflora of GIT may provide an environmental trigger (microorganisms, diet, infections, stress, NSAIDs smoking, antibiotics) to activate inflammation and are highly implicated in the development of IBD. Several genetic markers (antimicrobial peptides, autophagy, chemokines, cytokines) have been identified that occur more frequently in patients with IBD. This is identified as phase I or pre-disease stage.

In phase II-The inflammatory response with IBD may indicate abnormal regulation of the normal immune response or an auto-immune reaction to self antigens. Th1 cytokine activity is excessive in CD and increased expression of Interferon – gamma in the intestinal mucosa and production of IL -12 are features of immune response in CD. TNF- alpha is a pivotal pro-inflammatory cytokine that is increased in the mucosa and intestinal lumen of patients with CD and UC.

In Phase III-Chronicity or resolution. Antineutrophil cytoplasmic antibodies are found in a high percentage of patients with UC and less frequently with CD. Smoking appears to be protective for ulcerative colitis but associated with increased frequency of Crohn disease. The use of NSAIDs may trigger disease occurrence or lead to disease flares.

In phase IV-chronic inflammation sets in and further proceeds to fibrosis, stenosis, abscess, fistula, cancer and extra intestinal manifestations.

UC and CD differ in two general aspects. Anatomical sites and depth of involvement within the bowel wall. There is, however the overlap between the two conditions, with a small fraction of patients showing features of both diseases.

Ulcerative Colitis

- UC is confined to the colon and rectum and affects primarily the mucosa and submucosa. The primary lesions occur in the crypts of the mucosa (crypts of Lieberkuhn) in the form of a crypt abscess.
- Local complications (involving the colon) occur in the majority of the patients with UC. Relatively minor complications include hemorrhoids, anal fissures and perirectal abscesses.
- A major complication is toxic megacolon, a severe condition that occurs in upto 7.9% of UC patients admitted in hospitals. The patients with toxic megacolon usually have high fever, tachycardia, distended abdomen, elevated WBC count and a dilated colon.
- The risk of colonic carcinoma is much greater in patients with UC as compared with the general population. Approximately 11% of patients with UC have hepatobiliary complications, including fatty liver, pericholangitis, chronic active hepatitis, cirrhosis, sclerosing cholangitis, cholangio carcinoma and gall stones.
- Arthritis commonly occurs in patients with IBD and is typically asymptomatic and migratory. Arthritis typically involves one or a few large joints, such as the knees, hips, ankles, wrists and elbows.

- Ocular complications (iritis, episcleritis, and conjunctivitis) occur in 2% to 29% of patients. Skin and mucosal lesions associated with IBD include erythema nodosum, pyoderma gangrenosum, aphthous ulceration and sweet syndrome.

Crohn Disease [3]

- It is a transmural inflammatory process. The terminal ileum is the most common site of the disorder, but it may occur in any part of GIT. Most patients have some colonic involvement. Patients often have normal bowel separating segments of diseased bowel; that is, the disease is often discontinuous.
- Complications of Crohn disease may involve the intestinal tract or organs unrelated to it. Small bowel stricture with subsequent obstruction is a complication that may require surgery. Fistula formation is common (20% - 40% lifetime risk) and occurs much more frequently than with UC.
- Systemic complications of Crohn disease are common and similar to those found with UC. Arthritis, iritis, skin lesions, and liver disease often accompany Crohn disease.
- Nutritional deficiencies are common with Crohn disease (weight loss, iron deficiency, anemia, vitamin B12, deficiency, folate deficiency, hypoalbuminemia, hypokalemia, and osteomalacia).

Clinical Manifestation and Features

1. **Ulcerative Colitis:** There is a wide range of presentation in UC, ranging from mild abdominal cramping with frequent small volume bowel movements to profuse diarrhea. Many patients have disease confined to the rectum (proctitis).

   Most patients with UC experience intermittent bout of illness after varying intervals of no symptoms.

   Mild disease, which afflicts two third of patients, has been defined as fewer than four stools daily, with or without blood, with no systemic disturbance and a normal Erythrocyte Sedimentation Rate (ESR).

   Patients with moderate disease have more than four stools per day but with minimlal systemic disturbance.

   With severe disease, the patient has more than six stools per day with blood, with evidence of systemic disturbance as shown by fever, tachycardia, anemia or ESR greater than 30.

   Signs and Symptoms
   - Abdominal cramping
   - Frequent bowel movements often blood in the stool
   - Weight loss, Fever and tachycardia in severe disease
   - Blurred vision, eye pain and photophobia with ocular involvement.
   - Arthritis, Raised, tender, red nodules that vary in size from 1 cm to several centimeters.

Diagnosis with Algorithm [4]

Physical Examination:

Hemorrhoids, fissures or perirectal abscesses may be present

Iritis, uveitis, episcleritis and conjunctivitis with ocular involvement.

Dermatological findings with erythema nodosum, pyoderma gangrenosum or aphthous ulceration.

Laboratory Tests: Decreased hematocrit / hemoglobin

Increased ESR

Leucocytosis and hypoalbuminemia with severe disease

(+) perinuclear antineutrophil cytoplasmic antibodies

2. **Crohn Disease:** As with UC, the presentation of CD is highly variable. A patient may present with diarrhea and abdominal pain or a perirectal or perianal lesion.

The course of CD is characterized by periods of remission and exacerbation. Some patients may be free of symptoms for years, whereas others experience chronic problems despite medical therapy.

The Crohn Disease Activity Index (CDAI) and the Harvey Bradshw Index are used to gauge response to therapy and determine remission. Disease activity may be assessed and correlated by evaluation of serum C-reactive protein concentrations.

Signs and Symptoms:
- Malaise and fever, Abdominal pain
- Frequent bowel movement, Hematochezia, Fistula
- Weight loss and malnutrition, Arthritis

Physical Examination: Abdominal mass and tenderness

Perianal fissure or fistula

Laboratory Tests: Increased WBC count and Erthrocyte Sedimentation Rate (ESR)

Anti – *Saccharomyces cerevisiae* antibodies

Treatment

Goals of Treatment
- Resolution of acute inflammatory processes.
- Resolution of attendant complications (eg: fistulas or abscesses)
- Alleviation of systemic manifestations (eg: arthritis)
- Maintenance of remission from acute inflammation
- Surgical palliation or cure

Non Pharmacological Therapy

- Protein – energy malnutrition and sub-optimal weight is reported in upto 85% of patients with CD.
- Enteral supplementation advised. Parenteral nutrition is generally reserved for patients with severe malnutrition or those who fail enteral therapy, such as perforation, protracted vomiting, short bowel syndrome or severe intestinal stenosis.
- Probiotic formulas are effective for inducing and maintaining remission in UC.
- For UC, colectomy is indicated for patients with long standing disease (>8 to 10 years), and for patients with premalignant changes (severe dysplasia) on surveillance mucosal biopsies.
- The indications of surgeries with Crohn disease are not as well established as they are for UC, and surgery is usually reserved for the complication of the disease. There is a high recurrence rate of Crohn disease after surgery.

Pharmacologic Therapy [5]

- The major type of drugs used in IBD are aminosalicylates, glucocorticoids, immunosuppressive agents (Azathioprine, Mercaptopurine, Cyclosporine and Methotrexate), antimicrobials (Metronidazole and Ciprofloxacin), agents to inhibit TNF-α (Anti TNF –α antibodies) and leucocyte adhesion and migration (Natalizumab).
- Sulfasalazine combines a Sulfonamide (Sulfapyridine) antibiotic and Mesalamine (5- Amino salicylic acid) in the same molecule.
- Corticosteroids and adreno-corticotropic hormone have been widely used for the treatment of UC and are used in moderate to severe disease. Prednisolone is most commonly used. Immuno-sppressive agents such as Azathioprine and Mercaptopurine (a metabolite of Azathiprine) are used in the long-term treatment of IBD. These agents are generally reserved for patients who fail Mesalamine therapy or are refractory to or dependent on corticosteroids. Cyclosporine has been of short-term benefit in acute, severe UC when used in a continuous infusion.
- Methrotrexate given 25 mg intramuscularly once weekly is useful for treatment and maintenance of CD.
- Anti-microbial agents, particularly Metronidazole, are frequently used in attempts to control CD.
- Infliximab is an anti-TNF antibody that is useful in moderate to severe active disease and steroid dependent or fistulizing disease. Adalimumab is another anti-TNF antibody that is an option for patients with moderate to severe active Crohn disese or UC previously treated with Infliximab who have lost response. Natalizumab is a leukocyte adhesion and migration inhibitor that is used for patients with CD who are unresponsive to other therapies.

Treatment Approaches for Ulcerative Colitis

Disease Severity

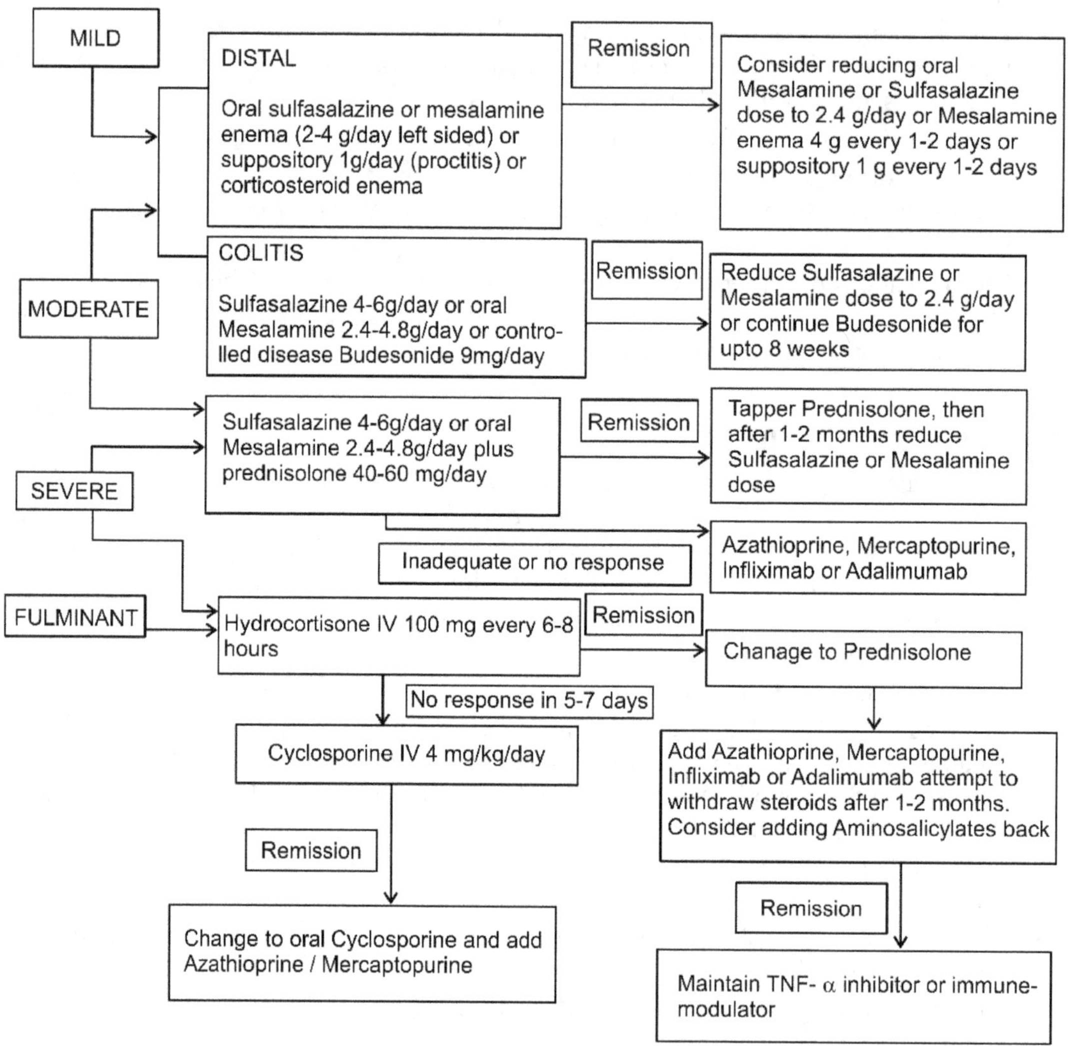

Fig. 58.1 Algorithm for management of Ulcerative colitis based on disease severity.

Source: Liehtens tein GR, Stein RB, Clinical Management of Ulcerative Wlitis, 2nd ed. Professional Communications. Inc. 2023.

(A) Mild to Moderate Disease: Most patients with mild to moderate active UC can be managed with oral or/and topical Mesalamine. When given orally usually 4g/day to 6g/day of Sulfasalazine is required to attain control of active inflammation. Sulfasalazine therapy should be instituted at 500 mg/day and increased every few days upto 4 g/day or the maximum tolerated.

Oral Mesalamine derivatives are reasonable alternatives to Sulfasalazine for treatment of UC as they are better tolerated.

(B) Moderate to Severe Disease: Steroids are used in the treatment of moderate to severe UC or in those who are unresponsive to maximal doses of oral and topical Mesalamine. Oral Prednisolone 40 to 60 mg daily is recommended for adult.

Infliximab is for patients with moderate to severe active UC who are unresponsive to steroids or other immune-suppressive agents.

(C) Severe or Intractable Disease: Patients with uncontrolled severe colitis or incapacitating symptoms require hospitalization for effective management. Most medication is given by the parenteral route.

IV Hydrocortisone 300 mg daily in three divided doses or Methyl Prednisolone 60 mg once daily is considered as first line agent. Patients who are unresponsive to parenteral Corticosteroids after 3 to 7 days can receive Cyclosporine or Infliximab. A continuous IV infusion of Cyclosporine 2 to 4 mg/kg/day is the typical dose range utilized.

(D) Maintenance of Remission: Once remission from active disease has been achieved, the goal of therapy is to maintain the remission.

Oral agents, including Sulfasalazine, Mesalamine and Balsalazide are all effective options for maintenance therapy. The optimal dose to prevent relapse is 2 to 2.4 g/day of Mesalamine equivalent with rates of relapse over 6 to 12 months reported as 40%.

Steroids do not have a role in the maintenance of remission with UC because they are ineffective. Steroids should be gradually withdrawn after remission is induced (over 2 to 4 weeks).

Treatment Approaches for Crohn Disease

Disease Severity

(A) Active Crohn Disease [6]: Mesalamine often tried as an initial therapy for mild to moderate CD.

Mesalamine derivatives (eg: Pentasa and Asacol) that release Mesalamine in the small bowel may be more effective than Sulfasalazine for ileal involvement.

Oral Corticosteroids such as Prednisolone 40 to 60 mg/day, are generally considered first line therapies and are frequently used for the treatment of moderate to severe Crohn disease. Budesonide (Entocort) at a dose of 9 mg daily is a viable first-line option for patients with mild-moderate ileal or right sided (ascending colonic)disease.

Metronidazole, given orally as 10 to 20 mg/kg/day in divided doses, may be useful in some patients with CD, particularly in patients with colonic or ileo-colonic involvement, those with perineal disease, or those who are unresponsive to Sulfasalazine.

Azathioprine and Mercaptopurine are not recommended to induce remission in moderate to severe CD; however they are effective in maintaining steroid-induced remission and are generally to use for patients not achieving adequate response to standard medical therapy or in the setting of steroid dependency. The usual doses of Azathioprine are 2-3 3 mg/kg/day and for Mercaptopurine 1 to 1.5 mg/kg/day. Starting doses are typically 50 mg/day and increased at 2 week intervals.

Patient deficient in Thiopurine S-Methyl Transferase (TPMT) are at greater risk of bone marrow suppression from Azathioprine and Mercaptopurine. Determination of TPMT or TPMT genotype is recommended to guide dosage.

Cyclosporine is not recommended for CD except for patients with symptomatic and severe peri-anal and cutaneous fistulas. The dose of Cyclosporine is important in determining efficiency. An oral dose of 5 mg/kg/day was not effective, whereas 7.9 mg/kg/day was effective.

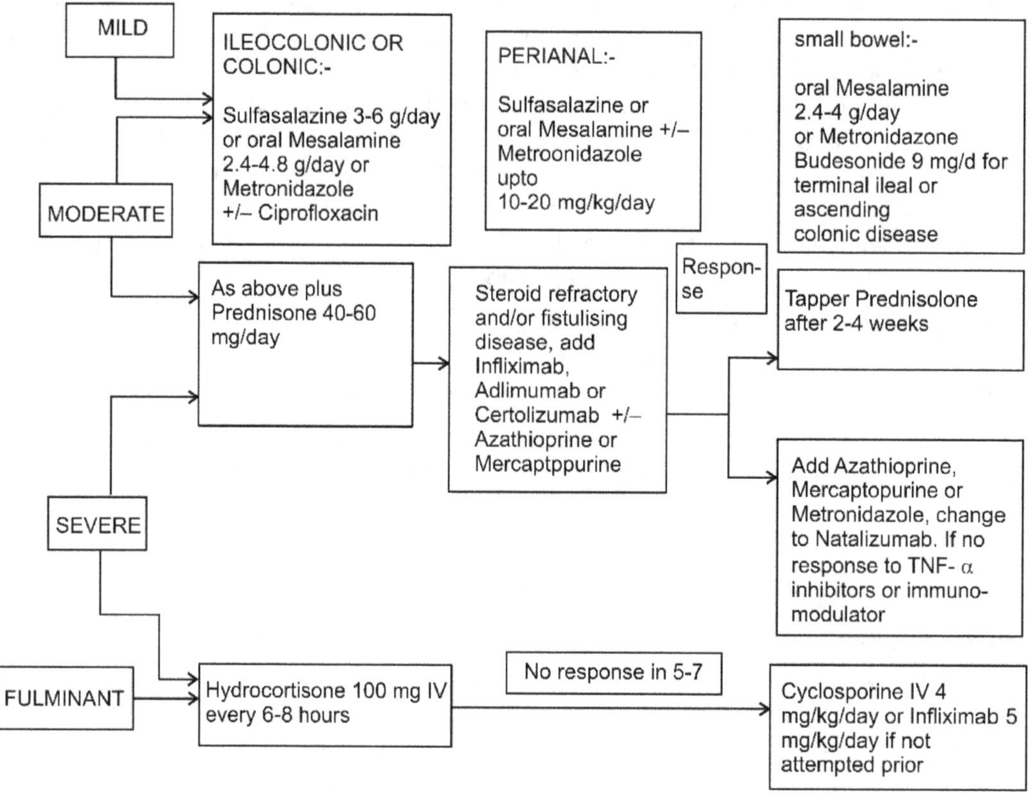

Fig. 58.2 Algorithm for management of Crohn's disease based on disease severity.

Source: Torres J, Bonovas S, Doherty G, Kucharzik T, Gisbert JP, Raine T et al., Ecco Buidelines on Therapeutics in Crohn's Disease: Medical treatment. J Crohn's Colities, 2020 Jan; 14(1): 4-22.

Methotrexate given as weekly injection of 25 mg has demonstrated efficacy for induction of remission in CD, as well as for maintenance therapy.

Infliximab is used for moderate to severe active CD in patients failing immuno-suppressive therapy, in those who are Corticosteroid dependent, and for treatment of fistulizing disease. A single 5 mg/kg infusion is effective when given everyday for 8 weeks. Additional doses at 2 and 6 weeks following the initial dose results in higher response rates. Patients may develop antibodies to Infliximab, which can result in serious infusion reactions and loss of drug response.

Adalimumab and Certolizumab are effective in patients with moderate to severe CD who have lost response to Infliximab. Natalizumab is reserved for patients who donot respond to steroids or the TNF inhibitors.

(B) Maintenance of Remission: Prevention of recurrence of disease is clearly more difficult with CD then with UC, Sulfasalazine and oral Mesalamine derivatives are effective in preventing acute recurrences in quiescent CD.

Azathioprine and MP are effective in maintaining remission in CD in upto 70% of patients, particularly in Infliximab or Steroid induced remission and therefore these drugs are generally considered first line drugs. Methotrexate, the TNF inhibitors are effective in maintaining remission in CD.

Selected Complications

(A) Toxic Megacolon: The treatment required for toxic megacolon includes general supportive measures to maintain vital functions, consideration for early surgical intervention and anti-microbials.

Aggressive fluid and electrolyte management are required for dehydration. When the patient has lost significant amount of blood (through rectum), blood replacement is also necessary.

Steroids in high dosages (Hydrocortisone 100 mg every 8 hours) should be administered IV to reduce acute inflammation.

Broad spectrum anti-microbials that include coverage for gram-negative bacilli and intestinal anaerobes should be used as preventive therapy in the event that perforation occurs.

(B) Systemic Manifestations: For arthritis Aspirin or another NSAID may be beneficial, as are Corticosteroids. However NSAID use may exacerbate the underlying IBD and predispose patients to GI bleeding.

Anemia secondary to blood loss from the GIT can be treated with oral ferrous sulfate. Vitamin B12 or Folic acid may also be required.

Agents for the Treatment of IBD

1. **Sulfasalazine**

   Brand name: Asulfidine

   MOA: It slows down the anti-inflammatory effects in the body. It also has immuno-suppressive actions.

   Initial dose: 500 mg to 1 g   Usual range: 4 to 6 g/day

   ADRs: Nausea, vomiting, headache, rash, anemia, pneumonitis, hepatotoxicity, nephritis, thrombocytopenia, lymphoma.

   Monitoring parameters: Folate, CBC, SCr, Liver function tests, BUN.

   Comments: Increase the dose slowly, over 1-2 weeks.

2. **Mesalamine**

   Brand names: Rowasa, Canasa, Asacol, Apriso, Lialda, Pentasa

MOA: Mesalamine belongs to a class of drugs known as Aminosalicylates. It works by decreasing swelling in colon.

Initial dose: 1 g (Suppository), 4 g (Enema), 1.2 – 2.4 g/day (Oral)

Usual range: 1 g daily, 3 times weekly (Suppository), 4 g daily to 3 times weekly (Enema), 1.2- 4.8 g/day once daily (Oral)

ADRs: Nausea, vomiting, headache

Monitoring parameters: GI disturbances

3. **Azathioprine**

Brand name: Imuran, Azasan

MOA: Azatioprine lowers body's immune system. It antagonizes purine metabolism. And may inhibit synthesis of DNA, RNA ans proteins. It inhibits mitosis.

Initial dose: 50-100 mg

Usual range: 1-2.5 mg/kg/day

ADRs: Bone marrow suppression, pancreatitis

Monitoring parameters: CBC

Comments: Check TMPT activity

4. **Mercaptopurine**

Brand name: Purinethol

MOA: MP competes with purine derivatives and convert itself to TIMP and interferes with glycoprotein synthesis.

Initial dose: 50-100 mg

Usual range: 1-2.5 mg/kg/day

ADRs: Liver dysfunction, rash, arthralgia

Monitoring parameters: Scr, BUN, LFT

5. **Methorexate**

Brand name: Trexall

MOA: It is a chemotherapy agent and immune system suppressant. It competitively inhibits DHFR, an enzyme that participates in the tetrahydrofolate synthesis.

Initial dose: 15-25 mg IM weekly

Usual range: 15-25 mg IM weekly

ADRs: Bone marrow suppression, pancreatitis, pneumonitis, pulmonary fibrosis, hepatitis.

Monitoring parameters: CBC, BUN, Liver function test, SCr

Comments: Check baseline pregnancy tests

6. **Prednisone**

Brand name: Deltasone

MOA: Prednisone is converted into Prednisolone in liver. It binds to cytoplasmic receptors and inhibit DNA synthesis.

Dose: 5-10 mg/week

ADRs: Hyperglycemia, dyslipidemia, osteoporosis, hypertension, edema, infection, myopathy, psychosis.

Monitoring parameters: GI disturbances, blood pressure, fasting lipid panel, glucose, vitamin D, bone density

Comments: Avoid long term use if possible or consider Budesonide (Initial dose: 9 mg; usual range: 6-9 mg daily)

7. **Cyclosporine**

   Brand name: Gengraf, Neoral, Sandimmune

   MOA: It lowers the activity of T –cells; it does so by Calcineurin-Phosphatase pathway and preventing mitochondrial peremeability transition pore from opening.

   Initial dose: 2-8 mg/kg/day oral; 2-4 mg/kg/day IV

   Usual range: 2-4 mg/kg/day IV

   ADRs: Gum enlargement, increased hair growth, convulsions' peptic ulcers, numbness, tingling, high BP, hyperkalemia.

   Monitoring parameters: B.P, Renal function test, Liver function test.

8. **Adalimumab**

   Brand name: Humira

   MOA: TNF inhibiting, anti-inflammatory drug

   Initial dose: 160 mg SC daily

   Usual range: 80 mg SC (day 15) and then 40 mg every 2 weeks

   ADRs: Heart failure, optic neuritis, demyelination, injection site reaction, signs of infection

   Monitoring parameters: Neurological exam, mental status

9. **Infliximab**

   Brand name: Remicade

   Initial dose: 5 mg/kg IV

   Usual range: 5 mg/kg weeks 2 and 6, 5-10 mg/kg every 8 weeks

   ADRs: Infusion-related reactions, infection

   Monitoring parameters: Heart rate, BP

   Comments: Need negative PPD and viral serologies.

10. **Certolizumab**

    Brand name: Cimzia

    Initial dose: 400 mg SC

    Usual range: 400 mg SC weeks 2 and 4; 400 mg SC monthly

    ADR: Lymphoma

    Monitoring parameters: Trough concentrations

11. **Natalizumab**

    Brand name: Tysabri

    MOA: It is humanized monoclonal antibody against the cell adhesion molecule α 4-integrin.

    Initial dose: 300 mg IV

Usual range: 300 mg IV every 4 weeks

ADRs: Infusion- related reactions

Monitoring parameters: Brain MRI, mental status, progressive multifocal leuko-encephalopathy.

Case Study of Adhesive Intestinal Obstruction

Summary

A 79 year old male patient came to the hospital with these symptoms. He had abdominal distension since one day and not passed flatus since morning He has no history of fever and jaundice and vomiting. He was admitted for further evaluation and management. He had problem of shortness of breath since one week. Anuria since a day. He had history of constipation and was on laxative. He had complaint of decreased urine output and decreased bowel sounds and decreased flatus. He is hypertensive and diabetic patient with seizure disorder and also has history of COPD and old CVA. He has been on medication for hypertension and diabetes and seizures. He underwent surgery choleystectomy five years back. His vitals are normal and showed the increase in blood pressure 200/176 and per abdomen status is distension positive. Complete blood count showed the increase in white blood cells 15800 cells/μ.mm. Normal value 4000-11000 cells/μ.mm and an increase in platelet count 3.8 lakhs/cmm and the peripheral smear of WBC showed leucocytosis. Serum electrolytes were within the normal range. Blood sugar test showed an increase in random blood sugar 394 mg /dl. CT scan of abdomen showed an impression of dilatation of the entire small bowel loops, duodenum and stomach noted with collapsed distal ileal loops noted in the right iliac forsa just proximal to the ileo cecal junction. Sub acute intestinal obstruction with possible adhesions. Air filled with dilated transfers colon with abrupt transition at the pelvic flexure. Simple cyst in segment VI of lower bilateral renal cortical scars, lumbar spondylosis.

Diagnosis: He was diagnosed with adhesive internal obstruction.

His Inpatient therapy included the following:

Trade name	Generic name	Route	Dose	Frequency
Stamlo	Amlodipine	Oral	5mg	STAT
Hai	Human atropine insulin	IV	16 Units	STAT
Nig	Nitroglycerine	IV	5mg per kg	STAT
Lasix	Furosemide	IV	40 mg	STAT
Monocef	Ceftriaxone	IV	1g	BD
Metrogyl	Metronidazole	IV	500mg	TID
Bronac	Acetyl cysteine	IV	1.5 g	
Pcm	Paracetamol	IV	1g	TID
Amlong	Amlodipine	RT	5mg	BD
Galvusmet	Metformin + vildaglipline	ORAL	50/500 mg	OD
Potklor	Chlozate	P/O	10 ml	TID
Cinod	Cilnidipine	P/O	10 mg	OD

The patient showed the improvement over time, passed the stools twice, urine output found to be good and diabetic levels were reduced. On the first day the patient did not pass stools and was nasuatic, has complaints of abdominal distension. On the second day the patient passed stools twice, urine output was good, distension reduced, BP and DM was under control. On the third day responding to verbal command, foley tube removed, he passed flatus. On the fourth day patient was conscious, passed stools, no fever, medicine for potassium correction. Then the patient was allowed to leave after all the check up and when test were found to be normal he was discharged with medications. Pan 40mg OD before breakfast for 5 days. Augmentin 625 mg BD after food for 5 days. Dolo 650 mg sos. Galvusmet 50/500 mg OD. Potklor 10 ml TID. Cinod 10 Mg OD. He has to do follow up after a week for serum electrolyte potassium, diabetic level, and then would be tested for ultra sound abdomen along with hypertensive level.

Patient Education

Intake of liquids on low fiber diet which is easily broken down into smaller fragments by digestive system

Maintain the glycemic levels

Intake of low salt which benefits in maintainance of BP

Should take the drugs prescribed without missing a dose

Take healthy diet

Assignment

1. **What causes small bowel obstruction?**

   Adhesions from previous abdominal surgery, Hernia containing bowel, Crohns disease causing adhesions or inflammatory strictures, Volvulus, Foreign bodies

   Neoplasmas beningn or malignant, Compression of the duodenum, Ischemic strictures

2. **What are the Signs and Symptoms Commonly Associated with Small Bowel Obstruction?**

   In small bowel obstruction the pain tends to be colicky (cramping and intermittent) in nature with spams lasting a few minutes. The pain tends to be central and mild abdominal Vomiting may occur without constipation. Dehydration, malaise, bloatting.

3. **Which lab tests are indicated in diagnosis?**

   Blood tests; X ray of abdomen, CT scan; Ultrasound, small bowel investigation with push endoscopy and laproscopy, colonoscopy

   Lab Studies: Serum chemistry: mildly elevated (vomiting)

   Bun: increased (dehydration), Serum lactate levels: increased levels (dehydration)

   Urine analysis, Prothrombine time, Lactate dehydrogenase

4. Which Medications are used in Initial Treatmnt of Small Bowel Obstruction?

1. Analgesics: Used for continuous pain
2. Anticholinergics: Scopoloamine butylbromide and Scopolamine hydrobromide. Used for Colicky pain.
3. Antisecretory agents: For nausea and vomiting
   Scopoloamine butylbromide: 40-120 mg/day
   Scopolamine hydrobromide:0.8-2.0mg/day
   Glycopyrrolate (0.1-0.2mg TID SC or IV   and/or
   Octrotide (0.2-0.9mg/day
4. Antiemetics: Metoclopramide
5. Neuroleptics: Haloperidol (5-15mg/day via SC infusion)
   Methotromeprazine (50-150mg/day via SC infusion)
   Prochlorperazine (25-75mg/day rectally)
   Chlorperazine (50-100mg/8h rectally or SC)
6. Antihistaminic agents: Cyclazine (100-150mg/day)
   Dimwnhydrinate (50-100mg/day SC)

5. Which Medications (a) Antibiotic (b) Anti Emetic (c) Analgesic Used In Treatment

(a)   Antibiotics: Cefazolin,cefoxitin,cefotetan,meropenam.
(b)   Antiemetic: Promethazine, ondansetron.
(c)   Analgesic: Morphine sulphate

6. Which abdominal surgeries are most commonly associated with obstruction?
Stent: A metal tube inserted into the intestine to open the area that is blocked.
Gastrostomy Tube: A tube inserted to the wall of the abdomen directly

7. What are the Risk Factors?

- Previous abdomen or pelvic surgery
- Previous radiation therapy
- May be part of the patient medical history
- Crohns disease which cause intestinal wall to thickened
- Cancer in abdomen

8. When is Surgical Intervention Indicated in Treatment of Small Bowel Obstruction?

If the obstruction does not clear on its own. Surgery may be needed to relieve the obstruction. Surgery typically involves removing the obstruction as well as any section of intestine that has damage.

References

1. Podolsky DK. Inflammatory bowel disease. N Engl J Med 2002;347:417–429.
2. Shanahan F. Pathogenesis of ulcerative colitis. Lancet 1993;342:407–411.

3. Gan SI, Beck PL. A new look at toxic megacolon: An update and review of incidence, etiology, pathogenesis, and management. Am J Gastroenterol 2003;98:2363–2371.

4. Collins P, Rhodes J. Ulcerative colitis: Diagnosis and management. BMJ 2006;333:340–343.

5. Kornbluth A, Sachar DB. Ulcerative practice guidelines in adults (update): American College of Gastroenterology, Practice Parameters Committee. Am J Gastroenterol 2004;99:1371–1385.

6. Hanauer SB, Sandborn W. Management of Crohn's disease in adults. Am J Gastroenterol 2001;96:635–643.

7. Schnüriger, B, Barmparas, G, Branco, B. "Prevention of postoperative peritoneal adhesions: a review of the literature". *Am J Surg.* vol. 201. 2011. pp. 111-21.

CHAPTER - 59

Viral Hepatitis

Introduction to Viral Hepatitis

Viral hepatitis can present as either an acute or chronic illness. Acute hepatitis is defined as an illness with a discrete date of onset with jaundice or increased serum aminotransferase concentrations >2.5 times the upper limit of normal. Acute viral hepatitis infection is a systemic process and lasts as long as, but not exceeding, 6 months. Chronic hepatitis is an inflammatory condition of the liver that involves ongoing hepatocellular necrosis for 6 months or more beyond the onset of acute illness.

This is mainly caused by hepatotrophic viruses. Hepatotrophic viruses are any of various microscopic organisms/ agents that infect living organisms, often causing diseases & that consist of a single or double strand DNA or RNA surrounded by a protein coat. Unable to replicate without a host cell, viruses are typically not considered living organisms.

Viruses involved are Hepatitis A, Hepatitis B, Hepatitis C, Delta Hepatitis and Hepatitis E.

Hepatitis A: (HAV)

HAV is often a self-limiting and acute viral infection to the liver poising a health risk. This infection is rarely fatal. Hepatitis A is a small nonenveloped, single stranded RNA virus, of Genus Hepatovirus, Family-Picornaviridae, with host as humans. Mode of transmission is Faecal – oral route. Virus is stable in the environment for at least a month, & required heating good to a minimum of 85C.for 1 Min (or) disinfecting with 1:100 dilution sodium hypochlorite in tap water for inactivation. Multiple genotype of the virus exist & although the clinical implications of infection by particular type are unknown. Type 1& 3 are the most commonly identified in human outbreaks.

Epidemiology: Various patient groups are at increased risk for infection with HAV. Children pose a particular problem with the spread of the disease because they often remain clinically asymptomatic. Children have infection for longer period of time than adults.

Etiology: Poor sanitary conditions and hygienic practices. For international travelers, longer lengths of stay in a country with a high rate of hepatitis A also correlates with increased risk. men who have sex with men, injecting drug users, and persons working with nonhuman primates. Both children and young adults can be infected from common-source outbreaks at day care centers.

Pathophysiology: HAV is usually acute, self-limiting and confers life long immunity. The natural history of the infection is divided into three stages based on viral serologic markers: incubation, acute hepatitis, and convalescence.

- HAV life cycle in the human beings with ingestion of the virus. Organism on entering the body enters into small intestine and circulation. Uptake of virus takes place in liver. In hepatocytes (target site of Hep − A) the replication takes place. The newly formed viral particles either enter Bile, Shred into small intestine or goes back to liver. After re-entering liver they continue with the replication and forms viral load, which causes hepatocyte degeneration.

- Acute hepatitis begins with a **preicteric phase** (before the onset of jaundice), which parallels initiation of the host immune response and occurs before significant liver cell injury. The preicteric phase is frequently associated with nonspecific influenza-like symptoms consisting of anorexia, nausea, fatigue, and malaise. Most patients with acute viral hepatitis develop only a few mild symptoms and minimal hepatocyte damage. This mild disease is called acute anicteric hepatitis. The minimal degree of liver cell damage is reflected by mild elevations of serum bilirubin, γ -globulin, and hepatic transaminase (alanine transaminase [ALT], aspartate transaminase [AST]) values to about twice normal. Subsets of patients experience enough hepatocyte destruction to produce significant liver dysfunction characterized by interruption of bilirubin metabolism and flow. This results in clinical jaundice and acute icteric hepatitis.

- **Icteric hepatitis** is generally accompanied by fever, right upper quadrant abdominal pain, nausea, vomiting, dark urine, acholic (light colored) stools, and worsening of systemic symptoms. Clinical symptoms are accompanied by elevations of the serum bilirubin, γ -globulin, and hepatic transaminases from 4 to 10 times above normal.

- Most patients with either acute anicteric or icteric hepatitis go through the convalescence stage to complete recovery without developing complications or chronic sequelae.

- Liver injury is immune mediated with cytolytic T cells maintaining the primary role in cell destruction. Death of hepatocytes results in viral elimination and eventual resolution of the clinical illness. Viremia begins soon after infection, continues and throughout the time liver enzymes are elevated.

Clinical Presentation of Acute Hepatitis A

Signs and Symptoms

- The preicteric phase brings nonspecific influenza-like symptoms consisting of anorexia, nausea, fatigue, and malaise
- Abrupt onset of anorexia, nausea, vomiting, malaise, fever, headache, and right upper quadrant abdominal pain with acute illness

- Icteric hepatitis is generally accompanied by dark urine, acholic (light-colored) stools, and worsening of systemic symptoms
- Pruritus is often a major complaint of icteric patients

Physical examination
- Icteric sclera, skin, and secretions
- Mild weight loss of 2 to 5 kg
- Hepatomegaly

Laboratory tests
- Positive serum IgM anti-HAV
- Mild elevations of serum bilirubin, γ-globulin, and hepatic transaminase (alanine transaminase [ALT], and aspartate transaminase [AST]) values to about twice normal in acute anicteric disease
- Elevations of alkaline phosphatase, γ-glutamyl transferase, and total bilirubin in patients with cholestatic illness

Treatment

Goal: Complete clinical resolution, reduce complication from the infection, other goals include normalization of liver function and reducing infectivity and transmission.

General Approach to treatment: General measures include a healthy diet, rest, maintaining fluid balance, and avoiding hepatotoxic drugs and alcohol.

Pharmacologic Therapy

In patient having liver failure, transplant is the only option.

Prevention of Hepatitis A: Highly effective inactivated vaccines against HAV have been available.

(a) **Immunoglobulin therapy:** Immunoglobulin (Ig) provides protection against HAV by passive transfer of concentrated antibodies (immunoglobulins) against HAV (anti-HAV). Ig is effective in modifying the course and preventing the spread of HAV in 85% or more of exposures when used within 2 weeks following the exposure. Ig therapy given through IV/IM but in HAV mostly IM is used. Dose: 0.02ml/kg – short term and 0.06ml/kg – long term. In special population, pregnant woman and infant the timerosal free formulation should be used. Anaphylaxis is reported in patients with IgA deficiency that have anaphylactic reaction to Ig should not receive it.

(b) **Vaccines to Prevent Hepatitis A:** Inactivated HAV vaccines, Havrix (SmithKline Beecham) and Vaqta (Merck) both demonstrate protective efficacy in 94% to 100% of vaccinees within 1 month after primary vaccination.

Groups at Increased Risk of Hepatitis A and Recommended for Preexposure Hepatitis A Vaccination

- Children living in states, counties, or communities where rates of hepatitis A are at least twice the national average ($\geq$20 cases per 100,000 populations).
- Persons traveling to or working in countries that have high or intermediate endemicity of infection.
- Men who have sex with men.
- Illegal-drug users.
- Persons who have occupational risk for infection (e.g., persons who work with HAV-infected primates or HAV in a research laboratory setting).
- Persons who have clotting-factor disorders.
- Persons who have chronic liver disease (e.g., persons with chronic liver disease caused by hepatitis B or C and persons awaiting liver transplants)

Table 59.1 Recommended doses of Havrix and Vaqta.

Vaccine	Age (yr)	Dose	No. of Doses	Schedule
Havrix	1-18	720 ELISA Units	2	0,6,12
	>19	1L440 ELISA Units	2	0,6,12
Vaqta	1-18	25 Units	2	0,6,18
	>19	50 Units	2	0,6,18

Hepatitis – B virus: It is a chronic and not self-limiting condition.

Epidemiology: HBV spread is predominantly by mother-to-infant perinatal transmission and by child-to-child transmission.

Mode of transmission:
- Mainly sexual, parenteral, prenatal (mother to child)
- Contagious disease.
- Very less concentrated in urine and saliva

Etiology: HBV is smallest known DNA virus. It is an enveloped double stranded DNA virus belonging to family – Hepadnaviridae. Mainly infects liver cells, and cause hepatic dysfunction cycles that lead to chronic hepatitis, cirrhosis and hepatocellular carcinoma. A small spherical and tubular particle known as HBsAg can be found circulating in the bloodstream of infected patients. Viral core contains a single molecule of partially doublestranded DNA referred to as the HBV core antigen (HBcAg). A DNA polymerase viral peptide is also found in the core and is referred to as the HBV e antigen (HbeAg). HBV has been classified into seven genotypes (A through G).

Pathogenesis: After the HBV enters the vascular compartment, it migrates to the liver, where primary replication occurs. The incubation period of HBV is 1 to 6 months—much longer than HAV. HBV replication occurs in liver cell nuclei, with HBsAg produced in the cell cytoplasm and expressed on the cell surface. These particles are also found circulating in the plasma of patients with acute HBV, the chronic carrier state, and chronic HBV infection.

Clinical Presentation of Acute Hepatitis B

- The duration of incubation is highly dependent on age and can vary between 6 and 24 weeks. Infants do not develop any symptoms and children between the ages of 1 and 5 years are asymptomatic in 85% to 95% of the cases
- Symptomatic infections vary in severity and include fever, anorexia, nausea, vomiting, jaundice, dark urine, clay-colored or pale stools, and abdominal pain.
- Acute HBV infection is diagnosed by the presence of anti-HBc IgM.

Clinical Presentation of Chronic Hepatitis B

Signs and symptoms

- Easy fatigability, anxiety, anorexia, and malaise
- Ascites, jaundice, variceal bleeding, and hepatic encephalopathy can manifest with liver decompensation
- Hepatic encephalopathy is associated with hyperexcitability, impaired mentation, confusion, obtundation, and eventually coma
- Vomiting and seizures

Physical examination

- Icteric sclera, skin, and secretions
- Decreased bowel sounds, increased abdominal girth, and detectable fluid wave
- Asterixis
- Spider angiomata

Laboratory tests

- Presence of hepatitis B surface antigen for at least 6 months
- Intermittent elevations of hepatic transaminase (alanine transaminase [ALT] and aspartate transaminase [AST]) and hepatitis B virus DNA greater than 105 copies/mL
- Liver biopsies for pathologic classification as chronic persistent hepatitis, chronic active hepatitis, or cirrhosis

Treatment:

Goals: No specific therapy is available for the management of acute HBV infection. The key goal of therapy for chronic HBV is to eradicate or permanently suppress HBV.

The short-term objective is to limit hepatic inflammation and to reduce the risk of fibrosis and/or decompensation.

The longitudinal goal is to prevent transaminase flares and the development of long-term complications, as well as to prolong survival.

Non- Pharmacological therapy:

- Counselling patient about disease
- Sexual and household contacts should be vaccinated

- Avoid alcohol consumption
- Immunize against HAV
- Herbal machines like phyllanthus, milk, thistle, glycgrrhizin can be taken.

Treatment algorithm based on the recommendations of the American GE association for chronic hepatitis B in adults and children

1. **Patients with HBeAg-positive chronic HBV:** ALT >2 times the upper limit of normal (ULN) or moderate to severe hepatitis on biopsy: Treatment may be initiated with either Lamivudine or Interferon-α ALT >2 times ULN: Treatment with Lamivudine or interferon-α should be limited to patients with significant necroinflammation on liver biopsy. Patients should have their ALT assessed every 3 to 6 months.

2. **Patients with HBeAg-negative chronic HBV:** Only patients with ALT >2 times ULN, HBV DNA >105 copies/mL, or moderate to severe hepatitis on biopsy should be considered for treatment with lamivudine or interferon-α.

3. Patients who fail to respond to a course of interferon-α and have ALT >2 times ULN, HBV DNA >105 copies/mL, or moderate to severe hepatitis on biopsy may be treated with a course of lamivudine.

4. Patients with decompensated cirrhosis: Interferon-α should not be used and lamivudine may be considered in these patients.

5. Patients in an inactive HBsAg carrier state: No treatment is indicated.

Pharmacological Therapy

Interferon: They have Antiviral, antiproliferative, iummunomodulatory properties. IFN-α2b should be administered by subcutaneous injection as 5 million units daily or 10 million units thrice weekly in adults. In children, thrice-weekly subcutaneous injections of 6 million units/m2 to a maximum of 10 million units per dose is recommended. Patients with HBV who are HBeAg-positive should be treated for 16 weeks, while HBeAg-negative patients should be treated for 12 month. IFN is replaced with pegylated INF (PEG-INF). PEG-INF will decrease the side effects.

Lamivudine: It is a Nucleoside analog that competitively inhibits viral reverse transcriptase and terminates proviral DNA chain extension. Because it does not affect host response, it suppresses viral replication but does not directly eliminate the virus from the hepatocytes. Dose: 100mg/day – 3 to 6months. Upon discontinuation of lamivudine HBV DNA tends to rebound, but to levels less than the original baseline. Virologic responses were maintained in about 75% of lamivudine-treated patients.

Adefovir: Adefovir is a nucleotide analog of deoxyadenosine monophosphate that is active against retroviruses (like HIV), herpes viruses, and hepadnaviruses. Adefovir dipivoxil 10 mg by mouth once daily for 48 weeks has been approved for use in adult patients with chronic HBV who are either treatment naïve or have lamivudine-resistant HBV. Dose: 10mg/day – for 1 year

Entecavir: It is a guanosine nucleosideanalogue. MOA: Acts by inhibiting HBV polymerase.

More potent than Lamivudine. Dose: 0.5mg/day for 48 weeks.

Telbivudine: It is HBV specific nucleoside analogue. MOA: acts as a competitive inhibitor of viral reverse transcriptase and DNA Polymerase. It inhibits HBV DNA synthesis with no activity against other viruses. It is more potent than lamivudine

Alternative therapy: Emtricitabine – is cytosine analogue approved for use in HIV and with activity against HBV

Tenofovir- is a nucleotide analogue approved for use in HIV and with activity against HBV

Special population: In Cirrhosis patient – Lamivudine, adefovir, entecavir

In HIV infected patient –tenofovir or lamivudine, entecavir

Recommended Schedule of Immunoprophylaxis to Prevent Perinatal or Sexual Transmission of HBV Infection

- **Infant born to HBsAg-positive mother:** Vaccine dose 1 HBIg (0.5 mL intramuscularly at a site different from that used for the vaccine). Within 12 hours of birth. Vaccine doses 2 and 3 months Usual schedule
- **Infant born to mother not screened for HbsAg:** Vaccine dose 1- HBIg (0.5 mL intramuscularly at a site different from that used for the vaccine). Within 12 hours of birth. If mother is found to be HBsAg-positive, administer dose to infant as soon as possible, but no later than 1 week after birth. Vaccine doses 2 and 3 months usual schedule
- **Sexual exposure:** HBIg (0.06 mL/kg intramuscularly at a site different from that used for the vaccine). Single dose within 14 days of sexual contact. Vaccine dose 1- At time of HBIg treatment, Vaccine doses 2 and 3 months usual schedule

Recommendations for Hepatitis B Prophylaxis Following Percutaneous or Permucosal Exposure

Vaccination Status of Exposed Person

(a) Unvaccinated: HBsAg-Positive: HBIG (one dose of 0.06 mL/kg IM), plus initiate vaccine

HBsAg-Negative- Initiate vaccine in the patient

(b) Previously vaccinated, known responder:

HBsAg-Positive: Test the exposed person for anti-HBs antibody level. No treatment if adequate, antibodies are present. If inadequate or titer unknown, one vaccine booster dose to be given to the patient.

HBsAg-Negative: no treatment needed

(c) Previously vaccinated, known nonresponder:

HBsAg-Positive: HBIg (two doses 1 month apart) or HBIg one dose, plus dose of vaccine

HBsAg-Negative: no treatment

(d) Previously vaccinated, response unknown:

HBsAg-Positive: Test the exposed person for anti-HBs antibody level. If inadequate, HBIg one dose + one vaccine booster dose. If adequate, no treatment is needed. If titer unknown, one vaccine booster dose to be given.

HBsAg-Negative: no treatment

Recommended Doses and Schedules of Currently Licensed Hepatitis B Vaccines

Recombivax HB

1. Infants, Children & Adolescents 0-19yrs of age 5 mcg (0.5 mL). 3 doses at 0, 1 and 6 months.
2. Adolescents (11-15 yrs of age): 10mcg (1.0 mL): 2 doses at 0 and 4-6 months.
3. Adults ($\geq$ 20 yrs of age): 10 mcg (1.0mL): 3 doses at 0, 1 and 6 months.
4. Predialysis and Dialysis patients: 40 mcg(1.0 mL): 3 doses at 0, 1 and 6 months.

Hepatitis – C

It is most common blood – borne pathogen. 40% of chronic liver disease is related to HCV.

Epidemiology: HCV is found worldwide and is transmitted primarily through injecting drug use and contaminated blood products. persons in their third and fourth decades of life have the highest prevalence of acute HCV, while chronic HCV has the highest prevalence rates in persons in the fifth and sixth decades of life.

Mode of Spread

Transmission may occur by sexual contact with multiple sex partners, transfusion of infected blood or its products; close contact with HCV infected, patient perinatal exposure.

Etiology: HCV is a enveloped, spherical, single-stranded RNA virus that belongs to the Flaviviridae family. There are six known genotypes (numbered 1 through 6) and greater than 50 subtypes (designated by letter: 1a, 1b, and so forth) of HCV. Genotype 1b often results in the 10 most aggressive form of liver disease.

Pathophysiology: The virus replicates mainly in the hepatocytes of the liver, where it is estimated that daily each infected cell produces approximately fifty virions. The virus may also replicate in peripheral blood mononuclear cells, potentially accounting for the high levels of immunological disorders found in chronically infected HCV patients. Because HCV does not replicate via a DNA intermediate, it does not integrate into the host genome.

After HCV gains access to the host, the virus enters hepatocytes. The virus then uncoats and releases the genome to begin replication. The viral genome serves as a template for translation of the polyprotein. The processed nonstructural protein forms a complex with the genome and begins synthesis for the negative strand. The negative strand functions as the template for synthesis of the positive strand. The RNA intermediate matures and interacts with the envelope and core proteins to assemble into new virus.

HCV is more likely to cause clinically chronic silent infection in immunocompetent people. . In acute HCV infection, specific T-cell receptors are activated and HCV-specific helper T cells assist with activation, differentiation, and induction of B cells, as well as stimulating virus-specific cytotoxic T cells. These effects are mediated by various immunoregulatory cytokines. CD8+ cytotoxic T cells recognize HCV peptides synthesized in infected cells, with resulting lysis of the infected cell.

Clinical Presentations:

Acute hepatitis C: Often asymptomatic, but they may have malaise, anorexia, and jaundice, which occur in up to 25% of cases. The mean incubation period of HCV is 50 days and viremia can be detected within 3 weeks of initial exposure.

Chronic hepatitis C: Fatigue, anxiety, anorexia, malaise, jaundice, ascites, varicel bleeding, hepatic encephalopathy, confusion, obtundation, vomiting and seizure. Peripheral neuropathy is the most common neurologic symptom in patients with HCV. Sensory loss may manifest bilaterally or may affect multiple isolated nerves.

Physical Examination:
- Icteric sclera, skin and secretions.
- Decreased bowel sound, increased abdominal girth, detectable fluid wave
- Asterixis (tremor of hand when the wrist is extended).
- Piderangiomata

Diagnosis:
- Presence of HBAg> 6 months
- RNA Viral Load
- LFT
- Elevation of hepatic transaminase (ALT&AST)
- HBV DNA > 20,000 IU/ml
- Live biopsies
- Culture sensitivity tests

Treatment:

Goal: To eradicate HCV infection. Resolving infection prevents the development of chronic HCV.

Non-Pharmacological therapy:
- HCV patient should be vaccinated against hepatitis A&B.
- Decreased alcohol consumption
- Reduce weight of obess
- Cessation of smoking

Contraindications to hepatitis C virus combination therapy:
- Autoimmune hepatitis
- Decompensated liver disease

- Patient whose female partner is pregnant
- Pt with hemoglobinopathies
- Pt with creatinine clearance<50,l/min
- Pt on haemodialysis
- Pt with CVS Disease

Pharmacological Therapy

Interferons: IFN-α2a and IFN-α2b are naturally occurring cytokines that have been manufactured using human recombinant techniques in Escherichia coli. In contrast, IFN alfacon-1 is a non–naturally occurring type 1 interferon also produced using human recombinant techniques. These gene products are responsible for the immunomodulatory, antiviral, and antiproliferative properties of these agents. Flu-like symptoms such as headache, fatigue, and chills occur in more than two thirds of patients.

Pegylated Interferons: Peginterferon-α2a (Pegasys) and peginterferon-α2b (PEG-Intron) are FDA approved for use as monotherapy and in combination with ribavirin for the treatment of chronic HCV in patients with compensated liver disease who are interferon-treatment–naïve.

Ribavirin: Ribavirin is a synthetic nucleoside antagonist that is administered orally in combination with α-interferons. Ribavirin has limited utility as monotherapy and should be administered twice daily with food when used in combination with α-interferons

Hepatits C has different genotype they are genotype 2, 3, 1

Non Specific HCV vaccination is available

Table 59.2 Recommended hepatitis C virus treatment dosing.

Genotype	Peg- INF Dose	Ribavirin dose	Duration
1	Peg-INF Alpha 2a 180 mcg/wk	<75kg/ 1,000mg	48 weeks
	Peg INF Alpha 2b 1.5 mcg/wk	>75kg/ 1200mg	48 weeks
2, 3	Pef INF Alpha 2a 180 mcg/ wk	800 mg	24 weeks
	Peg INF Alpha 2b 1.5 mcg/wk	800 mg	24 weeks

HCV infection treatment regimens based on the recommendations of the American GE Association

Genotype 1

Week 0	Initiate Therapy: Pegylated INF + wt based on ribavirin
Week 12	Check viral load for early virologic response (EVR) – if no EVR may consider stopping therapy if goal is viral eradication If EVR is present continue the therapy for 48 weeks.

Genotype 2 & 3

Week 0	Initiatetherapy: PEG – INF + wt based on ribavirin
Week 4	Check viral load
	If undetectable may consider stopping therapy
	If detectable continue the therapy for 24 weeks.

Table 59.3 AASLD/IDSA Recommended treatment regimens for treatment of naïve patients with HCV.

HCV Genotype	No Cirrhosis	Compensated Cirrhosis (CTP Class A)
1a	Elbasvi/ Grazoprevir x 12 weeks	Elbosvir/ Grazoprevir x 12 weeks
	Ledipasvir/ sofobovir x 12 weeks	Lediposvir. Sofosbuvir x 12 weeks
	Ombitasuir/ Paritaprevir/ ritonavir	Ledipasvir. Sofosbuvir x 12 weeks
	Dasabuvir / ribavirin x 12 week	Sotosbuvir/ Velapatasivir x 12 weeks
	Siimeprevir + sotobuvir x 12 weeks	
	Sofasbuvir/ Velpatasvir x 12 weeks	
	Daclatasvir + sotabuvir x 12 week	
1b	Elbasvir/ Erazoprevir x 12 weeks	Elbasvir/ Grazoprevir x 12 weeks
	Ledipasvir/ sotosbuvir x 12 week	Ledipasovir/ sotosbuvir x 12 weeks
	Ombitasvir/ partiprevir. Ritonavir	Ombitasvir/ Paritaprevir/ritonavir + daabuvir and ribavirin x 12 weeks
	Dactatasvir + sotosbuvir x 12 weeks	Sotosbuvi/velpatasvir x 12 weels
2	Sotosbuvir/relpatasvir x 12 weeks	Sotosbuvir/ relpatosvir x 12 weeks
3	Daclatasvir + sotosbuvir x 12 weeks	Sotosbuvir/ Velpatasvir x 12 weeks

Alternative Treatment:
- VX-950 and valopcitabine (NM283)
- VX-950 specific selective inhibitor of HCV replication
- Valopcitabine (NM283) – ribonucleoside it inhibits the viral replication

Special Population: Patient with normal ALT's: Should consider the risk and benefits of therapy

Patient with Decompensated cirrhosis: Liver transplantation is done therapy is not recommended.

Relapse Patient: IFN Monotherapy or IFN + ribavirin or PEF IFN + ribavirin

Non responders: Retreatment with PEG – IFN + ribavirin, IFN monotherapy and IFN + Ribavirin

Accidental neddle stick exposure: Prophylatic treatment is recommended. Treatment is considered for 24 weeks.

End Stage renal disease: IFN – monotherapy. PEG INF – monitor patient closely. Hemodialysis is CF in ribavirin treatment

HCV Coinfection: HCV+HIV patient- Ribavirin + diadanosin

Children: Children – 3 years INF Alpha 2b monotherapy in combination INF – 3 million cu/m$^{2/}$ ribavirin

Case Study of Hepatitis-C

Summary

A male patient of age 60 years was admitted to the male medical ward II with complaints of distension of the abdomen, SOB on exertion since a week and back pain. Past medical history: K/C/O DM and HTN. Past medication history: injection insulin (14U/BD), tab. Telsartan-H (OD). Patient is anaemic, leucocytic and had an elevated ESR (40mm/hr). RBS was elevated (209mg/dL). Prothrombin time was found to be increased (16.9 sec). APTT levels were also increased (49.8). HCV ELISA was reactive (+ve). Direct bilirubin (0.9mg/dl) and alkaline phosphatase enzyme (419IU/L) were also abnormally high. ECG revealed sinus tachycardia, short PR interval and left ventricular hypertrophy.

Diagnosis: The patient was diagnosed with Hepatitis – C with Liver Mass Ascites.

T/O R/O malignancy with HCC (metastasis to vertebrae).

The Inpatient therapy was:

Trade name	Generic name	Route	Dose	Frequency	D1	D2	D3	D4
Inj. LASIX	Furosemide	IV	20mg	OD	Y	Y	Y	Y
S. LACTULOSE	Lactose	Oral	30ml	H/S	Y	Y	Y	Y
Inj. INSULIN	Human insulin	SC	14 U	BD	Y	Y	Y	Y
T.TELSARTAN-H	Telmisartan	Oral	12.5/40mg	OD	N	Y	Y	Y

Assignment

1. **What are the physical findings, lab values and medical history information that suggest the presence of chronic HCV infection?**

   Increased: Prothrombin time (16.9), APTT (49.8), direct bilirubin (0.9mg/dl), alkaline phosphatase (419IU/L), neutrophils (91%) and leucocytes (20,500cells/cumm) and ESR (40mm/hr).

   The patient had 9.2 gm/dl of Hb and 3.7 million cells/cubicmm. I.e. the patient was anaemic.

   ECG findings indicated sinus tachycardia, borderline short PR interval and left ventricular hypertrophy.

   Ultrasound of the abdomen showed ascites. The main finding was the positive HCV ELISA test. It confirmed the presence of Hepatitis – C.

The signs and symptoms seen in this patient were – distension of the abdomen, SOB on exertion and back pain.

2. **What are the goals of treatment?**

The goals are:-

- To provide symptomatic relief.
- To improve the liver function and prevent further complications.
- To treat the co morbid conditions like hypertension and diabetes.
- To improve the health related quality of life.

3. **What are the non – pharmacologic measures that can be considered for this patient?**

The non-pharmacologic measures are –

- To avoid using syringes. If necessary use safe, sterile and disposable syringes.
- Improve personal health and hygiene.
- Take the vaccinations properly and on time.
- Maintain a healthy diet comprising of adequate electrolytes, vegetables like spinach and cabbage.

4. **What are the alternative pharmacotherapeutic regimens for the patient?**

Table 59.4 Therapies for Treatment-Naïve Patients, by HCV Genotype.

Geno type	Recommended Regimen	Alternative Regimen
1a	Ledipasvit/sofosbuvir *or* simeprevir + sofosbuvir with or without ribavirin *or* ombitasvir/paritaprevir/ritonavir + dasabuvir + ribavirin	None
1b	Ledipasvir/sofosbuvir Or simeprevir + sofosbuvir Or ombitasvir/paritaprevir + dasabuvir (+ ribavirin, if cirrhosis)	None
2	Sofosbuvir + ribavirin	None
3.	Sofosbuvir + ribavirin	Sofosbuvir + ribavirin + pegylated INF
4.	Ledipasvir/sofosbuvir Or ombitasvir/paritaprevir/ritonavir + dasabuvir + ribavirin Or Sofosbuvir + ribavirin	Sofosbuvir + ribavirin + pegylated INF *or* Sofosbuvir + simeprevir with or without ribavirin
5.	Sofosbuvir + ribavirin + pegylated INF	Ribavirin + pegylated INF
6.	Ledipasvir/sofosbuvir	Sofosbuvir + ribavirin + pegylated INF

Source: *Refer to the AASLD/IDSA/IASUSA guidelines for treatment duration and further details on specific regimens. AASLD: American Association for the Study of Liver Diseases: IAS-USA: International Antiviral Society-USA; DSA: Infectious Diseases Society of America; INF: interferon. Reference; AASLD/IDSA/IAS–USA. Recommendations for testing, managing, and treating hepatitis C. www.hcvguidelines.org.

5. **What actions can be taken if the patient develops intolerable adverse effects to the treatment recommended?**

    The actions to be taken are:

    1. Stop the drug and use an alternative drug.
    2. If the patient develops hypersensitivity reactions like fever, myalgia and malaise use NSAIDS like ibuprofen and acetaminophen.
    3. For vomitings use anti emetics like ondansetron.
    4. For symptoms suggestive to upper respiratory tract infections give cough medicines (anti tussives or expectorants), NSAIDS (for pain and inflammation) and antibiotics if necessary (penicillins) and nasal washing.
    5. Rehydration therapy: Drink lots of water and electrolytes.
    6. Rashes occur in half of the cases on oral Diphenhydramine and hydroxizine, to treat it hydrocortisone 1% or a moisturizing lotion.
    7. To treat diarrhoea loperamide 2mg is given.
    8. Immunomodulators like PEG-INF, INF-α are also given for hypersensitivity reactions.

6. **Outline a plan for vaccination for this patient against other forms of viral hepatitis.**

    There is no vaccine for hep-c but it is likely recommended for the patient to receive vaccines against hepatitis A and B viruses. These are separate viruses that can also cause liver damage and complicate the course of chronic hepatitis C.

7. **Compare PEG-INF and INF?**

    PEG-INF based regimens are superior to standard INF based regimens for the treatment of Chronic HEP-C.

    PEG-INF: It has polyethylene glycol (PEG) in the formulation. It lasts longer in the body. It is synthetic. There are types of these:

    1 PEG-INF-α-2a, 2 PEG-INF-α-2b, 3 PEG-INF-β-1a

    PEG INF is contraindicated in patients with hyperbilirubinemia.

    INF: Natural, released by host cell to heighten the anti viral defence. They bind to receptors and target cells which lead to expression of proteins that will prevent the virus from producing and replicating itself.

8. **What are the common extra hepatic manifestations of HCV infection?**

    They are:

    - Pain in abdomen/ Bleeding/ Bloating/ Fluid in abdomen
    - Nausea/ Diarrhoea / Vomiting/ Myalgia, hypersensitivity
    - Hepatic encephalopathy/ Anorexia and fatigue
    - Dark urine, light coloured stools.
    - Weight loss, depression, confusion and drowsiness.
    - Slurred speech and bruising.

9. What are the most common HCV genotypes and its prevalence?

HCV has 6 genotypes labelled from 1-6. They also have sub types like 1a and 1b. All genotypes cause the same amount of liver damage. Genotypes 1, 2 and 3 have worldwide distribution. Types 1a and 1b are the most common accounting for about 60% of global infections. Genotype 2 is less frequent.

CHAPTER - 60

Jaundice

Introduction to Jaundice

Jaundice, also known as Icterus. It is the yellowish discoloration of the tissues like skin, sclera and mucus membranes due to deposition of Bilirubin which occurs in presence of Hyperbilirubinemia.

Jaundice itself is not a disease, but rather a sign of one of many possible underlying pathologic processes that occur at same point along the normal physiological pathway of the metabolism of bilirubin in the blood.

- Normal serum bilirubin levels = 0.3-1.0mg/dl
- Conjugated = 0.1-0.3mg/dl
- Unconjugated = 0.2-0.7mg/dl

Equilibrium between bilirubin production and clearance is disturbed. Clinically, jaundice is evident when serum bilirubin crosses 3mg/dl and latent (non-evident) when serum bilirubin levels are between 1-3mg/dl.

When direct bilirubin level is less than 15% it is unconjugated bilirubinemia and when greater than 15% it is conjugated bilirubinemia.

Epidemiology

- Obstructive jaundice is the illness of elderly population and illness is higher among female population, and the most frequent cause of obstructive jaundice are gallstones (54.1% of patients). In 29.8% of patients the primary or secondary malignant disease was the cause of blockage in gall flow and subsequent jaundice, and the most frequent malignant cause of obstructive jaundice is pancreas cancer in 11.5% of patients.
- About 60% to 70% of healthy newborns develop hyperbilirubinemia in the first week of life. Severe hyperbilirubinemia (total serum bilirubin >95th percentile) occurs in 8% to 9% of neonates during the first week; approximately 4% after 72 hours of life. The risk for neonatal hyperbilirubinemia is higher in males and increases progressively with decreasing gestational age.

Etiopathogenesis [1]

Jaundice is either acquired or congenital. Bilirubin is synthesized within the body by the breakdown of aged red blood cell which causes the release of haemoglobin in the reticuloendothelial cell of liver, spleen and bone-marrow where iron is liberated from haemoglobin along with carbon monoxide and biliverdin which later gets converted by biliverdin reductase to bilirubin which remains in the body as a waste product. The liver usually filters out this bilirubin from the blood and then excreted out of the body through urine and faeces after being metabolized. Jaundice is either caused due to overproduction of bilirubin or inability of the liver to abandon it due to acute liver inflammation, bile duct inflammation, hemolytic anaemia, obstruction of the bile duct, cholestasis, and Gilbert's syndrome.

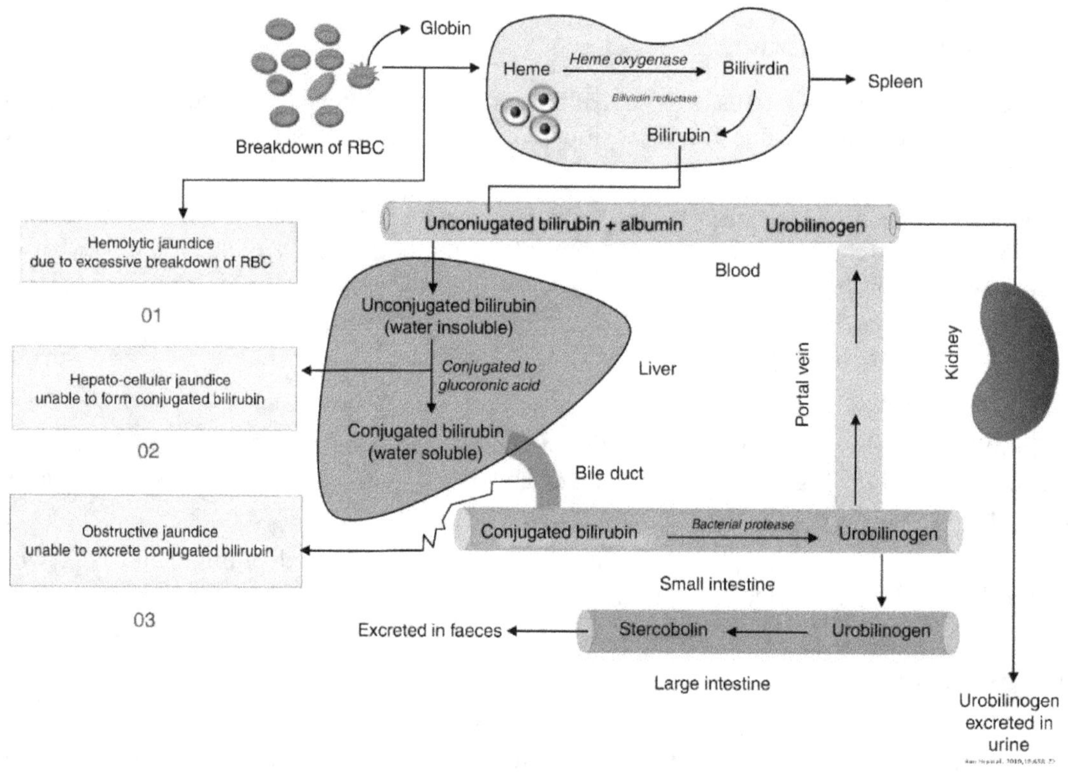

Fig. 60.1 Pathogenesis of Jaundice[2].

Three causes are-

1. Pre-Hepatic Jaundice

2. Hepatic Jaundice

3. Post-Hepatic Jaundice

I. Pre-Hepatic Jaundice: Also known as "Hemolytic Jaundice". It is due to excessive production of bilirubin due to breakdown of hemoglobin as in cases of anaemia.

Congenital causes of hepatic jaundice involve following [3]:
- Spherocytosis, Elliptocytosis
- Thalassemia, Sickle cell anemia
- GSH synthase deficiency
- Pyruvate kinase deficiency
- G6PD deficiency, Erythroblastosis fetalis

Acquired causes of pre-hepatic jaundice involve following:
- Resorption of extensive hematomas, Auto immune hemolysis, Transfusion reactions
- Trauma, Microangiopathy
- Hemolytic uremic syndrome
- Chemicals e.g. nitrites, aniline dyes, etc.
- Paroxysmal nightly hemoglobinuria
- Thrombotic thrombocytopenic purpura
- Vitamin B12 deficiency, Folic acid deficiency

In this type, an increase in RBC destruction (hemolysis) is responsible for an increase in bilirubin production. The increased breakdown of RBC leads to an increase in unconjugated bilirubin in the blood and deposition of unconjugated bilirubin in the liver Liver hepatocytes. In the liver, Uridine glucoronyl transferase converts unconjugated bilirubin into conjugated bilirubin. The transporter proteins MRP2 and MRP3 (multidrug resistant protein 2&3) of hepatocytes transport conjugated bilirubin to gallbladder and bile is stored. Little amount is stored in intestine, where intestinal microbes convert bile into urobilinogen. 80% eliminated and 20% is reabsorbed. 10% is eliminated through urine after absorption to kidney. 90% reabsorption to liver and process continues.

In case of excess hemolysis, increased amount of unconjugated bilirubin to conjugated bilirubin. Thus, more than required conjugated bilirubin is produced in the liver, where by chance of entering systemic circulation is more (entire amount of unconjugated bilirubin does not convert to conjugated bilirubin, thus, unconjugated bilirubin is also excess). When enters the systemic circulation, cannot be eliminated.

II. Hepatic Jaundice: This type of jaundice arises due to damage to hepatic cells and there is decreased Liver's ability to conjugate or excrete bilirubin and there is increased level of unconjugated bilirubin present. Due to hepatic damage, there is impairment of secretion of conjugated bilirubin into the bile, leading to an increase in plasma conjugated bilirubin.

Causes of Hepatic Jaundice
(i) Viral Hepatitis (HAV, HBV, HCV, HDV, HEV) & other viruses- Epsteinbarr, CBV, HSV.
(ii) Alcoholic Hepatitis (Balloon degeneration, fibrosis of parenchymal tissue), cirrhosis.
(iii) Drug toxicity- Acetaminophen, Isoniazid
(iv) Environmental toxins- vinyl chloride, kava kava, wild mushrooms, Jamaica bush tea-pyrrolizidine alkaloids.
(v) Autoimmune hepatitis.

(vi) Wilson's disease- hepatocellular degeneration due to copper accumulation in liver tissue.

(vii) Inherited conditions-

(i) Indirect Hyperbilirubinemia

1. Gilbert Syndrome - Enzyme deficiency (no UGT) – 10-33% activity only; increased unconjugated bilirubin.

2. Crigler Najjer Syndrome - Type 1(enzyme absent) and Type 2(0-10%activity); Increased Unconjugated Bilirubin.

(ii) Direct Hyperbilirubinemia [4]

1. Dubin Johnson Syndrome - Mutation in MRP2 gene. Defect in canalicular transport of organic anions.

2. Rotonsyndrome - Defect in bilirubin storage.

III. Post-Hepatic Jaundice: It is also known as obstructive jaundice and bilirubin formation rate is normal, any intrahepatic (or) extrahepatic condition leading obstruction to the flow of bile. Conjugation is normal = direct bilirubin. Due to obstruction in the bile duct, which prevents passage of bile containing conjugated bilirubin from liver or gall bladder to intestine. So there is an increase in conjugated bilirubin.

1. Intrahepatic Causes [5]-

(i) Viral hepatitis

(ii) Alcoholic hepatitis

(iii) Primary biliary cirrhosis

(iv) Primary sclerosing cholangitis

(v) Vanishing bile duct syndrome

(vi) Congestive hepatopathy and ischemic hepatitis

(vii) Inherited conditions

(viii) Cholestasis of pregnancy

(ix) Total parenteral nutrition

(x) Infections etc.

2. Extrahepatic Causes-

(a) Malignant Condition - Cholangiocarcinoma, Gallbladder carcinoma, Pancreatic Cancer, Ampullary Cancer,

-Malignant involvement of portal hepatislymphnodes

(b) Benign Condition - Choledocolithiasis

- Post operative biliary strictures

- Primary sclerosing cholangitis

- Chronic pancreatitis

- AIDS Cholangiopathy

- Ascariasis

Clinical Manifestation and Features

Signs and Symptoms

Early features	-	Yellowish discoloration, Pale/ clay colored stool
	-	Dark urine, Pruritis, Urticaria
Late features	-	Xanthelasma and xanthomas.
	-	Malabsorption- weight loss, steatorrhea, osteomalacia, increased bleeding tendency.
	-	Fever, rigor, pain (features of cholangitis)

(i) **Clinical presentations of pre-hepatic jaundice:** Patients with hemolytic jaundice are presented with Anemia, Yellowing of sclera, dark yellow-brown colored urine, yellowish skin and high bilirubin levels

(ii) **Clinical presentations of hepatic jaundice:** The clinical presentations of hepatic jaundice include abdominal pain, fever, vomiting and nausea along with the complications involving satiety, gastrointestinal bleeding, diarrhea, anemia, edema, weight-loss and associated weakness, if unchecked leading to mental disturbances like kernicterus, coma or even death.

(iii) **Clinical presentation of post-hepatic jaundice:** The clinical manifestations of obstructive jaundice are dark urine, pale stools and generalized pruritus. History of fever biliary colic, weight loss, abdominal pain and abdominal mass are also the representatives of obstructive jaundice. Obstructive Jaundice may lead to various complications including cholangitis, pancreatitis, renal and hepatic failure

Diagnosis

- Physical examination (yellowish discoloration)
- Liver function tests (abnormal Bilirubin, ALT, AST levels)
- Complete blood count (low blood count or anemia)
- Electrolyte panel, lipase levels.
- Hepatitis virus panel
- Liver biopsy
- Endoscopic retrograde cholangiopancreatography (ERCP)
- CT scan, MRI, Ultrasound
- Urine analysis

Differential Diagnosis

(i) Carotenoderma, discoloration is limited to palms, soles, forehead, nasolabial fold and not to sclera and inside of mouth; harmless condition.

(ii) Intake of drug Quinacrine (only yellowish of skin, eyes and urine)

(iii) Excessive exposure to phenols.

Complications

Hyperbilirubinemia due to unconjugated fraction may cause bilirubin to accumulate in the grey matter of CNS, potentially causing irreversible neurological damage leading to a condition known as "Kerincterus"; effects may range from clinically unnoticeable to severe brain damage and even death.

Treatment

✓ Treatment depends upon the cause of underlying condition leading to jaundice and any potential complications related to it.

✓ Treatment may consist of expectant management (watchful waiting) at home with rest.

✓ Medical treatment with IV fluids, medications, antibiotics or blood transfusions may be required.

✓ If a drug/toxin is the cause, they must be discontinued.

✓ In certain cases of newborn jaundice, exposing the baby to special colored lights (phototherapy) or exchange blood transfusions may be required to decrease elevated bilirubin levels

✓ Surgical treatment may be required incase of obstructive jaundice.

Other Medical Treatments

✓ Supportive case
✓ IV fluids in case of dehydrations
✓ Medications for Nausea/Vomiting and pain
✓ Antibiotics and Antivirals
✓ Blood Transfusions
✓ Steroids
✓ Chemotherapy/Radiation Therapy
✓ Phototherapy

Surgery: May be necessary in certain cases of cancer, congenital malformations, conditions that obstruct the bile ducts, gall stones and abnormalities of spleen.

✓ Sometimes, a liver transplant may be necessary

Neonatal Jaundice [6, 7, 8]

Jaundice is clinically detectable in the new born when the serum bilirubin levels ate greater than 35μmol/L. This occurs in approximately 60% of term infants and 80% of preterm infants.

Neonatal jaundice first becomes visible in the face and forehead. Blenching reveals the underlying color. Jaundice then gradually becomes visible on the trunk and extremities. Additional signs and symptoms that may be seen in newborn includes-

(i)   Poor feeding
(ii) Lethargy

(iii) Changes in muscle tone

(iv) High-pitched voice

(v) Seizures

Jaundice in Pregnancy

Intrahepatic cholestasis of pregnancy (ICP), also known as obstetric cholestasis, cholestasis of pregnancy, jaundice of pregnancy, and prurigogravidarum, is a medical condition in which cholestasis occurs during pregnancy. It typically presents with troublesome itching and can lead to complications for both mother and foetus.

Pruritus (itching) is a common symptom of pregnancy. Itching is caused by changes to the skin, that of abdomen, palms of the hands, soles of the feet. ICP occurs most commonly in the third trimester.

Treatement

Ursodeoxycholic Acid.

Vitamin K to avoid the risk of hemorrhage at delivery.

Patient Counselling

- ✓ Maintain adequate hydration by drinking fluids, and rest as needed.
- ✓ Take medications only as instructed and prescribed by a health care practitioner.
- ✓ Avoid medications, herbs or supplements which may cause detrimental side effects.
- ✓ Ensuring that you stick to the recommended daily alcohol (RAD) for alcohol consumption.
- ✓ Provide adequate milk intake for the body in cases of Breastfeeding Jaundice.
- ✓ If symptoms worsen or new symptoms arise, consult a health case practitioner.

Case Study of Neonatal Jaundice

Summary

A female patient of 5 days of age weighing 2.65kg was admitted in NICU with c/o yellowing of skin and cornea and increased serum bilirubin levels.

Physical examination- Colour –pink/yellow

Posture-flexed.

The following medications were given:

1. Inj.Vit K   IM   1mg   OD

2. Inj. Ampicillin IV 150MG   BD

Patient counseling: There's no real way to prevent newborn jaundice. During pregnancy, you can have your blood type tested.

After birth, your baby's blood type will be tested, if necessary, to rule out the possibility of blood type incompatibility that can lead to newborn jaundice. If your baby does have jaundice, there are ways you can prevent it from becoming more severe:

- Make sure your baby is getting enough nutrition through breast milk. Feeding your baby 8 to 12 times a day for the first several days ensures that your baby isn't dehydrated, which helps bilirubin pass through their body more quickly.
- If you're not breastfeeding feeding your baby formula, give your baby 1 to 2 ounces of formula every 2 to 3 hours for the first week. Preterm or smaller babies may take smaller amounts of formula, as will babies who are also receiving breast milk. Talk to your doctor if you're concerned your baby is taking too little or too much formula, or if they won't wake to feed at least 8 times per 24 hour.

Assignment

1. **Which factors increase the risk for neonatal jaundice?**
   - Sepsis; Foetal maternal blood group incompatibility
   - Pre maturity low birth weight; Cephalohematomas; Bruising
   - Trauma from instrumented delivery
   - Delayed meconium passage
   - Babies of diabetic mother.

2. **What is the difference between physiological and neonatal jaundice?**

   Physiological jaundice is caused by a combination of increased bilirubin production secondary to accelerated destruction of erythrocytues decreased excretory capacity secondary to low levels of ligandinin hepatocytes and low activity of the bilirubin conjugating enzyme uridine diphosphoglucoronyl transferase (UDPGT).

   Pathologic neonatal jaundice occurs when additional factors accompany the basic mechanisms described above. Examples include immune or non immune hemolytic anemia. Polycythemia and the presence of bruising or other extravasation of blood.

3. **Which conditions may require additional testing during evaluation of neonatal jaundice?**

   In infants who have hepatospleenomegaly, petechiae, thrombocytopenia or other findings suggestive of hepatobiliary disease, metabolic disorder or congenital infection, early measurement of bilirubin fractions is suggested.

   The same may apply to infants who remain jaundiced beyond the first 7-10 days of life and to infants whose total serum bilirubin levels repeatedly rebound following treatment.

4. What are recommended guidelines for the treatment of neonatal jaundice?

> **Phototherapy:** Absorption of light through the skin converts unconjugated bilirubin into bilirubin photoproducts that are excreted in the stool and urine.

> **Exchange transfusion:** Performed in infants with TSB levels in the range indicated by the nomogram, with TSB levels of 25mg per dl or greater and with jaundice and signs of acute bilirubin encephalopathy.

> **Modified breast feeding:** The American Academy of Pediatrics recommends promoting breast feeding for infants with jaundice assessing for the adequacy of breast feeding and increasing the frequency to 8-12 times per day.

> IV immunoglobulin.

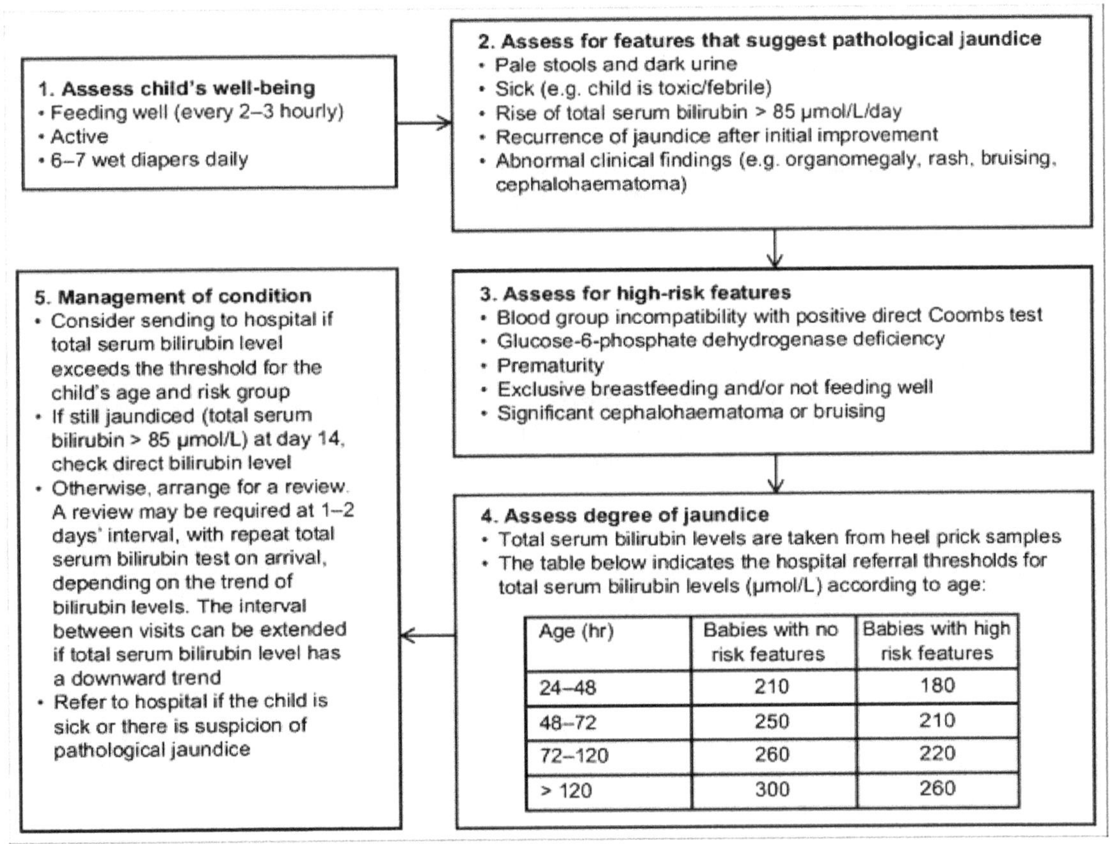

Age (hr)	Babies with no risk features	Babies with high risk features
24–48	210	180
48–72	250	210
72–120	260	220
> 120	300	260

Fig. 60.2 Algorithm for diagnosis of Neonatal Jaundice[9,10].

Souce: Mark Ng et al., When babies turn yellow. Singapore Medical Journal. Nov 2015; 56(11): 599-603.

5. Which medications are given for infants with physiologic neonatal jaundice?

Phenobarbital is inducer of hepatic bilirubin metabolism.

Reduces mean serum bilirubin values during 1st week of life.

6. What are the risk factors for hyperbilirubinemia in neonatal jaundice?
 ➢ Having siblings who had neonatal jaundice
 ➢ Having parents of East Asian or Mediterranean descent.
 ➢ Preterm babies, Poor feeding; Mother with diabetes
 ➢ Newborn with bruising or hematoma
 ➢ Blood type incompatibility; congenital infection.

References

1. W.A. Muhammad, T. Shamshad, A.A. Muhammad, J. Rukhsar. Jaundice: a basic review. Int J Res Med Sci, 4 (2016), pp. 1313-1319

2. Vandana Janghel et al., Plants used for the treatment of icterus (jaundice) in Central India; A Review Annals of hepatology, 2019; Vol 18(5): 658-672.

3. Vandana Janghel, Pushpendra Patel, Saket Singh Chandel. Plants used for the treatment of icterus (jaundice) in Central India: A review. Annals of hepatology. 2019; Vol 18 (5): 658-672.

4. Huang MJ, Kua KE, Teng HC, Tang KS, Weng HW, Huang CS. Risk factors for severe hyperbilirubinemia in neonates. *Pediatr Res*. 2004 Nov. 56(5):682-9.

5. Yusoff S, Van Rostenberghe H, Yusoff NM, et al. Frequencies of A(TA)7TAA, G71R, and G493R mutations of the UGT1A1 gene in the Malaysian population. *Biol Neonate*. 2006. 89(3):171-6.

6. Memon N, Weinberger BI, Hegyi T, Aleksunes LM. Inherited disorders of bilirubin clearance. *Pediatr Res*. 2015 Nov 23.

7. Watchko JF, Lin Z. Genetics of neonatal jaundice. Stevenson DK, Maisels MJ, Watchko JF. *Care of the jaundiced neonate*. New York: McGraw-Hill; 2012. 1-27.

8. Schutzman DL, Sekhon R, Hundalani S. Hour-specific bilirubin nomogram in infants with ABO incompatibility and direct Coombs-positive results. *Arch Pediatr Adolesc Med*. 2010 Dec. 164(12):1158-64

9. [Guideline] American Academy of Pediatrics Subcommittee on Hyperbilirubinemia. Management of hyperbilirubinemia in the newborn infant 35 or more weeks of gestation. *Pediatrics*. 2004 Jul. 114(1):297-316.

10. Mark Ng and choon How How. When babies turn yellow. Singapore medical journal. 2015; 56(11):599-603

CHAPTER - 61

Peptic Ulcer Disease

Introduction to Peptic Ulcer Disease

- It is a group of ulcerative disorders effecting the upper gastro intestinal tract due to abnormal acid or pepsin secretion
- Peptic ulcer disease (PUD) differs from gastritis and erosions in that ulcer extends deeper into the muscularis mucosa
- They could be gastric ulcers (can occur anywhere in the stomach) or duodenal ulcers (occur in the first part of duodenum)

Forms:

1. Helicobacter pylori (H. pylori) associated
2. NSAID induced
3. Stress ulcers (stress related mucosal damage) (or)   Stress gastritis

Epidemology

- Increased prevalence rate in H. pylori
- Mostly seen in men
- 10- 20% of the ulcers develop into peptic ulcer and 1% may change into cancer

Etiology and Risk Factors

H. pylori and NSAIDs are the two most common causes of chronic PUD. Most peptic ulcers occur in presence of acid and pepsin when *H. pylori*, NSAID or other factors disrupt mucosal defense and healing mechanism. Hypersecretion of acid is primary mechanism. Less common causes include hypersecretory states such as Zollinger-Ellison syndrome (ZES), viral infections (e.g., cytomegalovirus), radiation, and chemotherapy (e.g., hepatic artery infusion).

- o ***H. pylori***: It causes chronic gastritis in all infected individulas. Eradication of *H. pylori* decreases ulcer recurrence and recurrent bleeding. Prevalence rate is higher. Transmission can be through fecal-oral, oral-oral, gastro–oral (through inadequately sterilized endoscopes), but fecal-oral route is most common.

o **NSAID:** 15-30% of regular NSAID users may develop gastroduodenal ulcers within a week or with continued treatment (6 months or longer). They occur less frequently in oesophagus and colon. It is a dose related risk. The risk of GI bleeding increases when taken concurrently with anticoagulants, antiplatelet drugs and serotonin reuptake inhibitors, older than 60 years of age, concomitant use of steroids, chronic cardiovascular disease.

o **Cigarette smoking:** It can contribute to PUD due to delayed gastric emptying of solids and liquids, inhibition of pancreatic bicarbonate secretion, promotion of duodenogastric reflex or reduction in mucosal prostaglandin production. Smoking increases gastric acid secretion.

o **Diet:** Caffeine, tea, beer, cola act as acid stimulants and alcohol may cause acute mucosal damage at high concentrations and may lead to upper GI bleeding.

o Risk is more with Stress, corticosteroids, chronic diseases as chronic renal failure, hepatic cirrhosis, chronic pancreatitis, chronic pulmonary disease, and Crohn's disease.

Indications for Testing and Treating *Helicobacter Pylori* Infection [1]

Recommended (evidence established)

- Uninvestigated dyspepsia (depending on *H. pylori* prevalence)
- PUD (active gastric or duodenal ulcer)
- History of PUD (confirmed ulcer not previously treated for *H. pylori*)
- Gastric MALT lymphoma
- Following resection of early gastric cancer
- Reduce the risk of recurrent bleeding from gastroduodenal ulcer

Risk Factors for Nonsteroidal Anti-Inflammatory Drug-Induced Ulcer and Ulcer-Related Upper Gastrointestinal Complications [2]

- Confirmed prior ulcer or ulcer-related complication , Age >65 years,
- Multiple or high-dose NSAID use,
- Concomitant use of aspirin (including cardioprotective dosages)
- Concomitant use of an anticoagulant, corticosteroid, bisphosphonate, clopidogrel, or SSRI
- Selection of NSAID (selectivity of COX-1 vs. COX-2)

Pathophysiology

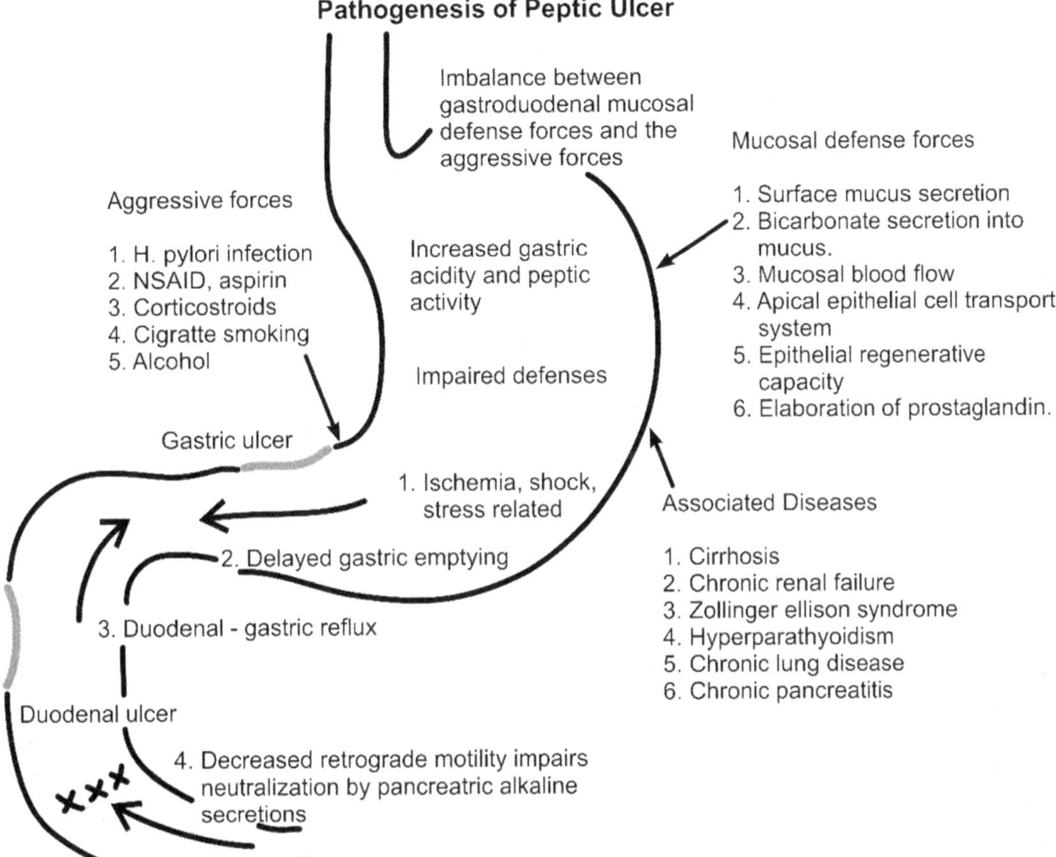

Fig. 61.1 Pathogenesis of Peptic ulcer disease.

Peptic ulcers occur due to an imbalance between aggressive factors (gastric acid, bile salts, *H.Pylori*, NSAIDs and pepsin) and protective factors (mucosal defense promoters- mucosal blood flow, mucus, mucus, mucosal bicarbonate secretion, mucosal cell restitution, and epitherlial cell renewal). Gastric acid is secreted by parietal cells that contain receptors for histamine, gastrin and acetylcholine. There is increased gastirc acid secretions due to their action on gastric parietal cells. Patients with Zollinger- Ellison's syndrome have gastric acid hypersecretion due to gastrin producing tumor. Pepsin is an important co factor that plays a role in proteolytic activity involved in ulcer formation. Pepsin is activated by acid (pH 1.8- 3.5), Destroyed irreversibly at pH7, Inactivated reversibly at pH 4. Mucosal defense and repair mechanism protects gastroduodenal mucosa from endogenous and exogenous substances. Mucous bicarbonate barrier of neutral pH protects the stomach from acidic contents in gastric lumen. Prostaglandins maintain mucosal integrity and repair the mucosa.

H. pylori: Spiral shaped, pH sensitive, gram negative bacteria. Resides between mucous layer and surface epithelial cells or any location where gastric like epithelium is found. Survival of bacteria in low pH: *H. pylori* release large amounts of urease, which *hydrolyzes* Urea in gastric juice and converts it into ammonia and CO_2. Ammonia acts as a local buffer creating a neutral environment surrounding the bacterium and protecting it from the acid. Production of acid inhibitory proteins also allow it to survive the low pH of stomach.

Mechanism: *H. pylori* attaches to gastric parietal cells by adherence pedestals (Prevents the organism from being shed during cell turnover and mucous secretion). Colonization of bacteria takes place and there is release of lipase, urease and bacterial enzymes. Decreased repair/ defense mechanism occur.

(A) Direct mucosal damage is produced by virulence factors such as Strains
   (a) Vacuolating cytotoxin (Vac A) consists of 50% of the cases
   (b) Cytotoxin associated gene protein (Cag A) causing duodenal ulcer, gastric ulcer consisting of Cag A -ve and Cag A +ve
(B) Damage of epithelial cells by bacteria is due to:
   (a) Ammonia in urease in toxic to gastric epithelial cell
   (b) Bacterial adherence enhances uptake of toxins
   (c) Infection alters host immune response and damages epithelial cells

NSAID induced ulcer mecahnism: Gastric mucosa is damaged by: Direct or topical irritation by gastric epithelium and Systemic inhibition of endogenous prostaglandin synthesis. Cyclooxygenase- I (found in stomach, kidney, intestine and platelets) which are responsible for producing protective prostaglandins and responsible for regulation of physiological process such as GI mucosal integrity. NSAIDs inhibit COX-1, so decreased production of prostaglandins which are usually responsible for mucus secretion in the GI lumen and prevents the acid form interacting with parieital cells with acid. Thus prostaglandins responsible for mucosal integrity are not present so results in ulcer formation. Inhibition of COX- I also causes decreased platelet aggregation, prolonged bleeding time, causing increased potential for upper and lower GI bleeding

Clinical Manifestation and Features

Varies depending on severity of pain and complication
- Epigastric pain, Dyspepsia
- Burning sensation, abdominal fullness, cramping
- Heart burn, Bloating accompanying pain
- Nausea, vomiting, Anorexia, weight loss
- Blood stools, Bleeding disorders

Complications
- Upper GI bleeding (10-15%), Perforation into abdominal cavity (7%), and gastric obstruction (2%).

- NSAID induced have most serious and life-threatening complications. Bleeding is due to erosion of ulcers into an artery (occurs in 10-15% of patient). It maybe hidden or present as melena (black coloured stools), hematemesis (vomiting of blood). Deaths occur in patients who rebleed after the initial bleed has stopped or who continue to bleed
- Perforation in peritoneal cavity occurs in 7% of patients, Higher mortality for perforated gastric ulcer
- Pain of perforation is sharp, severe, first in epigastrium and spreads to entire abdomen. Gastric outlet obstruction caused by scarring causing symptoms such as: Anorexia, Nausea, Vomiting, Weight loss

Diagnosis with Algorithm

If the patient is identified as NSAID-induced ulcer patient, discontinue NSAID. Initiate H2 receptor antagonists or PPI or sucralfate. Then *H.Pylori* culture testing has to be done.

- If *H.Pylori* positive –initiate either triple therapy or quadruple therapy.
- If *H.Pylori* negative- no treatment needed.
- If the patient is identified as NSAID –induced ulcer patient but unable to discontinue NSAID- continue NSAID at lowest effective dose and shortest duration; add PPI.
- Alternatively to reduce the risk of developing an NSAID-induced ulcer, switch to a selective COX-2 inhibitor of Misoprostal.

Diagnostic Tests for *Helicobacter pylori* Infection [3]

Tests Utilizing Gastric Mucosal Biopsy in Patients Undergoing Endoscopy

1. **Rapid Urease Test:**
   - Tests for active *H. pylori* infection; >90% sensitivity and >95% specificity.
   - Withhold H2RAs and PPIs 1 to 2 weeks prior to testing and antibiotics and bismuth salts 4 weeks prior to testing to reduce the risk of false negatives.
   - In the presence of *H.pylori* urease, urea is metabolized to ammonia and bicarbonate resulting in an increase in pH, which changes the color of a pH-sensitive indicator.
   - Results are rapid (usually within a few hours), and test is less expensive than histology or culture.

2. **Histology**
   - Considered "gold standard" for detection of *H. pylori* infection; >95% sensitivity and >95% specificity.
   - Permits further histologic analysis and evaluation of infected tissue (e.g., gastritis, ulceration, adenocarcinoma); tests for active *H. pylori* infection.
   - Results are not immediate; not recommended for intitial diagnosis; more expensive than rapid urease test.

3. **Culture**
   - Permits sensitivity testing to determine antibiotic choice or resistance; 100% specific.
   - Use usually limited to patients who fail several courses of eradication therapy; tests for active *H. pylori* infection.

> Results are not immediate; not recommended for initial diagnosis; more expensive than rapid urease test.

Tests that do not Utilize Gastric Mucosal Biopsy

1. **Urea Breath Test**
   - Tests for active *H. pylori* infection; >95% sensitivity and >95% specificity.
   - Radiolabeled urea with either C13 or C14 is given orally; urease secreted by *H. pylori* in the stomach (if present) hydrolyzes radiolabed urea to produce radiolabled CO_2, which is exhaled and then quantified from the expired breath; radiation exposure is minimal.
   - Withhold H2RAs and PPIs 1 to 2 weeks prior to testing and antibiotics and bismuth salts 4 weeks prior to testing to reduce the risk of false negatives.
   - Used to detect *H. pylori* prior to treatment and to document posttreatment eradicaton.
   - Results usually take about 2 days; less expensive than tests that utilize gastric mucosal biopsy but more expensive than serologic tests.

2. **Serologic Antibody Tests**
   - Detects IgG antibodies to *H. pylori* in serum, whole blood or urine; quantitative seriologic tests have a sensitivity of about 85% and specificity of about 79%.
   - Qualitative in office tests; provide results quickly (usually within 15 minutes) but yield more variable results.
   - Tests are widely available and inexpensive.
   - Not of benefit in documenting eradication, because antibodies to *H. pylori* remain positive for years following successful eradication of the infection.
   - Results not affected by H2RAs, PPIs, antibiotics, or bismuth.

3. **Fecal Antigen Test**
   - Identifies *H. pylori* antigen in stool; sensitivity and specificity comparable to the UBT for initial diagnosis.
   - H2RAs, PPIs, antibiotics, and bismuth may cause false-negative results but to a lesser exent than the UBT.
   - Considered an alterative to detecting *H. pylori* prior to treatment and documenting posttreatment eradicaton

Management

Goals:
- Relieving ulcer pain
- Healing the ulcer
- Preventing reoccurrence
- Reducing ulcer related complications
- Eradicate *H. pylori*

Non-pharmacological Therapy

- o Eliminate physiological stress, cigarette smoking, usage of NSAID
- o Avoid food that is spicy or beverages such as coke, alcohol, caffeine that causes dyspepsia or exacerbate ulcer symptoms
- o Alternate drugs such as acetaminophen, non-acetylated salicylate (e.g.: salsalate) or cox-2 inhibitors should be used for relief of pain
- o Surgeries include Vagotomy (inhibits vagal stimulation of gastric acid)

Pharmacological Therapy:

Algorithm:

Algorithm for Evaluation and Management of Ulcer Patients

Patient presents with dyspnoea and alarm symptoms present or age old than 55 years.

- If yes: Esophagogastroduodenoscopy (EGD) for barium studies. If EGD not feasible and ulcer present eradicate H.Pylori; administer antisecretory agents 4-8 weeks.
- If No: Detect and treat H.pylori infection. Advice discontinuation of NSAIDs, smoking, alcohol and drug abuse. Administer antisecretory agents with PPI preferably of H2 blocker for 4 weeks.
  - (a) Good clinical response: Long term mianteance with H2 blocker or PPI. If symptoms recur consider EGD.
  - (b) Persistent symptoms: continue H2 blocker or PPI for 4-8 weeks. If response is good consider maintenance therapy. If inadequate then poceed for EGD.

Mechanism of Action of Drugs:

1. **Proton Pump Inhibitors**: They bind to H^+/K^+ ATPase enzyme of gastric parietal cells and inhibit acid secretion. Inhibits basal and stimulated gastric acid secretion

   E.g.: Omeprazole, Pantoprazole, Rabeprazole

   ADR: Headache, nausea, vomiting, abdominal pain.
2. **H2 Receptor Antagonist**: Blocks H2 Receptors in parietal cells suppressing basal and meal-based secretion of gastric acid.

   E.g.: Cimetidine,   Famotidine,   Ranitidine,   Nizatidine
3. **Sucralfate:** Reacts with HCL in stomach forming cross links and paste like material and acts as acid buffer. Binds to proteins on surfaces of ulcer, forming stable insoluble complexes serving as protective barrier at ulcer surface.
4. **Prostaglandins analogue:** E.g.: Misoprostol. Synthetic E_1 analog. Inhibits acid secretion and enhances mucosal defense

   ADR: Diarrhea, abdominal cramping, flatulence, headache. Avoided in pregnant women as it produces uterine contractions.

5. **Bismuth Preparations**: E.g.: Bismuth subsalicylate. Bismuth subcitrate potassium. Acts as antibacterial. Local gastroprotective, Stimulates endogenous prostaglandins.
   ADR: Bleeding disorders, black coloured stool, tongue

6. **Antacids:** Neutralizes gastric acid. Inactivates pepsin Bind to bile salts. Aluminum containing antacid suppresses *H. pylori* and enhances mucosal defense.

   ADR: Constipation, diarrhea, hypophosphatemia (as they interfere with phosphate absorption). Caution: Magnesium containing antacids are avoided in patients with creatinine clearance less than 30ml/min. It interacts with drugs containing iron, tetracycline, warfarin, digoxin, isoniazid, ketoconazole, fluoroquinolones (interactions are avoided by giving a 2h hap between the drugs).

Table 61.1 Oral Drug Regimens Used to Eradicate Helicobacter Pylori Infection.

(i) Proton pump inhibitor based triple therapy:

Drug #1	Drug#2	Drug #3	Drug #4
Omeprazole – 20mg twice daily or lansoprazole- 30mg twice daily	Clarithromycin - 500mg BD	Amoxicillin- 1g BD or metronidazole -500mg BD	

(ii) Bismuth based quadruple therapy:

Omeprazole – 40mg twice daily or Pantoprazole- 40mg twice daily Or ulcer healing doses of H 2 receptor antagonist for 4-6 weeks	Bismuth Subsalicyalte- 525mg four time daily	Metronidazole 250-500mg four times daily	Tetracycline 500mg four times or Amoxicillin 500mg four times daily or Clarithromycin 250-500mg four times daily

(iii) Sequential therapy:

PPI once or twice daily on days 1-10	Amoxicillin 1g twice daily on day 1-5	Metronidazole 250-500mg twice daily on days 6-10	Clarithromycin 250-500mg daily on days 6-10

(iv) Second line (salvage) therapy for persistent infection:

PPI once or twice daily	Amoxicillin 1g twice daily	Levofloxacin 250mg twice daily	

Initial treatment failure:

Second line treatment should:
   (a) Use antibiotic that were not previously used during initial therapy
   (b) Using antibiotic that have no resistance problem
   (c) Drug that has topical effect such as bismuth

NSAID Induced Ulcer:

Prophylactic cotherapy is given or be switched to a cox- 2 inhibitor

Oral Drug Regimens to Heal Peptic Ulcers or Maintain Ulcer Healing

Duodenal or Gastric ulcer healing (mg)   Maintenance of gastric healing(mg)

- ➢ **PPI**

Omeprazole	20–40 daily	20–40 daily
Lansoprazole	15–30 daily	15–30 daily
Rabeprazole	20 daily	20 daily
Pantoprazole	40 daily	40 daily

- ➢ **Histamine-2 receptor antagonists**

Cimetidine 300 four times daily, 400–800 at bedtime; 400 twice daily 800 at bedtime
Famotidine 20 twice daily 20–40 at bedtime ;   20-40 at bedtime

Nizatidine 150 twice daily   150–300 at bedtime

    300 at bedtime

Ranitidine 150 twice daily   150–300 at bedtime

    300 at bedtime

- ➢ **Promote mucosal defense**

Sucralfate (g/dose) 1 g four times daily   1–2 g twice daily

    2 g twice daily   1g four times daily20–40 daily

Diagnosis and management of nonvariceal upper gastrointestinal hemorrhage: European Society of Gastrointestinal Endoscopy (ESGE) Guideline [4]

Main Recommendations

1. ESGE recommends immediate assessment of hemodynamic status in patients who present with acute upper gastrointestinal hemorrhage (UGIH), with prompt intravascular volume replacement initially using crystalloid fluids if hemodynamic instability exists (strong recommendation, moderate quality evidence).

2. ESGE recommends a restrictive red blood cell transfusion strategy that aims for a target hemoglobin between 7 g/dL and 9 g/dL. A higher target hemoglobin should be considered in patients with significant co-morbidity (e. g., ischemic cardiovascular disease) (strong recommendation, moderate quality evidence).

3. ESGE recommends the use of the GlasgowBlatchford Score (GBS) for pre-endoscopy risk stratification. Outpatients determined to be at very low risk, based upon a GBS score of 0–1, do not require early endoscopy nor hospital admission. Discharged patients

should be informed of the risk of recurrent bleeding and be advised to maintain contact with the discharging hospital (strong recommendation, moderate quality evidence).

4. ESGE recommends initiating high dose intravenous proton pump inhibitors (PPI), intravenous bolus followed by continuous infusion (80mg then 8mg/hour), in patients presenting with acute UGIH awaiting upper endoscopy. However, PPI infusion should not delay the performance of early endoscopy (strong recommendation, high quality evidence).

5. ESGE does not recommend the routine use of nasogastric or orogastric aspiration/lavage in patients presenting with acute UGIH (strong recommendation, moderate quality evidence). 6. ESGE recommends intravenous erythromycin (single dose, 250mg given 30–120 minutes prior to upper gastrointestinal [GI] endoscopy) in patients with clinically severe or ongoing active UGIH. In selected patients, pre-endoscopic infusion of erythromycin significantly improves endoscopic visualization, reduces the need for secondlook endoscopy, decreases the number of units of blood transfused, and reduces duration of hospital stay (strong recommendation, high quality evidence).

6. Following hemodynamic resuscitation, ESGE recommends early (≤24 hours) upper GI endoscopy. Very early (< 12 hours) upper GI endoscopy may be considered in patients with high risk clinical features, namely: hemodynamic instability (tachycardia, hypotension) that persists despite ongoing attempts at volume resuscitation; in-hospital bloody emesis/nasogastric aspirate; or contraindication to the interruption of anticoagulation (strong recommendation, moderate quality evidence).

7. ESGE recommends that peptic ulcers with spurting or oozing bleeding (Forrest classification Ia and Ib, respectively) or with a nonbleeding visible vessel (Forrest classification IIa) receive endoscopic hemostasis because these lesions are at high risk for persistent bleeding or rebleeding (strong recommendation, high quality evidence).

8. ESGE recommends that peptic ulcers with an adherent clot (Forrest classification IIb) be considered for endoscopic clot removal. Once the clot is removed, any identified underlying active bleeding (Forrest classification Ia or Ib) or nonbleeding visible vessel (Forrest classification IIa) should receive endoscopic hemostasis (weak recommendation, moderate quality evidence).

9. In patients with peptic ulcers having a flat pigmented spot (Forrest classification IIc) or clean base (Forrest classification III), ESGE does not recommend endoscopic hemostasis as these stigma ta present a low risk of recurrent bleeding. In selected clinical settings, these patients may be discharged to home on standard PPI therapy, e. g., oral PPI once-daily (strong recommendation, moderate quality evidence).

10. ESGE recommends that epinephrine injection therapy not be used as endoscopic monotherapy. If used, it should be combined with a second endoscopic hemostasis modality (strong recommendation, high quality evidence).

11. ESGE recommends PPI therapy for patients who receive endoscopic hemostasis and for patients with adherent clot not receiving endoscopic hemostasis. PPI therapy should be high dose and administered as an intravenous bolus followed by continuous infusion

(80mg then 8mg/hour) for 72 hours post endoscopy (strong recommendation, high quality evidence).

12. ESGE does not recommend routine second-look endoscopy as part of the management of nonvariceal upper gastrointestinal hemorrhage (NVUGIH). However, in patients with clinical evidence of rebleeding following successful initial endoscopic hemostasis, ESGE recommends repeat upper endoscopy with hemostasis if indicated. In the case of failure of this second attempt at hemostasis, transcatheter angiographic embolization (TAE) or surgery should be considered (strong recommendation, high quality evidence).

13. In patients with NVUGIH secondary to peptic ulcer, ESGE recommends investigating for the presence of Helicobacter pylori in the acute setting with initiation of appropriate antibiotic therapy when H. pylori is detected. Re-testing for H. pylori should be performed in those patients with a negative test in the acute setting. Documentation of successful H. pylori eradication is recommended (strong recommendation, high quality evidence).

14. In patients receiving low dose aspirin for secondary cardiovascular prophylaxis who develop peptic ulcer bleeding, ESGE recommends aspirin be resumed immediately following index endoscopy if the risk of rebleeding is low (e. g., FIIc, FIII). In patients with high risk peptic ulcer (FIa, FIb, FIIa, FIIb), early reintroduction of aspirin by day 3 after index endoscopy is recommended, provided that adequate hemostasis has been established (strong recommendation, moderate quality evidence).

References

1. Talley NJ, Vakil N. Practice Parameters Committee of the American College of Gastroenterology. Guidelines for the management of dyspepsia. Am J Gastroenterol 2005; 100: 2324.
2. Chey WD, Wong BCY. Practice Parameters Committee of American College of Gastroenterology. Guideline on the management of Helicobacter pylori infection. Am J Gastroenterol 2007; 102: 1808.
3. Dzierzanowska-Fangrat K et al. Diagnosis of Helicobacter pylori infection. Helicobacter 2006; 11(Suppl 1):6
4. Gralnek Ian M et al. Nonvariceal upper gastrointestinal hemorrhage: ESGE Guideline… Endoscopy 2015; 47: a1–a46
5. Amrish Kumar, VrishDhwaj Ashwlayan, Mansi Verma. Diagnostic approach & pharmacological treatment regimen of Peptic Ulcer Disease. Pharmacy and Pharmaceutical Research Open Access Journal. (2019); 1(1):1–12.

CHAPTER - 62

Anaemia

Introduction to Anemia

Anemia is a group of diseases characterized by a decrease in either hemoglobin or the volume of RBC resulting in decreased oxygen carrying capacity in blood.

WHO defines anemia as Hb levels:

For females: <12g/dl

For men: <13g/dl

Epidemiology [1]

A moderate degree of iron-deficiency anemia affected approximately 610 million people worldwide or 8.8% of the population. It is slightly more common in females (9.9%) than males (7.8%). Mild iron deficiency anemia affects another 375 million.

Classification of Anaemias Based on Morphology

1. Microcytic anemias (MCV<80 μm^3):
   - Iron deficiency anemia
   - Anemia of chronic disease
   - Thalassemia (I and II)
   - Sideroblastic anemia
2. Macrocytic anemias (MCV> 100 μm^3)
   (a) Megaloblastic anemia: Folate defiency/ Vitamin B12 defiency
   (b) Nonmegaloblastic anemia: liver disease/ alcoholism/ reticulocytosis/ drugs
3. Normocytic anemias (MCV 80-100 μm^3)
   Corrected reticulocyte count

If < 3%:
- ➤ blood loss< 1 week/Early stage iron deficiency / Early stage anemia chronic disease
- ➤ Renal disease/Malignancy

If ≥ 3%: (a) intrinsic RBC defect

> ➢ Membrane defects- hereditary spherocytosis/ hereditary elliptocytosis/
>
> ➢ Paroxysmal nocturnal hemoglobinuria
>
> ➢ Abnormal hemoglobins: sickle cell disease
>
> ➢ Deficient enzymes: G6PD deficiency/ pyruvate kinase deficiency

(b) Extrinsic RBC defect

> ➢ Blood loss > 1 week/ immune haemolytic anemias/ malaria/
>
> ➢ Micro/macroangiopathic haemolytic anemia

Etiological Clasification of Anemias

Anaemias due to impaired red cell production:

1. Anaemias due to deficiency of nutrients- iron deficiency anemias
   Megaloblastic anemia due to deficiency of folate or Vit B12
2. Anemia of chronic disease
3. Sideroblastic anemia
4. Aplastic anemia
5. Anemia of chronic disease
6. Anemia of endocrine disorders
7. Congenital dyserythropoietic anemia

Amemias due to red cell destruction (Hemolytic anemia)

1. Abnormally intrinsic to red cells
   (a) Defects in red cell membrane: hereditary spherocytosis, hereditary elliptocytosis
   (b) Defects in haemoglobin: thalasemias, sickle cell disease
   (c) Defects in enzymes: glucose -6-phosphate dehydrogenase deficiency, pyruvate kinase deficiency
2. Abnormally extrinsic to red cells
   (a) Immune haemolytic anemias: autoimmune, alloimmune, drug induced
   (b) Mechanical haemolytic anemias: microangiopathic, cardiac, hemoglobinuria
   (c) Direct action of physical, chemical or infectious agents
   (d) hypersplenism

1. **Microcytic Anemia:** It is caused by defects in haemoglobin synthesis.

   Iron deficiency anemia: Iron is the main component of hemoglobin, lack of iron results in decreased synthesis of hemoglobin, resulting in a reduction in the size of red blood cells. It can be due to decreased intake of iron, increased iron demand in the body (Pregnancy, infancy, lactation) decreased iron absorption (achlorhydria, gastric surgery, phytate, bran, drugs, celiac disease), chronic blood loss, in younger woman due to menstruation, in non menstruating women and in men due to gastrointestinal hemorrhage (esophageal varices, hiatus hernia, peptic ulcer, gastritis, neoplasm, hook worm infestation).

Anemia of chronic disease: Anemia of chronic disease is strongly associated with inflammatory diseases. In a chronic inflammatory state, the liver produces a protein called hepcidin. It works to stop iron absorption in the duodenum and prevents iron recycling by inhibiting the breakdown of old RBCs. Reduction in serum iron results in anemia of chronic disease. Causes are A) chronic inflammation- rheumatoid arthritis, systemic lupus erythematosus, chron's disease. B) chronic infection- tuberculosis, urinary tract infections, HIV, pneumonia. C) neoplasm- carcinoma, lymphoma, myeloma.

Sideroblastic anemia: Sideroblastic anemia occurs due to abnormalities in the synthesis of protoporphyrin, which results in decreased synthesis of hemoglobin. This happens because protoporphyrin along with iron makes heme (which combines with globular protein to make hemoglobin).

Iron accumulates in the cells because it is not being utilized to make heme due to the absence of protoporphyrin. This results in the characteristic ring sideroblast – iron-laden mitochondria making a ring around the nucleus of the RBC precursor cells.

Thalassemia: Thalassemia occurs due to abnormalities in the synthesis of the globular chains that attach to heme to make hemoglobin. There are two types of thalassemias:

Alpha thalassemia: Occurs because of gene deletion

3 gene deletion: HbH, this is because beta chains start making tetramers in the absence of alpha chains; symptoms are apparent after birth.

Beta thalassemia: Occurs due to gene mutation; there are 2 types:

Minor: Mild, asymptomatic

Major: Normal in fetus; severe anemia after birth

2. **Macrocytic Anemia:** In this type of anemia, the mean corpuscular volume is greater than 96 μm^3.

    Megaloblastic anemia: It is the most common form of macrocytic anemia and is caused specifically by vitamin B12 and/or folate deficiency.

    Vitamin B12 deficiency: Vitamin B12 is a water-soluble vitamin found in animal-derived proteins. The most common cause of vitamin B12 deficiency is pernicious anemia, which is autoimmune-mediated destruction of the parietal cells of the stomach that decreases the production of hydrochloric acid and intrinsic factor, both of which are needed for absorption of vitamin B12.

    Other causes include pancreatic insufficiency (as pancreatic enzymes are needed to free vitamin B12) and damage to the part of the small intestine (terminal Ileum) where vitamin B12 is absorbed.

    Folate deficiency: Folate is derived from green leafy vegetables like asparagus and broccoli. The body doesn't have large stores of folate so an increased demand or poor diet can result in folate deficiency within a month.

3. **Normocytic Anemia:** The mean corpuscular volume in normocytic anemia is within the range of **80–96 μm^3**.

    Extrinsic defect in red blood cells

This includes the following types of blood disorders:

1. **Immune hemolytic anemias:** IgG- or IgM-mediated destruction of RBCs; direct and indirect Coombs tests are used for diagnostic purposes.

Intrinsic defect in red blood dells

This includes membrane defects, abnormal hemoglobin, and enzymatic defects.

Membrane defects

Hereditary spherocytosis: Inherited defect in the proteins that maintain the integrity of the RBC membrane, leading to round, small cells with no central pallor; diagnosed with osmotic fragility test.

Abnormal hemoglobin

Sickle cell anemia is a genetic defect in the synthesis of hemoglobin chain. Glutamic acid gets substituted by valine, resulting in HbS, which sickles (polymerizes) when deoxygenated

Enzymatic defects

Glucose-6-phosphate dehydrogenase deficiency (G6PD deficiency) leads to reduced production of NADPH, which is needed to reduce oxidized glutathione. Glutathione is oxidized while protecting the RBCs from hydrogen peroxide. Therefore, G6PD deficiency results in destruction of RBCs by oxidative stress.

Etiology

Iron deficiency anemia: It can be due to decreased intake of iron, increased iron demand in the body (Pregnancy, infancy, lactation) decreased iron absorption (achlorhydria, gastric surgery, phytate, bran, drugs, celiac disease), chronic blood loss, in younger woman due to menstruation, in non menstruating women and in men due to gastrointestinal hemorrhage (esophageal varices, hiatus hernia, peptic ulcer, gastritis, neoplasm, hook worm infestation).

Megaloblastic anemias: The three major causes of vitamin B12 deficiency are inadequate intake, malabsorption syndromes, and inadequate utilization. Inadequate dietary consumption of vitamin B12 is rare. It usually occurs only in patients who are strict vegans and their breast-fed infants, chronic alcoholics, or elderly patients. Inability to absorb vitamin B12: after gastric surgery, lack of hydrochloric acid in gastric juice, lack of intrinsic factor due to auto antibodies to parietal cells.

Folate deficiency occurs due to- a) Inadequate intake: a poor diet, b) Old and bed ridden patients, ICU patients, c) over cooked food especially vegetable, d) Increased requirements- pregnancy and lactating mothers, Growing infants, e) Hemolytic anemic patients, e) drugs, f) Folic acid antagonists: Methotrexate, g) Chronic alcoholism: It inhibits folic acid absorption., It increases folate excretion through the urine, h) Inability to absorb folic acid: Following gastric surgery, chronic diarrhea

Hemolytic anemia

1. **Inherited haemolytic anemia:** 1.Enzymopathies: - G6PD deficiency. - Pyruvate kinase deficiency. 2. Membrane defect: - Hereditary spherocytosis. - Hereditary Ovalocytosis. 3. Haemoglobinopathies: - Thalassaemias: quantitative Hbpathies. - Qualitative Hbpathies: Hb S, C, D, E etc.

2. **Acquired haemolytic anemia:** Acquired Hemolytic anemias 1-Immune -warm antibody -cold antibody 2-Non immune -Microangiopathic hemolysis (Disseminated intravascular coagulation, Thrombotic thrombocytopenic purpura, Preeclampsia, eclampsia, HELLP, Drugs (mitomycin, cyclosporine), Valvular hemolysis -Infection - Paroxysmal nocturnal hemoglobinuria

Anemia of Chronic Disease

Diseases Causing Anemia of Chronic Disease

Common causes:

1. **Chronic infections:** Tuberculosis, Other chronic lung infections, Human immune-deficiency virus, subacute bacterial endocarditis, Osteomyelitis, Chronic urinary tract infections

2. **Chronic inflammation:** Rheumatoid arthritis, Systemic lupus erythematosus, Rheumatoid (collagen vascular) diseases, inflammatory osteoarthritis, Gout, Chronic inflammatory liver diseases.

3. **Malignancies:** Carcinoma Lymphoma, Leukemia, Multiple myeloma

Less common causes

Alcoholic liver disease, Congestive heart failure, Thrombophlebitis, Chronic obstructive lung disease, Ischemic heart disease.

Anemia in the Elderly

In the acute ward setting, the top three causes of anemia in the elderly have been identified as chronic disease (35%), unexplained cause (17%), and iron deficiency (15%), whereas in community-based outpatient clinics the most prevalent causes are unexplained (36%), infection (23%), and chronic disease (17%).

Pathogenesis

Iron Defiency Anemia: Inadequate dietary intake, inadequate gastrointestinal absorption, increased iron demand due to pregnancy etc leads to Iron deficiency anemia.

Megaloblastic Anemia: Lack of B12 allows folic acid to be trapped as nonfunctional methyl tetrahydrofolate. So deficiency of functional FH4 causes impairment of formation of deoxy thymidinemonophaospahte which is needed for DNA synthesis. As a result proerythroblast fails to divide rapidly to make mature RBC rather immature precursors of erythrocyte-blast cells appear to cause megaloblastic anemia.

Hemolytic Anemia: Inherited hemolytic anemia: Examples are
  (i)   sickle cell disease –defect in RBC shape
  (ii) hereditary spherocytosis- spherical shape of RBC
  (iii) thalasemia – defect in Hb synthesis
  (iv) Glucose 6 phosphate dehydrogenase deficiency- enzyme deficiency in RBC

Pathophysiology behind Normocytic Anemia

Defects in RBC's environment: Infection triggers/ immune system activation /autoimmune processes all these factors contribute to production of antibodies and immune complxes targeted against RBC surface antigens. Because of this immunoglobulin blood RBC's are marked for destruction by the immune system. This leads to destruction of RBC. Thrombocytopenic purpura TTP/ DIC-fibrin deposition blocking blood vessels/ artificial heart valve are the predisposing factors by which RBC's are sheared when they flow past an abnormal surface. This again leads to destruction of RBC.

Defects in RBC Membranes

Hereditary spherocytosis: In this condition there is mutation causing deficiency of RBC structural proteins like ankyrin or spectrin. Due to this RBC membranes become weakened and form belbs that break off. Now there is decreased RBC surface area while the volume remains constant. As a result RBC becomes spherical. These RBC are trapped in spleen during the blood circulation and then they are phagocytosed by spleenic macrophages because of abnormal shape. This again leads to destruction of RBC.

Defects in internal contents: This is seen in conditions like thalasemia, hemoglobinopathies, metabolic defects.

Sickle cell disease: There is a point mutation in hemoglobin (HgS) structure (Glutamine replaced with Valine). Due to the inappropriate HgS polymerization due to mutation, the RBC becomes rigid and forms a sickle shape. These inflexible RBC's become trapped in spleen. They are phagocytosed by spleenic macrophages leading to extravascular hemolysis.

Thalasemia: It is inherited disorder. Two types-

Alpha thalasemia: Mutation in HbA1 or HbA2 genes, resulting in decrease in alpha globulin chain production, and excess of beta chains. So they from unstable tetramers and alter the shape of RBC. These RBC with altered shape are less elastic and are sequestered and destroyed in spleen.

Beta thalasemia: Mutation in HbB gene, so no functional beta chains are produced. Excessive alpha chains are formed, due to which there is change in shape of RBC and become more fragile.

Glucose 6 phosphate dehydrogenase G6PD deficiency anemia: It is an X-linked disorder in which there is deficiency of enzyme G6PD. G6PD is involved in pentose phosphate pathway where NADPH is formed which is used for maintaining reduced glutathione levels (GSH). GSH is an antioxidant and protects RBC from oxidants. Because of the deficiency of this enzyme, due to oxidative stress in the body, RBC are more prone to oxidative damage and hemolysis occurs.

Beacuase of the above three mentioned mechanisms RBC destruction is greater than rate of bone marrow RBC synthesis. There is decrease in total number of RBC's leading to anemia.

Aplastic Anemia (Bone Marrow Depression): Pathogenesis

Ionizing radiation / chemicals like benzene cause direct chromosomal damage due to free radical formation. Because of this there will be premature death of hematopoietic progenitor cells leading to bone marrow failure.

In Genetic disorder like fanconi's syndrome there is impaired cellular response to DNA damage leading to premature death of hematopoietic progenitor cells leading to bone marrow failure.

Infection by viruses/ autoimmune disorder/ drugs like carbamazepine cause inappropriate T-cell activation. These t-cells attack bone marrow cells and cause lysis.

There is finally bone marrow failure due to which less blood cells are formed leading to a condition pancytopenia. Consequences are decreased platelet production which is thrombocytopenia. Platelets are responsible for hemostasis which is impaired. There will be mucocutaneous bleeding leading to epistaxis and petechia. Decreased RBC production leading to anemia. So there will be reduced oxygen carrying capacity of blood and dyspnoea, tachycardia and fatigue develops. Decreased WBC production there will be neutropenia and lymphopenia. There will be impaired immunity and phagocytosis. There will be impaired humoral and cell mediated immunity. The person succumbs to opportunistic infections and may also be prone to recurrent infections if he has any comorbidity.

Clinical manifestation and features:

(a) Anaemia of recent onset usually is manifested by cardiorespiratory symptoms such as
- Tachycardia
- Light headedness
- Breathlessness
- Chest tightness

(b) Chronic anaemia is manifested by fatigue, headache, vertigo, pallor, sensitivity, faintness and loss oof skin tone.

(c) Hb levels fall below 8-9g /dl.

(d) Iron deficiency anaemia is manifested by :
- Spooning of nails (koilonychias)

- Angular stomatis and glossitis
- Smooth tongue, brittle nails, cheilosis, dysphagia due to oesophageal webs. (plummer –vinson syndrome) and craving for substances not normally eaten (pica)

Vitamin B12 and folate deficiency anaemia are manifested by cardiorespiratory symptoms, anemia symptoms, neurological symptoms and gastro-intestinal complaints. Anemia symptoms include- weakness, palpitation, fatigue, lightheadedness, shortness of breath, premature graying of hair, jaundice and pallor. Severe pallor and slight jaundice combine to produce a telltale lemon-yellow skin in patient with megaloblastic anemia. Neurological symptoms. The syndrome usually begins with paraesthesiaθ (numbness and tingling) in the feet and fingers, difficulties in balance and walking. Vitamin B12 deficiency causes a demyelinizationθ of the peripheral nerves, the spinal cord, and the brain, resulting in more severe neurological symptoms. When it affects the spinal cord it causes spastic ataxia (stiffness of the muscles with uncoordinated movement). At the brain it results in dementia, psychotic depression and paranoid schizophrenia. This has been termed "megaloblastic madness. Gastro- intestinal complains: symptom include loss of appetite, glossitis (red, sore, smooth tongue) and diarrhoea.

Haemolytic anemia: Sudden Pallor, Jaundice, Red or dark urine due to Hemoglobinuria, Lasts usually for 2-6 days followed by spontaneous recovery, No organomegaly

Hereditary spherocytosis: jaundice, spleenomegaly, pigment gall stones

Clinical manifestations for sickle cell anaemia: Pneumonia or pain, Swelling of hands and feets, Splenomegaly, Pallor, weakness, Arthralgia, Fever, Anorexi, Sickle shaped RBC.

Complications: Renal problems, osteomyelitis, chronic ulcers, acute chest syndrome, cholelithiasis, heart and lung problems, risk of infections, restless legs syndrome, pregnancy related complications (post natal depression), weakness.

Diagnosis with Algorithm: Examination of RBC and peripheral blood smear

> **If MCV< 80** – It is considered as Microcytic anemia. Then check for serum iron studies. In the study if
>
>> (a) low iron and ferritin with high TIBC (Total iron binding capacity) it is considered as iron defiency anemia
>>
>> (b) low iron and ferritin with low TIBC-it is considered as anemia of chronic disesase
>>
>> (c) if MCV/RBC ratio is < 13 it is considered as Thalasemia
>
> **If MCV 80-100**- it is considered as normocytic anemia. Check for reticulocyte count.
>
>> (a) If < 2% hypoproliferative which may be due to leukemias/ aplastic anemia/ aplasia
>>
>> (b) If > 2% hypoproliferative which may be due to hemorrhage / haemolytic anemias.
>
> **If MCV >100**-It is considered as macrocytic anemia. Check for peripheral smear.
>
>> **(a) Megaloblastic anemia-** which may be due to Vit B12 or floate deficiency/ drug induced.
>>
>> **(b) Non-**megaloblastic anemia-which may be due to alcohol abuse/ liver disease/ congenital bone marrow failure syndromes

Laboratory evaluation:

1. **Hematocrit:** Proportion of the volume of red cells relative to the volume of blood • Rules of Three: – RBC X 3 = Hemoglobin – Hemoglobin X 3 = Hematocrit Packed cell volume (PCV) or Haematocrit (Hct) Men - 0.45 ± 0.05 l/l (40-50%) Women - 0.41 ± 0.05 l/l (38-45 % in non- pregnant women 36-42 % in pregnant women)

2. **Mean Corpuscular Volume:** Dividing the total volume of red cells by the number of red cells. Index for average size of red cells • Normal range - 92 ± 9 fl

$$\text{Mean cell volume MCV in femtoliters:} \quad \frac{\text{Packed cell volume} \times 10}{\text{Red cell count in million per cumm}}$$

3. **Mean Corpuscular Hemoglobin:** Average amount of haemoglobin in each red cell. It is expressed in picograms or pg. Normal range - 29.5 ± 2.5 pg

$$\text{MCH} = \frac{\text{Hemoglobin concentration} \times 10}{\text{Red cell count}}$$

4. **Mean Corpuscular Hemoglobin Concentration:** This represents the average concentration of haemoglobin in a given volume of packed red cells. Normal range – 330 ± 15 g/l. MCHC raised in hereditary spherocytosis. • Decreased in hypochromic anaemia.

$$\text{MCHC} = \frac{\text{Hemoglobin concentration}}{\text{Packed cell volume}} \times 100$$

5. **Red cell distribution width:** It is a measure of degree of variation in red cell size(anisocytosis) in a blood sample. Normal: As coefficient of variation (CV)- 11.6-14 % As Standard deviation(SD) – 39-46%

6. **Serum iron:** The level of serum iron is the concentration of iron bound to transferrin. Normally, transferrin is about one-third bound (saturated) to iron. There is also a 20% to 30% diurnal variation in serum iron levels (higher in the morning, lower in the afternoon) as well as a 20% to 25% day-to-day variation among individuals.

7. **Total Iron-Binding Capacity:** An indirect measurement of the iron-binding capacity of serum transferrin.

8. **Serum Ferritin:** The concentration of ferritin (storage iron) in the serum is proportional to total iron stores, and consequently is a reliable indicator of body iron stores. Ferritin levels indicate the amount of iron stored in the liver, spleen, and bone marrow cells.

9. **Schilling Test:** The purpose of the rarely used Schilling urinary excretion test is to diagnose vitamin B12 deficiency anemia caused by a B12 absorption defect resulting from a lack of intrinsic factor (pernicious anemia). The patient first receives an oral dose of radiolabeled vitamin B12. Two hours later, the patient receives a large intramuscular dose of nonlabeled vitamin B12 to saturate plasma transport proteins. Any excess vitamin B12 that is not taken up by the transport proteins or stored in the liver will be excreted in the urine. A 24-hour urine collection is then measured for radioactivity. If sufficient gastrointestinal intrinsic factor is being produced, the radiolabeled B12 will be absorbed.

10. **Coombs Test:** Antiglobulin tests, also called Coombs tests, indicate hemolytic anemia caused by an immune response. A direct Coombs test detects antibodies bound to erythrocytes, whereas an indirect Coombs test measures antibodies present in the serum. A positive finding in a direct Coombs test is usually indicative of antibody-mediated hemolysis.

Check for the normal levels below depending on the type of anaemia.

(a) Haemoglobin: male: 13.5 -17.5 g /dl.
     Female:12-16 g/ dl

(b) Haematocrit value (%): male: 41-53
     Female: 36 -46

(c) Mean corpuscular volume: 80-100fl

(d) Mean corpuscular haemoglobin concentrations: 31-37%

(e) Mean corpuscular haemoglobin :26-34 pg/cell

(f) RBC: 4.5 -5.9 million/cubic mm

(g) WBC: 4000-11000 cells/cubic mm

(h) Reticulocyte count (absolute): 0.5-1.5 %

(i) Serum iron: male: 50-160 microgram/dL
     Female: 40 -150 micro gram/dL

(j) Tot iron binding capacity: 250-400 microgram /dL

(k) Red blood cell distribution width :11-16 %

(l) Folate : 1.8 -16 nano gram/dL

(m) Erythropoietin : 0-19 mu/dL

(n) Vitamin B 12 : 100-900 pg/mL

(o) Ferritin : male : 15-200 ng/mL
     Female: 12-150 ng /mL

Diagnostic Tests

- **Complete Blood Count:** RBC indices, reticulocyte index and examination of the peripheral blood smear and of the total stool for occult blood.

Iron deficiency anemia

(a) Reduced transferrin saturation (<15%)

(b) Elevated free erythrocyte concentration.

(c) Elevated total iron binding capacity (> 400 micro gram/ dl).

(d) Decreased ferritin levels

(e) MCV decreased (Microcytic), MCH decreased (Hypochromic)

(f) Anisocytosis

Megaloblastic anemias:

(a) ↓ Hb/Hct, ↑ MCV, ↓ reticulocytes, ↓WBC, ↓Platelets, macroovalocytosis, anisocytosis, poikilocytosis, hypersegmentation of granulocytes. Also there may be variable thrombocytopenia.

(b) Bone marrow smear: Bone marrow examination reveals myeloid cell changes (giant bands, metamyelocytes and hypertsegmentation) and megakariocytes are decreased and show abnormal morphology.

(c) Biochemistry Test: hyperbilirubinemia ↑lactate dehrogenase (LDH)

(d) Schilling test: The Schilling test is used to determine whether there is faulty absorption of vitamin B12

Hemolytic anemias:

(a) **Blood Picture:** Variable anaemia, during the hemolytic episode, normal Hb between attacks. Red cell: normochromic, anisocytosis, some bitten cell (Blister cells) and marked polychromasia (markedly increased reticulocytes count). Denatured haemoglobin visible as Heinz bodies within the red cell cytoplasm.

(b) **Other Laboratory tests:** Hemoglobin in urine and plasma. Increased urine urobilinogen. Indirect hyperbilirubinaemia. Methemoglobin reduction test For G6PD deficiency (Screening test) Specific Assay for red cell G6PD.

Hereditary spherocytosis:

(a) The anemia is usually normocytic, with the characteristic morphology that gives the disease its name. A characteristic feature is an increase in mean corpuscular hemoglobin concentration (MCHC).

Thalassemia:

(a) *Beta-thalassaemia major (homozygotes):* Profound hypochromic anaemia, Evidence of severe red cell dysplasia, Erythroblastosis, Absence or gross reduction of the amount of haemoglobin A, Raised levels of haemoglobin F

(b) *Beta-thalassaemia minor (heterozygotes):* Mild anaemia, Microcytic hypochromic erythrocytes (not iron-deficient), Some target cells, Punctate basophilia, Raised haemoglobin A2 fraction, Evidence that one parents have thalassaemia minor

Sickle cell anemia:

- Diagnosis should be considered in any black person with haemolytic anemia especially if there is history of painful crisis, arthropathies, ankle ulcers or other clinical manifestations.

- Evaluation of a blood sample from a patient with sickle cell anemia will reveal reduced haemoglobin, increased reticulocyte count, usually increased platelet and leucocyte count and sickle forms on peripheral smear.

- Screening newborns is an important strategy but commonly used tests donot differentiate between sickle cell trait and anemia. This distictinction requires haemoglobin electrophoresis, isoelectric focussing, HPLC or DNA analysis.

Management

Goals of Treatment

- To alleviate signs and symptoms.
- Correct the underlying etiology (restore depleted stores of iron or other elements required for RBC Production).
- Prevent reoccurance of anemia.

Treatment

Algorithm for treatment of Iron deficiency anemia:

1. **After** iron defiency anemia is diagnosed, treat underlying cause and start oral iron therapy. If oral not tolerated start the IV iron therapy.

2. After the treatment, monthly CBC showing improved hematocrit and RBC indices, then continue therapy for 3 months. Evaluate hematocrit and ferritin levels, if they are normalised, discontinue oral iron.

   If monthly CBC has not shown improvement, revlauate for underlying cause. Consider IV iron therapy. Transfuse if symptomatic.

Iron Deficiency Anemia: Treatment include dietary supplementation and administration of iron preparations.

Oral Therapy: Therapy with soluble ferrous iron salts that are not enteric coated and not slow or sustained release is recommended at a daily dosage of 20mg.

- Ferrous sulphate : 60-65mg/300mg or 325mg tablet; elemental iron 20%
- Ferrous gluconate : 37-39 mg /300 or 325 mg tablet ; elemental iron 12%
- Ferrous fumarate 33 mg/100 mg tablet; elemental iron 33%
- Polysaccharide iron complex : 150mg capsule or 50mg tablet . elemental iron 100%
- Carbonyl iron   50mg tablet ; elemental iron 100%
- Iron is best absorbed from meat , fish and poultry.

Parenteral Iron Therapy: Incase of iron malabsorption and intolerance of oral iron therapy or non compliance.

1. **Iron dextran:** Given IM or IV by multiple slow injections of undiluted solution. Initial dose: 25mg IM or IV. Mechanism Of Action: Replacement of iron stores, found in haemoglobin, myoglobin and enzymes and works to transport oxygen. Kinetics: Plasma half life: 6 hours. Onset: 7-9 days; Peak plasma time: 10 days; Newer parenteral iron products, such as sodium ferric gluconate: 10-12.5mg/ml. Monitoring Paramters: Monitor for anaphylactic reactions, allergies for every 1 hour after initial dose.

2. **Sodium ferric gluconate:** Amount of elemental iron 62.5 mg iron/5 mL. Composition Ferric oxide hydrate bonded to sucrose chelates with gluconate in a molar rate of 2 iron molecules to 1 gluconate molecule. Indication Treatment of iron deficiency anemia in patients undergoing chronic hemodialysis who are receiving supplemental erythropoietin therapy. Usual dose 125 mg (10 mL) diluted in 100 mL normal saline, infused over 60 minutes; may also be administered as a slow IV injection (rate of 12.5 mg/min). Treatment 8 doses × 125 mg = 1,000 mg. Common adverse effects Cramps, nausea and vomiting, flushing, hypotension, rash, pruritus.

3. **Iron sucrose:** Amount of elemental iron- 20mg iron/ml. Treatment of iron deficiency anemia in patients undergoing chronic hemodialysis who are receiving supplemental epoetin alfa therapy.

Black box warning: anaphylactic-type reactions. Usual dose: 100 mg into the dialysis line at a rate of 1 mL (20 mg of iron) undiluted solution per minute. Up to 10 doses × 100 mg = 1,000 mg.

Adverse effects: Leg cramps, hypotension.

Equations for Calculating Doses of Parenteral Iron

In patients with iron defficiency anemia:

Adults + children over 15 kg

Dose (mL) = 0.0442 (desired Hgb − observed Hgb) × LBW + (0.26 × LBW)

LBW males = 50 kg + (2.3 × inches over 5 ft)

LBW females = 45.5 kg + (2.3 × inches over 5 ft)

Children 5–15 kg Dose (mL) = 0.0442 (desired Hgb − observed Hgb) × W + (0.26 × W) Hgb = hemoglobin mL = milliliter W = weight LBW = lean body weight

In patients with anemia secondary to blood loss (hemorrhagic diathesis or long-term dialysis): mg of iron = blood loss × hematocrit

where blood loss is in milliliters and hematocrit is expressed as a decimal fraction

Treatment for Vitamin B12 Deficiency Anemia

Replacement therapy with cyanocobalamin or hydroxycobalamin: 800-1000 microgram (IM) or deep SC, followed by 100-1000 microgram once a week until haemoglobin and haematocrit values return to normal. Followed by 100-1000 microgram once a month for lifetime. Oral vitamin b12 is indicated in patient with nutrition deficiency.

Oral cobalamin: 1000 microgram/day

For pernicious anemia: Mecobalamin or hydroxycobalamin of 30-50 microgram IM or SC for 14 days initially and total upto 1000microgram can be administered.

Mechanism of action of cobalamin:

5-deoxyadenosyl cobalamin is a type of Vitamin B_{12}. 5-Deoxyadenosyl cobalamin is a cofactor needed by the enzyme that converts L-methylmalonyl-CoA to succinyl-CoA. This conversion is an important step in the extraction of energy from proteins and fats. Furthermore, succinyl CoA is necessary for the production of hemoglobin, the substances that carries oxygen in red blood cells. Helps to treat anemia.

Monitoring parameters: Monitor closely if patient has celiac disease, crohn's disease or is a severe alcoholic. Also monitor plasma potassium levels after the initial doses of cobalamin.

Treatment for Folate Deficiency Anemia

Treatment is initiated with oral folate: 1-5mg daily for approximately 4months. Long term therapy is required only if the eitiology is chronic condition that cannot be corrected.

Mechanism of action: Folic acid is essential for the body to make DNA, RNA, and metabolise amino acids, which are required for cell divisionand also helps to synthezise RBC.

Monitoring parameters: Folate injection might contain aluminium which may reach toxic concentrations in patients with renal failure or in premature neonates.

Treatment for β-thalassaemia major

Allogenic HSCT from HLA-compatable sibling. Transfusion to maintain Hb > 100g/L; folic acid 5 mg daily; iron chelation therapy and splenectomy.

Anemia of Chronic Diseases and Renal Failure

Iron therapy is not effective when inflammation is present. RBC transfusions are effective but should be limited to episodes of inadequate oxygen carrying and haemoglobin of 8-10g/dl. Erythropoietin can be indicated because erythropoietin concentrations are low relative for severity of anemia. In patients with cancer, **epoetin alfa**, 150 U/kg three times weekly or 40,000 units once weekly SC, increased haemoglobin and decreased the need of transfusions.

Epoetin alfa reverses the anemia of chronic renal failure in essentially all patients, circumvents the inherent risks of RBC transfusions, and therefore has become the mainstay of treatment. Epoetinalfa should be initated at a dosage of 50-100 U/kg TID weekly until haematocrit value reaches 36%, the dosage should be titrated to maintain haematocrit values at 30-36%. Although epoetinalfa is administered IM or SC, oral ferrous sulphate may be used at sustained concentrations at a dose of 325 mg OD at bedtime.

Mechanism of action: To stimulate RBC and help to treat anemia. Ferrous sulphate replaces iron stores and helps to subside the symptoms of anemia.

Monitoring parameters: Check for muscle spasms and muscle pain with usage of epoetin alfa and closely monitor the blood pressure.

Treatment for Sickle Cell Anemia

Folic acid, 1mg daily is given empirically because of increased demand caused by accelerated erythropoiesis.

Mechanism: Folic acid helps cell proliferation and erythropoiesis and helps to prevent growth retardation in children with sickle cell anemia.

Monitoring parameters: Folate injection might contain aluminium which may reach toxic concentrations in patients with renal failure or in premature neonates. Patient with sickle cell anemia should receive pneumococcal and haemophilusinfluenzae type b conjugate vaccines at appropriate ages. In addition to vaccine prophylactic therapy with penicillin is recommended for children until they are 5 years old.

Penicillin V Potassium: 125 mg orally BD until 3 years of age then 250mg BD

Benzathinepenicillin: 600000 U IM every 4 weeks.

Mechanism: Penicillin inhibits activity of enzymes that are needed for the cross linking of peptidoglycans in bacterial cell walls, which is the final step in cell wall biosynthesis. It does this by binding to penicillin binding proteins with the beta-lactam ring, a structure found on penicillin molecules. This causes the cell wall to weaken, this results in cell lysis and death.

And used to prevent pneumococcal infections in children.

Hydroxyurea reduces the frequency of painful episodes of acute chest syndrome and reduces hospitalizations.

Mechanism: A gelation inhibitor, acts by increasing production of fetal haemoglobin, decreasing neutrophil, monocyte and reticulocyte levels and providing antioxidant properties.

Dose: Initial dose: 20mg/kg PO, monitor blood counts. Increase the dose to 25mg/kg depending upon the blood count and donot exceed 35mg/kg.

Monitoring parameters: Monitor serum creatinine levels, neutrophil, platelet and reticulocyte count closely. Additional strategies that are being considered to decrease gelation of sickle cells include **butyrate, clotrimazole, 5-aza-2-deoxycytidine** and a purified poloxamer known as **flocor.**

- **Pentoxifylline: dose:** 400 mg TID

Decreases number and severity of sickle cell crisis.

Treatment of Complications

Transfusion therapy may be beneficial in selected patients with life threatening complications such as sudden anemia in children with sequestration crisis, acute chest syndrome, surgery requiring general anaesthesia, complicated obstetric problems, refractory problems, refractory leg ulcers, and severe priapism. Transfusions help to prevent stroke reccurrence in children.

The risks of transfusion therapy include sensitization to transfusion products, acquired viral infection and iron overload. sickle cell haemolytic transfusion reaction syndrome is unique in this setting and is manifested by new onset or worsening of pain crisis and by post transfusion anemia, which may subside upon witholding of further transfusions.

Hematopoietic stem cell transplantation is potentially curative but is limited by toxicity and availability of donors. Candidates include patients younger than 16 years of age who have severe complications such as refractory pain, stroke or recurrent acute chest syndrome and who have matched donors.

Priapism has been treated with analgesics (morphine), anti- anxiety agents (hydroxyzine), vasoconstrictors to force blood out of the corpus cavernosum (phenylepinephrine ,epinephrine) and vasodilators to relax smooth muscle (beta agonists i.eterbutaline,hydralazine) .More invasive approaches include aspiration of the corpora cavernosa and surgery. Preventative measures include hydroxyurea, stilbestrol and gonadotropin releasing hormone analogue.

Recommended treatments for acute chest syndrome include frequent use of incentive spirometry; early use of broad spectrum antibiotics; and if indicated oxygen therapy.

Pregnancy induced Anemia

Any patient with HB < 11g/dL to 11.5g/dL at the start of pregnancy is treated as anemic. The reason is that as the pregnancy progresses, the blood is diluted and the woman will eventually become anemic. The dilution of blood in pregnancy is natural process and starts at approximately at 8th week of pregnancy and progresses until the 32nd to 34th week of pregnancy.

Complications:
- During pregnancy: pre-eclampsia, recurrent infection, heart failure preterm labor.
- During labor: uterine inerta, Post Partum Hemorrhage (PPH), cardiac failure, shock.
- During puerperium: puerperal sepsis, sub-involution, failing lactation.

Indications: To correct blood loss; to combat PPH; to prevent recurrence.

Treatment of anemia in pregnancy:
- Hospitalization, if Hb level is <7.5g/dL.
- Blood transfusions.
- Antibiotics for infective focuses.
- Balanced diet rich in proteins, vitamins and iron.
- Intramuscular: iron dextran and iron sorbital.

Case Study of Pancytopenia

Summary

A female patient of age 19 came to the hospital with the c/o fever on and off every 2/3 days since 2 months not associated with chills or rigors. Yellowish discoloration of eyes since 2 months. Generalized weakness (+) nausea (+) vomiting (-) skin itching (+). c/o easy fatigue ability, palpitations. Past medical history: Similar complaints 2 such episodes in past 3 years. Physical examination: Resp rate: 18 cycles/minute, CVS-S1S2(+), CVS-S1S2(+), Respiratory system-BAE (+), Temperature 99F, Complete blood picture: Hb(g/dL): 5.2, RBC: 1.4, lymphocytes: 52, basophills: 05, platelet count: 0.58, Peripheral smear: Microcytes, teardrop cells, pencil cells, RBCs: Anisocytes, ovarocytes, macrocytes, WBCs: Relative lympocytosis, Liver function test: Serum bilirubin total(0-1mg): 2.1mg, Other investigations: prothrombin time: Test-35 secs, control-31.9 secs. Radiological report: US Abd-mild hepatomegaly, iron-144.20 mg/dL, serum LDH-414 mgd/L, TIBC-105 mg/dL.

Final diagnosis: Pancytopenia with VITB12 deficiency.

Drug chart:

Trade name	Generic name	Route	Dose	Frequency	D1	D2	D3	D4	D5	
Tab. Doxy	Doxycycline	Oral	100mg	BD	✓	✓				
Tab. Lumerex	Artemether and lumefantriene	Oral	80mg	BD	✓	✓				

Contd...

Tab. Crocin	paracetamol	Oral	500mg	SOS	✓	✓	✓	✓	✓	
Tab. Udiliv	Ursodeoxychlic acid	Oral	300mg	BD	✓		✓			
Tab. Beplex forte	VITB and VITC and biotin	Oral	100-200mg	OD		✓	✓	✓		
Inj. Optineuron with 100 ml N/S	Vit B12 complex	IV	100ml	OD		✓	✓	✓	✓	
Folrite	Folate	Oral	5mg	OD		✓	✓			
Inj. Zofer	Ondasetron	IV	4mg	BD		✓	✓	✓		
Syp.Duphalac	Lactulose	Oral	15ml	H/S		✓	✓	✓	✓	

Assignment

1. **What is pancytopenia**?

A. pancytopenia is a medical condition in which there is reduction in the number of red and white blood cells, as well as platelets.

If only two parameters from the complete blood count are low, the term bicytopenia can be used.the diagnostic approach is same for both.

In the most extreme cases of pancytopenia, a person can have infections, the signs of the severe anemia, including fatigue and difficulty breathing and bleeding.

There are many different symptoms and degrees of severity of pancytopenia. sometimes it can be lead to symptoms that may be life threatening. most treatment depend on trying to find the underlying cause.

Causes

Pancytopenia is usually due to some disruption of the bone marrow's ability to produce new blood cells examples could include:

(i)   Cancer that destroys the bonemarrow cells.

(ii) Failure to make stem cells that turn into blood cells.

(iii) Fibrosis or scarring of bone marrow cells.

(iv) Immune system destroying healthy bone marrow cells.

(v)   Suppression of bone marrow function due to bone marrow function due to illness or medications

Some of the conditions that can cause pancytopenia include:

- Aplastic anemia, autoimmune conditions, cancer, chemotherapy treatments
- Exposure, infection, leukemia, which impacts bone marrow function.
- Megablastic anemia, deficiency of folate or vitamin B12 for making bone marrow
- Viruses, such as Epstein-bars, HIV or hepatitis C
- Medications-chlromphenicol, chemotherapy drugs,thiazide diuretics,anti epileptic drugs,colchicines,azathioprine and NSAIDS's.

2. **What are the complications of pancytopenia?**

A.complications from pancytopenia stem from lack of red blood cells,white blood cells are affected.

These problems can include:

- excess bleeding if bleeding are affected.
- increased risk for infectons if white blood cells are affected.
- severe pancytopenia can be life threatening.

3. **Describe the pathogenesis of pancytopenia?**

Decreased hematopoietic cell production

  (i) Bone marrow aplasia or hypoplasia: Drugs/ estrogens; infections; idiopathic or immune mediated

  (ii) Myelodysplasia: a) primary or b) secondary: immune-mediated; neoplasia/ infections/ drugs

  (iii) Bone marrow necrosis: septicemia; neoplasia; drugs; immune-mediated/ infections

  (iv) Bone marrow fibrosis/sclerosis: necrosis; neoplasia/ drugs/immune-mediated.

  (v) Myelopthisis: Neoplasia; granulomatous disease

Increased hematopoietic cell production

  (i) Sepsis

  (ii) Immune-mediated

  (iii) Hemophagocytic syndrome/hypersplenism: immune-mediated; myelodysplsia; neoplasia; infections

4. **What are the signs and symptoms?**

It is necessary to understand what each of the three different types of three different types of blood to clot, during wound healing or they may bleed easily. RBC carry oxygen, they may be prone to infection. Additional symptoms include: fast heart rate, pale skin color, rashes, unexplained fatigue, weakness, easy bruising.

A person should go or be taken to the emergency room immediately if they have have following symptoms- confusion, loss of consciousness, seizures, shortness of breath, significant blood loss

5. **How each of the complications of pancytopenia is managed?**

The goal of treating pancytopenia is to find and treat the underlying cause and treatment is aimed at minimizing the symptoms related to deficiency of blood cells.

Because there are so many different pancytopenia causes, the treatment vary widely from person to person.

- Blood transfusions to replace RBC, WBC and platelets.
- Bone marrow transplant or stem cell transplant which replaces damaged bone marrow with healthy stem cells that rebuild bone marrow.
- Antibiotics to treat an infection.
- Immune suppressive drugs if it is due to auto immune condition.

- drugs that stimulate bone marrow for chemotherapy induced and some other causes, the growth factors leukine, neupogen may be used to stimulate the formation of white blood cells for chemotherapy induced anemia, there are also medication to be considered based on condition.

6. What are the lab tests to identify pancytopenia?

Complete blood count:-

- ➢ anemia-haemoglobin <13.5g/dl (male) or 12g?dl(female)
- ➢ leucopenia-total white blood cell count <4.0*10^9/L. Decrease in all types of white blood cells (by differential count).
- ➢ thrombocytopenia-platelet count <150*10^9
- ➢ bone marrow aspiration and biopsy doctor uses a needle to remove a small amount of liquid and tissue from inside bone after the area has been numbered. The sample is sent to lab to examine under a microscope. the cells appearance can help identify the potential underlying cause of pancytopenia.
- ➢ Other tests-liver function tests, vitamin B12 levels, HIV and hepatitis testing.

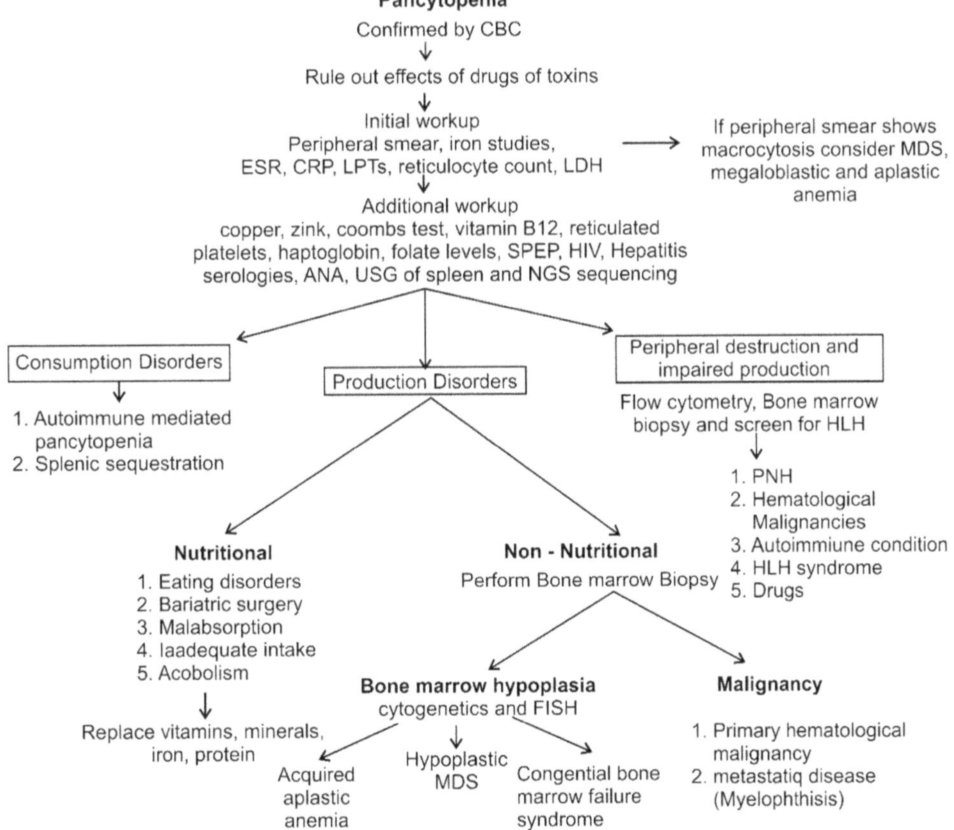

Fig. 62.1 Algorithm for the diagnosis of Pancytopenia [2].

References

1. Kossenko MM, Akleyev AA, Degteva MO, Kozheurov VP, Degtyaryova RC (August 1994). "Analysis of Chronic Radiation Sickness Cases in the Population of the Southern Urals (AD-A286 238)". DTIC. p. 5.
2. Jerome Gnanaraj et al., Approach to Panoytopenia: Diagnostic Algorithm for Clinical Hematologistis. Blood Reviews. Sep 2018; Vol 32(5); 361-367.

CHAPTER - 63

Epilepsy

Introduction to Epilepsy

- An epileptic seizure is a transient occurrence of signs and/or symptoms due to abnormal excessive or synchronous neuronal activity in the brain. Epilepsy is a disorder of the brain characterized by an enduring predisposition to generate epileptic seizures, and by the neurobiological, cognitive, psychological, and social consequences of this condition.
- An epileptic seizure is the clinical manifestation of an abnormal and excessive discharge of a set of neurons in the brain.
- The definition of epilepsy requires the occurrence of at least one epileptic seizure. Therefore, a seizure is the event and epilepsy is the disorder.
- By definition, one seizure does not make epilepsy, nor does a small series of seizures that have an immediate precipitating factor, for example, alcohol withdrawal seizures. The seizures must be spontaneous and recurrent to represent epilepsy.

Epidemiology [1]

Of the 70 million persons with epilepsy (PWE) worldwide, nearly 12 million PWE are expected to reside in India; which contributes to nearly one-sixth of the global burden. The overall prevalence (3.0-11.9 per 1,000 population) and incidence (0.2-0.6 per 1,000 populations per year) data from recent studies in India on general population are comparable to the rates of high-income countries (HICs) despite marked variations in population characteristics and study methodologies. There is a differential distribution of epilepsy among various sociodemographic and economic groups with higher rates reported for the male gender, rural population, and low socioeconomic status.

Etiology

Idiopathic seizures are those whose cause is unknown. Unfortunately, about 6 out of 10 seizures are idiopathic.

Common causes of seizures by age:

In Newborns:
- Brain malformations

- Lack of oxygen during birth
- Low levels of blood sugar, blood calcium, blood magnesium or other eletrolyte problems
- Inborn errors of metabolism
- Intracranial hemorrhage
- Maternal drug use
- **Prenatal injury.** Before birth, babies are sensitive to brain damage that could be caused by several factors, such as an infection in the mother, poor nutrition or oxygen deficiencies. This brain damage can result in epilepsy or cerebral palsy.

In Infants and Children:
- Fever (febrile seizures)
- Brain tumor (rarely)
- Infections: infections can cause inflammation and swelling in brain eg. Meningitis.

In Children and Adults:
- Congenital conditions (Down's syndrome; Angelman's syndrome; tuberous sclerosis and neurofibromatosis)
- Genetic factors
- Head trauma

In seniors:
- Stroke: because of brain damage it leads to epilepsy.
- Alzheimer's disease: increases the risk of epilpesy
- Trauma

Pathophysiology [2, 3]

Seizure activity is characterized by paroxysmal discharges occurring synchronously in a large population of cortical neurons. This is characterized on EEG as a sharp wave or spike. The basic physiology of a seizure episode is traceable to an unstable cell membrane or its surrounding supportive cells. The seizure originates from the gray matter of any cortical or perhaps subcortical area. Initially, a small number of neurons fire abnormally. Normal membrane conductances and inhibitory synaptic currents break down, and excess excitability spreads, either locally to produce a focal seizure or more widely to produce a generalized seizure. This onset propagates by physiologic pathways to involve adjacent or remote areas.

There is disruption of multiple systems in epilepsy involving neurons and astrocytes. Hyperexcitable neurons are associated with overactivation of voltage-gated Na+ channels and reduced activity of K+ channels, which generate an action potential that leads to increased release of glutamate (Glu). This activates AMPA and N-methyld-aspartate (NMDA) receptors on the postsynaptic membrane, causing excitatory synaptic potentials. Upregulated adenosine kinase (AdK) in reactive astrocytes increases the removal of extracellular adenosine, enhancing hyperexcitability. Decreased membrane transporters for K^+ and Glu (such as *GAT-1*) on reactive astrocytes further enhance hyperexcitability. Excessive Ca^{2+} intake in astrocytes even induces Glu release.

Selected neurotransmitters (e.g., glutamate, aspartate, acetylcholine, norepinephrine, histamine, corticotropin releasing factor, purines, peptides, cytokines, and steroid hormones) enhance the excitability and propagation of neuronal activity, whereas γ -aminobutyric acid (GABA) and dopamine inhibit neuronal activity and propagation. A relative deficiency of inhibitory neurotransmitters such as GABA or an increase in excitatory neurotransmitters such as glutamate would promote abnormal neuronal activity. Normal neuronal activity also depends on an adequate supply of glucose, oxygen, sodium, potassium, chloride, calcium, and amino acids. Systemic pH is also a factor in precipitating seizures. The different kinds of epilepsies probably arise from different neurophysiologic abnormalities.

Different parts of the brain control different parts and functions of the body. Therefore, the symptoms that occur during a seizure depend on where the abnormal burst of electrical activity occurs. Symptoms that may occur during a seizure can affect muscles, sensations, behaviour, emotions, consciousness, or a combination of these.

The type of seizure depends upon several factors. One of the most important factors is where in the brain the abnormal electrical discharge occurs. Strength and sensation are laid out along the border of the frontal and parietal lobes, with strength more toward the front (frontal) and skin sensation more toward the back (parietal) of the strip. In simple terms, if an abnormal electrical discharge originates in motor cortex: the patient will experience a motor seizure; if in sensory cortex: a sensory perception; if in visual cortex: lights, flashes, or jagged lines. Seizures in deep temporal lobe structures present with arrest of activities, loss of memory or awareness, and automatic (robot-like) behaviour. If a seizure spreads to all regions of brain, then a tonic-clonic (grand mal) seizure results, with loss of consciousness, stiffening and jerking.

Classification of Epileptic Seizures [4, 5]

I. Partial seizures (seizures begin locally)

    A. Simple (without impairment of consciousness)

        1. With motor symptoms

        2. With special sensory or somatosensory symptoms

        3. With psychic symptoms

    B. Complex (with impairment of consciousness)

        1. Simple partial onset followed by impairment of consciousness—with or without automatisms

        2. Impaired consciousness at onset—with or without automatisms

    C. Secondarily generalized (partial onset evolving to generalized tonic-clonic seizures)

II. Generalized seizures (bilaterally symmetrical and without local onset)

    A. Absence

    B. Myoclonic

    C. Clonic

    D. Tonic

    E. Tonic-clonic

    F. Atonic

III. Unclassified seizures

IV. Status epilepticus

1. **Partial seizures** have onset on one side of the brain, resulting in focal symptomatology such as twitching in an arm or face, a sensory change, or even the focal type of change in memory that occurs with temporal lobe seizures.

   Partial seizures are further divided into simple partial seizures with no alteration of consciousness or memory, or complex partial seizures with alteration of consciousness or memory.

   (a) Simple Partial Seizures: Simple partial seizures can be motor seizures with twitching, abnormal sensations, abnormal visions, sounds or smells, and distortions of perception. Seizure activity can spread to the autonomic nervous system, resulting in flushing, tingling, or nausea.

   (b) Complex Partial Seizures: Complex partial seizures previously were called "psychomotor seizures", "temporal lobe seizures" or "limbic seizures". Complex partial seizures may have an aura, which is a warning for the seizure, typically a familiar feeling (deja vu), nausea, heat or tingling, or distortion of sensory perceptions. About half of the patients do not have any remembered aura. During the complex partial seizure patients may fumble or perform automatic fragments of activity such as lip smacking, picking at their clothes, walking around aimlessly, or saying nonsense phrases over and over again. These purposeless activities are called automatisms.

   (c) Secondarily generalized (partial onset evolving to generalized tonic-clonic seizures): **Secondarily Generalized Seizures:** Seizures that begin focally can spread to the entire brain, in which case a tonic-clonic seizure ensues.

2. **Generalized Seizures**: Generalized seizures apparently start on both sides of the brain. "Generalized Seizures are further classified as:

   (a) Absence Seizures: Absence seizures previously were called **Petit mal seizures**. Absence seizures usually have onset in childhood, but they can persist into adulthood. Absence seizures present with staring spells lasting several seconds, sometimes in conjunction with eyelid fluttering or head nodding.

   (b) Tonic-Clonic Seizures: Generalized tonic-clonic seizures previously were called **Grand mal seizures.** These seizures start with sudden loss of consciousness and tonic activity (stiffening) followed by clonic activity (rhythmic jerking) of the limbs. The patient's eyes will roll up at the beginning of the seizure and the patient will typically emit a cry, not because of pain, but because of contraction of the respiratory muscles against a closed throat. Generalized tonic-clonic seizures usually last from one to three minutes. The seizure itself is called an ictus. After the seizure, the patient is "post-ictal": sluggish, sleepy and confused, variably for hours.

   (c) Atonic Seizures: Atonic seizures typically occur in children or adults with widespread brain injuries. People with atonic seizures suddenly become limp and may fall to the ground.

(d) Myoclonic Seizures A Myoclonic seizure is a brief un-sustained jerk or series of jerks, less organized than the rhythmic jerks seen during a generalized tonic-clonic seizure. Other specialized seizure types occasionally are encountered.

(e) Tonic Seizures: Tonic seizures involve stiffening of muscles as the primary seizure manifestation. Arms or legs may extend forward or up into the air. Consciousness may or may not be lost. By definition, the clonic (jerking) phase is absent.

3. **Unclassified Epileptic Seizures:** This category includes all seizures which cannot be classified because of inadequate or incomplete data, or seizures that defy classification in the categories as presently defined.

   - **Neonatal seizures:** brief episodes of apnoea, eye blinking, repetitive movements of arms and legs.
   - **Infantile spasms:** intense spasm of head, trunk and limbs and may also include sudden flexion of neck and abdomen with extension of limbs.

4. **Status Epilepticus**: Status epilepticus (SE) is a life-threatening condition in which the brain is in a state of persistent seizure. It is defined as one continuous, unremitting seizure lasting longer than 5 minutes, or recurrent seizures without regaining consciousness between seizures for greater than 5 minutes. A status epilepticus occurs whenever a seizure persists for at least 30 minutes, without full recovery of consciousness or is repeated so frequently that recovery between attacks does not occur. It is always considered a medical emergency. It is a dangerous condition which may result in brain damage (cerebral necrosis) with severe morbidity or death.

Clinical Presentation of Epilepsy

General

In most cases, the healthcare provider will not be in a position to witness a seizure. Many patients (particularly those with Complex partial (CP) or Generalised Toxic-Clonic (GTC) seizures) are amnestic to the actual seizure event. Obtaining an adequate history and description of the ictal event (including time course) from a third party (e.g., significant other, family member, or witness) is critically important. With treatment the typical clinical presentation of the seizure may change.

Symptoms

Symptoms of a specific seizure will depend on seizure type. Although seizures can vary between patients, they tend to be stereotyped within an individual.

- CP seizures can include somatosensory or focal motor features.
- CP seizures are associated with altered consciousness.
- Absence seizures can be almost nondetectable with only very brief (seconds) periods of altered consciousness.
- GTC seizures are major convulsive episodes and are always associated with a loss of consciousness.

Signs

Interictally (between seizure episodes), there are typically no objective or pathognomonic signs.

Diagnosis

Laboratory Tests

There are currently no diagnostic laboratory tests for epilepsy. In some cases, particularly following GTC (or perhaps CP) seizures, serum prolactin levels can be transiently elevated. Laboratory tests can be done to rule out treatable causes of seizures (e.g., hypoglycemia, altered electrolyte concentrations, infections, etc.) that do not represent epilepsy.

Other Diagnostic Tests

EEG is very useful in the diagnosis of various seizure disorders.

- An epileptiform EEG is found in only approximately 50% of the patients who have epilepsy.
- A prolactin serum level obtained within 10 to 20 minutes of a tonic-clonic seizure can be useful in differentiating seizure activity from pseudoseizure activity but not from syncope.
- Although magnetic resonance imaging (MRI) is very useful (especially imaging of the temporal lobes), a computed tomography (CT) scan typically is not helpful except in the initial evaluation for a brain tumor or cerebral bleeding.

Selected Epilepsy Syndromes [6]

1. Juvenile myoclonic epilepsy Myoclonic seizures often precede generalized tonic-clonic seizures. Myoclonic and generalized tonic-clonic episodes on awakening. Absence seizures also common. ↓ Sleep, fatigue, and alcohol commonly precipitate seizures. Valproate. Levetiracetam FDA approved as adjunct for myoclonic seizures. Phenytoin possibly an adjunct to valproate in resistant cases. Carbamazepine reported to exacerbate seizures in some patients.

2. Lennox-Gastaut syndrome generalized seizures: atypical absence, atonic/akinetic, myoclonic, and tonic most common. Abnormal interictal EEG with slow spike-wave pattern. Cognitive dysfunction and mental retardation. Status epilepticus common. Valproate and benzodiazepines may be effective. Lamotrigine and topiramate FDA-approved. Felbamate also may be effective, but potential hematologic toxicity limits use. Poorly responsive to AED

3. Childhood absence epilepsy (true petit mal) typical absences often in clusters of multiple seizures (pyknolepsy). Tonic-clonic seizures in ~40%. Onset usually between ages 4 and 8. Significant genetic component. EEG shows classic 3-Hz spike-wave pattern. Ethosuximide or valproate. Lamotrigine probably effective.

4. Temporal lobe epilepsy Complex partial seizures with automatisms. Simple partial seizures (auras) common; secondary generalized seizures occur in 50%. Carbamazepine, phenytoin, valproate, gabapentin, lamotrigine, topiramate, tiagabine, levetiracetam, oxcarbazepine, zonisamide, pregabalin

Management

Desired outcome

The goal of treatment is to control or reduce the frequency of seizures, minimize side effects, and ensure compliance, allowing the patient to live as normal a life as possible. Complete suppression of seizures must be balanced against tolerability of side effects, and the patient should be involved in defining the balance.

Nonpharmacological Treatment
1. Surgery is an extremely useful form of treatment in selected patients.
2. Dietary modification may be used for patients who cannot tolerate AED. Ketogenic diet- this low-carbohydrate, high-fat diet results in persistent ketosis
3. Vagus nerve stimulator (VNS) is approved for treatment of intractable partial seizures.

Treatment with Algorithm [7]
1. Seizures are classified if the patient is with new onset epilpesy or classify the epileptic syndrome
2. If the patient is with
   (a) Parital seizure with or without secondary generalisation, complex partial seizures or epilepsy syndrome – he is initiated with carbamazepine, oxcarbamazepine, phenytoin, valproate, or phenobarbitone.
   (b) If the patient is with generalised seizures or epilepsy syndrome-he is intiated with Valproate, phenytoin, phenobarbitone, carbamazepine, oxcarbazepine for generalised tonic-clonic seizures. Valproate, for GTCS, myoclonic jerks, absence seizures and generalised epilepsy syndromes.
   (c) If the patient is undetermined types like generalised or focal seiszures- he is intiated with Valproate, phenytoin, phenobarbitone, carbamazepine, oxcarbamazepine for generalised tonic-clonic seizures. Valproate, for GTCS, myoclonic jerks, absence seizures and generalised epilepsy syndromes.

Classification of Anti-Epileptic Drugs According to Mechanisms of Action [8]

1. Sodium Channel Blockers
Sodium channel blockade is the most common and best-characterized mechanism of currently available antiepileptic drugs (AEDs). AEDs that target sodium channels prevent the return of the channels to the active state by stabilizing the inactive form. The repetitive firing of the axons is prevented.

Phenytoin
Phenytoin is the most common inexpensive AED used by general physicians.

MOA: The primary site of action appears to be the motor cortex where spread of seizure activity is inhibited. Possibly by promoting sodium efflux from neurons, Phenytoin tends to stabilize the threshold against hyper-excitability caused by excessive stimulation or environmental changes capable of reducing membrane sodium gradient. Phenytoin reduces the maximal activity of brain stem centres responsible for the tonic phase of tonic clonic (grand mal) seizures.

Dose: Typical adult recommended dose is around 300 mg/day.

Side effects: Uunsteadiness and moderate cognitive problems. Long-term potential cosmetic (body/face hair growth, skin problems), and bone problems (osteoporosis). Phenytoin causes a rash rate of a few percent, sometimes even the dangerous rash called Stevens-Johnson syndrome.

Carbamazepine

Carbamazepine is considered an AED of first choice for newly diagnosed partial seizures and for primary GTC seizures that are not considered an emergency.

MOA: Carbamazepine affects sodium channels, and inhibits rapid firing of brain cells.

Dose: Typical adult dose is 400 mg TID.

Side effects: GI upset, weight gain, blurred vision, low blood counts, low blood sodium (hypo-natremia), Rash.

Oxcarbazepine

It is at least as effective, and may have fewer side effects, except for more risk for low blood sodium (hyponatremia). Oxcarbazepine does not produce the toxic 10,11epoxide metabolite, which is largely responsible for the adverse effects reported with Carbamazepine. It is more expensive than generic Carbamazepine. A typical adult dose is 600 mg twice a day. An immediate switch from Carbamazepine to full-dose Oxcarbazepine is possible in some cases.

Lamotrigine

Lamotrigine is a broad-spectrum alternative to Valproic acid, with a better side effect profile. LTG may not be as effective for myoclonic seizures. It is useful as both adjunctive therapy for partial seizures and as monotherapy. It may also be a useful alternative for primary generalized seizures, such as absence and as adjunctive therapy for primary GTC seizures.

MOA: Lamotrigine works by several mechanisms including blocking voltage-dependent sodium-channel conductance, blocking release of glutamate, the brain's main excitatory neurotransmitter.

Dose: Available as tablets and extended release forms with dosage of 25, 50, 100, 200, 250 and 500mg. Max dose-300-500mg/day

Side effects: Dizziness and fatigue, usually mild cognitive (thinking) impairment,.rash occurring in 5-10% of people. There-fore, it takes a couple of months to get up to the typical adult dose of 200 mg twice a day. Lamotrigine is also used for mood stabilization.

Zonisamide

MOA: Zonisamide exerts its mechanism of action by reduction of neuronal repetitive firing by blocking sodium channels and preventing neurotransmitter release. It also exerts influence on T-type calcium channels and prevents influx of calcium. ZNS exhibits neuroprotective effects through free radical scavenging.

Dose: Adult dose is 100-300 mg twice a day.

Side effects: nephrolithiasis, oligihydrosis

Lacosamide

Lacosamide is a new antiepileptic drug, for partial and secondarily generalized seizures. It is chemically related to the amino acid, serine.

MOA: They blocks sodium channels (but in a different way from other seizure medicines), and this block reduces brain excitability.

Side effects: Dizziness, headache, nausea or vomiting, double vision, fatigue, memory or mood problems. It may affect the internal organs, blood counts or heart rhythm, but these potentially serious side effects are infrequent. Atrial fibrillation, atrial flutter.

Dose: The recommended starting dose is 50 mg twice daily, increased each week by an extra 100 mg, to the recommended maintenance dosage of 100-200 mg twice a day.

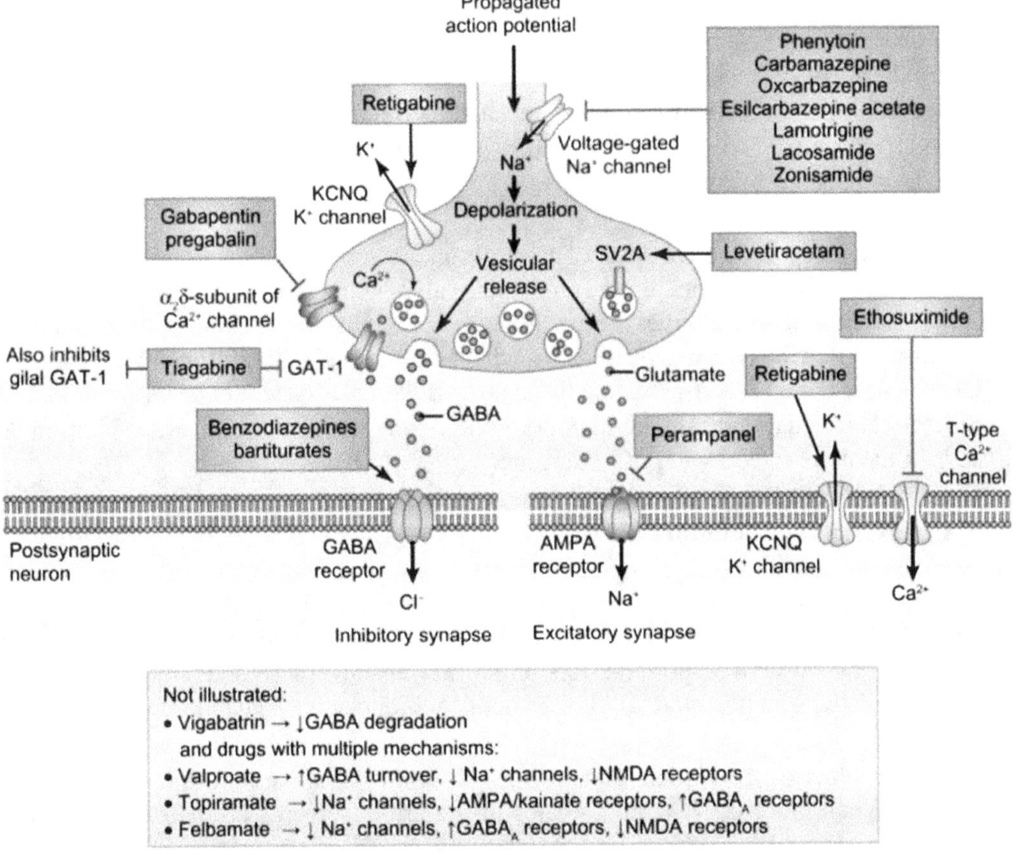

Fig. 63.1 Drug classification with mechanisms of action of drugs.

Souce: Jean Cshin et al., New Drug Classes for the treatment of partial onset epilepsy: Focus on peramipand. Therapeutics and clinical Risk management. 2013; 9(1): 285-93.

2. GABA Receptor Agonists

A seizure reflects an imbalance between excitatory and inhibitory activity in the brain, with an increment of excitation over inhibition. The most important inhibitory neurotransmitter in the brain is gamma-aminobutyric acid (GABA). There is a fascinating relationship between this most abundant and important inhibitory agent (GABA) and glutamate, the engine of excitation. GABA-A receptors have multiple binding sites for benzodiazepines, barbiturates, and other substances (e.g., neurosteroids). These drugs bind to different sites around the receptor to exert their action. The benzodiazepines most commonly used for treatment of epilepsy are lorazepam diazepam, midazolam, clonazepam, chlorazepate and clobazam.

Phenobarbital

MOA: Phenobarbital is a traditional, very inexpensive and effective in a single daily dose. Phenobarbital increases the effect of GABA, the main inhibitory neurotransmitter in the brain. Phenobarbital is used for tonic–clonic and partial seizures and may also be tried in atypical absence; atonic and tonic seizures. Phenobarbital is mildly addictive and requires slow withdrawal. During pregnancy, there is a significant rate of birth defects. Phenobarbital is the drug of choice for neonatal seizures, but in other situations it is reserved for patients who have failed other AEDs.

Dose: Adult dose is 100 mg per day. The target serum level is 10-40 mcg per ml.

Side effects: Sedation, thinking/memory problems and depression and also can cause long-term bone problems.

Clonazepam

MOA: Clonazepam is a member of the drug class known as benzodiazepines, to which diazepam, lorazepam, clorazepate, alprazolam also belongs. Benzodiazepines are used as anti-seizure drugs, sedatives, tranquilizers and muscle relaxants. Benzodiazepines increase the effectiveness of GABA, the brain's main inhibitory neurotransmitter. Clonazepam is more long-acting against seizures than are diazepam or lorazepam.

Side effects: Sedation, thinking/memory impairment, mood changes, and addiction. More so than most, its effects wear off over time.

Dose: Adult dose is 0.5-1.0 mg three times a day.

3. GABA Reuptake Inhibitors

Reuptake of gamma-aminobutyric acid (GABA) is facilitated by at least 4 specific GABA-A transporting compounds; these carry GABA from the synaptic space into neurons and glial cells, where it is metabolized. Nipecotic acid and Tiagabine (TGB) are inhibitors of these transporters; this inhibition makes increased amounts of GABA available in the synaptic cleft. GABA prolongs inhibitory postsynaptic potentials (IPSPs).

Tigabine

Tiagabine blocks inactivation (uptake) of the brain's main inhibitory neurotransmitter, GABA. When more GABA accumulates in the brain, seizures are harder to initiate and sustain. It is useful for partial and secondarily generalized seizures. It is not effective for absence or myoclonic seizures. It is considered second-line therapy for patients with partial seizures who have failed initial therapy.

Side effect: Sedation, abnormal thinking, and dizziness.

Dose: Adult dose begin with 4 mg at bedtime for a week, then increase 4 mg each week to 16-56 mg/d in two divided doses.

4. GABA Transaminase Inhibitors

Gamma-aminobutyric acid (GABA) is metabolized by transamination in the extracellular compartment by GABA-transaminase (GABA-T). Inhibition of this enzymatic process leads to an increase in the extracellular concentration of GABA. Vigabatrin (VGB) inhibits the enzyme GABA-T.

Vigabatrin

Vigabatrin blocks metabolism of GABA, the brain's main inhibitory neurotransmitter. It is a close structural analogue of GABA, binding irreversibly to the active site of GABA-T. It is effective for partial seizures, infantile spasms.

Dose: 500 mg twice a day and can increase over a month or two to 1500 mg twice a day.

5. AEDs with Potential GABA Mechanism of Action

The enzyme glutamic acid decarboxylase (GAD) converts glutamate into gamma-aminobutyric acid (GABA). Currently, Valproate (VPA) and Gabapentin have effect on this enzyme and thereby enhance the synthesis of GABA. VPA also blocks the neuronal sodium channel during rapid sustained repetitive firing. Gabapentin has a weak competitive inhibition of the enzyme GABA-T.

Gabapentin

It is a second-line agent for patients with partial seizures who have failed initial treatment. It may also have a role in patients with less severe seizure disorders, such as new-onset partial epilepsy, especially in elderly patients.

MOA: It acts by transportation of GABA and effects on calcium channels. It has no drug interactions, is not metabolized in the liver and it does not bind to blood proteins.

Side effects: Unsteadiness, weight gain, fatigue, dizziness.

Dose: Adult dose is 300-600 mg three times a, but doses can be up to 1200 mg three times a day. Gabapentin often is used also for chronic pains of certain types.

Pregabalin

It is more effective against seizures than Gabapentin. It is a second-line agent for partial seizures that have failed initial treatment.

MOA: Pregabalin does not alter GABA concentration in brain tissues or inhibit GABA transport in vitro. Pregabalin binds with high affinity to both the alpha2 delta-1 and alpha2delta-2 subtypes. Pregabalin has no drug interactions, no liver metabolism, no protein binding, and similar side effects to Gabapentin.

Dose: Typical adult dose is 150 - 600 mg bid.

Pregabalin often is used also for chronic pains of certain types.

Valproic Acid

It is first-line therapy for primary generalized seizures, such as absence, myoclonic, and atonic seizures, and is approved for adjunctive and monotherapy treatment of partial seizures. It can also be useful in mixed seizure disorders.

This is the standard broad-spectrum AED (treats all types of seizures) and no other AED is more effective for generalized seizure types. Valproate has effects on GABA, and a neurotransmitter called NPY to block seizures, and on calcium channels.

Side effects: Weight gain, tremor, hair loss, GI up-set, blood count decreases, hepatic or pancreatic injury, bone weakness over time (osteoporosis), birth defects in up to 10% (folic acid can help to prevent them).

Dose: Typical adult dose is 250 mg - 500 mg three times a day, but dose can be higher. An extended release form can be taken once a day.

6. **Glutamate Blockers**

Glutamate and aspartate are the most two important excitatory neurotransmitters in the brain. The glutamate system is a complex system that contains macromolecular receptors with different binding sites (i.e., alpha-amino-3-hydroxy-5-methylisoxazole-4-propionic acid [AMPA], kainate, N -methyl-D-aspartate [NMDA], glycine, and metabotropic sites). The AMPA and the kainate sites open a channel through the receptor, allowing sodium and small amounts of calcium to enter. The NMDA site opens a channel that allows large amounts of calcium to enter along with the sodium ions. This channel is blocked by magnesium in the resting state. The glycine site facilitates the opening of the NMDA receptor channel. The metabotropic site is regulated by complex reactions and its response is mediated by second messengers. NMDA antagonists have a limited use because they produce psychosis and hallucinations.

Felbamate

MOA: Felbamate has been proposed to a unique dual mechanism of action as a positive modulator of GABAA receptors and as a blocker of NMDA receptors, particularly isoforms containing the NR2B subunit.

It has efficacy against atonic seizures, as well as partial and secondarily generalized seizures. Felbamate has substantial drug interactions, which make it difficult to use in conjunction with other medications.

Dose: A typical adult dose of Felbamate is 400-1200 mg orally three times per day (total of 1200 - 3600 mg per day).

Topiramate

It is a first-line AED for patients with partial seizures. It is also approved for tonic-clonic seizures in primary generalized epilepsy.

MOA: Topiramate is a very potent anticonvulsant that is structurally different from other AEDs. Topiramate has multiple mechanisms of action. It exerts an inhibitory effect on sodium conductance, decreasing the duration of spontaneous bursts and the frequency of generated action potentials, enhances GABA by unknown mechanisms, inhibits the AMPA subtype glutamate receptor, and is a weak inhibitor of carbonic anhydrase. Blocking the enzyme carbonic anhydrase affects the acidity of brain tissue. More acidity (to a point) suppresses seizures.

Side effects: Thinking and memory problems in about 1/3rd, renal stones in 1-2%, rare cases of glaucoma (increased eye pressure) and weight loss.

Dose: Typical adult dose is 150-200 mg twice a day.

7. AEDs with Other Mechanisms of Action [9, 10]

Levetiracetam

Levetiracetam is one of the more used medicines in seizure clinics because it probably is effective for a broad-spectrum of seizures types, has a relatively low incidence of causing thinking/memory problems.

MOA: Action is possibly related to a brain-specific stereo-selective binding site, synaptic vesicle protein 2A (SV2A). SV2A appears to be important for the availability of calcium-dependent neurotransmitter vesicles ready to release their content. The lack of SV2A results in decreased action potential-dependent neurotransmission, while action potential independent neurotransmission remains normal. In addition, it reduces Bicuculline-induced hyperexcitability in rat hippocampal CA3 neurons, suggesting a mechanism that does not involve release of gamma-aminobutyric acid (GABA). LEV inhibits Ca2+ release from the inositoltrisphosphate (IP3)-sensitive stores without reducing Ca2+ storage, which could explain some of its antiepileptic properties. It has no drug interactions, is not metabolized in the liver and it does not bind to blood proteins.

Side effects: Dizziness, fatigue, insomnia, but the more troublesome problem can be irritability and mood changes. This may occur to some degree in up to a third of those taking the medicine. **Dose:** Adult dose is 500 - 1500 mg twice a day.

8. Benzodiazepines for epilepsy:

Clobazam:

iinitial 5 mg bid, titrated to 10mg bid on day 7.

Adverse effects: Stevens Johnson's syndrome

Clonazepam:

Dose: Initial: 0.5 mg tid; max 20mg daily in 3 divided doses; may titrate up 0.5-1mg every 3 days

Adverse effects: Paradoxical aggression or hyperactivity

Diazepam: Status epilepticus

Dose: initial: 5-10mg IV every 10-15min; max 30mg

Lorazepam: Status epilepticus

Dose: Initial 4 mg IV; 0.1mg/kg IV, may repeat once

9. Surgery

Medications can control seizures in most people with epilepsy, however it is ineffective and or intolerable in almost 30% of population, for them brain surgery may be an option. Surgery for epilepsy is performed either with a "curative" indication aiming to complete freedom of seizures or "palliative" aiming to decrease the frequency of occurrence of seizures. The type of surgery depends on the type of seizure and the area of the brain where the seizure start. The surgical options include lobe resection, lesionectomy, corpus callostomy, functional hemispherectomy, multiple subpial transaction, radiotherapy etc.

Initial Treatment

Initial treatment for epilepsy depends on the severity, frequency, and type of seizures and whether a cause for your condition has been identified. Medicine is the first and most common approach. Antiepileptic medicines do not cure epilepsy, but they help prevent seizures in well over half of the people who take them.

Ongoing Treatment

If epileptic seizures continue even though being treated, additional or other antiepileptic medicines may be tried. A thorough classification of drugs as per their mechanism of action can provide a better understanding for selection of treatment.

Antiepileptic Drugs (Aed) Useful For Various Seizure Types

Primarily generalised tonic-clonic

- Most Effective With Least Toxicity: Valproate, Phenytoin, Carbamazepine, Lamotrigine, Levetiracetam, Oxcarbazepine, Topiramate, Zonisamide
- Effective, but with unacceptable toxicity: Phenobarbital, Primidone, Felbamate
- Of little value: Ethosuximide. Trimethadone

Secondarily generalized tonic-clonic

- Most Effective With Least Toxicity: Carbamazepine, Phenytoin, Valproate, Gabapentin, Lamotrigine, Zonisamide, Levetiracetam,
- Effective, but with unacceptable toxicity: Phenobarbital, Primidone, Felbamate
- Of little value: Ethosuximide. Trimethadone

Simple or complex seizures

- Most Effective with Least toxicity: Carbamazepine, Oxcarbazepine, Phenytoin, Valproate, Lamotrigine, Levetiracetam, Topiramate, Zonisamide
- Effective, but with unacceptable toxicity: Clorazepate, Phenobarbital, Primidone, Felbamate
- Of little value: Ethosuximide. Trimethadone

Absence seizures

- Most Effective With Least Toxicity: Ethosuximode, Valproate, Lamotrigine
- Effective , but with unacceptable toxicity: Clonazepam, Trimethadone
- Of little value: Phenytoin, Carbamzepine, Phenobarbital, Primidone

Management of Adults presenting with an unprovoked first seizure

- Adults presenting with an unprovoked first seizure should be informed that the chance for a recurrent seizure is greatest within the first 2 years after the first seizure (21–45%).
- For evaluation, an EEG should be considered to be a part of the routine neurodiagnostic evaluation. Brain imaging using computed tomography (CT) or magnetic resonance imaging (MRI) should be ordered, preferably an MRI brain.
- Blood glucose, blood counts, and electrolyte panels (particularly sodium) may be helpful in specific clinical circumstances.
- Immediately AED therapy should be initiated.

Antiepileptic drug	Common side effects	Enzyme induction
Phenobarbital	Sedation, depression, and paradosical hyperactivity	Yes
Phenytoin	Nystagmus, ataxia, diplopia, gingival hyperplaysia, hirsutism, hepatoxicity, and lupus-like reactions	Yes
Carbamazepine	Nausea, rash, hyponatremia, leukopenia, and rare, hepatotoxicity	Yes
Oxcarbazepine	Hypontremia, fatigue, headaches, dizziness, ataxia, and rash	Yes
Lamotrigine	Stevens-Johnson syndrome, hypersensitivity, and rash	Yes
Topiramate	Impaired language fluency and cognitive dysfunction, paresthesias, metabolic acidosis, weight loss, renal calculi, and acute glaucoma	Yes (weak)
Zoniasamide	Rash, Stevens-Johnson syndrome, renal calculi, fatigue, and dizziness	No
Levetiracetam	Irritability and behaviour problems	No
Lacosamide	Dizziness, nausea	No
Eslicarbazepine	Dizziness, nausea, fatigue, and ataxia	Yes (weak)
Rufinamide	Fatigue, vomiting, and loss of appetite	Yes
Clobazam	Sedation	No
Perampenel	Dizziness, irritability, severe mood and behaviour changes, and homicidial ideations	No

0-5 minutes stabilization phase:

1. Stabilize patient (airway, breathing, circulation, disability - neurologic exam)
2. Time seizure from its onset, monitor vital signs
3. Assess oxygenation, give oxygen via nasal cannula/mask, consider intubation if respiratory assistance needed
4. Initiate ECG monitoring
5. Collect finger stick blood glucose. If glucose < 60 mg/dl then Adults: 100 mg thiamine IV then 50 ml D50W IV Children ≥ 2 years: 2 ml/kg D25W IV Children < 2 years: 4 ml/kg D12.5W IV
6. Attempt IV access and collect electrolytes, hematology, toxicology screen, (if appropriate) anticonvulsant drug levels

Does the seizure continue- if NO. If the patient is at baseline- then symptomatic medical care to be provided. But if seizure continues, then next initial therpay to be initiated.

5-20 Minutes Initial Therapy Phase: A benzodiazepine is the initial therapy of choice Choose one of the following 3 equivalent first line options with dosing and frequency:

- Intramuscular midazolam (10 mg for > 40 kg, 5 mg for 13-40 kg, single dose, or
- Intravenous lorazepam (0.1 mg/kg/dose, max: 4 mg/dose, may repeat dose once, or
- Intravenous diazepam (0.15-0.2 mg/kg/dose, max: 10 mg/dose, may repeat dose once,

If none of the 3 options above are available, choose one of the following:

- Intravenous phenobarbital (15 mg/kg/dose, single dose, or
- Rectal diazepam (0.2-0.5 mg/kg, max: 20 mg/dose, single dose, or
- Intranasal midazolam, buccal midazolam or

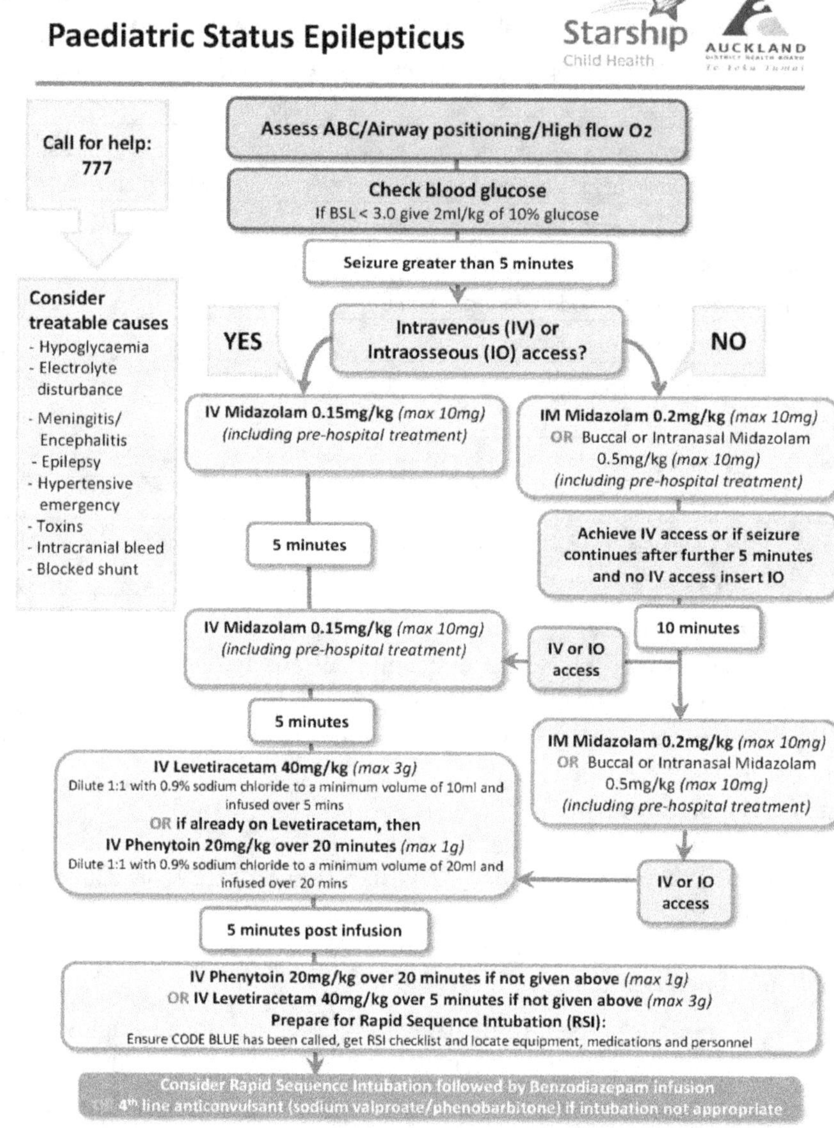

Fig. 63.2 Proposed Algorithm for Management of Convulsive Status Epilepticus.

Source: Lewana S et al., Emergency management of pediatric convulsive status epilepticus. Pediatric emergency care 2009; 25(2):83-7.

20-40 Minutes Second Therapy Phase: There is no evidence based preferred second therapy of choice (Level U): Choose one of the following second line options and give as a single dose

- Intravenous fosphenytoin (20 mg PE/kg, max: 1500 mg PE/dose, single dose, or
- Intravenous valproic acid (40 mg/kg, max: 3000 mg/dose, single dose, or
- Intravenous levetiracetam (60 mg/kg, max: 4500 mg/dose, single dose,

If none of the options above are available, choose one of the following (if not given already)

- Intravenous phenobarbital (15 mg/kg, single dose)

40-60 Minutes Third Therapy Phase: There is no clear evidence to guide therapy in this phase Choices include: repeat second line therapy or anesthetic doses of either thiopental, midazolam, pentobarbital, or propofol (all with continuous EEG monitoring)

Risk Factors Possibly Predicting Seizure Recurrence Following AED Withdrawal

- <2–6 yr seizure free before withdrawal
- Onset of seizures after age 12
- History of atypical febrile seizures
- Large number of seizures (>30) before control or total of >100 seizures
- Partial seizures (simple or complex)
- History of absence seizures
- Abnormal EEG persisting throughout treatment
- Slowing on EEG before medication withdrawal
- Organic neurologic disorder
- Moderate to severe mental retardation
- Withdrawal of valproate or phenytoin (higher rate of recurrence than withdrawal of other AED)

American Academy of Neurology Guideline for Discontinuing AEDs in Seizure-Free Patients

After assessing the risks and benefits to both patient and society from a recurrent seizure, the discontinuance of antiepileptic drugs may be considered by the physician and informed patient or parent/guardian if the patient meets the following profile:

- Seizure-free 2 to 5 years on AEDs (mean, 3.5 years)
- Single type of partial seizure (simple partial, complex partial, or secondary generalized tonic-clonic seizure) or single type of primary generalized tonic-clonic seizures
- Normal neurologic examination/normal IQ
- EEG normalized with treatment

References

1. Sridharan R, Murthy BN. Prevalence and pattern of epilepsy in India. Epilepsia. 1999; 40:631–6.

2. P.A. Dekker, M.D. Epilepsy – A Manual to Medical & Clinical Officers in Africa. Revised 2nd edition. World Health Organization, Geneva 2002.

3. Browne T.R. & Holmes G.L., Philadelphia, PA, Lippincott Williams & Wilkins. Handbook of Epilepsy. 2000; 2nd Ed. 42-55, 91-94.

4. Commission on Classification and Terminology of the International League against Epilepsy. Proposal for revised clinical and electroencephalographic classification of epileptic seizures. Epilepsia. 1981; 22:489–501.

5. Engel Jr. Classifications of the International League against Epilepsy: time for reappraisal. Epilepsia. 1998; 39:1014–1017.

6. Dreifuss FE. The epilepsies: clinical implications of the international classification. Epilepsia 1990;31(Suppl 3):S3

7. Mrinal kanti roy et al., Indian guidelines on epilepsy. Neurology. Chapter 116. 2015.

8. Cramer JA, Fisher R, Ben-Menachem E, et al: New anti-epileptic drugs: comparison of key clinical trials. Epilepsia 1999; 40:590–600.

9. K.P. Sampath Kumar et al. Recent Advances in Epilepsy drug therapy and management disease. International Journal of PharmTech Research. 2010, 2(1).

10. Spencer SS, Berg AT, Vickrey BG, et al. Initial outcomes in the Multicenter Study of Epilepsy Surgery. Neurology. 2003; 61 (12): 1680–5.

11. Pellock JM. Efficacy and adverse effects of antiepileptic drugs. Pediatr Clin North Am 1989;36: 435.

12. Jean C Shih et al., New drug classes for the treatment of partial onset epilepsy: Focus on perampanel. Therapeutics and Clinical Risk Management. 2013, 9(1):285-93.

CHAPTER - 64

Headache Disorders

Introduction to Headache Disorders [1,2]

International Headache Society Classification System: Focus on Migraine Headache

Migraine

Migraine without aura

Migraine with aura

   Typical aura with migraine headache (aura lasting less than 1 hour)

   Typical aura with nonmigraine headache

   Typical aura without headache Familial hemiplegic migraine

   Sporadic hemiplegic migraine

   Basilar-type migraine

Childhood periodic syndromes that are commonly precursors of migraine

   Cyclical vomiting (self-limiting episodic condition)

   Abdominal migraine (episodic midline abdominal pain attacks lasting 1 to72 hours)

   Benign paroxysmal vertigo of childhood (brief episodic vertigo)

Retinal migraine (repeated attacks of monocular visual disturbance)

Complications of migraine

   Chronic migraine (occurring on 15 or more days per month for more than 3months)

   Status migrainosus (debilitating attack lasting for more than 72 hours)

   Persistent aura without infarction (symptoms persisting for more than 1 week)

   Migrainous infarction (aura symptoms associated with an ischemic brain lesion)

   Migraine-triggered seizure

Probable migraine

Probable migraine without aura

Probable migraine with aura

Probable chronic migraine

Tension-type headache

Cluster headache and other trigeminal autonomic cephalalgias

Other primary headaches

Headache attributed to head and/or neck trauma

Headache attributed to cranial or cervical vascular disorder

Headache attributed to non-vascular intracranial disorder

Headache attributed to a substance or its withdrawal

Headache attributed to infection Headache attributed to disorder of homeostasis

Headache or facial pain attributed to disorder of cranium, neck, eyes, ears, nose, sinuses, Teeth, mouth, or other facial or cranial structures

Headache attributed to psychiatric disorder cranial neuralgias and central causes of facial Pain. Other headache, cranial neuralgia, central or primary facial pain.

Most recurrent headaches are the result of a benign chronic primary headache disorder. Less often, headaches are symptomatic of a serious underlying medical condition, such as infection, cerebral haemorrhage, or brain mass lesion. The peak prevalence of tension-type and migraine headache, the most common of the primary headache disorders, occurs during the most productive years of life (20 to 55 years of age).

Migraine Headache

Migraine is a common, recurrent, primary headache of moderate to severe intensity that interferes with normal functioning and is associated with GI, neurologic, and autonomic symptoms

Epidemiology [3]:
- Before the age of 12 years, migraine is more common in boys than in girls, but prevalence increases more rapidly in girls after puberty. After age 12, females are two to three times more likely than males to suffer from migraine.
- Prevalence is highest in both men and women between the ages of 35 and 45 years.
- A number of neurologic and psychiatric disorders, including stroke, epilepsy, major depression, and anxiety disorder, show increased comorbidity with migraine.

Etiopathogenesis [4]:
- Migraine aura is caused by intracerebral arterial vasoconstriction that is followed by reactive extracranial vasodilation and associated headache. Although studies of regional

blood flow in the brain do not support the vascular hypothesis, the aura phase of migraine is associated with a reduction in cerebral blood flow that begins in the occipital region and moves across the cerebral cortex at a rate of 2 to 3 mm/min. The neurologic changes of the aura parallel those which occur during spreading depression, a neuronal event characterized by a wave of depressed electrical activity that advances across the brain cortex at a rate that is consistent with the spread of aura symptoms.

- Migraine without aura is a neurobiologic disorder.
- Migraine pain is believed to result from activity within the trigeminovascular system, a network of visceral afferent fibers that arises from the trigeminal ganglia and projects peripherally to innervate the pain-sensitive intracranial extracerebral blood vessels, dura mater, and large venous sinuses.
- These fibers also project centrally, terminating in the trigeminal nucleus caudalis in the brain stem and upper cervical spinal cord, and thus provide a pathway for nociceptive transmission from meningeal blood vessels into higher centres of the central nervous system (CNS).
- Activation of trigeminal sensory nerves triggers the release of vasoactive neuropeptides, including calcitonin gene–related peptide (CGRP), neurokinin A, and substance P, from perivascular axons.
- The released neuropeptides interact with dural blood vessels to promote vasodilation and dural plasma extravasation, resulting in perivascular inflammation.
- Orthodromic conduction along trigeminovascular fibers transmits pain impulses to the trigeminal nucleus caudalis, where the information is relayed further to higher cortical pain centers.
- Continued afferent input may result in sensitization of these central sensory neurons, producing a hyperalgesic state that prolongs and intensifies headache pain as the attack progresses.
- Activity within the trigeminovascular system may be regulated in part by noradrenergic and, most important, serotonergic neurons within the brain stem. Thus the pathogenesis of migraine may be related to an imbalance in the activity of serotonin-containing neurons and/or noradrenergic pathways in brain stem nuclei that modulate cerebral vascular tone and nociception.
- This imbalance may result in vasodilation of intracranial extracerebral blood vessels and consequent activation of the trigeminovascular system. Future research may further delineate the role of the brain stem as the "migraine generator.
- Genetic factors appear to play an important role in an individual's susceptibility to migraine attacks. Studies in monozygotic twins suggest that up to 50% of the contribution to the common migraine variants is genetically based, with a substantial influence from environmental factors.
- The hyper responsiveness of the migrainous brain may be the result of an inherited abnormality in P/Q-type calcium channels that regulate cortical excitability through the release of serotonin and other neurotransmitters. Low levels of magnesium or dopamine, increased levels of excitatory amino acids, and alterations in levels of endogenous opioids also may affect the migraine threshold.

- Serotonin (5-hydroxytryptamine, or 5-HT) has long been implicated as an important mediator of migraine headache.

Hypothesized Sequence of Events in Migraine

Modulating factors like drugs, environment, gender, hormone, genes, ionic or metabolic disturbances contribute to disturbance of cortical and ot brainstem excitability. This leads to

(i) activation of cortical waves- cortical spreading depression which causes increase in BBB permeability and generation of AURA (Visual, sensory, cognitive changes).

(ii) Activation of brainstem leading to activation of trigeminal nucleus caudalis, pons, central sensitisation. From here the stimulus is forwarded and there is activation of pain receptors. Now there is release of nociceptive messengers like Substance P, NO, Atrial natruretic peptide; vasoactive peptides like CGRP(Calcitonin Gene Related Peptide), NKA (Neurokinin A), SP which cause neurogenic inflammation, vasodilation and protein extravasation events.

(iii) There is activation of sensory pathways- nausea, vertigo, photophobia, cutaneous allodynia

(iv) All these events converge to initiate and propagate the pain.

Clinical manifestations and features:

General

Migraine is a common, recurrent, severe headache that interferes with normal functioning. It is a primary headache disorder divided into two major subtypes, migraine without aura and migraine with aura.

Symptoms

Migraine is characterized by recurring episodes of throbbing head pain, frequently unilateral, that when untreated can last from 4 to 72 hours. Migraine headaches can be severe and associated with nausea, vomiting, and sensitivity to light, sound, and/or movement. Not all symptoms are present at every attack.

Neurologic symptoms (phonophobia, photophobia, hyperosmia, difficulty concentrating) are most common, but psychological (anxiety, depression, euphoria, irritability, drowsiness, hyperactivity, restlessness), autonomic (e.g., polyuria, diarrhea, constipation), and constitutional (e.g., stiff neck, yawning, thirst, food cravings, anorexia) symptoms may also occur.

Signs

A stable pattern, absence of daily headache, positive family history for migraine, normal neurologic examination, presence of food triggers, menstrual association, long-standing history, improvement with sleep, and subacute evolution are all signs of migraine headache. Aura may signal the migraine headache but is not required for diagnosis.

Diagnosis [5, 6]

Diagnostic approach to the patient with frequent headaches
1. **Identify** the most probable headache diagnosis; assess for serious underlying condition.
    (a) High probability: urgent assessment and intervention
    (b) Low probability: diagnosis unclear: reassess and consider consult
    Probably migraine or tension type headache: assess for medciation overuse headache-treat if present
    Possibly trigeminal autonomic cephalalgia: perform imaging assessment
2. **Implement individualized management plan**
    (a) Acute and prophylactic therapies
    (b) Behavioral and physical therapies
    (c) Counsel patient about medication adherence and appropiraite medication use.
    (d) Reduce risk factors, triggers, and exacerbating factors
    (e) Promote healthy lifestyle
    (f) Manage comorbidities
    (g) Provide headache education for patient and family menbers

Laboratory Tests

In selected circumstances and secondary headache presentation, serum chemistries, urine toxicology profiles, thyroid function tests, lyme studies, and other blood tests such as a complete blood count, antinuclear antibody titer, erythrocyte sedimentation rate, and antiphospholipid antibody titer may be considered.

Diagnostic Tests

Perform a general medical and neurologic physical examination. Check for abnormalities: vital signs (fever, hypertension), funduscopy (papilledema, hemorrhage, and exudates), palpation and auscultation of the head and neck (sinus tenderness, hardened or tender temporal arteries, trigger points, temporomandibular joint tenderness, bruits, nuchal rigidity, and cervical spine tenderness), and neurologic examination (identify abnormalities or deficits in mental status, cranial nerves, deep tendon reflexes, motor strength, coordination, gait, and cerebellar function). Consider neuroimaging studies in patients with abnormal neurologic examination findings of unknown etiology and in those with additional risk factors warranting imaging.

- The migraine *aura,* a complex of positive and negative focal neurologic symptoms that precedes or accompanies an attack.
- The aura typically evolves over 5 to 20 minutes and lasts less than 60 minutes. Headache usually occurs within 60 minutes of the end of the aura. Occasionally, aura symptoms begin at the onset of headache or during the attack.
- Visual auras vary in their complexity and can include both positive (scintillations, photopsia, teichopsia, or fortification spectrum) and negative (scotoma, hemianopsia) features. Sensory and motor aura symptoms, such as paresthesias or numbness involving the arms and face, dysphasia or aphasia, weakness, and hemiparesis.

- Migraine headache may occur at any time of the day or night but occurs most often in the early morning hours on awakening. Pain is usually gradual in onset, peaking in intensity over a period of minutes to hours and lasting between 4 and 72 hours in adults. Pain may occur anywhere in the face or head but most often involves the frontotemporal region.
- Gastrointestinal symptoms include nausea, emesis. Other systemic symptoms include anorexia, food cravings, constipation, diarrhea, abdominal cramps, nasal stuffiness, blurred vision, diaphoresis, facial pallor, and localized facial, scalp, or periorbital edema.

International Headache Society (HIS) Diagnostic Criteria for Migraine

Migraine without Aura

- At least five attacks
- Headache attack lasts 4 to 72 hours (untreated or unsuccessfully treated)
- Headache has at least two of the following characteristics:
  Unilateral location
  Pulsating quality
  Moderate or severe intensity
  Aggravation by or avoidance of routine physical activity (i.e., walking or climbing stairs)
- During headache at least one of the following:
  Nausea, vomiting, or both
  Photophobia and phonobhobia
- Not attributed to another disorder

Migraine with Aura (Classic Migraine)

At least two attacks

Migraine aura fulfils criteria for typical aura, hemiplegic aura, or Basilar-type aura

Not attributed to another disorder

Typical Aura: Fully reversible visual, sensory, or speech symptoms (or any combination) but no motor weakness.

Homonymous or bilateral visual symptoms including positive features (e.g., flickering lights, spot, lines) or negative features (e.g., loss of vision) or unilateral sensory symptoms including positive features (e.g., visual loss, pins and needles) or negative features (i.e., numbness), or any combination.

At least one of the following:

- At least one symptom that develops gradually over a minimum of 5 minutes or different symptoms that occur in succession or both;
- Each symptom lasts for at least 5 minutes and for no longer than 60 minutes;
- Headache that meets criteria for migraine without aura begins during the aura or follows aura within 60 minutes.

Pound Mnemonic for Diagnosis of Migraine

Clinical features:

Pulsatile quality of headache

Oneday duration of headache (4-72 hrs if untreated or unsuccessfully treated)

Unilateral headache

Nausea or vomiting

Disabling intensity of headache

Management: Migraines [7]

Desired outcomes:

Treatment strategies must:

- Address both immediate and long term goals.
- Acute migraine therapies should provide consistent, rapid relief and enable the patient to resume normal activities.
- Recurrence of symptoms and treatment-related adverse effects should be minimal.

Goals of Therapy in Migraine Management

Goals of Long-Term Migraine Treatment

- Reduce migraine frequency, severity, and disability
- Reduce reliance on poorly tolerated, ineffective, or unwanted acute pharmacotherapies
- Improve quality of life
- Prevent headache
- Avoid escalation of headache medication use
- Educate and enable patients to manage their disease
- Reduce headache-related distress and psychological symptoms.

Goals for Acute Migraine Treatment

- Treat migraine attacks rapidly and consistently without recurrence
- Restore the patient's ability to function
- Minimize the use of backup and rescue medications.
- Optimize self-care for overall management
- Be cost-effective in overall management
- Cause minimal or no adverse effects

Non pharmacologic Treatment:

- Apply ice to the head and recommend periods of rest or sleep, usually in a dark, quiet environment.
- Identify and avoid triggers of migraine attacks
- Behavioural interventions (relaxation therapy, biofeedback, and cognitive therapy) may help patients who prefer non drug therapy or when drug therapy is ineffective or not tolerated.

Treatment algorithm for migraine headaches:
- Once the diagnosis of migraine is confirmed, the patient education regarding a general wellness program and avoidance of trigger factors. Later Assess headache severity and degree of associated disability- Consider prophylactic pharmacotherapy.
- But if the patient is associated with severe nausea or vomiting, pretreat with antiemetic: consider use of suppository, parenteral or intranasal formulation.
- Based on the severity: If the patient is presented with **mild to moderate symptoms-** Simple analgesic: acetaminophen, acetaminophen/aspirin/caffeine NSAIDs: aspirin, ibuprofen, naproxen is to be initiated.

If the response in inadequate- Combination analgesics: Midrin, acetaminophen, or aspirin/ butalbital/caffeine are to be initiated.

- If the patient is presented with **severe symptoms-**a) triptans OR b) Dihydroergotamine or ergotamine tartrate is to be initiated.
- If inadequate response is seen after the respective initial treatment- Opioid combination analgesics, butorphanol nasal spray has to be started.
- For adults with a severe intractable migraine, or status migrainosus (ie, a debilitating attack lasting for more than 72 hours), a combination of intravenous fluids plus parenteral medications, including ketorolac and a dopamine receptor blocker (eg, prochlorperazine, metoclopramide, chlorpromazine) is advised. Other options include valproate and/or dihydroergotamine; some patients may require admission for persistent disabling symptoms.
- For patients who present to the hospital emergency department with moderate to severe migraine, particularly if the migraine is accompanied by vomiting or significant nausea, subcutaneous sumatriptan 6mg+intravenous(IV) metoclopramide (10mg)
  or prochlorperazine (10 mg) and adjunct use of diphenhydramine (12.5 to 25 mg IV every hour up to two doses) to prevent akathisia and other dystonic reactions.
  https://www.uptodate.com/contents/acute-treatment-of-migraine-in-adults#H25

Pharmacologic Treatment of Acute Migraine [8]:
- Administer acute migraine therapies at the onset of migraine
- Pre-treatment with an anti-emetic (e.g., metoclopramide, chlorpromazine, or prochlorperazine) 15 to 30 minutes before oral or non-oral migraine treatment may be advisable when nausea and vomiting are severe. Metoclopramide also helps reverse gastroparesis and enhances absorption of oral medications.
- Frequent or excessive use of acute migraine medications can result in increasing Headache frequency and drug consumption known as medication-overuse headache.

Analgesics and anti inflammatory drugs [9]:
- Simple analgesics and nonsteroidal anti-inflammatory drugs (NSAIDs) are first-line treatments for mild to moderate migraine attacks; some severe attacks are also responsive. Aspirin, diclofenac, ibuprofen, ketorolac, naproxen sodium, tolfenamic acid, and the combination of acetaminophen plus aspirin and caffeine are effective.
- NSAIDs appear to prevent neurogenically mediated inflammation in the trigeminal-vascular system by inhibiting prostaglandin synthesis.

- Acute NSAID therapy is associated with gastrointestinal (e.g., dyspepsia, nausea, vomiting, and diarrhea) and CNS side effects (e.g., somnolence, dizziness). NSAIDs should be used cautiously in patients with previous ulcer disease, renal disease, or hypersensitivity to aspirin.

Ergot Alkaloids and Derivatives

- Ergot alkaloids are useful for moderate to severe migraine attacks. They are nonselective 5HT1 receptor agonists that constrict intracranial blood vessels and inhibit the development of neurogenic inflammation in the trigemino vascular system. Venous and arterial constriction occurs. They also have activity at dopaminergic receptors.
- Side effects: Nausea, vomiting, abdominal pain, weakness, fatigue, paresthesias, muscle pain, diarrhea, and chest tightness, painful extremities; continuous paresthesias; diminished peripheral pulses; and claudication.
- Contraindications: Renal and hepatic failure; coronary, cerebral, or peripheral vascular disease; uncontrolled hypertension; sepsis; and women who are pregnant or nursing.

Table 64.1 Dosage regimen for the management of Migraine.

Drug	Dosage	Comments
1. Analgesics Acetaminophen	1000mg at onset; repeat every 4-6 hours as needed	Maximum daily dose is 4g
Acetaminophen 250mg/ aspirin 250mg/ caffeine 65mg	2 tablets at onset and every 6 hours	Available OTC as Excedrin Migraine
Aspirin or acetaminophen with butalbital, caffeine	1-2 tablets every 4-6 hrs	Limit dose to 4 tablets/day and usage to 2 days/week
Isometheptene 65mg/ dichloralphenazone 100mg/ acetaminophen 325mg(Midrin)	2 capsules at onset; repeat 1 capsule every hour as needed.	Maximum of 6 capsules/ day and 20 capsules/month
2. Nonsteroidal Anti-Inflammatory Drugs Aspirin	500-1000mg every 4-6hrs	Max daily dose is 4g
Ibuprofen	200-800mg every 6 hrs	Avoid doses >2.4g/day
Naproxen sodium	550-825mg at onset; can repeat 220mg in 3-4hrs	Avoid doses >1.375g/day
Diclofenac(Cataflam, Voltaren)	50-100mg at onset; can repeat 50 mg in 8hours.	Avoid doses >150mg/day
3. Ergotamine tartrate Oral tablet(1mg) with caffeine 100mg (cafergot)	2mg at onset; then 1-2mg every 30mins as needed	Max dose is 6mg/day or 10mg/wk; consider pre-treatment with an anti- emetic.
4.Dihydroergotamine Injection 1mg/ml	0.25-1mg at onset IM, IV or subcutaneous; repeat every hour as needed	Max dose is 3 mg/ day or 6 mg/wk.

Contd....

Drug	Dosage	Comments
5.Serotonin agonists(triptan) Sumatriptan Injection	6 mg SC at onset; may repeat after 1 hour if needed	Maximum daily dose is 12 mg.
Oral tablets	25, 50, or 100 mg at onset; may repeat after 2 hours if needed	Optimal dose is 50–100 mg; maximum daily dose is 200 mg.
Nasal spray	5, 10, or 20 mg at onset; may repeat after 2 hours if needed	Optimal dose is 20 mg; maximum daily dose is 40 mg; single-dose device delivering 5 or 20 mg; administer one spray in one nostril.
Zolmitriptan	2.5 or 5 mg at onset as regular or orally disintegrating tablet; may repeat after 2 hours if needed	Optimal dose is 2.5 mg; maximum dose is 10 mg/day Do not divide ODT dosage form.
Naratriptan	1 or 2.5 mg at onset; may repeat after 4 hours if needed	Optimal dose is 2.5 mg; maximum daily dose is 5 mg.
Rizatriptan	5 or 10 mg at onset as regular or orally disintegrating tablet; may repeat after 2 hours if needed	Optimal dose is 10 mg; maximum daily dose is 30 mg; onset of effect is similar with standard and orally disintegrating tablets; use 5-mg dose (15 mg/day max) in patients receiving propranolol.
Almotriptan	6.25 or 12.5 mg at onset; may repeat after 2 hours if needed	Optimal dose is 12.5 mg; maximum daily dose is 25 mg.
Frovatriptan	2.5 or 5 mg at onset; may repeat in 2 hours if needed	Optimal dose 2.5–5 mg; maximum daily dose is 7.5 mg (3 tablets).
6.Miscellaneous Butorphanol nasal spray	1 spray in 1 nostril (1 mg) at onset; repeat in 1 hour if needed	Limit to 4 sprays/day; consider use only when non opioid therapies are ineffective or not tolerated.
Metoclopramide	10 mg IV at onset	Useful for acute relief in the office or emergency department setting.
Prochlorperazine	10 mg IV or IM at onset	Useful for acute relief in the office or emergency department setting.

Serotonin Receptor Agonists (Triptans) [10, 11]

- The triptans are appropriate first-line therapies for patients with mild to severe migraine or as rescue therapy when nonspecific medications are ineffective.
- They are selective agonists of the 5HT1B and 5HT1D receptors. Relief of migraine headache results from (1) normalization of dilated intracranial arteries, (2) inhibition of vasoactive peptide release, and (3) inhibition of transmission through second-order neurons ascending to the thalamus.

- Second-generation triptans (all except sumatriptan) have higher oral bioavailability and longer half-lives than oral sumatriptan, which could theoretically reduce headache recurrence.
- Side effects: Paresthesias, fatigue, dizziness, flushing, warm sensations, and somnolence.
- Chest tightness; pressure; heaviness; or pain in the chest, neck, or throat.
- Contraindications: Ischemic heart disease, uncontrolled hypertension, cerebrovascula disease, hemiplegic and basilar migraine, and pregnancy.

Opioids

- Opioids and derivatives (e.g. meperidine, butorphanol, oxycodone, and hydromorphone) for patients with moderate to severe infrequent headaches in whom conventional therapies are contraindicated or as rescue medication after failure to respond to conventional therapies.

β-adrenergic antagonists [12]

- Propranolol, timolol, and metoprolol reduce the frequency of migraine attacks by 50% in more than 50% of patients. Atenolol and nadolol are probably also effective.
- Side effects include drowsiness, fatigue, sleep disturbances, vivid dreams, memory disturbance, depression, sexual dysfunction, bradycardia, and hypotension.
- Use with caution in patients with heart failure, peripheral vascular disease, atrioventricular conduction disturbances, asthma, depression, and diabetes.

Antidepressants

- The tricyclic antidepressants (TCA) amitriptyline and venlafaxine are probably effective for migraine prophylaxis.
- Increased appetite and weight gain can occur. Orthostatic hypotension and slowed
- atrio ventricular conduction are occasionally reported.
- Phenelzine has been used for refractory headache,

Anticonvulsants [9]

- Valproic acid, divalproex sodium (a 1:1 molar combination of valproate sodium and valproic acid), and topiramate can reduce the frequency, severity, and duration of headaches.
- Side effects of valproic acid and divalproex sodium include nausea (less common with divalproex sodium and gradual dosing titration), tremor, somnolence, weight gain, hair loss, and hepatotoxicity (the risk of hepatotoxicity appears to be low in patients older than 10 years on monotherapy). The extended-release formulation of divalproex sodium is administered once daily and is better tolerated than the enteric-coated formulation. Valproate is contraindicated in pregnancy and patients with a history of pancreatitis or chronic liver disease.
- Fifty percent of patients respond to topiramate. Paresthesias (~50% of patients) and weight loss (9%–12% of patients) are common. Other side effects include fatigue, anorexia, diarrhea, difficulty with memory, language problems, taste perversions, and nausea. Kidney stones, acute myopia, acute angle-closure glaucoma, and oligohidrosis have been infrequently reported.

Nonsteroidal Antiinflammatory Drugs

- Nonsteroidal anti-inflammatory drugs (NSAIDs) are modestly effective for reducing the frequency, severity, and duration of migraine attacks, but potential GI and renal toxicity limit daily or prolonged use.
- They may be used intermittently to prevent headaches that recur in a predictable pattern (e.g., menstrual migraine). Treatment should be initiated 1 or 2 days before the time of headache vulnerability and continued until vulnerability is passed.
- For migraine prevention, evidence for efficacy is strongest for naproxen and weakest for aspirin.

Other Drugs

- Verapamil has been widely used, but evidence for efficacy is inadequate.
- Frovatriptan is effective for prophylaxis of menstrual migraine, and naratriptan and zolmitriptan are probably effective.
- Other medications that may be effective include Petasites, riboflavin (vitamin B2), extract of feverfew, subcutaneous histamine, lisinopril, candesartan, clonidine, guanfacine, and coenzyme Q10, but additional research is needed to confirm efficacy.

Treatment algorithm for prophylactic management of migraine headaches:

If the patient meets the criteria for prophylactic pharmacotherapy

- Headaches recur in other agents ineffective predictable pattern (e.g., menstrual migraine)-NSAID at the time of vulnerability
- Healthy or comorbid hypertension, angina, or anxiety: β-adrenergic antagonist (verapamil if β-adrenergic antagonist contraindicated or ineffective)
- Comorbid depression or insomnia: Tricyclic antidepressant
- Comorbid seizure disorder or manic-depressive illness: Divalproex sodium to be initiated. But if ineffective - β-adrenergic antagonist (verapamil if β-adrenergic antagonist contraindicated or ineffective)
- Other agents ineffective- Methysergide can be given.

Prophylaxis of Patients' Migraine Attacks

First Line Medications for Migraine Preventive Therapy [13]

1. **Anticonvulsants:**

   Topiramate: Oral route; 25-50mg/d upto 400mg/dl

   SE: Sedation and cognitive effects as confusion, GI upset

   Valproic acid: 250 mg BID; ↑ by 250 mg/day at weekly intervals to effect or adverse effects; most should benefit from 1,000–2,000 mg/day

   SE: Lethargy, depression, weight gain, alopecia

2. **Beta blockers:**

   Propranolol: Oral route; 60-120mg/d 20 mg BID–TID; gradually ↑ dose at weekly intervals to effect or max of 320 mg/day

   SE: Dizziness, insomnia, fatigue, GI upset, respiratory distress

Atenolol: Oral route; 25-50mg/d

SE: Fewer respiratory effects than propranolol

Metoprolol: Oral route ; 25-100mg/d

SE: Fewer respiratory effects than propranolol

3. **Tricyclic antidepressants:**

   Amitryptilline: 10–25 mg HS; ↑ by 10–25 mg/day at weekly intervals to max 150 mg/day; most should benefit from 50–75 mg/day

   SE: Sedation, insomnia, weight gain, dry mouth and constipation

   Doxepin: Oral ; 10mg at bedtime; titrate upto 25-50mg/d ; Max dose- 150mg/d

   SE: Similar to amitryptilline

4. **NSAIDs:**

   Naproxen: Oral route; 500-550mg/d; max dose 1000-1100mg/d

   SE: GI side effects, but more preffered for menstrual migraine in young patients

5. **Calcium channel blockers:**

   Verapamil: oral 80 mg TID. If needed, ↑ dose gradually to max of 480 mg/day

   SE: Constipation.

   May be combined with other first line medications

Second Line Medications for Migraine Preventive Therapy [14]

1. **Anti-seizure medication:**

   Gabapentin: Oral route; 600-2400mg/d; for some patients 100-300mg/

   SE: Sedation and dizziness.

   Pregabalin: Oral route; 25mg BID to 150mg

   SE: Weight gain

2. *Muscle relaxants:* Cyclobenzaprine: oral route; 5-10mg/d

   SE: Sedation

   Tizanidine: Oral route; 2-4mg every night SE-dry mouth, sedation

   Can be used as needed for minor headaches, neck or back pain

3. *Antidepressants:* The antidepressants with dual mechanisms are more effective for pain and headache than the SSRI's

   Duloxetine: Oral route; 30-60mg/d

   Venlafaxine: Oral; 75-225mg/d

Tension-Type Headache

- Tension-type headache, the most common type of primary headache, is more common in women than men. Pain is usually mild to moderate and nonpulsatile. Episodic headaches may become chronic in some patients.

Pathophysiology

- The pain of episodic tension-type headache is thought to originate from the myofascial tissues, although central mechanisms also may be involved.
- Following activation of supraspinal pain perception structures, a self-limiting headache results in most individuals owing to central modulation of the incoming peripheral stimuli.
- Chronic tension-type headache may evolve from episodic tension-type headache in predisposed individuals owing to a disturbance of central nociceptive processing and subsequent sensitization of the CNS.

Clinical Presentation

- Premonitory symptoms and aura are absent, and pain is usually mild to moderate, bilateral, nonpulsatile, and in the frontal and temporal areas, but occipital and parietal areas can also be affected.
- Mild photophobia or phonophobia may occur. Pericranial or cervical muscles may have tender spots or localized nodules in some patients.

Diagnosis

Criteria for diagnosis

(i) **Headache** lasting for hours

(ii) headache with atleast 2 of the following characteristics:
- Bilateral location
- Pressing or tightening quality
- Mild to moderate intensity
- Not aggravated by routine physical activity

(iii) both of the following
(a) No more than 1 of photophobia, phonophobia or mild nausea
(b) neither moderate or severe nausea nor vomiting

(iv) not attributed to any ither disorder

(v) pericranial tenderness on bimanual palpation may be increased

Treatment

- Nonpharmacological therapies include reassurance and counselling, stress management, relaxation training, and biofeedback. Physical therapeutic options (e.g., heat or cold packs, ultrasound, electrical nerve stimulation, massage, acupuncture, trigger point injections, and occipital nerve blocks) have performed inconsistently.
- Simple analgesics (alone or in combination with caffeine) and NSAIDs are the mainstay of acute therapy. Acetaminophen, aspirin, diclofenac, ibuprofen, naproxen, ketoprofen, and ketorolac are effective.
- High-dose NSAIDs and the combination of aspirin or acetaminophen with butalbital, or rarely, codeine are effective options. Avoid the use of butalbital and codeine combinations when possible.

- Give acute medication for episodic headache no more often than 3 days (butalbital-containing), 9 days (combination analgesics), or 15 days (NSAIDs) per month to prevent the development of chronic tension-type headache.
- Consider preventive treatment if headache frequency is more than two per week, duration is longer than 3 to 4 hours, or severity results in medication overuse or substantial disability.
- The TCAs are used most often for prophylaxis of tension headache, but venlafaxine, mirtazapine, gabapentin, and topiramate may also be effective.

Prophylactic Management of Tension Type Headache [15]:

Acute management:

Acetaminophen 1000mg

Ibuprofen 200-400mg

Naproxen sodium 375-550 mg

Ketoprofen 25-50mg

Diclofenac potassium 50-100mg

Prophylactic management:

Amitrypyline 10-75 mg/day

Mirtazapine 30mg/day

Cluster Headache [16]

- Cluster headache, the most severe of the primary headache disorders, is characterized by attacks of severe, unilateral head pain that occur in series lasting for weeks or months (i.e., cluster periods) separated by remission periods usually lasting months or years.
- Cluster headaches may be episodic or chronic.

Pathophysiology

- Similar to migraine headache, the head pain of cluster attacks is thought to involve activation of trigeminovascular neurons with resulting release of vasoactive neuropeptides and the development of sterile, neurogenic inflammation.
- The periodicity and regularity of attacks may implicate hypothalamic dysfunction and resulting alterations in circadian rhythms in the pathogenesis of cluster headache.
- Hypothalamus-induced changes in cortisol, prolactin, testosterone, growth hormone, β-endorphin, and melatonin have been demonstrated during periods of cluster headache attack.
- Neuroimaging studies performed during acute cluster headache attacks have demonstrated activation of the ipsilateral hypothalamic gray area.

- Because serotonergic systems modulate activity in both the hypothalamus and trigeminovascular neurons, 5-HT may play a significant role in cluster headache pathophysiology.

Clinical Presentation

- Attacks occur in cluster periods lasting 2 weeks to 3 months in most patients, followed by long pain-free intervals.
- Attacks occur suddenly, with pain peaking quickly after onset and generally lasting 15 to 180 minutes. The cluster headache attacks occur at night in more than 50% of patients.
- Auras are not present with cluster headaches.
- The pain is excruciating and penetrating but usually non throbbing and is most often unilateral in orbital, supraorbital, and temporal locations.
- These features are present on the pain side and include conjunctival injection, lacrimation, and nasal stuffiness or rhinorrhea. Ipsilateral scalp and facial tenderness, ptosis, miosis, and periorbital swelling also are described.

Diagnosis

Diagnostic criteria for cluster headache [17]

1. Associated symptoms- atleast one ipsilateral symptom in the eye, nose or face, restlessness or agitation
2. Duration : 15 to 180 minutes
3. Frequency: one episode every other day to eight episode per day
4. Location: unilateral in temporal od periorbiatl area
5. Pain quality: severe, suicide headache

Treatment: [18, 19]

As in migraine, therapy for cluster headaches involves both abortive and prophylactic therapy. Abortive therapy is directed at managing the acute attack. Prophylactic therapy is intended to shorten the duration of episodic cluster attacks, in addition to reducing the frequency and severity of attacks in both episodic and chronic cluster headache. Prophylactic therapies are started early in the cluster period and administered daily until the patient is headache-free for at least 2 weeks. The medication is then tapered but may be restarted with the next cluster period. Patients with chronic cluster headache may require prophylactic medications indefinitely.

Abortive Therapy

Oxygen: The standard acute treatment of cluster headache is inhalation of100% oxygen by facial mask at a rate of 7–10 L/min for 10 to 15 minutes. Repeat administration may be necessary because of recurrence because oxygen appears merely to delay, rather than abort, the attack in some patients. No side effects have been reported with the use of oxygen.

Ergotamine Derivatives: Intravenous or intramuscular dihydroergotamine provides effective relief for acute attacks of cluster headache. Repeated intravenous administration of dihydroergotamine for 3 to 7 days can break the cycle of frequent cluster headache attacks with minimal side effects.

Triptans: Subcutaneous and intranasal sumatriptan is considered safe and effective treatment for acute cluster headaches. Adverse events reported in cluster headache patients are similar to those seen in migraineurs. Sumatriptan has been used in the management of cluster headaches for up to 1 year without evidence of tachyphylaxis or increased toxicity.

Prophylactic Therapy

Verapramil: Verapamil, the preferred calcium channel blocker for the prevention of cluster headaches. Effective doses usually range from 240 to 360 mg/day for episodic attacks, but higher doses may be necessary to control chronic cluster headache.

Lithium: Lithium carbonate is effective against episodic and chronic cluster headache attacks, with beneficial effects often appearing during the first week of therapy. The usual dose of lithium for cluster headache is 600 to 900 mg/day administered in divided doses. Tachyphylaxis to lithium has been reported occasionally during prolonged therapy. Initial side effects are mild and include tremor, lethargy, nausea, diarrhea, and abdominal discomfort. Lithium should be administered with caution to patients with significant renal or cardiovascular disease, dehydration, pregnancy, or concomitant diuretic use.

Ergotamine: Ergotamine can be an efficacious agent for prophylactic as well as abortive therapy of cluster headaches. A 2-mg bedtime dose is often beneficial for the prevention of nocturnal headache attacks. Daily use of 1 to 2 mg ergotamine alone or in combination with verapamil or lithium may provide effective headache prophylaxis in patient's refractory to other agents with little risk of ergotism or rebound headache.

Methysergide: In patients unresponsive to other therapies, methysergide 4 to 8 mg/ day in divided doses is usually effective in shortening the course of cluster headaches. Response to treatment usually occurs within 1 week of initiation of the drug.

Corticosteroids: Corticosteroids are useful for chronic cluster headaches refractory to verapamil, lithium, ergotamine, and methysergide or combinations of these agents. Therapy is initiated with 40 to 60 mg/day prednisone and tapered over approximately 3 weeks. Relief appears within 1 to 2 days of initiating therapy. To avoid steroid-induced complications, long-term use is not recommended. Headaches may recur when therapy is tapered or discontinued.

Miscellaneous Agents: Other therapies that have been used in the acute management of cluster headache include intranasal lidocaine, intranasal capsaicin, and intramuscular leuprolide. Neurosurgical intervention may be necessary for patients with chronic cluster headache that is resistant to all medical therapies.

Pharmacotherapy of Acute Cluster Headache

1. **Oxygen:** 100% via nonrebreather face mask at 12 to 15 L per minute for 15 to 20 minutes. No adverse effects
2. **Sumatriptan:** 6mg SC, may repeat once atleast one hour later
   20mg nasal spray; maximum of 40mg per day
   Adverse effects: injections-dizziness, fatigue, parasthesias
3. **Zolmitriptan:** 5 mg nasal spray; may be repeated once after 2 hours
   5mg orally, maximum of 10mg per day
   Adverse effects- nasal-bad taste, nasal cavity discomfort, somnelence
   Tablets: dizziness, heaviness, chest tightness
4. *Octrotide:* 100mcg SC
   Adverse effects: Bloating, diarrhoea, lethargy
5. **Ergotamine:** 2 mg sublingually, may repeat dose every 30 minutes to maximum of 6 mg per day
   Adverse effects: Angina, prurirtis

Case Study of Migraine

Summary

A 65 year old man came to the hospital with these complaints. Left side headache since 3 months in temporal region with vomiting and nausea along with sweating. He had complaint of giddiness and vertigo. He had no complaint of fever ear discharge and ear pain. He is hypertensive patient and on medication his vitals are normal. Liver function test, serum bilurubin total showed the increase in the level i.e 15mg/dL. Serum electrolytes showed - decrease in serum sodium levels i.e, 128(135-155). CT scan of abdomen showed the presence of acute/ subacute. On the calculation of MIDAS score (migraine disability assessment) it was found to be 6 grade 2 (mild disability).

Diagnosis: He was diagnosed with migraine

The patient therapy includes the following;

Inj. Pan	(pantaprazole)	iv	40 mg	bd
Inj. Stugeron plus	(Cinnarazine+dimenhydrinate)	iv	20mg + 40mg	bd
Inj. Stemetil	(Prochlorperazine)	im	1ml/5mg	sos
Inj. Piptaz	(Pieracillin+tazobactam)	iv	4.5g	tid
T. Flucan	(Fluconazole)	p/o	150mg	od
T. Dolo	(Paracetmol)	p/o	650mg	sos
T. Becosules-z	(Multivitamin)	p/o	1 tab	od
Inj. Zofer	(Ondansetron)	iv	4mg	bd

Progress Chart

- The patient slowed the improvement over time symptoms were reduced and relieved.
- On the first day patient was unstable with pain in left sided head.
- On the second day medications given to relieve the pain and any infection
- On the third day pain was decreased and kept under observation ,vitals were normal
- Then the patient was kept under observation to maintain the vitals

Patient Education:

To relieve the stress; Psychotherapy

Try to identify any in attacks it may help to find triggering factors, enough sleep

Avoid alcohol, cheese and other food that trigger; Exercise often

Assignment

1. **Calculate the patients MIDAS score and describe the severity of her migraine headache MIDAs -** migraine disability assessment. According to **MIDAs** the severity of the patient is grade 2
2. **What clinical information is consistent with a diagnosis of migraine in patient?**
   The clinical information is consistent with a diagnosis of migraine in the elevated patient count.
3. **Could any of the patients problems have been caused or exacerbated by his drug therapy?**
   No none of his medications in drug therapy either caused or exacerbated patients problems
4. **What are the goals of therapy?**
   - To reduce the pain and relieve the patient from headache
   - To prevent the recurrent attacks of headache
   - To improve the patient condition of headache does not create any interruption in day to day life
   - The regimen provided should not excaudate any of its condition
5. **What pharmacotherapeutic regimen is available for?**
   (a) Treatment of patient's migraine attacks

Table 64.2 Acute treatment options for migraine headache.

Modification	Dosage	Route	Comments
			Antidopaminergics
Metoclopranide	10 mg	IV	Diphenhydramine indicated to prevent akathisia
Prochlorperazine	10 mg	IV	Diphenhydramine indicated to prevent akathisia
Chlorpromazine	0.1 mg/kg	IV	Max dosage: 25 mg; diphenhydramine indicated to prevent akathisia
			Anticholinergic
Diphenhydramine	25 mg	IV	Uses for ADR management, not for headache treatment

Contd...

Modification	Dosage	Route	Comments
			Triptans
Sumatriptan	6 mg	SC	May repeat in 1 h if no response: max dosage: 12 mg/24h; faster onset of action than 1N route
	5 mg, 10 mg	IN	May repeat in 2 h if no response; max dosage: 40 mg/24 h
Zolmitriptan	2.5 mg, 5 mg	IM	May repeat in 2 h if no response; max dose: 10 mg/24h
			NSAID
Ketoralac	30 mg	IV	Max dosage: 120 mg/24 h; in patients >65y, max dosage: 60 mg/24 h; max duration of therapy: 5 days
			Certicesteroid
Dexamethasone	10 mg	IV	Used to reduce headache recurrence after ED discharge

ADR: adverse drug reaction: ED: emergency department: IN: intranasal: max: maximum: NSAID: nonsteroidal anti-inflammatory drug.

Source: Friedman B. Managing migraine. *Ann Emerg Med.* 2017; 69(2):202-207.

6. Describe the agents used for aborting migraines

Dihydro ergotamine is an ergot derivative that is more effect and has side effects than erogotamine it also less likely to lead medication overused headaches.

Sodium valproate; primarily used to prevent migraine headaches it has few side effects feeling sleepy weight gain feeling risk.

7. Write about MIDAs score evaluation for headaches

MIDAS group	definition	score
One	little / nodisability	0-5
Two	mild disability	6-10
Three	moderate disability	11-20
Four	severe disability	21plus

References

1. *Adapted with permission from Headache Classification Committee of the International Headache Society. The international classification of headache disorders, 2nd ed. Cephalalgia 2004;24(Supp1):1–151.*

2. IHS, International Headache Society. *Adapted with permission from Headache Classification Committee of the International Headache Society. The international classification of headache disorders, 2nd ed. Cephalalgia 2004;24(Suppl):1–151.*

3. Lipton RB, Bigal ME. The epidemiology of migraine. Am J Med 2005;18(Suppl 1):S3–10.

4. Gardner KL. Genetics of migraine: An update. Headache 2006;46(Suppl 1):S19–24.

5. Silberstein SD, Lipton RB, Dalessio DJ. Overview, diagnosis, and classification of headache. In: Silberstein SD, Lipton RB, Dalessio DJ, eds. Wolff's Headache and Other Head Pain, 7th ed. New York: Oxford University Press, 2001:6–26.

6. Silberstein SD, Lipton RB, Goadsby PJ. Headache in Clinical Practice. London: Martin Dunitz, 2002:21–33, 69–128.

7. Ramadan NM. Targeting therapy for migraine. Neurology 2005;64(Suppl 2):S4–8.

8. Ferrari MD. Migraine. Lancet 1998;351:1043–1051.

9. Goadsby PJ, Lipton RB, Ferrari MD. Migraine: Current understanding and treatment. N Engl J Med 2002;346:257–270.

10. Silberstein SD. Practice parameter: Evidence-based guidelines for migraine headache (an evidence-based review). Neurology 2000;55:754–763.

11. Silberstein SD, Goadsby PJ. Migraine: Preventive treatment. Cephalalgia 2002;22:491–512.

12. Diamond S. A fresh look at migraine therapy. Postgrad Med 2001;109(1):49–60.

13. Mathew NT, Rapoport A, Saper J, Magnus L, et al. Efficacy of gabapentin in migraine rophylaxis. Headache. 2001;41(2):119-128.

14. Robbins L. Robbins Headache Clinic. http://www.headachedrugs.com.

15. Golden L. Peters, PharmD, BCPS. Pharmacotherapy for Primary Headache Disorders in the Emergency Department. *US Pharm.* 2018;43(3):HS2-HS8.

16. McGeeney, BE. Cluster headache pharmacotherapy. Am J Ther 2005;12(4):351–358.

17. Headache Classification Subcommittee of the International Headache Society. The international classification of headache disorders: 2nd edition. *Cephalalgia.* 2004;24 (suppl 1):9–160.

18. Francis GJ, Becker WJ, Pringsheim TM. Acute and preventive pharmacologic treatment of cluster headache. *Neurology.* 2010;75(5):463–473.

19. Rozen TD. Inhaled oxygen for cluster headache: efficacy, mechanism of action, utilization, and economics [published ahead of print January 29, 2012]. Curr Pain Headache Rep.

CHAPTER - 65

Pain Management

Types of Pain

1. **Pain** is an unpleasant sensory and emotional experience that is associated with actual or potential tissue damage.
2. **Acute pain** lasts 30 days longer than the usual healing process for that type of injury, and occurs after muscle strains and tissue injury, such as trauma or surgery. The pain is usually self-limiting, decreasing with time as the injury heals.
3. **Chronic pain** is persistent or episodic pain of a duration or intensity that adversely affects the function or well-being of the patient and can persist after the resolution of an injury. Some define it as lasting more than 6 months. **Chronic non-malignant pain** may be a complication of acute injury in which the healing process does not occur as expected or may be caused by a disease such as a rheumatological disorder (e.g., osteoarthritis, rheumatoid arthritis, fibromyalgia).
4. **Chronic cancer pain** occurs in 60% to 90% of patients with cancer. Its characteristics are similar to those of chronic non-malignant pain. Tumour causes of pain include bone metastasis, compression of nerve structures, occlusion of blood vessels, obstruction of bowel, or infiltration of soft tissue.
5. **Neuropathic pain** is a result of an injury or malfunction of the nervous system. Neuropathic pain is described as aching, throbbing, burning, shooting, stinging, and tenderness or sensitivity of the skin.

Basic Mechanism of Pain [1]

1. Stimulation. Noxious stimulus sensitizes and/or stimulates nociceptors and causes the release of neural chemicals that also sensitize and/or stimulate nociceptors. This activation leads to the production of an action potential.
2. Transmission. The action potential continues from the site of noxious stimulus to the dorsal horn of the spinal cord and then ascends to higher centers in the CNS. Transmission takes place in at least five pathways: a. Spinothalamic tract b. Spinoreticular tract c. Spinomesencephalic tract d. Dorsal column postsynaptic spinomedullary pathway e. Propriospinal multisynaptic ascending systems

3. Perception. Conscious experience of pain.

4. Modulation. Inhibition of nociceptive impulses. Neurons from the brain stem descend to the spinal cord and release substances such as endogenous opioids, serotonin, and norepinephrine that inhibit transmission of nociceptive impulses

Clinical Presentation of Pain

Acute pain

General

- Often obvious distress (e.g., trauma)

Symptoms

- Can be described as sharp, dull, shock-like, tingling, shooting, radiating, fluctuating in intensity, and varying in location (these occur in a timely relationship with an obvious noxious stimuli)

Signs

- Hypertension, tachycardia, diaphoresis, mydriasis, and pallor, but these signs are *not diagnostic*
- In some cases there are no obvious signs
- Comorbid conditions usually not present
- Outcome of treatment generally predictable

Laboratory Tests

- Pain is always subjective
- There are *no* specific laboratory tests for pain
- Pain is best diagnosed based on patient description and history

Chronic pain

General

- Can appear to have no noticeable suffering

Symptoms

- Can be described as sharp, dull, shock-like, tingling, shooting, radiating, fluctuating in intensity, and varying in location (these often occur *without* a timely relationship with an obvious noxious stimuli). Over time, the pain stimulus may cause symptoms that completely change (e.g., sharp to dull, obvious to vague)

Signs

- Hypertension, tachycardia, diaphoresis, mydriasis, and pallor are seldom present
- In most cases there are NO obvious signs. Comorbid conditions often present (e.g., sleep problems, depression, relationship problems)
- Outcome of treatment often unpredictable

Diagnosis

Laboratory Tests
- Pain is always subjective
- Pain is best diagnosed based on patient description and history
- There are *no* specific laboratory tests for pain; however, history and/or diagnostic proof of past trauma (e.g., computed tomography) or present disease state (e.g., autoantibodies) may be helpful in diagnosing etiology

Principles of management [2]
1. **Comprehensive pain assessment** should determine the characteristics of the patient's pain complaint, clinical status, and pain management history.
   (a) Assessment of the pain complaint should include chronology and symptomatology of the presenting complaint such as information about onset, location, intensity, duration, quality, distribution, provocative factors, temporal qualities, severity, and pain history.
   (b) Assessment of clinical status should include the extent of underlying trauma or disease. Also, the patient's physical, psychological, and social conditions should be determined.
   (c) Assessment of pain management history includes drug allergies, analgesic response, onset, duration, and side effects.
2. **Appropriate pain management targets** should be established.
   (a) The primary pain management goal is to improve patient comfort.
   (b) For acute pain management, improved comfort can aid the healing and rehabilitation process.
   (c) For chronic pain, the specific objectives are to break the pain cycle (i.e., erase pain memory) and minimize breakthrough pain.
   (d) Other targets for chronic pain management include improvement of general well-being, sleep, outlook, and self-esteem, activities of daily living, support, and mobility.
3. **Individualized pain management regimens** should be determined and initiated promptly.
   (a) The optimal analgesic regimen, including dose, dosing interval, and mode of administration, should be selected.
   (b) Additional pharmacological adjuncts and nonpharmacological therapies should be added if needed.
   (c) The most common regimens for acute pain include intermittent (as needed) dosing, patient controlled analgesia (PCA), or epidural infusions with narcotic or nonnarcotic agents.

(d) Nonnarcotic analgesics and nonpharmacological management usually are maximized. Narcotic use may be appropriate for certain patients being treated for chronic non-malignant pain. Pain management specialists often include these agents in their plans.

(e) For chronic cancer pain, an individualized around-the-clock analgesic regimen is established, using a long-acting analgesic. An intermittent, as-needed regimen for breakthrough pain, using a short-acting analgesic, is also determined.

4. **Monitoring** the pain management regimen and **reassessment** of the patient's pain should occur ona continuous, timely basis. Any changes in analgesic, dose, dosing interval, or method of administrationshould be noted in the patient's medical record and carried out in a timely fashion.

5. **Effective analgesic therapy** begins with an accurate assessment of the patient. The Pain Intensity and Pain Distress Scales can help clinicians assess pain. When obtaining a pain history, it is important to gather details about the pattern, duration, location, and character of the pain. Pain intensity should be measured using an appropriate pain scale according to the patient's ability to communicate.

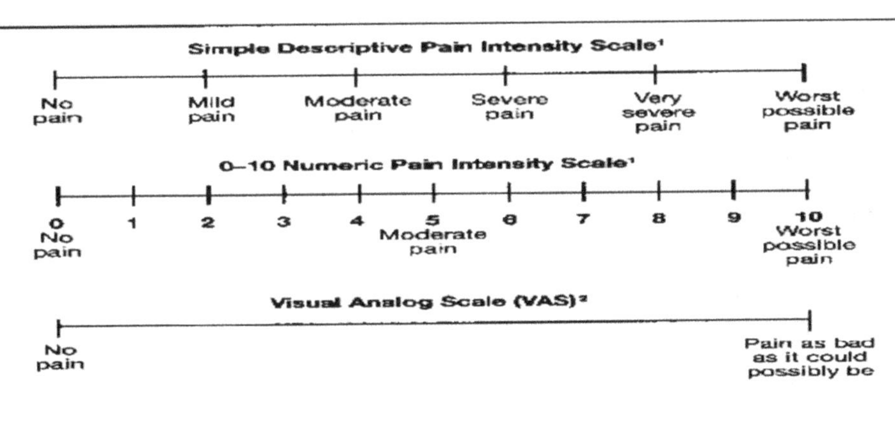

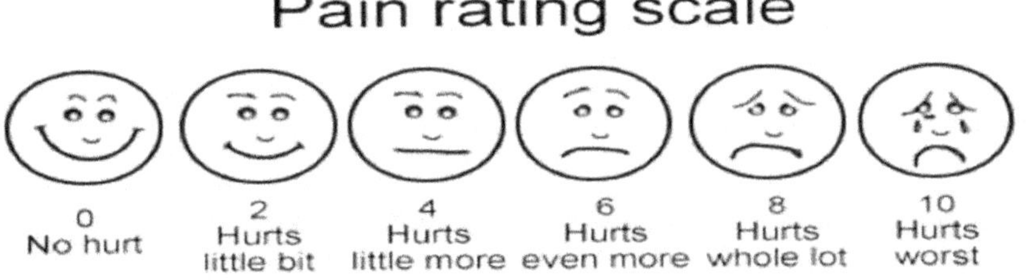

Souce: Childs JD, Piva SR, Fritz JM. Responsiveness of the numeric pain rating Scale in patients with low back pain spine 2015; 30:1331-4

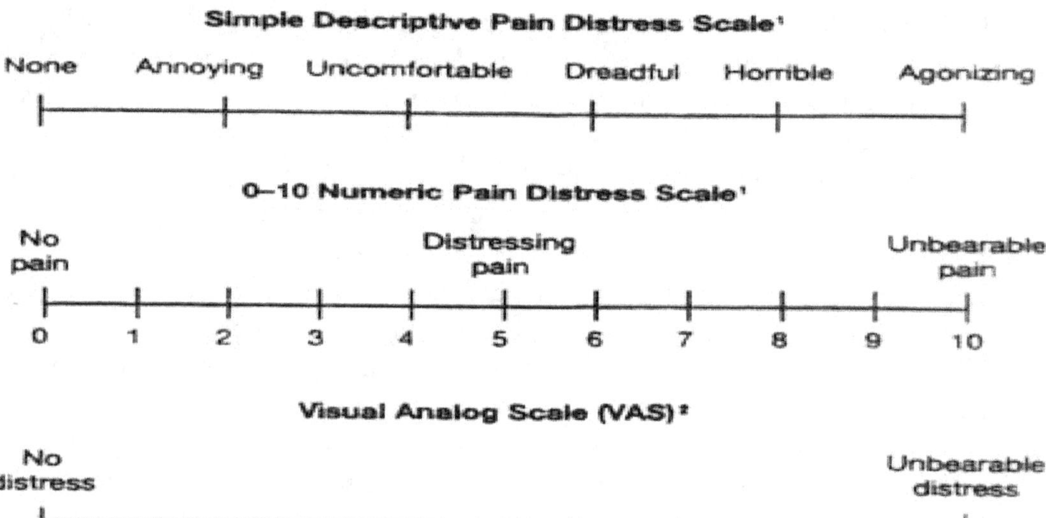

Source: Delado et al., 2018. Validation of digital visual analog scale pain scoring with a traditional paper loased visual analog scale in adults. H Am Academic Orthio surg Glob. Res. Rev 2m e088.

Treatment:

Nonpharmacological therapy:

Stimulation therapy-Transcutaneous electrical nerve stimulation (TENS) has been used in managing both acute and chronic pain (e.g., surgical, traumatic, low back, arthritis, neuropathy, fibromyalgia, and oral-facial pain).

Psychological Intervention: Relaxation training, imagery, and hypnosis, have proven effective in the management of postprocedure pain and in cancer-related pain

- The elderly and the young are at a higher risk for undertreatment of pain because of misunderstanding about the pathophysiology of their pain.

Pharmacological Therapy

Non-Opioid Agents

- Analgesia should be initiated with the most effective analgesic with the fewest side effects.
- The nonopioids are preferred over the opioids for mild to moderate pain. The salicylates and nonsteroidal anti-inflammatory drugs(NSAIDs) reduce prostaglandins produced by the arachidonic acid cascade,thereby decreasing the number of pain impulses received by the CNS.
- NSAIDs may be particularly useful for management of cancer-related bone pain.
- NSAIDs are more likely to cause GI side effects. The salicylate salts causefewer GI side effects than aspirin and do not inhibit platelet aggregation.

- Aspirin-like compounds should not be given to children or teenagers with influenza or chickenpox, as Reye's syndrome may result.
- Acetaminophen has analgesic and antipyretic activity but little anti-inflammatoryaction. It is highly hepatotoxic on overdose.

Adult FDA-Approved Nonopioid Analgesics

Salicylates

Acetylsalicylic acid   usual dose range mg- 0.25 325–1,000 every 4–6 h

Acetaminophen   usual dose range mg- 325–1,000 every 4–6 h

Mefenamic acid   usual dose range mg- Initial 500; 250 every 6 h (maximum 7 days)

Ibuprofen   usual dose range mg- 200-400 every 4-6h

Opioid Agents [3, 4, 5]

- With oral opioids, the onset of action usually takes about 45 minutes; and peak effect usually is seen in about 1 to 2 hours.
- Partial agonists and antagonists compete with agonists for opioid receptorsites and exhibit mixed agonist-antagonist activity. They may have selectivity for analgesic receptor sites and cause fewer side effects.
- In the initial stages of acute pain treatment, analgesics should be givenaround the clock. As the painful state subsides, as-needed schedules can beused. Around-the-clock administration is also useful for management ofchronic pain.
- Patients with severe pain may receive very high doses of opioids with no unwanted side effects, but as pain subsides, patients may not tolerate even low doses.
- Most of the itching or rash reported with the opioids is due to histamine release and mast cell degranulation, not to a true allergic response.
- When allergies occur with one opioid, a drug from a different structuralclass of opioids may be tried with caution. For these purposes, the mixedagonist/antagonist class behaves most like the morphine-like agonists.

Morphine dose 10 mg

Levorphanol dose 2 mg IM

Mepiridine dose 75 mg IM

Tramadol dose 50-100mg PO

Dosing guidelines

- NSAIDs/acetaminophen/aspirin- Used in mild-to-moderate pain. May use in conjunction with opioid agents to decrease doses of each. Regular alcohol use and high doses of acetaminophen may result in liver Toxicity
- Morphine- Drug of choice in severe pain. po 5–30 mg q 3–4 h
- Hydromorphone- Use in severe pain. po 2–4 mg q 3–6 h

- Hydrocodone- po 5–10 mg q 4–6 h. Use in moderate/severe pain. Most effective when used with NSAIDs, aspirin, or acetaminophen. Only available as combination product with other ingredients for pain and/or cough.
- Fentanyl IV 25–50 mcg/hour Used in severe pain. Transmucosal for "breakthrough" cancer pain in patients already receiving or tolerant to opioids
- Methadone- Effective in severe chronic pain. IM 2.5–10 mg q 8–12 h (acute) Sedation can be major problem. Some chronic pain PO 5–20 mg q 6–8 h (chronic patients can be dosed every 12 h)
- Butarphanol: Second-line agent for moderate to severe pain. May precipitate withdrawal in opiate-dependent patients. IM 1–4 mg q 3–4 h; IV 0.5–2 mg q 3–4 h; Intranasal 1 mg (1 spray) q 3–4 hb If inadequate relief after initial spray, may repeat in other nostril × 1 in 30–60 minutes
- Buprenorphine- IM 0.3 mg q 6 h. Second-line agent for moderate-to-severe pain. Slow IV 0.3 mg q 6 h - May precipitate withdrawal in opiate-dependent patients. May repeat ×1, 30–60 min after initial dose- Naloxone may not be effective in reversing respiratory depression.
- Tramadol po 50–100 mg q 4–6 h*a* Maximum dose for nonextended-release, 400 mg/24 h; maximum for extended release, 300 mg/24 h If rapid onset not required, start 25mg/day and titrate over several days. Extended release po 100 mg q 24 h Decrease dose in patient with renal impairment and in the elderly

Major Adverse Effects of the Opioid Analgesics

Effect   **Manifestation**

Mood changes: Dysphoria, euphoria

Somnolence: Lethargy, drowsiness, apathy, inability to concentrate

Stimulation of chemoreceptor trigger zone: Nausea, vomiting

Respiratory depression: Decreased respiratory rate

Decreased gastrointestinal motility: Constipation

Increase in sphincter tone: Biliary spasm, urinary retention (varies among agents)

Histamine release: Urticaria, pruritus, rarely exacerbation of asthma (varies among agents)
Tolerance: Larger doses for same effect

Dependence: Withdrawal symptoms upon abrupt discontinuation

Initial Regimens for Different Pain Levels Based on Guidelines from the World Health Organization (WHO)

- **Mild pain:** 1-3 score for typical corresponding numerical rating scale. Non-opiod analgesics- Acetaminophen 650 mg every 4 hr ; Acetaminophen 1,000 mg every 6 hr;

Ibuprofen 600 mg every 6 hr. Consider adding adjunct analgesic or using an alternate regimen if pain not reduced in 12 days. Consider step up if pain not relieved by two different regimens. [paracetamol+/- NSAID]

- **Moderate pain: 4-6 score on** typical corresponding numerical rating scale. Add opioid for moderate pain (e.g., moderate potency analgesic). Use on a schedule, not as needed. Acetaminophen 325 mg/codeine 60 mg every 4 hr ; Acetaminophen 325 mg/Oxycodone 5 mg every 4 hr; Tramadol 50 mg every 6 hr. Consider adding adjunct analgesic or using an alternate regimen if pain not reduced in 12 days. Consider step up if pain not relieved by two different regimens.[paracetamol+/-NSAID + tramadol or codeine]

- **Severe pain**: **7-10 score on** typical corresponding numerical rating scale. Switch to a high potency (strong) opioid; administer on a regular schedule. Morphine 15 mg every 4 hr; Hydromorphone 4 mg every 4 hr; Morphine controlled release 60 mg every 8 hr. Consider alternate regimen (e.g., different strong opioid) if pain not reduced in 12 days. Consider increased dose of strong opioid, or addition of nonopioid agents, if pain not adequately relieved by two regimens [paracetamol+/- NSAID + morphine].

- Morphine is an effective treatment for many types of severe pain. Its analgesic effect is dosedependent. Its adverse effects have often been exaggerated and should not be an obstacle to its use.

- The most serious adverse effect of morphine is respiratory depression, which may be fatal. This adverse effect results from overdose. It is, therefore, important to increase doses gradually. Respiratory depression is preceded by drowsiness, which is a warning to monitor respiratory rate.

  The Respratory rate should remain equal to or greater than the thresholds indicated below:

  Children 1 to 12 years: RR≥ 25 respirations/ minute

  Children 1 to 2 years: RR ≥ 20 respirations/minute

  Children 2 to 5 years: RR ≥ 20 respirations/minute

  Children > 5 years and adults: RR ≥ 20 respirations/minute

  Respiratory depression must be identified and treated quickly: verbal and physical stimulation of the patient; administration of oxygen; respiratory support (bag and mask) if necessary. If no improvement, administer **naloxone** (antagonist of morphine) in bolus to be repeated every minute until RR normalises and the excessive drowsiness resolves: 5 micrograms/kg in children and 1 to 3 micrograms/kg in adults.

- Morphine and codeine always cause constipation. A laxative should be prescribed if the opioid treatment continues more than 48 hours. **Lactulose** PO is the drug of choice: children < 1 year: 5 ml daily; children 1-6 years: 5 to 10 ml daily; children 7-14 years: 10 to 15 ml daily; adults: 15 to 45 ml daily. If the patient's stools are soft, a stimulant laxative (**bisacodyl** PO: children > 3 years: 5 to 10 mg once daily; adults: 10 to 15 mg once daily) is preferred.

- **For chronic pain in late stage disease** (cancer, AIDS etc.), morphine PO is the drug of choice. It may be necessary to increase doses over time according to pain assessment. Do not hesitate to give sufficient and effective doses.

Treatment of nociceptive pain in pregnant and breast-feeding women

- Paracetamol: it is the first choice drug for 0-5 months, from 6th month and in breast feeding also.
- Aspirin: it is to be avoided in 0-5 months; contra-indicated from 6th month and to be avoided in breast feeding.
- Ibuprofen: it is to be avoided in 0-5 months; contra-indicated from 6th month and possibly taken in breast feeding.
- Codeine: it is possible to be taken in 0-5 months; from 6th - The neonate may develop withdrawal symptoms, respiratory depression and drowsiness in the event of prolonged administration of large doses at the end of the thirdtrimester. Closely monitor the neonate. During breast feeding- Use with caution, for a short period (2-3 days), at the lowest effective dose.
- Tramadol: The child may develop drowsiness when the mother receives tramadol at the end of the thirdtrimester and during breast-feeding. Administer with caution, for a short period, at the lowest effective dose, and monitor the child.
- Morphine: The child may develop withdrawal symptoms, respiratory depression and drowsiness when the mother receives morphine at the end of the third trimester and during breast-feeding. Administer with caution, for a short period, at the lowest effective dose, and monitor the child.

Neuropathic pain

- **Amitriptyline** PO

  Adults: 25 mg once daily at bedtime (Week 1); 50 mg once daily at bedtime (Week 2); 75 mg once daily at bedtime (as of Week 3); max.150 mg daily. Reduce the dose by half in elderly patients.

- **Carbamazepine** PO

  Adults: 200 mg once daily at bedtime (Week 1); 200 mg 2 times daily (Week 2); 200 mg 3 times daily (as of Week 3)

Management of Cancer Pain in Adult Patients: Esmo Clinical Practice Guidelines

1. **Treatment of mild pain**
   - Analgesic treatment should start with drugs indicated by the WHO analgesic ladder appropriate for the severity of pain.
   - There is no significant evidence to support or refute the use of paracetamol alone or in combination with opioids for mild to moderate pain.

- There is no significant evidence to support or refute the use of NSAIDs alone or in combination with opioids for mild to moderate pain.

2. Treatment of mild to moderate pain

- For mild to moderate pain, weak opioids such as tramadol, dihydrocodeine and codeine can be given in combination with non-opioid analgesics.
- As an alternative to weak opioids, low doses of strong opioids could be an option, although this recommendation is not currently part of WHO guidance.
- There is no evidence of increase in adverse effects from the use of low-dose strong opioids instead of the standard step 2 approach with weak opioids.

3. Treatment of moderate to severe pain

- The opioid of first choice for moderate to severe cancer pain is oral morphine
- The average relative potency ratio of oral to i.v. morphine is between 1:2 and 1:3
- The average relative potency ratio of oral to s.c. morphine is between 1:2 and 1:3
- Oxycodone or hydromorphone, in both immediate-release and modified-release formulations for oral administration, and oral methadone are effective alternatives to oral morphine
- Fentanyl and buprenorphine (via the t.d. or i.v. route) are the safest opioids in patients with chronic kidney disease stages 4 or 5 (estimated glomerular filtration rate < 30 mL/min).

References

1. Twycross RG. Pain and analgesics. Curr Med Res Opin 1978;5:497–505.
2. American Pain Society. Principles of Analgesic Use in the Treatment of Acute Pain and Chronic Cancer Pain, 5th ed. Glenview, IL: American Pain Society, 2003.
3. Landau R. One size does not fit all: Genetic variability of mu-opioid receptor and postoperative morphine consumption. Anesthesiology 2006;105:334–337.
4. Gutstein HB, Akil H. Opioid analgesics. In: Brunton LL, Lazo AS, Parker KL, eds. The Pharmacological Basis of Therapeutics, 11th ed. New York: McGraw-Hill, 2006:547–590.
5. Pasero C, Portenoy RK, McCaffery M. Opioid analgesics. In: McCaffery M, Pasero C, eds. Pain. St. Louis: Mosby, 1999:161–299.

CHAPTER - 66

Parkinsonism

Introduction to Parkinsonism

Parkinsonism is a progressive neurological disorder of muscle movement, characterized by tremors, muscular rigidity, bradykinesia (slowness in initiating and carrying out voluntary movements), and postural and gait abnormalities. Most cases involve people over the age of 65, among whom the incidence is about 1 in 100 individuals.

Epidemiology

It is an age related disorder and about 1% of persons suffer from this disease at the age of 65 yrs. The incidence rises from 20 per 100,000 persons in fifth decade of life to about 90 per 100,000 persons in seventh decade of life. Males and females are equally affected. Symptoms start appearing after 70-80% dopaminergic neurons are lost.

Etiology

Parkinsonism may be caused by genetic and toxin exposure (Intrinsic and Extrinsic).

- Histopathophysiologic feature is degeneration of dopaminergic neurons in substanstia nigra that project to striatum (nigrostriatal pathway).
- There by neuronal vulnerability spreads to spinal cord, autonomic ganglia, basal ganglia, neocortex.
  1. **Genetic factors**: particularly if the disease starts before the age of 50. Mutations in some genes such as mutations of α-syniclein, and parkin genes.
  2. **Environmental factors:** Chronic exposure to pesticides, heavy metals (iron and manganese), rural living, drinking water. MPTP is a toxic chemical which is selectively taken up dopaminergic neurons of substantia nigra and produces impairment in mitochondrial energy metabolism to destry neurons. Exposure to MPTP like molecules may contribute to PD.
  3. **Endogenous oxidative stress due to dopamine metabolism:** Intrinsically substantia nigra pars compacta is a region characterized by high levels of oxidative stress because of free radicals generated by dopamine autooxidation due to MAO-B.
  In normal conditions, these free radicals are neutralized by anti-oxidants. There may be accumulation of free radicals due to decrease in anti-oxidant mechanism like

decrease in reduced glutathione, ascorbic acid or Superoxide dismutase. An increase in free radicals may produce neurodegeneration.

4. **Drug induced parkinsonism**: some drugs whose exposure may produce symptoms similar to that of parkinson's disease. Eg. Anti-psychotics

5. **Presence of lewy bodies:** Neuronal cytoplasmic filamentous aggregates composed of presynaptic protein alpha synuclein in the SNc neurons.

Stages of Parkinsonism depending on severity of disease

1. **Stage I:** Unilateral involvement
2. **Stage II:** bilateral involvement, with no postural defect
3. **Stage III:** bilateral involvement with mild postural defects, but person leads independent life
4. **Stage IV:** bilateral involvement with postural instability and requires help
5. **Stage V:** person is restricted to bed or chair and is in very severe condition

Pathophysiology

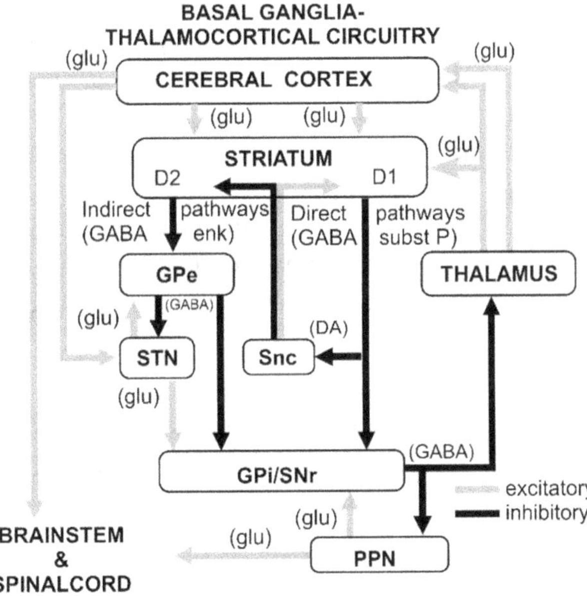

Fig. 66.1 Schematic illustration of the basal ganglia-thala-mocortical "motor" circuit and its neurotransmitters. "Indirect" and "direct" pathways from the striatum to basal ganglia output nuclei are represented by the arrows. GPe, globus pallidus pars externa; GPi, globus pallidus pars interna; STN, subthalamic nucleaus; SNr, substantia nigra pars reticulata; SNc, substantia nigra pars compacta; PPN, pedunculopontine nucleus; glu, glutamate; GABA, gammaaminobutyric acid; enk, enkephalin; subst P, substance P. Dopamine (DA) receptor subtypes 1 and 2 are represented as D1 and D2, respectively.

Source: Watts RL, Koller WC, eds. Movement Disorders: Neurologic Principles and Practice. New York: McGraw-Hill, 1997:240

Substantia nigra: The substantia nigra, part of the extrapyramidal system, is the source of dopaminergic neurons that terminate in the striatum. Each dopaminergic neuron makes thousands of synaptic contacts within the neostriatum and, therefore, modulates the activity of a large number of cells. These dopaminergic projections from the substantia nigra fire tonically rather than in response to specific muscular movements or sensory input. Thus, the dopaminergic system appears to serve as a tonic, sustaining influence on motor activity rather than participating in specific movements.

Neostriatum (Corpus striatum): Normally, the neostriatum is connected to the substantia nigra by neurons that secrete the inhibitory transmitter GABA at their termini in the substantia nigra. In turn, cells of the substantia nigra send neurons back to the neostriatum, secreting the inhibitory transmitter dopamine at their termini. This mutual inhibitory pathway normally maintains a degree of inhibition of the two separate areas.

The cause of Parkinson's disease is unknown for most patients. The disease is correlated with destruction of dopaminergic neurons in the extrapyramidal system. The extrapyramidal system is responsible for fine control of motor activity and posture maintenance. This pathway consists of basal ganglia, which contains caudate putamen, and putamen nuclei and these are collectively called as "corpus striatum" (neostriatum). Globus pallidus is another nucleus present in basal ganglia. Dopamine is the main neurotransmitter in this extrapyramidal system, particularly in the nigrostriatal tract that originates from substantia nigra and then innervates neostraiatum. Substantia nigra has two parts, substantia nigra pars compacta and substantia nigra pars reticulate. The primary defect in PD is the detruction of dopaminergic neurons of substantia nigra pars compacta and thus, the input from substantia nigra to stiatum is reduced. There is direct correlation between the extent of nigrostiatal dopamine loss and clinical features.

The increase in acetyl choline levels in neostraitum region is responsible for some of symptoms as tremors. An excessive cholinergic activity has been linked to decrease in dopaminergic activity. In normal conditions dopamine inhibits acetylcholine neurons in the striatum, therefore the degeneration of nigrostriatal dopamine neurons results in a relative increase of striatal cholinergic interneuron activity.

Clinical Manifestation and Features [1]

General Features -For clinically probable PD, the patient exhibits at least two of the following: resting tremor, rigidity, or bradykinesia.

Asymmetric onset (unilaterality) of these features is usual. Postural instability (difficulty with maintaining balance) is more common in advanced IPD.

- Motor Symptoms -The patient experiences decreased manual dexterity, difficulty arising from a seated position, diminished arm swing during ambulation, dysarthria (slurred speech), dysphagia (difficulty with swallowing), festinating gait (tendency to pass from a walking to a running pace), flexed posture (axial, upper/lower extremities), "freezing" at initiation of movement, hypomimia (reduced facial animation), hypophonia (reduced voice volume), and micrographia (diminution of handwritten letters/ symbols) .

- Autonomic and Sensory Symptoms -The patient experiences bladder and anal sphincter disturbances, constipation, diaphoresis, fatigue, olfactory disturbance, orthostatic blood pressure changes, pain, paresthesia, paroxysmal vascular flushing, seborrhea, sexual dysfunction, and sialorrhea (drooling).
- Mental Status Changes - The patient experiences anxiety, apathy, bradyphrenia (slowness of thought processes), confusional state, dementia, depression, hallucinosis/psychosis (typically drug-induced), and sleep disorders (excessive daytime sleepiness, insomnia, obstructive sleep apnea, and rapid eye movement sleep behavior disorder.

Diagnosis with Algorithm

Clinically probably PD is diagnosed when at least two of the following are present: limb muscle rigidity, resting tremor (at 3 to 6 Hz and abolished by movement), or bradykinesia.

Definite PD is diagnosed when there is at least two of the following: resting tremor, rigidity, bradykinesia, and a positive response to antiparkinson medication.

Laboratory Tests -No laboratory tests are available to diagnose IPD.

Other Diagnostic Tests: Genetic testing is not routinely helpful.

Neuroimaging may be useful for excluding other causes of Parkinsonism.

Medication history should be obtained to rule out drug induced Parkinsonism.

Rating scales for assessing the symptoms of condition

1. **Unified Parkinson's disease Rating Scale (UPDRS)**: The UPDRS combines elements of several scales to produce a comprehensive and flexible tool to monitor the course of Parkinson's and the degree of disability. Part I: Evaluation of mental activity, behaviour and mood; Part II: Self-evaluation of activities of daily living, Part III: Evaluation of motor function, Part IV: Evaluation of complications of therapy.
2. **The Hoehn and Yahr Scale is** used to measure how Parkinson's symptoms progress and the level of disability.
   - Stage 0 - No signs of disease
   - Stage 1 - Symptoms on one side only (unilateral)
   - Stage 1.5 - Symptoms unilateral and also involving the neck and spine
   - Stage 2 - Symptoms on both sides but no impairment of balance
   - Stage 2.5 - Mild symptoms on both sides, with recovery when the 'pull' test is given (the doctor stands behind the person and asks them to maintain their balance when pulled backwards)
   - Stage 3 - Balance impairment, mild to moderate disease, physically independent

- Stage 4 - Severe disability, but still able to walk or stand unassisted
- Stage 5 - Needing a wheelchair or bedridden unless assisted.

3. **Schwab and England Activites of Daily Living (ADL) Scale**: The Schwab and England ADL Scale is a means of measuring a person's ability to perform daily activities in terms of speed and independence through a percentage figure.

- 100% - Completely independent. Able to do all activities without slowness, difficulty or impairment
- 90% - Completely independent. Able to do all activities with some slowness, difficulty or impairment. Activities may take twice as long to complete
- 80% - Independent in most activities, but activities take twice as long. Conscious of difficulty and slowing
- 70% - Not completely independent. More difficulty with activities, which may take three to four times as long. May take large part of day for chores
- 60% - Some dependency. Can do most activities, but very slowly and with much effort, but some chores are impossible
- 50% - More dependent. Help required with half of chores. Difficulty with everything
- 40% - Very dependent. Can assist with all chores but can manage few alone
- 30% - With effort, now and then does a few chores alone or begins alone. Much help needed
- 20% - Cannot do anything alone. Can give some slight help with some chores. Severe invalid
- 10% - Totally dependent, helpless
- 0% - Vegetative functions such as swallowing

Diagnostic criteria with algorithm [2]

- When the patient is presented, first physical exercises are checked for all the patients. They are categorized as
  - (a) No functional impairment- no treatment or Rasagiline
  - (b) Low functional impairment-rasagiline
  - (c) Moderate functional impairment-consider the age.

    If age<65 yrs and risk factor ICD- low dose of DA+ Rasagiline

    If no risk factor for ICD-DA + rasagiline

    If age> 65 yrs and No cognitive impairment and prominent neuropsychiatric non motor symptoms are present- use DA+ rasagiline. Levodopa can be added in case of suboptimal therapeutic response.

Goals of therapy:

The goals of treatment are

- To minimize symptoms, disability, and side effects
- Maintaining quality of life.

- Education of patients and caregivers is critical,
- exercise and proper nutrition are essential

Non-Pharmacological Treatment

Occupational and physical therapy

- Offering persons newly affected by Parkinson's disease (PD) rehabilitation treatment based on physical therapy is recommended.
- It would be advisable to include physical therapy techniques as part of the interdisciplinary approach to PD, placing special emphasis on the functional rehabilitation of the patient.
- The use of exercise programmes for strengthening/stretching/functioning, supervised aerobic exercise, low-intensity treadmill running, and progressive endurance exercises are recommended in patients with PD.
- Occupational therapy must be available for persons with PD. Special attention should be given to:
- Maintaining jobs and family roles, instrumental and advanced daily life, domestic, and leisure activities
- Improving and maintaining movement and mobility
- Improving personal care activities such as eating, drinking, washing, and dressing.
- The aspects of the environment to improve safety and motor functions.
- Cognitive evaluation and appropriate intervention.

Speech therapy

- Improvement of voice volume and tone range, including speech therapy programs

Nutrition and Diet

- Supplementation with vitamin D (as part of the diet, through enriched foods, food supplements, or medication) helps to prevent fractures in patients with PD who do not ingest a sufficient quantity, or who have a deficit of exposure to sunlight or have a greater need for vitamin D.
- It may be advisable to inform patients to keep protein intake within the recommended dietary requirements (≈ 0.8 g/kg/day) when beginning treatment with Levadopa

Pharmacotherapy

Strategy of treatment [3]

In addition to an abundance of inhibitory dopaminergic neurons, the neostriatum is also rich in excitatory cholinergic neurons that oppose the action of dopamine. Many of the symptoms of parkinsonism reflect an imbalance between the excitatory cholinergic neurons and the greatly diminished number of inhibitory dopaminergic neurons. Therapy is aimed at restoring dopamine in the basal ganglia and antagonizing the excitatory effect of cholinergic neurons, thus reestablishing the correct dopamine/acetylcholine balance. Because long-term treatment with *levodopa* is limited by fluctuations in therapeutic responses, strategies to maintain CNS dopamine levels as constant as possible have been devised.

Monotherapy usually begins with a monoamine oxidase-B (MAO-B) inhibitor, or if the patient is physiologically young, a dopamine agonist.

- When additional relief is needed, the addition of levodopa (L-dopa) should be considered. With the development of motor fluctuations, addition of a catechol-O-methyltransferase (COMT) inhibitor should be considered to extend L-dopa duration of activity.
- For management of L-dopa–induced dyskinesias, the addition of amantadine should be considered.

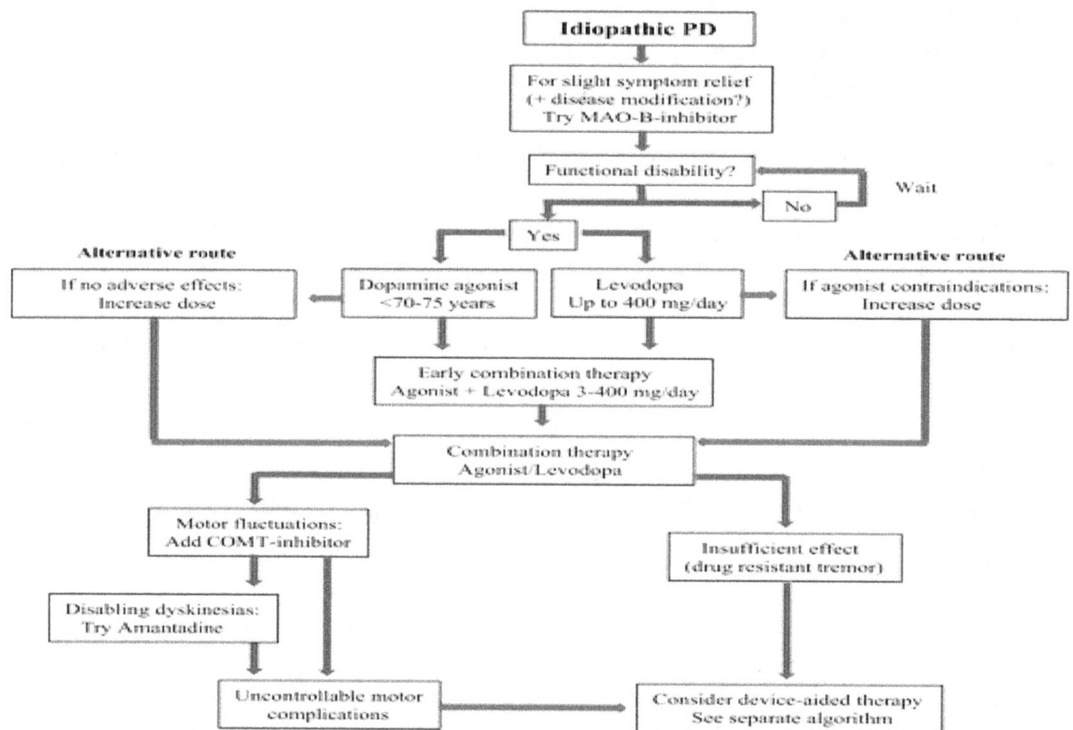

Fig. 66.2 Algorithms for the treatment of motor problems in Parkinson's disease.

Source: E.Dietrichs, P.Odin, Algorithms for the treatment of motor problems in Parkinson's disease. Acta Neurologica, 2017; 136(5):378-385.

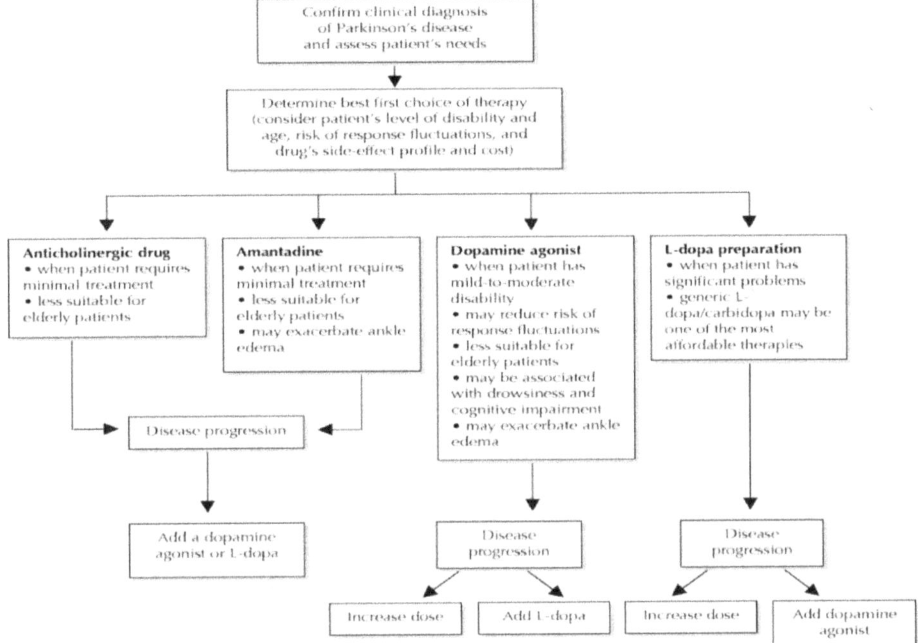

Fig. 66.3 Treatment algorithm for the management of the early stages of Parkinson's disease.

Source: Mark Guttman et Al., Current Concepts in the Diagnosis and Management of Parkinson's Disease Candian Medical Association Journal. 2003; 168(3):293-301.

Algorithm for treating advanced IPD [4]

- If the patient is diagnosed with advanced disease, comprehensive physical, occupational, and speech therapy evaluation is to be done.
- If the patient is on dopamine agonists- increase the dose. Observe for response, and then add carbidopa/ l-dopa. If no adequate response increase dose and/or frequency OR
  - (a) Change to carbidopa/l-dopa CR and/or
  - (b) Add selegiline and/or
  - (c) Add COMT inhibitor and/or
  - (d) Add amantadine and/or
  - (e) Consider surgery.
- If the patient is already on carbidopa/l-dopa and no adequate response, increase dose and/or frequency
  - (a) Change to carbidopa/l-dopa CRand/or
  - (b) Add selegiline and/or
  - (c) Add COMT inhibitor and/or
  - (d) Add amantadine and/or
  - (e) Consider surgery.

Pharmacological Management of Parkinsonism

Surgical Therapy

- The most effective surgical technique is deep brain stimulation (DBS) of the STN, which decreases outflow from this region (as shown in Fig. 57–2B) and thus reduces input to the thalamus.
- Thalamic DBS and thalamotomy (a focal destructive lesion of the thalamus) can reduce disabling tremor
- Pallidotomy (a focal destructive lesion of the GPi) and GPi DBS can help with severe dyskinesias and on/off fluctuations but is not as helpful for bradykinesia.

Anticholinergic Medications [5, 6]

- Anticholinergic drugs effective for tremor and dystonic features in some patients but rarely show substantial benefit for bradykinesia or other disabilities. They can be used as monotherapy or in conjunction with other antiparkinsonian drugs.
- Anticholinergic side effects include dry mouth, blurred vision, constipation, and urinary retention. More serious reactions include forgetfulness, sedation, depression, and anxiety.

Amantadine

- Amantadine is often effective for mild symptoms, especially tremor. It may also decrease dyskinesia at relatively high doses (400 mg/day).
- Adverse effects - sedation, vivid dreams, dry mouth, depression, hallucinations, anxiety, dizziness, psychosis, and confusion.

Levodopa and Carbidopa/Levodopa

L-dopa is the precursor of dopamine. It crosses the blood–brain barrier, whereas dopamine does not.

In the CNS and elsewhere, L-dopa is converted by L-amino acid decarboxylase (L-AAD) to dopamine. In the periphery, L-AAD can be blocked by administering carbidopa or benserazide, which does not cross the blood–brain barrier.

Carbidopa therefore increases the CNS penetration of exogenously administered L-dopa and decreases adverse effects (e.g., nausea, vomiting, cardiac arrhythmias, postural hypotension, vivid dreams) from peripheral L-dopa metabolism to dopamine.

- Starting L-dopa at 300 mg/day (in divided doses) maximal dose of L-dopa is 800 to 1,000 mg/day.
- 75 mg of carbidopa is required to effectively block L-AAD,
- Carbidopa/L-dopa is most widely used in a 25-mg/ 100-mg tablet, but 25-mg/250-mg and 10-mg/100-mg dosage forms are also available.
- Meals delay gastric emptying, but antacids promote gastric emptying. L-dopa is absorbed primarily in the proximal duodenum by a saturable large neutral amino acid transport system.

- L-dopa is not bound to plasma proteins, and the elimination half-life is about 1 hour. The addition of carbidopa can extend the half-life to 1.5 hours, and the addition of a COMT inhibitor (e.g., entacapone) can extend it to about 2 to 2.5 hours.
- Bedtime administration of carbidopa/L-dopa CR or ropinirole CR or Rotigotine transdermal patch help to reduce nocturnal off episodes and improve functioning upon awakening.
- "Delayed-on" can result from delayed gastric emptying or decreased absorption in the duodenum. Crushing the tablet of carbidopa/Ldopa and taking with a glass of water or using the orally disintegrating tablet formulation on an empty stomach can help.
- "Freezing," a sudden, episodic inhibition of lower extremity motor function may be worsened by anxiety and may increase the risk of falls.
- "Off-period dystonia," sustained muscle contractions that occur more commonly in distal lower extremity (e.g., foot), occur often in the early morning hours. They may be treated with bedtime administration of sustained-release products, use of baclofen, or selective denervation with botulinum toxin.

Monoamine Oxidase B Inhibitors [7]

At therapeutic doses, selegiline and rasagiline are unlikely to induce a "cheese reaction" (hypertension, headache) unless excessive amounts of dietary tyramine (400 mg or greater) are ingested. Selegiline and rasagiline may be neuroprotective.

Selegiline (deprenyl; Eldepryl) is an irreversible MAO-B inhibitor that blocks dopamine breakdown and can modestly extend the duration of action of L-dopa (up to 1 hour). It often permits reduction of L-dopa dose by as much as one-half. Selegiline also increases the peak effects of L-dopa and can worsen preexisting dyskinesias or psychiatric symptoms such as delusions and hallucinations. Other adverse effects include insomnia, jitteriness.

Rasagiline, another MAO-B inhibitor, has similar effects as selegiline in enhancing L-dopa effects and modest beneficial effect as monotherapy.

Catechol-O-Methyltransferase Inhibitors [8]

Tolcapone (Tasmar) and entacapone (Comtan) are used only in conjunction with carbidopa/L-dopa to prevent the peripheral conversion of L-dopa to dopamine

COMT inhibition is more effective than controlled-release carbidopa/Ldopa in providing consistent extension of effect and avoids the delay in time to maximal effect seen with controlled-release L-dopa products.

Tolcapone 100 mg three times daily + carbidopa/L-dopa. Side effect is fatal liver toxicity.

Dopamine Agonists [9]

Ergot derivative- bromocriptine

> Nonergots-   pramipexole
>
> > Rotigotine
> >
> > Ropinirole

They are beneficial adjuncts in patients with deteriorating response to L-dopa, those experiencing fluctuation in response to L-dopa, and those with limited clinical response to L-dopa due to inability to tolerate higher doses.

They decrease the frequency of "off" periods and provide an L-dopa-sparing effect.

The nonergots are safer and are effective as monotherapy in mild-moderate PD as well as adjuncts to L-dopa.

Bromocriptine is not commonly used because of an increased risk of pulmonary fibrosis and reduced efficacy compared to the other agonists.

Side effects: Nausea, confusion, hallucinations, lightheadedness, lower-extremity edema, postural hypotension, sedation, and vivid dreams.

Pramipexole: 0.125 mg three times daily and increased every 5 to 7 days as tolerated. It is primarily renally excreted; initial dose must be adjusted in renal insufficiency.

Rotigotine: Transdermal patch once-daily, initiated at 2 mg/day and increased by 2 mg/day on a weekly basis to a maximum of 6 mg for early PD.

Ropinirole: 0.25 mg three times daily and increased by 0.25 mg three times daily on a weekly basis to a maximum of 24 mg/day.

Apomorphine: Nonergot dopamine agonist., subcutaneous apomorphine triggers an "on" response within 20 minutes, and duration of effect is up to 100 minutes. Most patients require 0.06 mg/kg.

Motor Fluctuations of levodopa therapy and Possible Interventions in PD

Effect with Possible Treatments

- **End of dose deterioration** ("wearing off"): Increase frequency of doses; controlled-release carbidopa/L-dopa; consider dopamine agonists, selegiline, COMT inhibitors, or amantadine; duodenal or intravenous L-dopa infusions; carbidopa/L-dopa oral solution; subcutaneous apomorphine infusions; transdermal dopamine agonists
- **Delayed onset of response** Give on empty stomach before meals; crush or chew and take with a full glass of water; reduce dietary protein intake; antacids; morning standard-release carbidopa/L-dopa if on sustained-release carbidopa/L-dopa; infusions of L-dopa; dopamine agonists

- Drug-resistant "off" periods Increase carbidopa/L-dopa dose and/or frequency; give on empty stomach before meals; crush or chew and take with a full glass of water; infusions of L-dopa or dopamine agonists; apomorphine subcutaneous injection; consider deep brain stimulation
- Random oscillations ("on/off") Dopamine agonists; controlled-release carbidopa/L-dopa, selegiline; COMT inhibitors; infusions of L-dopa or dopamine agonists; consider drug holiday and deep brain stimulation
- Start hesitation ("freezing") Increase carbidopa/L-dopa dose; dopamine agonists; gait modifications (tapping, rhythmic commands, stepping over objects, rocking)
- Peak-dose dyskinesia (I-D-I responsea) Smaller more frequent doses of carbidopa/L-dopa; controlled-release carbidopa/L-dopa; dopamine agonist; consider amantadine, propranolol, fluoxetine, buspirone, clozapine, deep brain stimulation
- Diphasic dyskinesias (D-I-D responseb) Reduce anticholinergic medication
- Dystonia Baclofen; nighttime carbidopa/L-dopa; morning standard-release carbidopa/L-dopa if on sustained-release carbidopa/L-dopa; dopamine agonists; anticholinergics; selective denervation with botulinum toxin
- Myoclonus Decrease nighttime L-dopa doses; clonazepam
- Akathisia Benzodiazepines; propranolol; dopamine agonists; gabapentin

Stepwise Approach to Drug-Induced Psychosis in Parkinson's disease

1. General measures such as evaluating for hypoxemia, infection (especially encephalitis, systemic sepsis, or urinary tract infection), or electrolyte disturbance (especially hypercalcemia or hyponatremia).
2. Simplify the antiparkinsonian regimen as much as possible by discontinuing the medications with the highest risk-benefit ratio first.
   (a) Discontinue anticholinergics, including other nonparkinsonian medications with anticholinergic activity such as antidepressants, e.g., amitriptyline.
   (b) Discontinue selegiline.
   (c) Taper and discontinue dopamine agonists.
   (d) Taper and discontinue amantadine, being aware that amantadine withdrawal delirium has been reported.
   (e) Consider reduction of levodopa (especially at the end of day) and discontinuation of COMT inhibitors.
3. Consider atypical antipsychotic medication if psychosis persists. a. Quetiapine 12.5–50 mg at bedtime and gradually increased upward by 12.5–25 mg per week until psychosis controlled, or b. Clozapine 12.5–50 mg at bedtime and gradually increased upward by 12.5 mg per week until psychosis controlled (requires weekly monitoring for leukopenia).

Treatment of complications of Parkinson's according to NICE guidelines

- Excessive sleepiness is common in those with Parkinson's and may represent a risk for driving. If this symptom is troublesome, the guideline recommends consideration of the drug modafinil, which then requires regular monitoring by a specialist.

- Rapid eye movement sleep behaviour disorder is characterised by abnormal movements during sleep, often associated with vivid dreaming, which may be violent. NICE recommends consideration of clonazepam or melatonin for this condition.
- Orthostatic hypertension (drop of blood pressure on standing) is a common problem in Parkinson's, worsened by medication. It may require adjustment of medication and the use of the unusual hypertensive agent, midodrine.
- Dementia is common as the disease advances. NICE's recommendations of cholinesterase inhibitors for this problem

Case Study of Parkinsonism

Summary

A 65 year female patient was admitted to the hospital with chief complaints of drowsiness and difficulty in walking since 2 days, tremors since 2 years, general weakness since two days, history of SOB and wheezing. She has a Know case of Parkinsonism and is on resperidone + trihexphas (T. rhize plus). She has a family h/o (husband) DM. She underwent cataract two years back and hysterectomy 30 years back. Her vitals were stable with normal temperature, BP of 120/80 mmHg, pulse: 84 bpm. Her CBP reports showed a decrease in Hb that is 10.3 mg/dL. Her urine analysis showed presence of numerous pus cells and albumin. Her Liver Function test (LFT) showed a slight increase in SGOT (39 IU/L). Her biochemical investigations showed an increase in serum creatinine (2.2mg/dL) and blood urea (70mg/dL). 2D echo showed AV sclerosed, grade 1 diastolic dysfunction. MRI of brain showed age related cerebral atrophy with periventricular ischaemic changes. ECG showed sinus tachycardia and low T wave.

Diagnosis

By the above subjective and objective data the patient was diagnosed to be suffering with Parkinsonism.

Her therapy involved.

Drug	Drug	Route	Dose	Frequency
Inj. Nootropil	Piracetam	IV	15ml	TID
Inj. Pan	Pantaprazole	IV	40mg	OD
Inj. Citizac	Citicoline	IV	2ml	BD
Inj. Re xite plus	Multivitamin	IM	1 amp	OD
Inj. Zofer	Ondansetron	IV	4mg	SOS
Tab. phylline	Acebrophylline	PO	100mg	BD
Neb duolin and budecort	Levosalbutamol+ Ipratropium	Nasal	1 resp	TID
Inj. Monocef	Ceftriaxone	IV	1g	BD
Syp. Citralka	Dosodium hydrogen citrate	Oral	2 tsp	TID
T. Nepro hp powder	Protein powder	PO	2tsp	TID

On day1, the patient was admitted with chief complaints of difficulty in walking. On day 3 the patient is on liquid diet. On day 5 patients vitals were checked. On day 6, no fresh complaints. Patient was discharged.

Patient counselling:

- Take enough rest; Conserve your energy; Exercise for strength and moving around.
- Eat a healthy diet; eat a lot of fresh fruits; Breathe fresh air.
- Practice yoga; Keep your mind calm.

Discharge medications:

Inj. Nootropil (piracetam) (TID)

Tab phylline 100 mg acebrophylline (BD)

T. Monocef ceftriaxone (BD)

Inj. Pan pantaprazole (OD) 40mg

Syp citralka pantaprazole 2 tsp (TID).

She was asked to review after one week.

Assignment

1. **List and assess each of patient's complaints.**
   - Patient was admitted in to hospital with chief complaints of drowsiness and difficulty in walking since 2 days, tremors since 2 years, general weakness since two days, history of SOB and wheezing.
   - MRI Of brain showed age related cerebral atrophy with peri ventricular ischemic changes.rbances
   - The patient was assessed with Parkinsonism.

2. **List the cardinal motor and non motor symptoms of Parkinsonism.**
   - Cardinal motor symptoms include tremors, rigidity, and bradykinesia.
   - Non motor symptoms include neuropsychiatric disturbances, sleep and autonomic disturbances.

3. **According to Hoehn-yahr scale, What stage is the patient's disease ?**
   The Hoehnyahr scale is used to describe the symptom progression in parkinsons disease. It was originally described in 1967 and included stage 1-5. It has been modified with addition of stages 1.5 and 2.5 for the intermediate course of parkinsonism.
   Stage 0: no sign of disease.
   Stage 1: symptoms are very mild, unilateral involvement only.
   Stage 1.5: unilateral and axial involvement.
   Stage 2: bilateral involvement without impairment of balance.
   Stage 2.5: mild bilateral disease with recovery on pull test.

Stage 3: mild to moderate bilateral disease; some postural instability physical independence.

Stage 4: severe disability; still able to walk and stand unassisted.

Stage 5: wheel chair bound or bed ridden unless aided.

The patient was found to be suffering with stage 1 Parkinsonism

4. **What are the goals of therapy of patients with PD?**
   - To reduce the complaints.
   - To improve the condition.
   - To improve the quality of life .
   - To reduce tremors and drowsiness.

5. **What non pharmacological alternatives may be beneficial for treatment of PD?**
   - Healthy eating, eating foods high in fiber , and drinking adequate amount of fluids.
   - Balanced diet also provides nutrients such as omega 3 fatty acids.
   - Exercising may increase your muscle strength , flexibility and balance.
   - Try not move quickly and look in front but not directly down while walking.
   - Avoid walking backwards.
   - Massage may reduce muscle tension and promote relaxation.

6. **What drug, drug dosage form, dose, schedule and duration of therapy are best?**

Drug class	Examples	Intial dose	Usual dose	Side effects
L-dopa (combined with carbidopa or benserazide)	Regular (immediate-release) Sinamet® or Prolopa® 100/25 mg	½ tablet TID.	1-2 tablets TID	Peripheral dopaminergic side effects (anorexia, nausea, vominiting, OH); confusion, hallucinations, MRC with long-term therapy (see text)
Non-ergot dopamine agonists	Pramipexole (Mirapex®) (Rotigotine skin patch has recently been released in the U.S. but is not available in Canada)	0.125 mg TID 0.25 mg TID	0.5-1.5 mg TID 3-8 mg TID	Higher incidence compared to L-dopa of: Peripheral dopaminergic side effects: confusion, hallucinations: EDS/SAs: ICDs: peripheral edema. Lower incidence of MRC compared to L-dopa
Selective MAO-B inhibitors	Selegiline Rasagiline (Azilect)	5 mg/d	5 mg BID	Generally well-tolerated; Theoretic risk of serotonin syndrome when combined with SSRI, but extremely rare in practice

Contd....

Drug class	Examples	Intial dose	Usual dose	Side effects
NMDA antagonist	Amantadine (Symmetrel®)	100mg/d	100 mg 2-4x/d	Generally well-tolerated; Possible side effecte include confusion, hallucinations, livedo reticularis, peripheral edema. Avoid or dose in renal impairment (as mostly excreted unchanged in urine)
Antiholinergic agents	Trihexyphenidyl/benzhexol (Artane®)	1 mg TID	2 mg TID	Confusion, hallucinations, dry mouth, blurred vision, angle-closue glaucoma, urinary retention, constipation

Slow titration starting with low doses, is recommended to minimize adverse effects. Persistent peripheral dopaminergic side effects may be treated with domeridone (10-20 mg t.i.d)

Abbreviations: EDS, excessive daytime somnolence; ICDs, impulse control disorders, MAO-B, monamine oxidase B; MRC, motor response complications; NMDA, N-methyl-D=aspartate, OH, Orthostatic hypotension; SAs sleep attacks; SSRIs, selective serotonin-reuptale inhibitors

7. **Which monitoring parameters should be used to evaluate the patients response to medications and to detect adverse effects?**

   Patients with PD must have regular follow up to ensure adequate treatment if motor and behavioral abnormalities, once patients are stable on medication regimen, provide follow up care for atleast 3-6months. Patients need to be monitored for adverse events such as somnolence, sudden onset of sleep, impulse control disorder and pyshcosis. In addition people must be evaluated and treated for emergence of clinically relevant non motor symptoms including dementia, mood and sleep disorders.

8. **Which medications are used to control the motor symptoms of PD?**

   Levodopa + peripheral decarboxylase inhibitor such as carbedopa remains the gold standard of symptomatic treatment of motor features of PD. It provides the greatest anti parkinsonian benefit with the fewest ADRS in the short term. However long term use is associated with development of fluctuations and dyskinesia.

9. **Which medications are commonly used to control motor symptoms in early PD?**

   Medications commonly include levodopa, MAO-B inhibitor and dopamine agonist.

10. **How is resting tremor, rigidity, bradykinesia, postural instability, speech tendencies assessed in patients with PD?**

    Resting tremor is assessed by having patients relax their arms in their seated position, having patients count aloud backwards from 10 may help to bring out the tremor. The arm should be observed in an outstretched position to assess postural tremor and kinetic tremor.

    Rigidity refers to an increase in resistance to passive movements above the joint. The resistance can be either smooth (lead pipe) or oscillating (cog wheeling). Cog wheeling is thought to reflect tremors rather than rigidity and may be present with tremors. Rigidity is usually tested by flexing and extending the patient's relaxed wrist and can be made more obvious by having the patient perform voluntary movements such as tapping with a contra lateral limb.

Bradykinesia refers to slowness of movements but also includes reduced spontaneous movements and decreased amplitude of movement. It is also expressed as micrographia (small hand writing), hypomimia (decreased facial expressions), decreased blink rate and hypophonia (soft speech). Thus the patient's blink rate and facial expression should be observed.

In addition speech amd amplitude of movements is assessed by having patient open his or her hand and tap his/her thumb and index finger repeatitively, trying to perform the movement as big and as fast as possibe. Similarly the patient should be asked to tap the toes of each foot as big and as fast as possible. The patient is then observed while walking to assess stride length and speed as well as arms swing.

Postural stability refers to imbalance and loss of righting reflexes. Postural stability is typically assessed by having patients stand with their eyes open and then pulling their shoulders back towards the examiner side. Patients are told be ready for the displacement and to regain balance as quickly as possible. Taking one or two steps backward to balance is considered normal. The examiner should be ready to catch the patients if they are unstable.

As the patient is speaking, the vocal loudness, intonation and quality including fluidity of speech and articulation should be assessed. Sustaining vowel phonation (ex : 'ah') for maximum duration, counting 50 and reading a passage that tests articulation provide reasonable speech samples.

A soft, monotonic voice, vocal tremor, poor articulation, variable speech is characteristic of PD.

References

1. Hauser RA, McDermott MP, Messing S. Factors associated with the development of motor fluctuations and dyskinesias in Parkinson disease. Arch Neurol 2006;63:1756–1760.

2. Chloe Laurencin et al., Initial treatment of Parkinson's disease in 2016: The 2000 consensus conference revisited. Revue Neurologique 2016; 172; (8-9)

3. Management of Parkinson's disease: An evidence-based review. Mov Disord 2002;17 Suppl 4:S1–S166.

4. Mark Guttman, Stephen J. Kish, Yoshiaki Furukawa. Current concepts in the diagnosis and management of Parkinson's disease. CMAJ February 04, 2003 168 (3) 293-301

5. Miyasaki JM, Martin W, Suchowersky O, et al. Practice parameter: Initiation of treatment for Parkinson's disease: An evidence based review. Report of the Quality Standards Subcommittee of the American Academy of Neurology. Neurology 2002:58;11–17.

6. Pahwa R, Factor SA, Lyons KE, et al. Quality Standards Subcommittee of the American Academy of Neurology. Practice Parameter: Treatment of Parkinson disease with motor fluctuations and dyskinesia (an evidence- based review): Report of the Quality

Standards Subcommittee of the American Academy of Neurology. Neurology 2006;66:983–995.

7. Chen JJ, Swope D. Clinical pharmacology of rasagiline: A novel, second-generation propargylamine for the treatment of Parkinson disease. J Clin Pharmacol 2005;45:878–894.

8. Ruottinen HM, Rinne UK. COMT inhibition in the treatment of Parkinson's disease. J Neurol 1998;245(suppl 3):25–34.

9. Zanettini R, Antonini A, Gatto G, et al. Valvular heart disease and the use of dopamine agonists for Parkinson's disease. N Engl J Med 2007;356:39–46.

10. Dietrichis E and odin P. algorithms for the treatment of motor problems in parkinson's disease. Acta Neurol Scand. 2017;136:378–385.

11. Shen –Yang Lim. An Update on the Management of Parkinson's Disease, Geriatrics and Aging. 2008;11(4):215-222.

CHAPTER - 67

Alzheimer's Disease

Introduction to Alzheimer's Disease [1]

Alzheimer's disease is a chronic neurodegenerative disorder, characterized by progressive cognitive decline including memory loss, disorientation, and impaired judgment and learning. Pathologic hallmarks of the disease in the brain include **neurofibrillary tangles** and **neuritic plaques (senile plaques)** made up of various proteins, which result in a shortage of the neurotransmitter acetylcholine.

Alzheimer's disease (AD) is a non-reversible, progressive dementia manifested by gradual deterioration in cognition and behavioral disturbances. AD profoundly affects the family as well as the patient.

Epidemiology

The prevalence of AD increases with age and it is most prevalent in person's age 65 years and older. The mean survival time of persons with AD is reported to be approximately 6 years from the onset of symptoms until death.

Etiology

The exact etiology of AD is unknown; however, age, gender, several genetic and environmental causes have been explored as potential causes of AD.

1. **Gender:** The disease is more prevalent in women than men and women have 1 in 6 chance of developing Alzheimer's disease as compared to 1 in 11 chances for women. It is reported that 60% of Alzheimer's patients are women at the age of 65.
2. **Genetic factors:** Genetics is an important factor that predisposes to AD development in both early and late onset AD
   (i) ***Early onset AD:*** Alterations in chromosomes 1,14 and 21 have been associated with early onset AD. In majority of cases, the mutations in presenelin 1 (PSEN 1) gene located on chromosome 14 is responsible for development of dementia. PESN1 of chromosome 14 encodes for protein presenelin 1. Presenelin 2 (PSEN 2) gene located on chromosome 1 encodes for protein presenelin 2. APP genes located on chromosome 21 encode for amyloid precursor protein (APP). Both

presenelin 1 and presenelin 2 are part of "gamma secretase enzyme complex and are involved in processing of amyloid precursor protein. In early onset AD, mutation followed by overexpression of any one of three genes (Presenelin 1, 2 or APP) results in overproduction of beta-amyloid protein.

(ii) *Late onset AD:* The development of late-onset AD is controlled by genes responsible for production of apolipoprotein E, which are located on chromosome 19. The development of late onset AD is associated with an inheritance of apo E4 allele.

3. **Age:** Age is most important contributing factor and incidence increases with age.
4. **Environmental factors:** Stressful life, anxiety, alcohol abuse, head trauma etc.

Risk Factors

Family history. However, it is unknown how other factors such as environment – small head circumference, repeated or severe head trauma contribute and interact with the genetic predisposition for AD.

Female gender: Mitochondria from young females are protected against amyloid-beta toxicity, generate less reactive oxygen species, and release less apoptogenic signals than those from males. However, all this advantage is lost in mitochondria from old females. Since estrogenic compounds protect against mitochondrial toxicity of amyloid-beta, estrogenic action may be important in protecting cells from amyloid-beta toxicity.

Smoking: It increases the risk of vascular problems including smaller bleeds in brain. Toxins in smoke increase oxidative stress and inflammation which are linked to alzheimer's.

Diabetes: Because of insulin resistance, the cells do not get the energy due to ineffective use of insulin. So brain cannot work in the right manner. As blood glucose levels are increased, over time it can cause harmful fatty deposits in the blood vessels. Increased levels of insulin cause imbalance in the neurotrnasmitters of brain. Inflammation cause damage to blood vessels leading to alzheimer's.

Down syndrome: The presence of extra genetic material found among persons with Down syndrome may lead to abnormalities in the immune system and a higher susceptibility to certain illnesses, such as *Alzheimer's*.

Hypertension: Older people with *high blood pressure*, or hypertension, were more likely to have biomarkers of Alzheimer's in their spinal fluid.

Heart disease, high LDL, low HDL: Alzheimer's and heart disease share a genetic link: the apolipoprotein E gene known as APOE. The APOE gene provides instructions for making a protein that transports cholesterol in the bloodstream. Having at least one copy of the undesirable e4 variant of APOE increases blood levels of both harmful LDL cholesterol and triglycerides. Variant seems to hamper the clearance of amyloid plaque, the clumps of protein found in the brains of people with Alzheimer's. Amyloid plaque is thought to destroy brain cells, causing the disease's devastating symptoms.

Pathoenesis [2]

Structural Changes

AD is defined by both neuropathologic and clinical criteria. Neuropathologically, AD destroys neurons in the cortex and limbic structures of the brain, particularly the basal forebrain, amygdala, hippocampus, and cerebral cortex. These areas are responsible for higher learning, memory, reasoning, behavior, and emotional control.

Anatomically, four major alterations in brain structure are seen: cortical atrophy, degeneration of cholinergic and other neurons, presenceof neurofibrillary tangles (NFTs), and the accumulation of neuritic plaques.

NFTs and neuritic plaques are considered the signature lesions of AD; without them AD does not occur. Plaques and tangles may also be present in other diseases, even in normal aging, but there is a much higher concentration of plaques and tangles in patients with AD.

1. **Cortical atrophy:** Significant shrinkage of cerebral cortex, due to which size of brain reduces significantly in AD. The cortical atrophy is associated with loss of gyri and sulci in the temporal lobe, parietal lobe and parts of the frontal cortex.

2. **Presence of neurofibrillary tangles:** NFTs are comprised of paired helical filaments that aggregate in dense bundles. Paired helical filaments are formed from tau protein. Tau protein provides structural support to microtubules, the cell's transportation and skeletal support system. When tau filaments undergo abnormal phosphorylation at a specific site, they cannot bind effectively to microtubules, and the microtubules collapse. Without an intact system of microtubules, the cell cannot function properly and eventually dies. Overactivity of kinases such as microtubule affinity-regulating kinase, or underactivity of phosphatases could theoretically produce or prevent breakdown of abnormally phosphorylated tau protein.

3. **Presence of Neuritic plaques (amyloid or senile plaques):** Neuritic plaques (also termed amyloid or senile plaques) are extracellular lesions found in the brain and cerebral vasculature (amyloid angiopathy). Plaques are comprised of βAP, and an entwined mass of broken neurites (axon and dendrite projections of neurons). Many of these broken neurites contain neuropil filaments made up of the abnormally phosphorylated tau protein found in NFTs. Two types of glial cells, astrocytes and microglia, are also found in plaques. Among other functions, glial cells secrete inflammatory mediators and serve as scavenger cells, which may be important in causing the inflammatory processes that occur in the development of AD.

   βAP is derived from faulty cleavage of APP. It is normally cleaved by α-secretase and then by an enzyme γ-secretase to produce soluble and harmless metabolites. But during pathological process it is first cleaved by *β-secretase* and then γ-secretase to form insoluble βAP fragment. The accumulation of βAP in the extracellular space leads to its accumulation in the form of neuritic or senile plaques.

4. **Inflammatory Mediators:** Inflammatory mediators and other immune system constituents are present near areas of plaque formation, suggesting that the immune system plays an active role in the pathogenesis of AD. Cytokines (IL-1 and IL-6) and components of classical complement pathway are found in βAP deposited area.

5. **Acetylcholine:** The neurotransmitter acetylcholine (Ach) is responsible for transmitting messages between certain nerve cells in the brain. In AD, the plaques and tangles damage these pathways, leading to a shortage of Ach, resulting in learning and memory impairment. The loss of Ach activity correlates with the severity of AD. The basis of pharmacologic treatment of AD has been to improve cholinergic neurotransmission in the brain. **Acetylcholinesterase** is the enzyme that degrades Ach in the synaptic cleft. Blocking this enzyme leads to an increased level of Ach with a goal of stabilizing neurotransmission.

6. **Glutamate:** Glutamate is the primary excitatory neurotransmitter in the central nervous system (CNS) involved in memory, learning, and neuronal plasticity. It acts by providing information from one brain area to another and affects cognition through facilitation of connections with cholinergic neurons in the cerebral cortex and basal forebrain. In AD, one type of glutamate receptor, N-methyl-D-aspartate (NMDA), is less prevalent than normal. There also appears to be overactivation of unregulated glutamate signaling. This results in a rise in calcium ions that induces secondary cascades which lead to neuronal death and an increased production of APP. The increased production of APP is associated with higher rates of plaque development and hyperphosphorylation of tau protein. The drug memantine is a non-competitive NMDA antagonist which targets this pathophysiologic mechanism. Memantine is presently the only agent in this class that is approved for the treatment of AD.

7. **Cholesterol:** Increased cholesterol concentrations have been associated with AD. The cholesterol increases β-amyloid protein synthesis which can lead to plaque formation. Also, the apo E4 allele is thought to be involved in cholesterol metabolism and is associated with higher cholesterol levels.

8. **Deficits that exist in other pathways are:** Serotonergic neurons of the raphe nuclei and noradrenergic cells of the locus ceruleus are lost. Monoamine oxidase type B activity is increased.

Stages of Alzheimer's disease [3]

The Mini-Mental Status Exam is a commonly used scale that measures orientation, recall, short-term memory, concentration, constructional praxis, and language. The MMSE is scored from 0 to 30, with a score of 10–26 typical of mild to moderate Alzheimer's disease

1. **Mild (MMSE score 26–18):** Patient has difficulty remembering recent events. Ability to manage finances, prepare food, and carry out other household activities declines. May get lost while driving. Begins to withdraw from difficult tasks and to give up hobbies. May deny memory problems.

2. **Moderate (MMSE score 17–10):** Patient requires assistance with activities of daily living. Frequently disoriented with regard to time (date, year, season). Recall for recent events is severely impaired. May forget some details of past life and names of family and friends. Functioning may fluctuate from day to day. Patient generally denies problems. May become suspicious or tearful. Loses ability to drive safely. Agitation, paranoia, and delusions are common.

3. **Severe (MMSE score 9–0):** Patient loses ability to speak, walk, and feed self. Incontinent of urine and feces. Requires care 24 hours a day, 7 days a week.

Stages of Cognitive Decline: The Global Deterioration Scale (GDS)

- **Stage 1- Normal:** No subjective or objective change in intellectual functioning.
- **Stage 2- Forgetfulness:** Complaints of losing things or forgetting names of acquaintances. Does not interfere with job or social functioning. Generally a component of normal aging.
- **Stage 3- Early confusion:** Cognitive decline causes interference with work and social functioning. Anomia, difficulty remembering right word in conversation, and recall difficulties are present and noticed by family members. Memory loss may cause anxiety for patient.
- **Stage 4- Late confusion (early AD):** Patient can no longer manage finances or homemaking activities. Difficulty remembering recent events. Begins to withdraw from difficult tasks and to give up hobbies. May deny memory problems.
- **Stage 5- Early dementia (moderate AD):** Patient can no longer survive without assistance. Frequently disoriented with regard to time (date, year, season). Difficulty selecting clothing. Recall for recent events is severely impaired; may forget some details of past life (e.g., school attended or occupation). Functioning may fluctuate from day to day. Patient generally denies problems. May become suspicious or tearful. Loses ability to drive safely.
- **Stage 6- Middle dementia (moderately severe AD):** Patients need assistance with activities of daily living (e.g., bathing, dressing, and toileting). Patients experience difficulty interpreting their surroundings; may forget names of family and caregivers; forget most details of past life; have difficulty counting backward from 10. Agitation, paranoia, and delusions are common.
- **Stage 7- Late dementia:** Patient loses ability to speak (may only grunt or scream), walk, and feed self. Incontinent of urine and feces. Consciousness reduced to stupor or coma

Clinical Manifesation and Features

The onset of AD is almost imperceptible, without abrupt changes in cognition or function. Deficits occur progressively over time, affecting multiple areas of cognition. For treatment and assessment purposes, it is helpful to divide Alzheimer's symptoms into two basic categories: cognitive symptoms and noncognitive (behavioral) symptoms. Cognitive symptoms are present throughout the illness, whereas behavioral symptoms are less predictable

General

The patient may have vague memory complaints initially, or the patient's significant other may report that the patient is "forgetful."

Cognitive decline is gradual over the course of illness. Behavioral disturbances may be present in moderate stages. Loss of daily function is common in advanced stages.

Symptoms

Cognitive: Memory loss (poor recall and losing items); aphasia (circumlocution and anomia); apraxia; agnosia; disorientation (impaired perception of time and unable to recognize familiar people); impaired executive function

Noncognitive: Depression, psychotic symptoms (hallucinations and delusions), behavioral disturbances (physical and verbal aggression, motor hyperactivity, uncooperativeness, wandering, repetitive mannerisms and activities, and combativeness)

Functional: Inability to care for self (dressing, bathing, toileting, and eating)

Diagnosis with Algorithm

Natinal Institute of Neurological and Communicable Disorders and Stroke (NINCDS) Alzheimer's Disease and Related Disorders Association (ADRDA) Criteria and Diagnostic Work-Up for Probable Alzheimer's disease [4]
1. History of progressive cognitive decline of insidious onset
   In-depth interview of patient and caregivers
2. Deficits in at least two or more areas of functioning
3. No disturbance of consciousness
   Confirmation with use of dementia rating scale (e.g., Mini-Mental Status Exam [MMSE] or Blessed Dementia Scale)
4. Age between 40 and 90 years (usually >65 years)
5. No other explainable cause of symptoms
   - Normal laboratory tests including hematology, full chemistries, B12 and folate, thyroid function tests, Venereal Disease Research Lab test (to rule out venereal disease or syphilis)
   - Normal electrocardiogram and electroencephalogram
   - Normal physical exam, including thorough neurologic exam
   - Neuroimaging: CT or MRI scanning: No focal lesions signifying other possible causes of dementia are present. Abnormalities which are common, but not diagnostic for AD include general cerebral wasting, widening of sulci, widening of the ventricles, and lesions of white matter surrounding the ventricle deep in the brain

Evaluation of neuropsychological symptoms according to standard criteria's [5]
1. **Cognitive deficits:** NINCDS-ADRDA criteria: Memory decline and impairment in atleast one other cognitive domain.
   Diagnostic and Statistical Manual for Mental Disorders (DSM-IV) criteria: Memory decline and atleast one of aphasia, apraxia, agnosia, executive dysfunction
   ICD-10 criteria: Memory decline and deterioration in judgement and thinking
2. **Confirmation:** NINCDS-ADRDA criteria: MMSE or similar and neuropsychological testing
   Diagnostic and Statistical Manual for Mental Disorders (DSM-IV) criteria:
   ICD-10 criteria:

3. **Functional impairment:**
   NINCDS-ADRDA criteria:
   DSM-IV criteria: Impairment of social or occupational functioning
   ICD-10 criteria: Impairment of activities of daily living
4. **Course:**
   NINCDS-ADRDA criteria: progressive worsening
   DSM-IV criteria: gradual onset and continuing decline
   ICD-10 criteria: gradual onset and slow deterioration
5. **Exclusions:**
   NINCDS-ADRDA criteria: age at onset < 40 or > 90 years
   DSM-IV criteria: substance abuse or other major mental disorder
   ICD-10 criteria: sudden onset or focal neurological signs

Laboratory Tests

Rule out vitamin B12 and folate deficiency

Rule out hypothyroidism with thyroid function tests

Other Diagnostic Tests [6]

CT or MRI scans may aid diagnosis
1. In MRI scan there is decreased volume of hippocampus and other temporal lobe structures. There is also tissue loss and neurodegeneration seen.
2. In PET scan using 13F-fluorodeoxyglucose PET- there is decreased uptake in posterior cingulated –precuncus and temporoparietal cortex. Glucose hypometabolism and neurodegeration also observed. Where as in 13C-PiB and fluorinated tracers for amyloid PET testing- increased cortical retention observed due to deposition of Beta amyloid in the cortex.
3. CSF examination shows the decreased concentration or ratio of Aβ42 due to abnormal metabolism of β-amyloid. There is increased concentration of total tau and hypophosphorylated tau protein which is due to neuronal damage and accumulation of tau, hyperphosphorylated tau in the brain areas.

Management

Desired Outcome
1. To maintain functioning as long as possible
2. To treat psychiatric and behavioural symptoms.

Nonpharmacologic Therapy
- Sleep disturbances, wandering, urinary incontinence, agitation, and aggression should be managed with behavioral interventions whenever possible.
- On initial diagnosis, the patient and caregiver should be educated on the course of illness,

available treatments, legal decisions, changes in lifestyle that will be necessary with disease progression, and other quality of life issues.

Basic Principles of Care for the Alzheimer's Patient

Keep requests and demands of the patient simple, and avoid complex tasks that might lead to frustration.

Avoid confrontation, and defer requests that lead to frustration.

Remain calm, firm, and supportive if the patient becomes upset.

Maintain a consistent environment and avoid unnecessary changes.

Provide frequent reminders, explanations, and orientation cues.

Recognize declines in capacity and adjust expectations for patient performance.

Bring sudden declines in function and the emergence of new symptoms to professional attention

Classification of Drugs for the Treatment

Based on Pathological Hallmarks of the Disease and their Targets [7]

1. **Acetylcholine decrease:** Cholinesterase inhibitors/ influence on serotonin transmission/ influence on histamine transmission/ increasing Ach response
2. **Glutamate increase:** NMDA blockers or glutamate release inhibitors
3. **Increased Amyloid plaques:** BACE inhibitors/ increasing (Amyloid β) clearance/γ-secretase inhibitors
4. **Increased neurofibrillary tangles:** Increasing Tau stabilisation/ Tau aggregation inhibitors/ increasing p-Tau clearance
5. **Increased neuroinflammation:** Microglial activation inhibitors

Proposed treatment algorithm for cognitive impairment

- After the Patient is diagnosed with AD according to NINCDS-ADRDA criteria, assess all comorbid medical disorders and drug therapies that may affect cognition.
- Rule out comorbid depression. Now evaluate the pharmacotherapy based on illness stage
  (a) **Mild to moderate AD:** Cholinesterase inhibitor or memantine + vitamin E. Observe the therapy is effective by MMSE score. If stable MMSE (< 4 point decline over 1 year), continue the regimen.

    Donepezil 5mg once daily; titrate to 10mg once daily

    Galantamine (oral tablets/solution) 4 mg twice daily titrate to 8 mg twice daily

    Galantamine ER capsules 8mg one daily ; titrate to 16mg twice daily

    Rivastigmine oral 1.5mg twice daily; titrate to 6mg twice daily

    Rivastigmine patch 4.6mg once daily; titrate to 9.5mg daily

(b) Moderate to severe AD: Cholinesterase inhibitor, memantine, or combination cholinesterase inhibitor and memantine + vitamin E. Observe the therapy is effective by MMSE score. If deteriorating MMSE (> 4 point decline over 1 year), alternative drugs with higher dose + VIT E should be initiated.

Donepezil 5mg once daily; titrate to 10mg once daily

Rivastigmine patch 4.6mg once daily; titrate to 9.5mg daily

Memantine 5mg once daily; titrate to 10mg twice daily

Combination CHEI + memantine 7mg twice daily or 10mg once daily ER; titrate to 10mg twice daily or 28mg once daily ER (extended Release)

Proposed treatment algorithm for Concomitant Psychiatric or Behavioral Symptoms

- If the patient is identified with Psychiatric symptoms after assessment- Address medical co-morbidities; later Address concomitant drug therapy for potential side effects
- advice the patient about nonpharmacological approaches
- if the patient is identified with
  - **(a) Depression:** Citalopram or sertraline can be initiated as first line therapy. Fluoxetine, paroxetine, venlafaxine or mirtazepine can be used as alternatives.
  - **(b) Psychoses:** Olanzapine, or risperidone can be initiated as first lone therapy. Quetiapine or haloperidol can be used as alternatives.
  - **(c) Other agitation:** Olanzapine, or risperidone can be used as first line drugs. Citalopram or carbamazepine as alternatives. Diazepam, buspirone, trazodone or selegiline as next alternatives.

Pharmacotherapy for Cognitive Symptoms [8]

Cholinesterase Inhibitors

Donepezil: Donepezil is a piperidine cholinesterase inhibitor with specificity for inhibition of acetylcholinesterase as compared to butyrylcholinesterase. This specificity is claimed to result in fewer peripheral side effects (such as nausea, vomiting, and diarrhea) than with nonspecific cholinesterase inhibitors such as tacrine.

Dose: Donepezil should be initiated at a 5-mg/day dose in the morning and titrated to 10 mg/day after 4 to 6 weeks if it is well tolerated.

Rivastigmine: Butyrylcholinesterase is thought to play an important role in acetylcholine degradation following the depletion of acetylcholinesterase. Acetylcholinesterase is also found in two forms: globular G4 and globular G1. The highest concentrations of globular G1 can be found in the hippocampus and cortex, two regions known to be affected in AD. By blocking this particular form of the acetylcholinesterase enzyme, higher concentrations of acetylcholine may be obtained Rivastigmine has central activity at acetylcholinesterase and butyrylcholinesterase, but low activity at these sites in the periphery

Dose: Rivastigmine should be initiated at a dose of 1.5 mg twice daily and titrated upward at a minimum of 2-week intervals to a maximumdaily dose of 12 mg.

Galantamine. Galantamine is the fourth approved cholinesterase inhibitor, and it also has activity as an allosteric nicotinic receptor agonist.

Dose: Though galantamine has been shown to be efficacious at dosages of 16 mg/day, 24 mg/day, and 32 mg/day, the maximum dosage recommended is 24 mg/day Galantamine should be initiated at 8 mg/day with dosage titration of 8 mg/day occurring at 4-week intervals.

Antiglutamatergic Therapay

Memantine: Memantine, an NMDA-antagonist, is a novel agent for treating AD. By blocking NMDA receptors, excitotoxic reactions, which ultimately lead to cell death, may be prevented. It is indicated for treatment of moderate to severe AD.

Dose: Memantine should be initiated at 5 mg once a day and increased weekly by 5 mg a day to the effective dose of 10 mg twice daily. It may be given with or without food. Dosing of 10 mg daily is recommended in patients with creatinine clearance of 40 to 60 mL/min and patients with severe renal impairment (creatinine clearance <40 mL/min) should not receive memantine.

Other Potential Treatment

Vitamin E and Selegiline: Vitamin E is often recommended as adjunctive treatment for AD patients.

Estrogen: Two studies evaluating the potential benefit of conjugated estrogens as a treatment for cognitive decline did not show any benefit; behavioral and functional outcomes were not improved either.

Lipid-Lowering Agents: Interest in the potential protective effects in AD patients of lipid-lowering agents, particularly the 3-hydroxy-3-methylglutaryl-CoA (HMG-CoA)-reductase inhibitors.

Ginkgo Biloba: An extract of ginkgo biloba, is claimed to improve memory. Although it is thought to be an antioxidant and to affect inflammation and neuromodulation,

Pharmacotherapy of Noncognitive Symptoms

These symptoms can be roughly divided into three categories: psychotic symptoms, inappropriate or disruptive behavior, and depression. Effective management of these problems is important because behavioral symptoms are distressing to both the patient and the caregiver. Strategies for treatment of psychotic or behavioral symptoms should include both environmental and pharmacologic interventions (e.g., antipsychotics, antidepressants, mood stabilizers, and anxiolytics).

Antipsychotics

Antipsychotic medications have traditionally been used to treat disruptive behaviors and psychosis in AD patients. Symptoms responding to antipsychotics include assaultiveness, extreme agitation, hyperexcitability, hallucinations, delusions, suspiciousness, hostility, and uncooperativeness; whereas withdrawal, apathy, cognitive deficits, wandering, and incontinence are not responsive.

Antipsychotics Psychosis: They target symptoms like hallucinations, delusions, suspiciousness Disruptive behaviors: agitation, aggression

Olanzapine 2.5–10 mg

Quetiapine 12.5–200 mg

Risperidone 0.25–2 mg

Haloperidol 0.5–4 mg

Antidepressants

Apathy, decreased initiative and socialization, decreased concentration, psychomotor retardation, agitation, and changes in appetite and sleep patterns are all symptoms intrinsic to both dementia and depression.

Antidepressants Depression: They target symptoms like poor appetite, insomnia, hopelessness, anhedonia, withdrawal, suicidal thoughts, agitation

Fluoxetine 5–20 mg

Mirtazapine 15–45 mg

Paroxetine 10–40 mg

Sertraline 50–200 mg

Trazodone 75–400 mg

Venlafaxine 37.5–150 mg

Citalopram 10–20 mg

Anticonvulsants: They target agitation and aggression.

Carbamazepine: 200-600mg/day

Valproaic acid: 500-1000 mg/day

Others: They target disruptive behaviors

Buspirone   10-45mg

Selegiline   10mg

Oxazepam   10-60mg

References

1. Alzheimer's Association. 2017 Alzheimer's disease facts and figures,. Alzheimers Dement. 2017;13:325-373.
2. Jicha GA, Parisi JE, Dickson DW, et al. Alzheimer's and Lewy body pathology in

centenarian case series. Neurology 2005;6(Suppl 1):A275.

3. Lleó A, Greenberg SM, Growdon JH. Current pharmacotherapy for Alzheimer's disease. Annu Rev Med 2006;57:513–533.

4. McKhann G, Drachman D, Folstein M, et al. Clinical diagnosis of Alzheimer's disease: Report of the NINCDS-ADRDA work group under the auspices of the department of health and human services task force on Alzheimer's disease. Neurology 1984;34:939–944

5. Elsonn storey et al., The neuropsychological diagnosis of Alzheimer's disease. Journal of Alzheimer's disease: 2001, 3(3):261-285.

6. https://www.alzheimer-clarity.info/en/healthcare-professionals/section-5-new-criteria-diagnosis-alzheimers-disease-ad-using-biomarkers

7. Shih-ya-hung et al., Drug candidates in clinical trials for Alzheimer's disease. Journal of Biomedical Science. 2017; 24(1).

8. Grossberg GT, Desai AK. Management of Alzheimer's disease. J Gerontol A Biol Sci Med Sci 2003;58A:331–353.

CHAPTER - 68

Anxiety Disorders

Introduction to Acute Renal Failure

Anxiety is an emotional state commonly caused by the perception of real or perceived danger that threatens the security of an individual. It allows a person to prepare for or react to environmental changes.

Anxiety can produce uncomfortable and potentially debilitating psychological (e.g., worry or feeling of threat) and physiological arousal (e.g., tachycardia or shortness of breath) if it becomes excessive. Anxiety disorders are among the most frequent mental disorders encountered in clinical practice.

Types of Anxiety Disorders [1]:

- Generalized anxiety disorders [GAD]
- Panic disorder
- Social anxiety disorder [SAD]
- Post traumatic stress disorder

Etiology

1. The differential diagnosis of anxiety disorders includes medical and psychiatric illnesses.
2. Certain drugs like
   - Anticonvulsants: carbamazepine
   - Antidepressants: selective serotonin reuptake inhibitors, tricyclic antidepressants
   - Antihypertensives: felodipine
   - Antibiotics: quinolones, isoniazid
   - Bronchodilators: albuterol, theophylline
   - Corticosteroids: prednisone
   - Dopa Agonists: levodopa
   - Herbals: ma huang, ginseng, ephedra
   - Nonsteroidal anti-inflammatory drugs: ibuprofen
   - Stimulants: amphetamines, methylphenidate, caffeine, cocaine

- Sympathomimetics: pseudoephedrine
- Thyroid hormones: levothyroxine
- Toxicity: anticholinergics, antihistamines, digoxin
- Withdrawal: alcohol, sedatives

3. Behavioral inhibition, characterized by wariness, decreased social interaction, and withdrawal, is a genetic trait that may contribute to SAD (Social Anxiety disorder)
4. Parental dysfunction and abuse are potential risk factors for developing SAD.

❖ **Medical Diseases Associated with Anxiety Disorders**

Common Medical Illnesses Associated with Anxiety Symptoms
- Cardiovascular disorders
- Endocrine and Metabolic Cushing's disease,
- Hyperparathyroidism
- Thyroid disorders
- Hypoglycemia
- Hyponatremia, Hyperkalemia, Pheochromocytoma
- vitamin B12 or Folate deficiencies
- Neurologic disorders
- neoplasms
- poor pain control
- Respiratory system disorders
- Others include Anemias, systemic lupus Erythematosus, Vestibular dysfunction.

❖ **Pathophysiology [2, 3]**

❖ The modulation of normal and pathologic anxiety states is associated with multiple regions of the brain and abnormal function in several neurotransmitter systems, including norepinephrine (NE), γ-aminobutyric acid (GABA), and serotonin (5-HT)

❖ Female gender due to hormonal factors, less internal locus of control; genetics (persons with positive family history) have more predisposition to anxiety. There is an imbalance and/or abnormal functioning of NE, 5-HT, DA, and GABA. This causes a threat to hippocampus and cingulated gyrus. Environmental stress also poses a threat to hippocampus. Because of the threat amygdala gets activated and activates fear responses. Now under the influence of amygdala there is a) activation of hypothalamus-pituitary – adrenal cortex axis and b) activation of autonomic nervous system and adrenal medulla. There is release of cortisol and epinephrine from their respective centres. These stress hormones which are released due to stress interact with the different brain areas and body organs to show pathological mechanisms. Hippocampus shrinks in size and due to chronic activation of stress hormones over time causes death of neurons in hippocampus. Consequences which develop are anxiety disorders-an emotional state causing fear, worry and excessive stress. The symptoms which develop in the persons are characterized as physiological arousal, unpleasant tension, apprehension, mood dysregulation, memory impairment, and decrease in brain derived neurotrophic factor (which correlates with degree of neuronal loss in hippocampus).

Neurochemical Theories

Noradrenergic Model

> In response to threat or fearful situations, LC (Locus Ceruleus) serves as an alarm center activating NE release and stimulating the sympathetic and parasympathetic nervous systems.

> Chronic central noradrenergic overactivity downregulates α2-adrenoreceptors in patients with GAD. This receptor is hypersensitive in some patients with panic disorder.

> Patients with Society Anxiety Disorders (SAD) appear to have a hyperresponsive adrenocortical response to psychological stress. Drugs with anxiogenic effects (e.g., yohimbine [an α2-adrenergic receptor antagonist]) stimulate LC firing and increase noradrenergic activity. NE in turn increases glutamate release (an excitatory neurotransmitter).

> This produces subjective feelings of anxiety and can precipitate a panic attack in those with panic disorder, but not in normal volunteers or those with other psychiatric illnesses.

> Drugs with anxiolytic or antipanic effects (e.g., benzodiazepines, antidepressants, and clonidine) inhibit LC firing, decrease noradrenergic activity, and block the effects of anxiogenic drugs

Gaba Receptor Model

There are two superfamilies of GABA protein receptors: $GABA_A$ and $GABA_B$. Drugs to reduce anxiety and produce sedation target the $GABA_A$ receptor. The $GABA_B$ receptor Is a G-protein coupled receptor postulated to be involved in the presynaptic inhibition of GABA release. $GABA_A$ receptors are ligand-gated ion channels. The opening of the channel is composed of five peptide subunits (i.e., α, β, γ, δ, or ρ subunits) that surround a central pore that crosses the neuronal cell membrane and is permeable to chloride.

> Benzodiazepine ligands either enhance or diminish the inhibitory effects of GABA.

> GABA, the major inhibitory neurotransmitter in the CNS, has a strong regulatory or inhibitory effect on the 5-HT, NE, and dopamine (DA) systems.

> When GABA binds to the GABAA receptor, chloride ion channel opens and permits the influx of negatively charged chloride ions, results in hyperpolarization of the cell membrane and decreases nerve cell excitability.

Serotonin Model

> 5-HT is primarily an inhibitory neurotransmitter that is used by neurons originating in the raphe nuclei of the brain stem and projecting diffusely throughout the brain.

> Abnormalities in serotonergic functioning through release and uptake at the presynaptic autoreceptors (5-HT1A/1D), the serotonin reuptake transporter site (SERT), or effect of 5-HT at the postsynaptic receptors (e.g., 5-HT1A, 5-HT2A, and 5-HT2C) may play a role in anxiety disorders.

Greater 5-HT activity reduces the NE activity in the Locus Cerulus. Inhibition of defense/escape response occurs via the periaqueductal gray region. There is decrease in hypothalamic release of corticotropin-releasing factor. This is responsible for panic and anxiety.

- ➢ Low 5-HT activity may lead to a dysregulation of other neurotransmitters. NE and 5-HT systems are closely linked, and interactions between the two are reciprocal and vary.
- ➢ NE may act at presynaptic 5-HT terminals to decrease 5-HT release, and its activity at post synaptic receptors can cause increased 5-HT release. Stimulation of the postsynaptic 5-HT2A receptors in the limbic system results in anxiety and avoidance behavior.
- ❖ Generalized Anxiety Disorders

    The onset,course of illness, and comorbid conditions of GAD are important considerations. GAD has a gradual onset with an average age of 21 years; however, there is a bimodal distribution. If GAD is the primary disorder, the patient can present in their teens. If it develops secondary to another anxiety disorder, the onset can be as late as age 30 years and even extend into the mid-50s. [4]

Clinical Presentations [5, 6, 7, 8]

Psychological and cognitive symptoms

- ➢ Excessive anxiety
- ➢ Worries that are difficult to control
- ➢ Feeling keyed up or on edge
- ➢ Poor concentration or mind going blank

Physical symptoms :

- ➢ Restlessness
- ➢ Fatigue
- ➢ Muscle tension
- ➢ Sleep disturbance
- ➢ Irritability

Impairment :

- ➢ Social, occupational, or other important functional areas
- ➢ Poor coping abilities

Screening questions

- ➢ What is going on in your life?
- ➢ How do you feel about it?
- ➢ What troubles you the most?

Diagnostic Criteria for Generalized Anxiety Disorder

1. Unrealistic or excessive anxiety and worry about life circumstances for a period of at least 6 months, during which the person has been bothered more days than not by these concerns
2. Person has difficulty controlling anxiety and worry

3. Anxiety and worry are associated with at least three of the following symptoms:

(a) Restlessness or feeling keyed up or on edge b. Easy fatigue

(b) Difficulty concentrating or mind going blank d. Irritability

(c) Muscle tension f. Sleep disturbances

4. If another psychiatric disorder is present, the focus of the anxiety and worry is unrelated to it

5. Anxiety, worry, or physical symptoms cause significant distress or impairment in social, occupational, or some other important aspect of functioning

6. Disturbance is not due to the direct effects of a substance, medication, or general medical condition and does not occur only during the course of a mood disorder, psychotic disorder, or pervasive developmental disorder

Management

Non-Pharmacology Therapy

> GAD include psycho education, short-term counseling, stress management, psychotherapy, meditation,orexercise.

> Psycho education includes information on the etiology and management of GAD.

> Anxious patients should be instructed to avoid caffeine, nonprescription stimulants, diet

> pills, and excessive use of alcohol.

> Most patients with GAD require psychological therapy, alone or in combination with antianxiety drugs, to over come fears and to learn to manage their anxiety and worry.

> Cognitive behavioral therapy (CBT) is the most effective psychological therapy in GAD patients.

Algorithm for pharmacotherapy of GAD [9]

- After the patient is diagnosed and

- If acute relief is needed, start with BZ for 2-6 weeks. If adequqte response is not obtained, start with venlafaxine or SSRI.

- If acute relief is not needed, therapy is started with venlafaxine or SSRI. If adequate response is obtained continue the therapy for 3-10 months. If adequate response is not obtained, switch to another anxiolytic- SSRI or imipramine or buspirone or hydroxyzine

- If adequate response is obtained, continue the therapy for 3-10 months. If not add BZ for somatic symptoms for 2-4 weeks.

Pharmacological Therapy

Nonbenzodiazepine Anti-anxiety Agents

1. Antidepressants

Venlafaxine Xr: Dose: 37.5 OR 75mg per day; Dose Range: 75-225 mg/day

Paroxetine: Dose: 20 mg per day; Dose Range: 20-50 mg/day

Escitalopram: Dose: 10mg per day; Dose Range: 10-20 mg/day
Imipramine: dose 50mg per day; dosage range: 75-200mg

2. **Azapirones**
   Buspirone dose: 7.5mg twice per day
3. **Diphenylmethane**
   Hydroxyzine 25 or 50 mg 4 times daily   dosage range: 200-400mg/day

Buspirone

Mechanism of action: Buspirone is a 5-HT1A partial agonist that lacks anticonvulsant, muscle relaxant, sedative-hypnotic, motor impairment, and dependence-producing properties.

Anxiolytic agent. The drug does not act on benzodiazepine receptors.It enhances the activity of specific noradrenergic & dopaminergic pathways & reduces activity of serotonin & acetylcholine.

Indications: Short term management of anxiety disorders and the relief of symptoms of anxiety with or without accompanying depression.

Dosage: Initial 5 mg 2-3 times daily, dose may be increased every 2-3 days. Maint 15 mg-30 mg daily. Max 45 mg daily.

Contra-Indications: Hypersensitivity, epilepsy, severe renal & hepatic disease, pregnancy & lactation.

Special Precautions: History of renal or hepatic impairment, alcoholics.

Side Effects: Dizziness, headache, nervousness, light headedness, excitment and nausea. Rarely tachycardia, palpitations, chest pain, drowsiness, confusion, dry mouth, fatigue, sweating.

Benzodiazepine Anti-anxiety Agents [10]

Alprazolam: It is a triazolo analogue of benzodiazepine, which is indicated as an anti-anxiety drug in various disorders associated with anxiety. Drug has a dose related depressant effect on central nervous system varying from mild impairment of task performance to hypnosis.

Indications: Anxiety disorders and short term relief of symptoms of anxiety. Anxiety associated with depression.

Dosage: Starting dose is 0.25-0.5 mg 3 times daily. Max 3-4 mg daily in divided doses.

Contra-Indications: Hypersensitivity to benzodiazepines. Acute narrow angle glaucoma.

Special Precautions: C.N.S. depressants. Paediatrics: Not recommended. Pregnancy: Contraindicated. Lactation: Contraindicated. Elderly: Dose should be reduced.

Side Effects: Drowsiness or light headedness, withdrawal seizures, anorexia, transient amnesia or memory impairment, loss of coordination, slurred speech, musculo skeletal weakness, pruritus.

Chlordiazepoxide

It is first benzodiazepines to be used clinically. It is slowly absorbed, produces a smooth long lasting effect; preferred in chronic anxiety states but has poor anticonvulsant action.

Indications: Anxiety, tension. Behavioural disorders. Insomnia, emotional disturbances. Pre & post operative apprehensions.

Dosage: 10 mg 2-4 times daily. Children 10 mg daily or as required. Elderly 10 mg daily.

Contra-Indications: Hypersensitivity to benzo-diazepines, jaundice, acute narrow angle glaucoma.

Special Precautions: Pregnancy, lactation, alcoholics, hepatic or renal impairment. Paediatrics: Contraindicated below the age of6 years. Pregnancy: Contraindicated. Lactation: Contraindicated. Elderly: Reduced dose may be necessary.

Side Effects: Drug dependence & abuse, drowsiness, dizziness, impaired liver function & blood counts

Clonazepam: Dose: 0.25 mg

Clorazepate: Dose: 7.5–60 mg:

Diazepam: Dose: 2–40 mg

Lorazepam: Dose: 0.5–10 mg

Oxazepam: Dose: 30-120 mg

Adverse effects: Tolerance usually develops to this effect. Other side effects are disorientation, psychomotor impairment, confusion, aggression, excitement, and anterograde amnesia.

Clinical Practice Guidelines for the Management of Generalised Anxiety Disorder (GAD)

The drug treatment of GAD is sometimes is seen as a 6-12 month treatment, some evidence indicate that treatment should be long term.

Goals: Reduce psychological and autonomic symptoms and other co morbid conditions. Improve occupational and social functioning.

1. **BDZ is the drugs of choice:** Can be prescribed on as needed basis, so that patients take a rapidly acting BZD when they feel particularly anxious. Alternatively, BZDs prescribed for a limited period, during which psychosocial approaches are implemented. Some may fail to respond, and tolerance and dependence may occur. Treatment for most anxiety conditions lasts for about 4 to 6 weeks, followed by 1 to 2 weeks of tapering drug use before it is discontinued.

2. **SSRIs:** Effective in anxious patients with co morbid depression; also useful in anxious patients without depression, as they have strong anxiolytic effects, especially seen after 6-8 weeks of treatment. Fluoxetine transiently increases anxiety; hence sertraline and

paroxetine may be preferred. Begin with SSRI's and BZDs and taper the latter after 2-3 weeks of use.

3. **Venlafaxine:** Works both on serotonin and norepinephrine. Improves insomnia, poor concentration, restlessness, irritability and excessive muscle tension

4. **Buspirone:** Takes 2 to 3 weeks for its action and patient may be lost for treatment. Has been found to be useful in 60 to 80% patients with GAD Evidences indicate that it improves cognitive symptoms.

5. **Psychotherapy:** Cognitive behaviour therapy and behavioural techniques like meditation, yoga.

Social Anxiety Disorders

Clinical Presentation:

Signs and Symptoms:

- **Fears:** Being scrutinized by others, Being embarrassed, Being humiliated
- **Some feared situations:** Addressing a group of people, Eating or writing in front of others, Interacting with authority figures, Speaking in public, Talking with strangers, Use of public toilets
- **Physical symptoms:** Blushing, "Butterflies in the stomach", Diarrhea, Sweating, Tachycardia, Trembling

Types

- Generalized type: fear and avoidance extend to a wide range of social situations
- Nongeneralized type: fear is limited to one or two situations

Diagnostic Criteria for Phobic Disorders

Social Anxiety Disorder (Social Phobia)

1. Marked and constant fear of one or more social situations in which the person is exposed to unfamiliar people or possible scrutiny by others and the person fears humiliation or embarrassment.
2. Exposure to the situation provokes an immediate anxiety response
3. Person realizes the fear is excessive or unreasonable (not required in children)
4. Feared situation is avoided or endured with intense anxiety or distress
5. Fear or avoidance significantly interferes with the person's normal routine or activities or causes marked distress
6. In individuals younger than 18 years of age, the duration of the fear is at least 6 months
7. Anxiety or phobic avoidance are not better accounted for by another psychiatric disorder (e.g., fear of having a panic attack, obsessions that accompany OCD, trauma related to PTSD)

Management

Goals: In the acute phase of treatmen are to reduce physiological symptoms of anxiety. In the continuation phase are to extend the therapeutic benefits of the acute phase, especially the patient's ability to participate in social activities, and improve QOL. This phase usually lasts 3 to 6 months.

Nonpharmacologic Therapy

- Patients should be educated about SAD, the symptoms they experience, and effective therapeutic options.
- CBT for SAD consists of exposure therapy, cognitive restructuring, relaxation training techniques, and social skills training. Through CBT, patients learn to overcome anxiety in social situations and change the beliefs and responses that maintain this behavior

Treatment algorithm for pharmacotherapy of SAD

1. If the patient is diagnosed with generalized social anxiety disorder- and
   (a) If present with comorbid depression, second anxiety disorder, or substance abuse- paroxetine, sertraline, or venlafaxine XR can be initiated.
   (b) If response is good-continue for 12 months.
   (c) If no response is seen- switch to another SSRI or venlafaxine XR can be given
   If partial response is seen- Consider augmentation with buspirone
   If after the treatment still inadequate response is observed-switch to phenelzine.
   (a) if nonresponse is observed- consider gabapentin therapy
   (b) if response is good –continue for 12 months.
2. If the patient is in urgency to be treated and has no substance abuse- start with BZ.
   (a) If inadequate response SSRI + BDZ Benzodiazepines
   (b) Response is good –continue for 12 months

Pharmacology therapy:

1. **First line drugs:**
   - Escitalopram : Dose : 5mg/day; Dose Range :10-20mg/day
   - Fluvoxamine : Dose : 50mg/day Dose Range: 150-300mg/day
   - Paroxetine : Dose : 10mg/day ;   DoseRange : 10-60mg/day
   - Sertraline : Dose:25-550mg/day; DoseRange : 50-200 mg/day
   - Venlafaxine XR: Dose : 75 mg/day; Dose Range : 75-225 mg/day
2. **Second line drugs:**
   - Citalopram: Dose: 20 mg/day; Dosage Range : 20-40 mg/day
   - Clonazepam : Dose : 0.25 mg/day; Dose Range : 1-4 mg/day
3. **Third line drugs:**
   - Buspirone: Dose : 10mg twice per day; Dose range : 45-60 mg/day
   - Gabapentin Dose: 100mg TID
   - Mirtazapine: Dose : 15 mg at bed time ; Dose Range : 30 mg/day

- Phenelzine: Dose : 15mg at bed time ;   Dose Range : 60-90 mg/day
- Pregabalin: Dose : 100mg three times a day ; Dose Range : 600 mg/day

Post Traumatic Stress Disorder

Clinical Presentation:

Signs and symptoms:

Reexperiencing symptoms
- Recurrent, intrusive distressing memories of the trauma
- Recurrent, disturbing dreams of the event
- Feeling that the traumatic event is recurring (e.g., dissociative flashbacks)
- Physiologic reaction to reminders of the trauma

Avoidance symptoms
- Avoidance of conversations about the trauma
- Avoidance of thoughts or feelings about the trauma
- Avoidance of activities that are reminders of the event
- Avoidance of people or places that arouse recollections of the trauma
- Inability to recall an important aspect of the trauma
- Anhedonia
- Estrangement from others
- Restricted affect
- Sense of a foreshortened future (e.g., does not expect to have a career, marriage)

Hyperarousal symptoms
- Decreased concentration
- Easily startled
- Hypervigilance
- Insomnia
- Irritability or angry outbursts

Subtypes
- Acute: duration of symptoms is less than 3 months
- Chronic: symptoms last for longer than 3 months
- With delayed onset: onset of symptoms is at least 6 months posttrauma

Screening questions
- Have you ever experienced a significant trauma in your life?
- Did this experience have a lasting negative impact or change your life?

Diagnostic Criteria for Post Traumatic Stress Disorder (PTSD)

1. Person has experienced a traumatic event in which the individual witnessed, experienced, or was confronted with actual or threatened death, or serious injury to self or others, and to which the person responded with intense fear, helplessness, or horror
2. Traumatic event is re-experienced persistently in some way (e.g., dreams, nightmares, flashbacks, recurrent thoughts or images), or intense distress is experienced on exposure to stimuli associated with the traumatic event
3. Persistent avoidance of stimuli associated with the event and numbing of general responsiveness involving at least three of the following: a. Efforts to avoid thoughts, feelings, or conversations related to the trauma b. Efforts to avoid people, places, or activities that are reminders of the trauma c. Impaired recall of the traumatic event d. Decreased interest or participation in activities e. Feelings of detachment f. Restricted range of affect g. Sense of foreshortened future
4. Persistent symptoms of increased arousal (not present before the event) that include at last two of the following: a. Sleep disturbances b. Irritability or anger outbursts c. Difficulty concentrating d. Hypervigilance e. Exaggerated startle response
5. Duration of the disturbance (2–4) of at least 1 month 6. Disturbance causes significant impairment in some aspect of daily functioning

Management:

Goals:

- The short-term goal of therapy in the management of PTSD is reduction in core symptoms (i.e., intrusive re-experiencing, avoidance, and hyperarousal). Patients should also have improvements in disability, comorbid conditions, and QOL.
- The long-term goal in PTSD is remission

Nonpharmacological therapy

- Psychotherapy can be used when a patient suffers from mild symptoms for anxiety management.
- CBT (e.g., exposure therapy, cognitive processing therapy, and eye movement desensitization reprocessing), insight-oriented therapies (e.g., psychodynamic therapy, and hypnosis), and psychoeducation.

Treatment algorithm for PTSD

1. Start with SSRI. If good response is seen-continue for 12-24 months.
2. If no response is observed-change to Triacylic antidepressants (TCA).
3. If response is good – continue for 12-24 months
4. If response is not good change to phenelzine or lamotrigine

Pharmacology Therapy

1. Selective Serotonin Reuptake Inhibitors:

Escitalopram

Indications: Treatment of major depressive disorder, anxiety disorder.

Dosage: 10mg once daily, increased, if necessary to 20mg once daily.

Contra Indications: Concomitant use with MAOIs, hypersensitivity to escitalopram or citalopram.

Special Precautions: Mania, seizure disorders, works requiring mental alertness e.g. operating hazardous machinery, including automobiles; severe renal impairment; hepatic impairment.

Side Effects: Nausea, diarrhoea, increased sweating, insomnia, impotence, ejaculation disorder, fatigue, somnolence.

- Citalopram: Dose: 20 mg per day; Dose Range: 20–60 mg/day
- Fluoxetine: Dose: 10–20 mg per day; Dose range: 10–80 mg/day
- Fluvoxamine: Dose: 50 mg per day; Dose range: 100–250 mg/day
- Paroxetine: Dose: 10–20 mg per day; Dose Range: 20–50 mg/day
- Sertraline: Dose: 25–50 mg per day; Dose Range: 50–200 mg/day

Common side effects: Somnolence, nausea, ejaculation disorders, decreased libido, dry mouth, insomnia, and fatigue.

2. Other Agents

- Amitriptyline: Dose: 25–50 mg per day; DoseRange: 50–300 mg/day
- Imipramine: Dose: 25–50 mg per day; Dose range: 50–300 mg/day
- Mirtazapine: Dose: 15 mg at bedtime; Dose range:15–45 mg/day
- Phenelzine: Dose:15 mg every night; DoseRange:15–90 mg/day
- Venlafaxine Extended Release: Dose: 37.5 mg per day
- Dose Range: 37.5–225 mg/day

PANIC ATTACK

Clinical Presentation [11, 12]

Signs and symptoms:

Psychological symptoms

- Depersonalization, Derealization, Fear of losing control
- Fear of going crazy, Fear of dying

Physical symptoms

- Abdominal distress, Chest pain or discomfort, Chills, Dizziness or light-headedness
- Feeling of choking, Hot flushes, Palpitations, Nausea, Paresthesias
- Shortness of breath, Sweating, Tachycardia, Trembling or shaking

Diagnostic Criteria for Panic Disorder

1. Presence of at least two unexpected panic attacks, characterized by at least four of the following symptoms, which develop abruptly and reach a peak within 10 minutes:

a. Palpitations, pounding heart, or accelerated heart rate b. Sweating c. Trembling or shaking d. Sensations of shortness of breath or smothering e. Feeling of choking f. Chest pain or discomfort g. Nausea or abdominal distress h. Feeling dizzy, unsteady, lightheaded, or faint i. Derealization or depersonalization j. Fear of losing control or going crazy k. Fear of dying l. Numbness or tingling sensations m. Chills or hot flushes

2. At least one of the attacks has been followed by at least one of the following symptoms for a duration of at least 1 month:

   a. Persistent concern about having another attack b. Worry about the implications or consequences of the attack c. Significant change in behavior because of the attack

3. Symptoms are not due to the direct effects of a medication, substance, or general medical condition

4. Panic attacks are not better accounted for by another psychiatric or anxiety disorder (e.g., phobias, obsessive-compulsive disorder)

5. May occur with or without agoraphobia

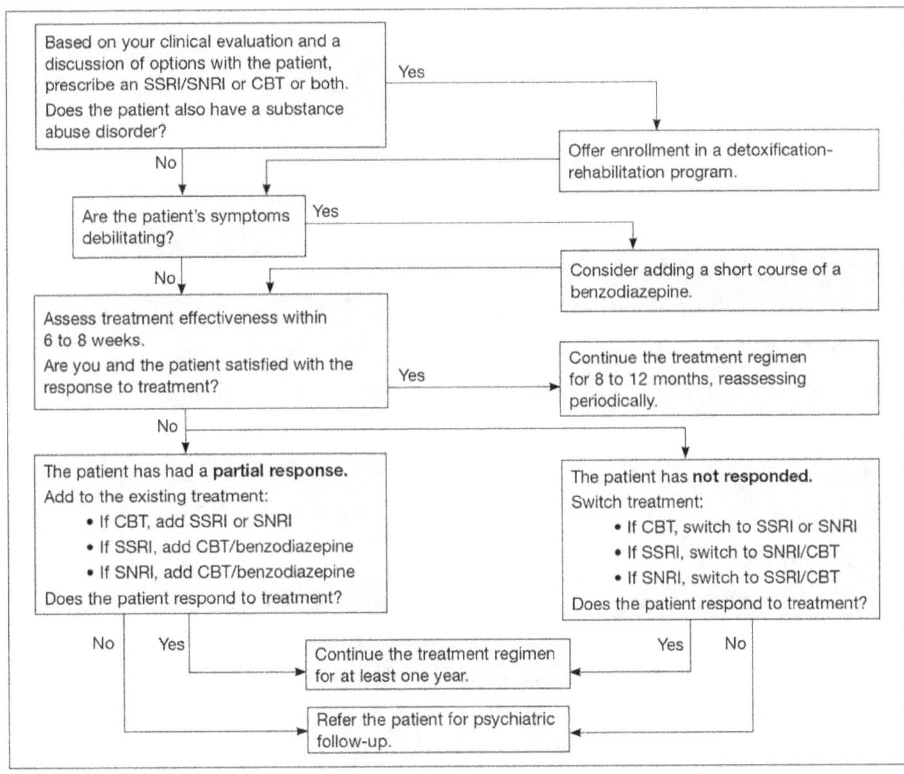

Fig. 68.1 Algorithm for the management of Panic disorder.

Source: Stein MB, Goin MRK, Pollack MH et al., Practice guideline for the treatment of patients with panic disorder 2nd ed. Washing DC; American Psychiatric Association 2010.

Management

Goals: Remission and free of panic attacks. have no or minimal anticipatory anxiety and agoraphobic avoidance, and no functional impairment

General Approach to Treatment

Therapeutic options include single or combined pharmacologic agents, concurrent psychotherapy, or psychotherapy followed by pharmacotherapy

Nonpharmacologic Therapy

1. Patients should be educated to avoid substances that can precipitate panic attacks, including caffeine, drugs of abuse, and nonprescription stimulant
2. CBT focuses on the correction of a patient's maladaptive thoughts and behaviors that initiate, perpetuate, or exacerbate panic symptom
3. CBT alone is certainly indicated. CBT is associated with short-term improvement in 80% to 90% of patients and 6-month improvement in 75% of patients.

Pharmacological Therapy

1. **Selective Serotonin Reuptake Inhibitors**
   - Citalopram: Dose:10 mg per day; Dose Range: 20–60 mg/day
   - Escitalopram: Dose: 5 mg per day; Dose Range: 10–20 mg/day
   - Fluoxetine: Dose: 5 mg per day; Dose Range: 10–30mg/day
   - Fluvoxamine: Dose: 25 mg per day; Dose Range: 100–300mg/day
   - Paroxetine: Dose: 10 mg per day; Dose Range: 20–60 mg/day
   - Paxil: Dose: 12.5 mg per day; Dose Range: 25–75mg/day
   - Sertraline: Dose: 25 mg per day; Dose Range: 50–200mg/day

   Adverse effects: Nausea, vomiting, diarrhea,headache, insomnia, fatigue, and sexual dysfunction.

2. **Serotonin Norepinephrine Reuptake Inhibitors**
   - Venlafaxine Xr: Dose: 37.5 mg per day; Dose Range: 75–225 mg/day

3. **Benzodiazepines**
   - Alprazolam: Dose: 0.25 mg three times a day; Dose Range: 4–10mg/day
   - Xanax XR: Dose: 0.5–1 mg per day; Dose Range:1–10mg/day
   - Clonazepam: Dose: 0.25 mg once or twice per day; Dose Range: 1–4 mg/day
   - Diazepam; Dose: 2–5 mg three times a day; Dose Range: 5–20 mg/day
   - Lorazepam; Dose: 0.5–1 mg three times a day; Dose Range: 2–8mg/day

4. **Tricyclic Antidepressants**
   - Imipramine: Dose:10 mg per day; Dose Range:75–250 mg/day
   - Adverse effects: Dry mouth, blurred vision, constipation, urinary retention, tachycardia, memory impairment, and delirium)

5. Monoamine Oxidase Inhibitor
- Phenelzine: Dose:15 mg per day; Dose Range: 45–90 mg/day
- Adverse effects: Postural hypotension

Case Study of Panic Disorder

Case summary: A male patient of age 49 years was admitted in the male psychiatry ward with the chief complaints of chest pain, palpitations, SOB, sweating, fear of loss of control, fear of dying (2-3 episodes) since last 6 months.

Mood- depressed, sad, disturbed sleep

Family history- not significant

Medications prescribed: Tab. Paridep-CR (paroxetime) -12.5md-OD

Inj. Lorazepam-IM-1amp-SOS.

Patient education: There's no sure way to prevent panic attacks or panic disorder. However, these recommendations may help.
- Get treatment for panic attacks as soon as possible to help stop them from getting worse or becoming more frequent.
- Stick with treatment plan to help prevent relapses or worsening of panic attack symptoms.
- Get regular physical activity, which may play a role in protecting against anxiety.
- Avoid smoking and caffeine

Assignment

1. What are the DSM-5 diagnostic criteria for panic disorder?

The individual experiences recurrent unexpected panic attacks, which are abrupt feelings of intense fear or discomfort that reach great heights within minutes, during a time in which atleast four of the following symptoms occur-
- Palpitations, Abnormal sweating, Trembling, SOB, Feeling of choking
- Chest pain, Nausea/ abdominal pain, Chills or hot flushes
- Numbness/ tingling sensations, Derealization / depersonalization
- Fear of losing control, Fear of death

One or more of the attacks were followed by a month of one or both of the following:
- Persistent worry about having more panic attacks and or their consequences
- Abnormal change in behavior in response to attack.

The disturbance cannot be attributed to physiological effects of drug or substance or medical condition.

The disturbance cannot be explained by other mental disorders.

2. What are the complications of panic disorder?

- Hindrance in lifestyle, Problems with employment, Depression
- Alcohol abuse or dependence, Suicidality

3. What educational information about panic disorder should be provided to patients and their family?

- Teach the patients breathing techniques that can be used to help and keep the patients calm during the stress of a panic attack.
- Cognitive behavioural therapy(CBT) focuses on the importance of both behavioural and thought processes in understanding and controlling anxiety and panic attacks.
- Avoid smoking and caffeine
- Yoga, meditation and muscle relaxation exercises can help the patients to cope with stress in their life.
- Advice the families of patients with panic disorder to provide special care to the patients.

4. What are the types of panic attacks?

- Anxiety; Generalized anxiety disorder; Obsessive compulsive disorder
- Phobias; Social anxiety disorder; Post- traumatic stress disorder.

5. What standardized mental status screening tests are used for patients with panic disorder?

For the diagnosis of panic disorder, the diagnostic and statistical manual of mental disorders (DSM-5), published by the American psychiatric association, lists these points:

- You have frequent, unexpected panic attacks
- Atleast one of the attacks has been followed by one month or more of ongoing worry about having another attack, continued fear of consequences of attack such as losing control, heart attack, significant changes in behavior.
- Panic attacks are not caused by drugs or other substance or medical conditions or any other mental health condition.

6. What are the American Psychiatric Association (APA) recommendations on the evaluation of treatment for panic disorder?

According to DSM-IV criteria, patients have been defined as panic free if they donot have a sufficient number of panic symptoms to meet the diagnostic criteria of panic disorder.

7. Describe the treatment approach in the patient.

<u>Non-pharmacological</u>: CBT; Psychotherapy, also called talk therapy.

<u>Pharmacological</u>:

- Selective serotonin reuptake inhibitors(SSRIs)- fluoxetine,paroxetime, setraline.
- Serotonin and norepinephrine reuptake inhibitors(SNRIs)- venlafaxine
- Benzodiazepines- alprazolam(xanax) and clonazepam(klonopin).

8. How are persistent or recurrent symptoms managed in treatment of panic disorder?

- Increasing the dose of agent being used is a simple first step towards assuring adequate intensity of treatment
- This can be followed by augmentation with another antidepressant or other agent.
- If there is a total lack of response after 6 wks, it seems prudent to switch to another agent.

References

1. Chen J, Reich L, Chung H. Anxiety disorders. West J Med 2002;176:249–253.
2. Condren RM, O'Neill A, Ryan MC, et al. HPA axis response to a psychological stressor in generalised social phobia. Psychoneuroendocrinology 2002;27:693–703.
3. Kent JM, Mathew SJ, Gorman JM. Molecular targets in the treatment of anxiety. Biol Psychiatry 2002;52:1008–1030.
4. Roy-Byrne PR, Wagner A. Primary care perspectives on generalized anxiety disorder. J Clin Psychiatry 2004;(65 Suppl 13):20–26.
5. Data from American Psychiatric Association. Diagnostic and Statistical Manual of Mental Disorders, 4th ed., text revision.Washington, DC: American Psychiatric Association, 2000:429–484; and Baldwin DS, Anderson IM, Nutt DJ, et al. Evidence-basedguidelines for the pharmacological treatment of anxiety disorders: Recommendations from the British Society for Psychopharmacology.J Psychopharmacology 2005;19:567–596.
6. Data from American Psychiatric Association. Diagnostic and Statistical Manual of Mental Disorders, 4th ed., text revision.Washington, DC: American Psychiatric Association, 2000:429–484; Baldwin DS, Anderson IM, Nutt DJ, et al. Evidence-basedguidelines for the pharmacological treatment of anxiety disorders: Recommendations from the British Society for Psychopharmacology.J Psychopharmacology 2005;19:567–596; and Katon WJ. Panic disorder. N Engl J Med 2006;354:2360–2367.
7. Data from American Psychiatric Association. Diagnostic and Statistical Manual of Mental Disorders, 4th ed., text revision.Washington, DC: American Psychiatric Association, 2000:429–484; Schneier FR. Social anxiety disorder. N Engl J Med2006;355:1029–1036; and Ballenger JC, Davidson JRT, Lecrubier Y, et al. Consensus statement on social anxiety disorder from the International Consensus Group on Depression and Anxiety. J Clin Psychiatry 1998;59(Suppl 17):54–60.
8. Data from American Psychiatric Association. Diagnostic and Statistical Manual of Mental Disorders, Fourth Edition, Text Revision.Washington, DC: American Psychiatric Association, 2000:429–484; and Ballenger JC, Davidson JRT, Lecrubier Y, et al. Consensus statement update on posttraumatic stress disorder from the International Consensus Group on Depression and Anxiety. J Clin Psychiatry 2004;65(Suppl 1):55–62.
9. Ballenger JC, Davidson JRT, Lecrubier Y, et al. Consensus statement on generalized anxiety disorder from the International Consensus Group on Depression and Anxiety. J Clin Psychiatry 2001;62(Suppl 11):53–58
10. Baldwin DS, Anderson IM, Nutt DJ, et al. Evidence-based guidelines for the pharmacological treatment of anxiety disorders: Recommendations from the British Society for Psychopharmacology. J Psychopharmacology 2005;19:567–596.
11. Katon WJ. Panic disorder. N Engl J Med 2006;354:2360–2367.

12. Ballenger JC, Davidson JRT, Lecrubier Y, et al. Consensus statement on social anxiety disorder from the International Consensus Group on Depression and Anxiety. J Clin Psychiatry 1998;59(Suppl 17):54–60.
13. Eric H. Berko **and** Gabriela Feier. Panic disorder: ensuring prompt recognition and treatment. Clinician reviews. 2018; 28(3): 24-28, 28.

CHAPTER - 69

Schizophrenia

Introduction to Schizophrenia

Schizophrenia is one of the most complex and challenging of psychiatric disorders. It represents a heterogeneous syndrome of disorganized and bizarre thoughts, delusions, hallucinations, inappropriate affect, and impaired psychosocial functioning.

Epidemiology

Lifetime prevalence of schizophrenia ranges from 0.6% to 1.9%, with an average of approximately 1%. Schizophrenia most commonly has its onset in late adolescence or early adulthood and rarely occurs before adolescence or after the age of 40 years. Although the prevalence of schizophrenia is equal in males and females, the onset of illness tends to be earlier in males. Males most frequently have their first episode during their early twenties, whereas with females it is usually during their late twenties to early thirties.

Etiology

Although the etiology of schizophrenia is unknown, research has demonstrated various abnormalities in brain structure and function. Numerous studies have shown neuropsychologic abnormalities and impairment in reaching normal motor milestones and abnormal movements in young children who later develop schizophrenia. Abnormalities in brain function occur long before the onset of psychotic symptomatology and provide empiric evidence for schizophrenia, being a neurodevelopmental disorder.

Genetics [1]

Although the risk of developing schizophrenia is 0.6% to 1.9% in the general population, the risk is approximately 10% if a first-degree relative has the illness and 3% if a second-degree relative has the illness. If both parents have schizophrenia, the risk of producing a schizophrenic offspring increases to approximately 40%. Twin studies in dizygotic twins report that the risk of the second twin developing schizophrenia if one twin has the illness is between 12% and 14%.

However, in monozygotic twins the risk increases to 48%. Dysbindin is a neurodevelopmental protein gene that is found on chromosome 6. Alleles associated with decreased dysbindin RNA in the dorsolateral prefrontal cortex have been reported in patients with schizophrenia and their families.

Pathogenesis

Genetics, dopamine level dysregulation, social factors (social stress or isolation), psychological factors (cognitive biases) biological factors predispose to schizophrenia. There are abnormalities of neurotransmitter dopamine transmission in various regions of brain. As a consequence of this there is a) increased dopaminergic transmission in mesolimbic projection and b) decreased dopaminergic transmission in mesocortical projection. Dopaminergic neurons from mesolimbic region project into limbic system which is responsible for behaviors and emotions. Due to abnormal dopamine transmission here is thought to cause the positive symptoms of schizophrenia. Dopaminergic neurons from mesocortical region project into cerebral cortex-frontal lobes which are responsible for thinking, decision making, language production and mood. Abnormal dopamine transmission here is thought to cause negative symptoms of schizophrenia.

Computed axial tomography (CAT) scans and magnetic resonance imaging (MRI) studies show increased ventricular size, particularly in the third and lateral ventricles dopaminergic hyperactivity in the head of the caudate nucleus and dopaminergic hypofunction in the frontotemporal regions. PET studies using Dopamine-2 (D2)-specific ligands suggest increased densities of D2 receptors in the head of the caudate nucleus with decreased densities in the prefrontal cortex. PET studies assessing Dopamine-1 (D1) function suggest that subpopulations of schizophrenics may have decreased densities of D1 receptors in the caudate nucleus and the prefrontal cortex. Hypofrontality can be associated with lack of volition and cognitive dysfunction, core features of schizophrenia [2].

The positive symptoms are possibly more closely associated with DA-receptor hyperactivity in the mesocaudate, whereas negative symptoms and cognitive impairment are most closely related to DA-receptor hypofunction in the prefrontal cortex. Presynaptic D1 receptors in the prefrontal cortex are thought to be involved in modulating glutamatergic activity. The glutamatergic system is one of the most widespread excitatory neurotransmitter systems in the brain. Alterations in its function, either hypo- or hyperactivity, can result in toxic neuronal reactions [3].

Dopaminergic innervation from the ventral striatum decreases the limbic system's inhibitory activity (through γ-aminobutyric acid [GABA] interneurons); thus, dopaminergic stimulation increases arousal. The corticostriatal glutamate pathways have the opposite effect, inhibiting dopaminergic function from the ventral striatum, therefore allowing the limbic system to have increased inhibitory activity.

Serotoninergic receptors are present on dopaminergic axons, and stimulation of these receptors decreases DA release, at least in the striatum.

Table 69.1 Dopaminergic Tracts and Effects of Dopamine Antagonists.

Dopamine Tract	Origin	Innervation	Function
Nigrostriatal	Substantia nigra (A9 area	Caudate nucleus Putamen	Extrapyramidal system, movement
Mesolimbic	Midbrain ventral tegmentum (A10 area)	Limbic areas (e.g., amygdala, olfactory Arousal, memory, tubercle, septal nuclei), cingulate GYRUS	stimulus processing motivational behaviour
Mesocortical	Midbrain ventral tegmentum (A10 area)	Frontal and prefrontal lobe cortex	Cognition, communication, social function, response to stress
Tuberoinfundibular	Hypothalamus	Pituitary gland	Regulates prolactin release Increased prolactin concentrations

Glutamatergic dysfunction. A deficiency of glutamatergic activity produces symptoms similar to those of dopaminergic hyperactivity and possibly symptoms seen in schizophrenia.

- *Serotonin (5-HT) abnormalities.* Schizophrenic patients with abnormal brain scans have higher whole blood 5-HT concentrations, and these concentrations correlate with increased ventricular size.

Clinical manifestations and features

- Symptoms of the acute episode may include the following: being out of touch with reality; hallucinations (especially hearing voices); delusions (fixed false beliefs); ideas of influence (actions controlled by external influences); disconnected thought processes (loose associations); ambivalence (contradictory thoughts); flat, inappropriate, or labile affect; autism (withdrawn and inwardly directed thinking); uncooperativeness, hostility, and verbal or physical aggression; impaired self-care skills; and disturbed sleep and appetite.
- After the acute psychotic episode has resolved, the patient typically has residual features (e.g., anxiety, suspiciousness, lack of volition, lack of motivation, poor insight, impaired judgment, social withdrawal, difficulty in learning from experience, and poor self-care skills). Patients often have comorbid substance abuse and are nonadherent with medications.

DSM-IV-TR Diagnostic Criteria for Schizophrenia

A. Characteristic symptoms: Two or more of the following, each persisting for a significant portion of at least a 1-month period:

1. delusions
2. hallucinations

3. disorganized speech
4. grossly disorganized or catatonic behavior
5. negative symptoms

Note: Only one criterion A symptom is required if delusions are bizarre or if hallucinations consist of a voice keeping a running commentary on the person's behavior or two or more voices conversing with each other.

B. Social/occupational dysfunction: For a significant portion of the time since onset of the disorder, one or more major areas of functioning such as work, interpersonal relations, or self-care are significantly below the level prior to onset.

C. Duration: Continuous signs of the disorder for at least 6 months. This must include at least 1 month of symptoms fulfilling criterion A (unless successfully treated). This 6 months may include prodromal or residual symptoms.

D. Schizoaffective or mood disorder has been excluded.

E. Disorder is not due to a medical disorder or substance use.

F. If a history of a pervasive developmental disorder is present, there must be symptoms of hallucinations or delusions present for at least 1 month.

The *Diagnostic and Statistical Manual of Mental Disorders,* specifies the following criteria for the diagnosis of schizophrenia:

✓ Persistent dysfunction lasting longer than 6 months

 Two or more symptoms (present for at least 1 month), including hallucinations, delusions, disorganized speech, grossly disorganized or catatonic behavior, and negative symptoms

✓ Significantly impaired functioning (work, interpersonal, or self-care)

The *Diagnostic and Statistical Manual of Mental Disorders,* classifies symptoms as positive or negative.

- Positive symptoms (the ones most affected by antipsychotic drugs) include delusions, disorganized speech (association disturbance), hallucinations, behavior disturbance (disorganized or catatonic), and illusions.
- Negative symptoms include alogia (poverty of speech), avolition, affective flattening, anhedonia, and social isolation.
- Cognitive dysfunction is another symptom category that includes impaired attention, working memory, and executive function.

Differential Diagnosis for Schizophrenia (DSM-IV-TR)
- **Drug-induced Psychoses**
  Amphetamine, Cocaine, Cannabis (marijuana), Phencyclidine (PCP), Lysergic acid diethylamide (LSD), Anticholinergics
- **Primary Psychiatric Disorders**
  Brief psychotic disorder, Schizophreniform disorder, Bipolar affective disorder, manic type, Mood disorder with psychotic features

- **Personality Disorders**
  Schizotypal , Schizoid, Paranoid

Diagnosis with algorithm [4, 5]

> If the patient is identified with Psychotic features: Consider differential diagnosis like

i)	Organic mental conditions
ii)	Acute and transient psychotic disorder
iii)	Persistent delusional disorder
iv)	Schizoaffective disorder
v)	Severe depression with psychotic symptoms
vi)	Drug induced psychosis

> Establish the diagnosis of schizophrenia

Assessment:

  a) Severity of illness; risk of harm to self and others; comorbid substance use/dependence; level of functioning; detilaed physical examination; record-BP, weight,BMI and waist circumference; Mental status examination

  b) Investigations: hemogram; liver function test; renal function test; fasting blood glucose, ECG

  c) Treatemtn history: response to previous medications, compliance, side effects etc.

  d) Assessment of social support, coping

  e) Assesswment of caregivers burden, coping and distress

> Decision about treatment setting: consider inpatient care in case of suicidality, severe agitation and violence, malnutrition, catatonia, patient unable to care for self.

1. Pharmacological management: Choose an anti-psychotic based on past treatment response, past history of side effects, cost, comorbidity, patient/family preference, preffered route of administration, current medication profile, past history of compliance, treatment resistance.
2. Electroconvulsive therapy: if the patient has catatonia, affective symptoms, rapid control of symptoms, suicidality, past response to ECT, augmentation etc.
3. Non-pharmacological manangeemnt: psychoeducation, psychosocial intervention

Management

Goals of therapy

1. Alleviation of target symptoms
2. Avoidance of side effects, improvement in psychosocial functioning and productivity
3. Compliance with the prescribed regimen, and involvement of the patient in treatment planning.

Nonpharmacological therapy: Psychotherapeutic approaches may be divided into three categories: individual, group, and cognitive behavioral. Psychotherapy is a constantly evolving therapeutic area. Emerging psychotherapies include meta-cognitive training, narrative therapies, and mindfulness therapy. Nonpharmacological should be used as an addition to medications, not as a substitute for them. Nonpharmacological therapies fill in gaps in pharmacological treatments; they help to ensure that patients remain adherent to their medications. Nonadherence rates in schizophrenia range from 37% to 74%.

Comprehensive Care Elements in the Treatment of Schizophrenia

Medication treatment
   Individual supportive therapy
   Cognitive and psychosocial therapies
   Family psychoeducation and support
   Social support
   Case management
   Housing
   Financial support
   Vocational support

Options for the management for schizophrenia

1. First generation antipsychotic medications (oral/ parenteral/ depot or ling acting-preparations)
2. Second generation anti-psychotic medications(oral/ parenteral/ depot or ling acting-preparations)
3. Somatic treatments : Electroconvulsive therapy
4. Adjunctive medications: anti-cholinergics; anti-depresssants; benzodiazepines; hypnotic-sedatives; anti-covulsants; lithium carbonate
5. Psychosocial interventions: family intervention, cognitive behavioral therapy, social skills training, cognitive remediation, individual therapy, group therapy, vocational rehabilitation, early intervention programmes, case management, community mental-health teams, crisis resolution teams
6. Othermeasures: lifestyle and dietary modifications

Factors that influence selection of antipsychotics

- Past treatment response
- Cost of treatment, affordability, psychiatric comorbidity
- Medical comorbidity and side effects
- Preferred route of administration
- Concomitant medications
- Non-adherance
- Treatment resistance

Clinical Practice Guidelines treatment algorithm for Management of Schizophrenia [6]

- Patient given an adequate antipsychotic trial (adequate dose for atleast 6 weeks duration)
  - (a) If adequate response is seen, continue with the same dose of anti-psychotic medication and keep on monitoring the side effects.
  - (b) If non-response to treatment given: then re-evaluate the diagnosis and assess the medication compliance.
- If true non-response is observed-change the anti-psychotic medication
  - (a) If adequate response is seen –continue the same dose and keep on monitoring the side effects

(b) If again failure of 2 adequate trials of anti-psychotic, one of which is SGA-consider clozapine

(c) If still inadequate response to clozapine: consider combining clozapine with ECT or another antipsychotic medication. More intensive psychosocial intervention

- If pseudo nonresponse due to poor compliance: evaluate the causes, address the same and ensure compliance. Incase of poor compliance due to intolerable side effects-consider change of antipsychotic

The Texas Medication Algorithm Project (TMAP) has provided a six-stage pharmacotherapeutic algorithm for the treatment of schizophrenia.

Stage 1: It is first-line monotherapy with an SGA. If the patient shows little or no response, he or she should proceed to stage 2,

Stage 2: It onsists of monotherapy with either another SGA or an FGA. If there is still no response, the patient should move to stage 3,

Stage 3: This consists of clozapine monotherapy with monitoring of the white blood cell (WBC) count. If agranulocytosis occurs, clozapine should be discontinued. If stage-3 therapy fails to elicit a response, the patient should proceed to stage 4,

Stage 4: It combines clozapine with an FGA, an SGA, or electroconvulsive therapy (ECT). If the patient still shows no response to treatment,

Stage 5: Calls for monotherapy with an First Generation-psychotics (FGA) or an Second Generation Antipsychotics (SGA) that has not been tried. Finally, if stage 5 treatment is unsuccessful,

Stage 6: Consists of combination therapy with an SGA, an FGA, ECT, and/or a mood stabilizer

Recommended therapeutic dose ranges of antipsychotics

First generation anti-psychotics (FGAs)

Chlorpromazine	300-800mg/day	max dose 800/day
Haloperidol	20-60mg/week	250mg/week
Perphenazine	12-64 mg	64mg
Pimozide	4-10mg	10mg
Thioridazone	300-800 mg	800mg

Second generation anti-psychotics (SGAs)

Amisulpiride	50-800 mg	1200 mg
Aripiprazole	10-30 mg	30mg
Clozapine	150-600mg	900mg
Olanzapine	10-30mg	30mg
Quetiapine	300-800mg	800mg
Risperidone	2-8mg	16mg
Ziprasidone	75-300mg	300mg

Pharmacological management [7, 8]

In the event of an acute psychotic episode, drug therapy should be administered immediately. During the first seven days of treatment, the goal is to decrease hostility and to attempt to return the patient to normal functioning (e.g., sleeping and eating). At the start of treatment, appropriate dosing should be titrated based on the patient's response.

Treatment during the acute phase of schizophrenia is followed by maintenance therapy, which should be aimed at increasing socialization and at improving self-care and mood. Maintenance treatment is necessary to help prevent relapse. The incidence of relapse among patients receiving maintenance therapy, compared with those not receiving such therapy, is 18% to 32% versus 60% to 80%, respectively. Drug therapy should be continued for at least 12 months after the remission of the first psychotic episode.

According to the American Psychiatric Association, second-generation (atypical) antipsychotics (SGAs)—with the exception of clozapine—are the agents of choice for first-line treatment of schizophrenia. Clozapine is not recommended because of its risk of agranulocytosis. SGAs are usually preferred over first-generation (typical) antipsychotics (FGAs) because they are associated with fewer extrapyramidal symptoms. However, SGAs tend to have metabolic side effects, such as weight gain, hyperlipidemia, and diabetes mellitus. These adverse effects can contribute to the increased risk of cardiovascular mortality observed in schizophrenia patients.

Initial therapy

The goals during the first 7 days are decreased agitation, hostility, anxiety, and aggression and normalization of sleep and eating patterns. IM antipsychotic administration (e.g., ziprasidone 10 to 20 mg, olanzapine 2.5 to 10 mg, or haloperidol 2 to 5 mg) can be used to calm agitated patients. Intramuscular (IM) lorazepam , 2 mg, as needed in combination with the maintenance antipsychotic may actually be more effective in controlling agitation than using additional doses of the antipsychotic.

Stabilization therapy

During weeks 2 and 3, the goals should be to improve socialization, self care habits, and mood. Improvement in formal thought disorder may require an additional 6 to 8 weeks.

- Most patients require a dose of 300 to 1,000 mg of CPZ equivalents (of FGAs) daily or SGAs in usual labeled doses. Dose titration may continue every 1 to 2 weeks as long as the patient has no side effects.
- If symptom improvement is not satisfactory after 8 to 12 weeks, a different strategy should be tried.

Maintenance Therapy

- Medication should be continued for at least 12 months after remission of the first psychotic episode. Continuous treatment is necessary in most patients at the lowest effective dose.
- Antipsychotics (especially FGAs and clozapine) should be tapered slowly before discontinuation to avoid rebound cholinergic withdrawal symptoms.

Depot Antipsychotic Medications

Risperidone Consta is the first SGA to be available as a long-acting injectable. The recommended starting dose is 25 mg. Usual dosing range is 25 to 50 mg deep IM every 2 weeks **fluphenazine decanoate**, an esterified formulation in sesame seed oil, the simplest conversion is the Stimmel method, which uses 1.2 times the oral daily dose for stabilized patients, rounding up to the nearest 12.5-mg interval, administered IM in weekly doses for the first 4 to 6 weeks.

Haloperidol decanoate, an esterified formulation in sesame seed oil, a factor of 10 to 15 times the oral daily dose is commonly recommended, rounding up to the nearest 50-mg interval, administered IM in a once monthly dose with oral haloperidol overlap for 1 month.

Management of Treatment-Resistant Schizophrenia [9]

Symptomatic improvement with clozapine often occurs slowly in resistant patients, and as many as 60% of patients may improve if clozapine is used for up to 6 months.

Augmentation therapy involves the addition of a non-antipsychotic drug to an antipsychotic in a poorly responsive patient, while combination treatment involves using two antipsychotics simultaneously.

Mood stabilizers (e.g., lithium, valproic acid, and carbamazepine) used as augmentation agents may improve labile affect and agitated behavior.

Selective serotonin reuptake inhibitors have been used with FGAs with improvement of negative symptoms

Propranolol, pindolol, and nadolol have been used for antiaggressive effects, especially in organic aggressive syndrome. 20 mg three times daily.

Adverse Effects [10]

Autonomic Nervous System

- Anticholinergic (ACh) side effects include impaired memory, dry mouth, constipation, tachycardia, blurred vision, inhibition of ejaculation, and urinary retention. Elderly patients are especially sensitive to these side effects. Low potency FGAs, clozapine, and olanzapine are most likely to cause ACh effects.

Central Nervous System

Extrapyramidal System

Dystonia

- Dystonias are prolonged tonic muscle contractions, with rapid onset (usually within 24 to 96 hours of dosage initiation or dosage increase); they may be life threatening (e.g., pharyngeal-laryngeal dystonias). Dystonic reactions occur primarily with FGAs. Risk factors include younger patients (especially males), use of high-potency agents, and high dose.

- Treatment includes IM or IV AChs or benzodiazepines-Benztropine mesylate, 2 mg, or Diphenhydramine , 50 mg, may be given IM or IV, or diazepam , 5 to 10 mg slow IV push, or Lorazepam , 1 to 2 mg IM, may be given.

Akathisia

- Symptoms include subjective complaints (feelings of inner restlessness) and/or objective symptoms (pacing, shuffling, or tapping feet). Diazepam may be used (5 mg three times daily), but efficacy data are conflicting.
- Propranolol (up to 160 mg/day) and metoprolol (up to 100 mg/day) are reported to be effective.

Tardive Dyskinesia

The classic presentation is buccolingual-masticatory movements (BLM). Symptoms may become severe enough to interfere with chewing, wearing dentures, speech, respiration, or swallowing. Facial movements include frequent blinking, brow arching, grimacing, upward deviation of the eyes, and lip smacking. Involvement of the extremities occurs in later stages (restless choreiform and athetotic movements of limbs.

Sedation and Cognition

- Administration of most or all of the daily dose at bedtime can decrease daytime sedation and may eliminate the need for hypnotics.

Thermoregulation

- In temperature extremes, patients taking antipsychotics may experience their body temperature adjusting to ambient temperature (poikilothermia)

Neuroleptic Malignant Syndrome

- Neuroleptic malignant syndrome occurs in 0.5% to 1% of patients taking FGAs. It may be more frequent with high-potency FGAs, injectable, or depot antipsychotics; in dehydrated patients; or in those with organic mental disorders. Symptoms develop rapidly over 24 to 72 hours and include body temperature exceeding 38°C (100.4°F), altered level of consciousness, autonomic dysfunction (tachycardia, labile blood pressure, diaphoresis, tachypnea, urinary or fecal incontinence), and rigidity.

Endocrine System

- Antipsychotic-induced elevations in prolactin levels with associated galactorrhea and menstrual irregularities are common. These effects may be dose related and are more common with the use of FGAs and risperidone. • Possible management strategies for galactorrhea include switching to an SGA (e.g., olanzapine, quetiapine, aripiprazole, or ziprasidone).

Cardiovascular system

Low-potency piperidine phenothiazines (e.g., thioridazine), clozapine, and ziprasidone are more likely to cause ECG changes.

- ECG changes include increased heart rate, flattened T waves, ST-segment depression, prolongation of QT and PR intervals, and torsade de pointes. Torsade de pointes has been reported with thioridazine, which may be a cause of cardiac sudden death.

- Ziprasidone prolonged the QTc interval about one-half as much as thioridazine. Ziprasidone's effect on the ECG is probably without clinical sequelae except in patients with baseline risk factors.
- It has been recommended to discontinue a medication associated with QTc prolongation if the interval consistently exceeds 500 msec.
- QTc prolongation may lead to the development of ventricular tachyarrhythmias such as torsades de pointes and ventricular fibrillation, which can cause syncope, cardiac arrest, or sudden cardiac death.
- Comparision of QTc changes with antipsychotics: Thioridazone> ziprasidaone> Quetiapine> risperidone> olanzapine> haloperidol

Lipid Effects
- Some SGAs and phenothiazines cause elevations in serum triglycerides and cholesterol.

Ophthalmologic Effects
- Impairment in visual accommodation results from paresis of ciliary muscles. Photophobia may also result. If severe, pilocarpine ophthalmic solution may be necessary.

Hepatic System
- Liver function test abnormalities are common. Cholestatic hepatocanalicular jaundice can occur in up to 2% of patients receiving phenothiazines.

Genitourinary System
- Urinary hesitancy and retention are commonly reported, especially with low-potency FGAs and clozapine.

Hematologic System
- Transient leukopenia may occur with antipsychotic therapy

Some indications for inpatient care during acute episodes
- Presence of suicidal behaviour which puts the life of the patient at risk.
- Presence of svere agitation or violence which puts the life of others at risk
- Refusal to eat which puts the liefe of patint at risk
- Severe malnutrition
- Patient unable to care for self to the extent that she/he requires cobstabt supervision or support
- Catatonia
- Presence of general medical or comorbid psychiatric conditions which make magenet unsafe and ineffective in the outpatient setting

Possible indications of use of ECT in patients of schizophrenia
- Catatonic symptoms; Affective symptoms; Refusal to eat
- Need for rapid control of symptoms
- Presence of suicidal behaviour
- Patients not responding to adequate trial of anti-psychotic medications
- Clozapine resistant schizophrenia; Presence of severe agitation or violence

Common Rating Instruments for Schizophrenia and Antipsychotics

Psychosis

Brief Psychiatric Rating Scale (BPRS)

Positive and Negative Symptom Scale for Schizophrenia (PANSS)

Scale for Assessment of Positive Symptoms (SAPS)

Scale for Assessment of Negative Symptoms (SANS)

Movement Disorders—Tardive Dyskinesia

Abnormal Involuntary Movement Scale (AIMS)

Dyskinesia Identification System Condensed User Scale (DISCUS)

Movement Disorders—Parkinsonism

Simpson Angus Scale for Extrapyramidal Symptoms

Movement Disorders—Akathisia

Barnes Akathisia Scale

Agents to treat acute agitation
1. Lorazepam   1-2mg   PO, IM, IV
2. Typical anti-psychotics: Haloperidol   5-10mg   PO , IM, IV
3. Atypical anti-psychotics:
   Olanzapine PO (tablet), IM, ODT 10 mg
   Risperidone PO (tablet, liquid), ODT 2 mg
   Ziprasidone PO (tablet), IM 20 mg
   Aripiprazole PO (tablet, liquid), IM 9.75 mg

Agents used to treat extrapyramidal side effects
1. Antimuscarinics: Benztropine Biperidena Trihexyphenidyl
2. Anithistaminic: Diphenhydramine
3. Dopamine agonist: Amantadine
4. Benzodiazepines: Lorazepam, Diazepam, Clonazepam
5. β-Blockers: Propranolol

Guidelines for Response to Clozapine-Induced White Blood Cell Abnormalities

(i)   **Do Not Initiate Clozapine**
       Initial WBC count < 3500/mm3
       Initial ANC <2000/mm3
       History of myeloproliferative disorder
       History of agranulocytosis or granulocytopenia related to clozapine

(ii)   **WBC<2000/mm3 and or ANC < 1000/mm3**
       Discontinue clozapine immediately Do not rechallenge patient Monitor WBC and differential: until normal and for at least 4 weeks

(iii) WBC 2000/mm3 – 3000/mm3 or ANC 1000/mm3-1500/mm3

Discontinue clozapine

Monitor WBC and differential

May restart clozapine when: —if no symptoms of infection present

(iv) WBC Drops to 3,000–3,500/mm3; > 3000/mm3 over 1-3 weeks; immature WBCs present: Repeat WBC with differential and confirm

Case Study of Schizoprenia

Summary: A female patient of age 26 years was admitted in the female psychiatry ward with the chief complaints: case of speaking to herself since 7 days after 3 months of third delivery. Fear of trying to kill her. Body pains. Decreased sleep since 2 days, decreased social interaction since 7 days. Gets up from sleep, walks some distance and comes back and sleep and again does the same for around 10 min during night, hearing other voices. Past medical history: similar complaints 3 yrs ago after 6 months of 2nd delivery. Had hallucinations, delusions and anger. Past medication history: used medication for 30 days and then stopped since 3 yrs. No social history and no allergies. Vitals are normal.

Final diagnosis: Schizophrenia

Medication chart:

Tab qutipin (Quotepine) PO 50mg OD

Inj. Serenace +Inj phenergan (Haloperidol+Promethazine) SOS

Inj optineuron(Vit B complex) IV 100ml   OD

Tab pacitane (Trihexyphenidyl) PO 2 mg OD

Tab zerodol-SP (aceclofenac+paracetamol)   PO 300mg BD

Tab Xycal-5 (levocetrizine) PO 5mg OD

Pharmacist interventions: Drug interactions: Promethazine and haloperidol-both increase QTc interval.

Patient education: There's no sure way to prevent attacks. However, these recommendations may help.

Stick with treatment plan to help prevent relapses or worsening of symptoms.

Get regular physical activity, which may play a role in protecting against anxiety.

Assignment

1. **What information (signs, symptoms, lab values) indicates the presence or severity of an acute exacerbation of schizophrenia, paranoid type?**

   Signs and symptoms: Psychomotor excitation, or impulse control, tension, in cooperation, increased sympathetic tone, dehydration, disorganized thinking, and negative thoughts.

Lab Values:
- Abnormal lab values during psychomotor excitation were frequent like,
- Increased WBC count, low serum potassium levels, high levels of fasting blood sugar, lactace dehydrogenase and uric acid.
- Abnormal triglyceride levels were found significantly more frequent in patients receiving Olanzapine than Risperidone.
- Usage of psychoactive drugs that effect mind and mental process which may trigger symptoms in those who are susceptible.

2. **What Non drug therapy is indicated in the patient?**

Psycho Social Interventions:
- Individual therapy: psychotherapy may help to normalize thought pattern and also learning to cope with stress and identify early warning signs of relapse can help people with schizophrenia manage their illness.
- Social skills training: focuses on improving communication and social interactions and improving ability to participate in daily activities.
- Family therapy: provides support and education to family dealing with schizophrenia.
- Vocational rehabilitation and support employment
- Cognitive behavioral therapy: can help person to change their thinking and behavior ability.
- Cognitive enhancement therapy: cognitive remediation

3. **What drug, dosage form, dose schedule, duration of therapy is best for patient.**

Tab. Qutupin

Generic name	: Quetiapine
Route	: PO
Dose	: 50 mg
Dosage form	: tablet
Frequency	: OD
Duration of therapy	: daily (as prescribed by the physician)
Category	: Atypical Antipsychotic.

Tab. Oleanz

Generic name	: Olanzapine
Route	: PO
Dose	: 5 mg/10 mg
Dosage form	: tablet
Frequency	: OD
Duration of therapy	: for 2 days (as prescribed by the physician)
Category	: Antipsychotic.

Tab. Pacitone

Generic name	: Trihexyphenidyl
Route	: PO

Dose	: 2 mg
Dosage form	: tablet
Frequency	: BD
Duration of therapy	: daily
Category	: Ant parkinsonism agent

Inj. Optineuron

Generic name	: Vitamin B Complex
Route	: IV
Dose	: 100 ml
Dosage form	: IV infusion
Frequency	: OD
Category	: Vitamin

4. What is the alternative therapy if initial therapy fails?

Electro convulsive therapy is used as an alternative therapy if the initial therapy is failed. Course of ECT therapy involves 2 to 3 treatments per week for several weeks.

In this process, electrodes are attached to patients scalp and under general anaesthesia; small electrodes are sent to the brain which each shock causes controlled seizures. A series of treatment over time improves in mood and thinking ability.

5. What clinical and laboratory parameters are indicated for diagnosis?

- CT Scan; MRI Scan
- Physiological tests: Cognitive testing; Personality testing; Behavior; Thinking and learning ability
- **Laboratory tests:** Physical examination; Blood tests; Blood sugar levels

To Detect or Prevent Adverse Effects: Early warning signs of relapse:

- Trouble sleeping; Eating less; Trouble concentrating or being disorganized
- Mood changes or nervousness
- Having strong ideas or disorganized thinking
- Delusion ,aggression and suicidal thoughts

6. Atypical antipsychotics likely to cause more weight gain. Why?

Most antipsychotics cause weight gain. The risk appears to be highest with Olanzapine and Clozapine. Weight increases rapidly in initial period after starting anti psychotics. Patients continue to gain weight in long term.

Antipsychotics likely to cause less weight gain

Antipsychotics	Weight Gain
Aripiprazole	low
Lurasidone	low
Ziprasidone	low
Haloperidone	low

7. Name the drugs causing change in Qtc interval

Typical: Thioridazine increases the QTC interval from baseline by 30.1 ms

Haloperidol increases it by 7.1 ms

Atypical: Ziprasidone and Ilopeudone are considered to have potential to cause clinical significant increases in QTC interval.

References

1. McDonald C, Murphy KC. The new genetics of schizophrenia. Psychiatr Clin North Am 2003;26:41–63.
2. Mathalon DH, Sullivan EV, Lim KO, Pfefferbaum A. Progressive brain volume changes and the clinical course of schizophrenia in men: A longitudinal magnetic resonance imaging study. Arch Gen Psychiatry 2001;58:148–157.
3. Harrison P. The neuropathology of schizophrenia. A critical review of the data and their interpretation. Brain 1999;122:593–624.
4. Lieberman JA, Bymaster F, Mahadik SP, Weinberger DR. Neurobiology of schizophrenia and antipsychotic effects. Biol Psychiatry, Narendran R, Frankle WG, Keefe R, et al. Altered prefrontal dopaminergic function in chronic recreational ketamine users. Am J Psychiatry 2005;162:2352–2359.
5. American Psychiatric Association. Schizophrenia and other psychotic disorders. In: Diagnostic and Statistical Manual of Mental Disorders, 4th ed., Text Revision. Washington, DC: American Psychiatric Association, 2000:297–319.

6. Sandeep grover et al., Clinical Practice Guidelines for Management of Schizophrenia. CLINICAL PRACTICE GUIDELINES. 2017; 59(5): 19-33.
7. Lehman AF, Lieberman JA, Dixon LB, et al. American Psychiatric Association Practice Guidelines; Work Group on Schizophrenia. Practice guideline for the treatment of patients with schizophrenia, 2nd ed. Am J Psychiatry 2004;161(2 Suppl):1–56.
8. Jones P, Buckley P. Schizophrenia. London: Mosby, 2006.
9. Moore TA, Buchanan RW, Buckley PF, et al. The Texas Medication Algorithm Project antipsychotic algorithm for schizophrenia: 2006 update. J Clin Psychiatry 2007;68:1751–1762.
10. Van Putten T, Marder SR. Behavioral toxicity of antipsychotic drugs. J Clin Psychiatry 1987;48(Suppl 9):13–19.

CHAPTER - 70

Sleep Disorders

Introduction to Sleep Disorders

Changes in sleeping patterns or habits that can negatively affect health.

Sleep Physiology

Sleep Cycles

1. Non–rapid eye movement (NREM) sleep and
2. Rapid eye movement (REM) sleep.

Humans typically experience four to six cycles of NREM and REM sleep, with each cycle lasting between 70 and 120 minutes.

There are four stages of NREM sleep: There are four stages of NREM sleep. Healthy sleep will typically progress through the four stages of NREM sleep prior to the first REM period. From wakefulness, sleep typically progresses quickly through stages 1 and 2. During stages 3 and 4 NREM, both metabolic activity and brain waves slow. This slow-wave sleep occurs most frequently early in the sleep cycle. After stage 4, the first REM cycle occurs and typically lasts between 5 and 7 minutes. REM cycles tend to lengthen in the later stages of the sleep cycle.2 REM sleep involves a dramatic physiological change from stage 4 NREM slow-wave sleep, to a state in which the brain becomes electrically and metabolically activated. REM occurs in bursts, and is accompanied by a 62% to 173% increase in cerebral blood flow, generalized muscle atonia, poikilothermia, vivid dreaming, and fluctuations in respiratory and cardiac rate.

Circadian Rhythm

At birth human infants spend up to 20 hours a day sleeping, and it is not until between 3 and 6 months of age that differentiation between REM and NREM sleep occurs. By age 3, the ultradian sleep-wake rhythm changes to a circadian pattern, with most sleep occurring at night. The suprachiasmic nucleus of the brain serves as the biological clock and paces the circadian rhythm. Although the length of a day is 24 hours, in environments devoid of light cues, the sleep-wake cycle lasts 24hours.Without environmental cues (zeitgebers) such as alarm clocks and lights, it would be difficult to set our internal clocks. In midlife, there is a gradual decline in sleep efficiency and sleep time. In the elderly, sleep is lighter in depth and more fragmented, with intermittent arousals, shifts in the sleep stages, and a gradual disappearance of slow wave sleep.

Neurochemistry

The neurochemistry of sleep is complex since sleep cannot be localized to either a specific area of the brain or a specific neurotransmitter. NREM sleep appears to be controlled by the basal forebrain, the area surrounding the solitary tract in the medulla and the dorsal raphenucleus, which is primarily serotonergic. Sleep is reduced when there are decreases in serotonin or destruction of the dorsal raphe nucleus in the brain stem. REM sleep appears to be turned off by the dorsal raphe nucleus, the locus ceruleus, and the nucleus peribrachialislateris, the latter two of which are primarily noradrenergic. The ascending reticular activating system and the posterior hypothalamus facilitate arousal and wakefulness. Dopamine has an alerting effect. Drugs that increase dopamine in the brain cause increased wakefulness, and those that decrease dopamine cause sleepiness. Neurochemicals involved in wakefulness include norepinephrine and acetylcholine in the cortex and histamine and neuropeptides such as substance P and corticotropin-releasing factor in the hypothalamus.

Electrophysiology

Sleep is typically measured and observed in sleep laboratories by electroencephalograms (EEGs), electro-oculograms (EOGs) of each eye, and electromyograms (EMGs) of the mentalis and submentalis muscles. This information in total is used to evaluate the character of sleep. The EEG is characterized during wakefulness by low-voltage, rapid-frequency alpha (8 to 13 Hz) and beta rhythms (>13 Hz).

Stage 1 of NREM sleep is the stage between wakefulness and sleep during which alpha waves evolve into slower theta waves (4 to 7 Hz). Individuals describe this experience as being awake, being drowsy, or as being asleep.

Stage 2 is characterized by theta rhythms with sleep spindles (brief bursts of electrical activity at 12 to 14 Hz) and K complexes (an electronegative wave followed by an electropositive wave).

Stage 3 and stage 4 sleep is called delta sleep since more than 20% to 50% of the sleep is characterized by high-amplitude slow activity known as delta waves (0.5 to 3 Hz). In this stage eye movements are absent and muscle tone is atonic.

REM sleep is characterized by a low-amplitude, mixed frequency EEG, absence of muscle tone, and bursts of bilateral rapid eye movements. Dreaming occurs during REM sleep, and if an individual is awakened during or at the end of one of these periods, 80% to 90% can report the content of their dream.

Classification of Sleep Disorders (DSM-IV-TR)

Primary Sleep Disorders

Dyssomnias

Primary insomnia

Primary hypersomnia

Narcolepsy

Breathing-related sleep disorder

Circadian rhythm sleep disorder

Delayed sleep phase type

Jet lag type

Shift work type

Unspecified type

Dyssomnia not otherwise specified

Parasomnias

Nightmare disorder

Sleep terror disorder

Sleepwalking disorder

Parasomnia not otherwise specified

Sleep disorders related to another mental disorder:

Insomnia related to another mental disorder

Hypersomnia related to another mental disorder

Other sleep disorders:

Sleep disorder due to a general medical condition

Substance-induced sleep disorder

Insomnia

Insomnia is defined as a complaint of difficulty falling asleep, difficulty maintaining sleep, or experiencing non restorative sleep (Sleeping but not feeling rested) that lasts at least 1 month. This sleep disorder causes distress, frequently due to fear that they may not be able to fall asleep at bedtime, or impaired occupational functioning due to daytime fatigue or drowsiness. While young adults are more likely to complain that they have difficulty falling asleep, middle-aged and elderly adults are more likely to complain that they have middle-of-the-night awakening or early morning awakening. It is important to evaluate insomnia based on its duration. A sleep complaint lasting two or three nights is considered to be transient insomnia. Short-term insomnia usually resolves in less than 3 weeks, and is typically due to illness, jet lag, or stress. According to the Diagnostic and Statistical Manual, insomnia lasting longer than 1 month is considered chronic.

Epidemiology

Insomnia is the most common complaint in general medical practice settings. Primary insomnia usually begins in young adulthood or middle age, and is rare in childhood or adolescence. More than 50% of the population complains of insomnia in their lifetime.

Etiologies of Insomnia: Situational: Work or financial stress, Interpersonal conflicts, Major life events, Jet lag or shift work

Medical: Cardiovascular (angina, arrhythmias, heart failure); Respiratory (asthma, sleep apnea); Chronic pain; Endocrine disorders (diabetes, hyperthyroidism); Gastrointestinal (gastroesophageal reflux disease, ulcers); Neurologic (delirium, epilepsy, Parkinson's disease); Pregnancy

Psychiatric: Mood disorders (depression, mania); Anxiety disorders (generalized anxiety disorder, obsessive-compulsive disorder, or panic disorder); Substance abuse (alcohol or sedative-hypnotic withdrawal)

Pharmacologically induced: Anticonvulsants, Central adrenergic blockers, Diuretics, Selective serotonin reuptake inhibitors, Steroid Stimulants

Pathogenesis: Due to the precipitating event or stressor, there is development of genetic vulnerability (Family history, neurotransmitter genes). Over the time it leads to abnormalities in neurobiological processes. Age, sex, race, medical comorbidities, medications also predispose to abnormal processes. One of the important is simulataneous co-activation of wake and sleep promoting genes. There is an also reduced cortical GABA level in brain. Normaaly, there is a balance between neurophysiologic hyperarousal and psychological and behavioral processes. Precipitating factors for hyperarousal are increased high-frequency EEG, increased sensory information processing, increased REM EEG arousals. Precipitating factors for behavioral processes are increased attention to sleep and sleep related threat cues, increased intention and effort to sleep, increased worry and arousal. Imbalance between these processes to regulate sleep and wake cycle due to above mentioned various stressors leads to insomnia. Over the time sleeplessness leads to adverse health outcomes like mental health-depression, physical health-cardiometabolic disturbances happen.

Clinical Manifestations and Features

Signs and Symptoms

Difficulty falling asleep at night, waking up during the night, waking up too early, not feeling well-rested after a night's sleep, day time tiredness or sleepiness, irritability, depression or anxiety, difficulty paying attention, ongoing worries about sleep

Diagnosis with algorithm:

Evaluation pattern in the patient:

1. When Patient complains of sleep problems
   (a) Difficulty going to sleep or laying asleep with impairment of daytime functioning. Assessment of sleep habits have to be done. If sleep habits and sleep schedules are normal and the person complains of above problems, then assessment of intake of sleep disturbing substances has to be evaluated. If there is no intake of any abuse drugs, it is confirmed as insomnia.
   (b) Excessive daytime sleepiness, heavy snoring, restless legs, sudden sleep attacks or catalepsy seen in the patient, then referred to a sleep specialist and advised about sleep habits, lifestyle and circadian rhythm disorder has to be evaluated.
   (c) Unusual behaviours at night, injurious or distressing, he has to be referred to a sleep specialist.

Treatment: Insomnia

Nonpharmacologic Therapy [1]:

Nonpharmacologic Recommendations for Insomnia (cognitive behavioral therapy)

Stimulus control procedures
1. Establish regular times to wake up and to go to sleep (including weekends).
2. Sleep only as much as necessary to feel rested.
3. Go to bed only when sleepy. Avoid long periods of wakefulness in bed. Use the bed only for sleep or intimacy; do not read or watch television in bed.
4. Avoid trying to force sleep; if you do not fall asleep within 20–30 minutes, leave the bed and perform a relaxing activity (e.g., read, listen to music, or watch television) until drowsy. Repeat this as often as necessary.
5. Avoid daytime naps.
6. Schedule worry time during the day. Do not take your troubles to bed.

Sleep hygiene recommendations
1. Exercise routinely (three to four times weekly), but not close to bedtime because this may cause arousal.
2. Create a comfortable sleep environment by avoiding temperature extremes, loud noises, and illuminated clocks in the bedroom.

3. Discontinue or reduce the use of alcohol, caffeine, and nicotine.
4. Avoid drinking large quantities of liquids in the evening to prevent nighttime trips to the restroom.
5. Do something relaxing and enjoyable before bedtime

Management with Algorithm

1. When the Patient Is Diagnosed with Insomnia-behavioural interventions has to be done.
2. If the person is suffering with any associated medical conditions have to be addressed.
3. If the symptoms resolve, reinforce intervention and continue.
4. If the symptoms do not resolve, then the type of insomnia has to be assessed.
   (a) Sleep onset insomnia- melatonin controlled release (or) Eszopiclone OR Zaleplon OR Zolpidem treatment has to be initiated.
   (b) sleep-maintenance insomnia- Eszopiclone OR Doxepin OR Zolpidem has to be initiated
   (c) insomnia in older adults—Doxepin OR Melatonin controlled release OR Ramelton have to be started
   (d) depression and insomnia—Doxepin OR Mirtazepine has to started

Pharmacological Therapy [2, 3]

- Behavioral and educational interventions that may help include short-term cognitive behavioral therapy, relaxation therapy, stimulus control therapy, cognitive therapy, sleep restriction, paradoxical intention, and sleep hygiene education.
- Management includes identifying the cause of insomnia, educating about sleep hygiene, managing stress, monitoring for mood symptoms, and eliminating unnecessary pharmacotherapy.
- Transient and short-term insomnia should be treated with good sleep hygiene and careful use of sedative-hypnotics if necessary. Chronic insomnia calls for careful assessment for a medical cause, non pharmacologic treatment, and careful use of sedative-hypnotics if necessary.
- Antihistamines (eg, diphenhydramine, doxylamine, and pyrilamine) are less effective than benzodiazepines, but side effects are usually minimal. Their anticholinergic side effects may be problematic, especially in the elderly.
- Amitriptyline, doxepin, and nortriptyline are effective, but side effects include anticholinergic effects, adrenergic blockade, and cardiac conduction prolongation.
- Trazodone, 25 to 100 mg, Side effects include serotonin syndrome, oversedation, α-adrenergic blockade, dizziness, and, rarely, priapism.
- Ramelteon is a melatonin receptor agonist selective for the MT1 and MT2 receptors. The dose is 8 mg at bedtime. It is well tolerated, but side effects include headache, dizziness,

and somnolence. It is not a controlled substance. It is effective for patients with chronic obstructive pulmonary disease and sleep apnea.

- Valerian, a herbal product, is available without a prescription. The recommended dose is 300 to 600 mg. Purity and potency concerns are an issue. It may cause daytime sedation.
- The benzodiazepine receptor agonists are the most commonly used drugs for insomnia. They carry a caution regarding anaphylaxis, facial angioedema, complex sleep behaviors (eg, sleep driving, phone calls, and sleep eating). They include the newer non benzodiazepine γ-aminobutyric acid A (GABA$_A$) agonists and the traditional benzodiazepines, which also bind to GABA.

Benzodiazepine Hypnotics

- Benzodiazepines have sedative, anxiolytic, muscle relaxant, and anticonvulsant properties. They increase stage 2 sleep and decrease REM and delta sleep.
- Triazolam is distributed quickly because of its high lipophilicity and thus has a short duration of effect. Erythromycin, nefazodone, fluvoxamine, and ketoconazole reduce the clearance of triazolam and increase plasma concentrations.
- The effects of flurazepam and quazepam are long because of active metabolites

  Zaleplon : 5-10mgPOat bedtime Half-life: 1 hr

  Zolpidem: 5-10mgPOat bedtime Half-life-1.5-4.5hr

  Zopiclone 7.5-15 mgPO at bedtime Half-life: 3.5-6 hr

Benzodiazepines

  Clonazepam 0.5 mg PO at bedtime

  Estazolam 1-2 mg PO at bedtime

  Lorazepam 1-4mg PO at bedtime

  Oxazepam 15-30 mg PO at bedtime

Benzodiazepine Adverse Effects

- Side effects include drowsiness, psychomotor incoordination, decreased concentration, cognitive deficits, and anterograde amnesia which is minimized by using the lowest dose possible.
- Tolerance to daytime CNS effects (eg, drowsiness, decreased concentration) may develop in some individuals.
- Rebound insomnia occurs frequently with high doses of triazolam, even when used intermittently.
- Rebound insomnia is minimized by using the lowest effective dose and tapering the dose upon discontinuation.

Nonbenzodiazepine GABA$_A$ Agonists

Zaleplon

- Effects: Similar hypnotic effects to benzodiazepines but side effects tend to be less. Does not alter normal sleep patterns and is not associated with tolerance or rebound insomnia

Zolpidem

- Effects: Similar hypnotic effects to benzodiazepines but side effects tend to be less
- Does not alter normal sleep patterns and is usually not associated with rebound insomnia
- Tolerance and dependence has occurred in some patients
- Has been used for up to 6 month usually without withdrawal issues or rebound insomnia upon discontinuation

Zopiclone

- Effects: Decreases sleep latency when compared to placebo and generally increases sleep duration without changing normal sleep patterns
- Rebound insomnia has occurred but not as severe as with benzodiazepines
- Recommended for short-term use limited to maximum 4 weeks duration

Stepwise Approach to Selecting A Hypnotic for Insomnia

Step 1. Determine type of insomnia: DFA, DMS, EMA; duration.

Step 2. Consider possible causes: medical, psychiatric, drug; treat causes.

Step 3. CBT and sleep hygiene ineffective or only partially effective; significant insomnia persists.

Step 4. Assess type of patient: age, size, diagnosis, organ function, drug interactions, abuse potential.

   (i) **Anti depressants:** Can be used for DFA and EMA. Duration of therapy: Chronic use in depressive diagnosis. Onset and duration of effects: Intermediate to long onset.

   (ii) **Chloral hydrate:** Duration of therapy: Short-term use, 2–7 days Onset and duration of effects: Rapid onset; intermediate duration Pharmacokinetic considerations: Major metabolite, trichloroethanol, is active Clinical considerations: GI side effects; rapid tolerance; no EEG effects; drug interactions

   (iii) **Flurazepam or quazpam:** Used for DFA and DMS. Duration of therapy: Short term and chronic. Onset and duration of effects: Rapid onset; long duration. Pharmacokinetic considerations: Active metabolite. Clinical considerations: Efficacy long term

   (iv) **Temazepam:** Duration of therapy: Short term and chronic Onset and duration of effects: Long onset; moderate duration Pharmacokinetic considerations: No hepatic metabolism.

   (v) **Zolpidem, zaleplon, or triazolam:** Duration of therapy: Short-term use, 7–10 days for triazolam, 2–4 weeks for zaleplon and several months for zolpidem Onset and duration of effects: Rapid onset; short duration Pharmacokinetic considerations: Short half-life Clinical considerations: Rebound insomnia; CNS side effects.

Sleep Apnea

Sleep apnea is defined as the cessation of airflow at the nose and mouth lasting at least 10 seconds. Sleep apnea is quantified using polysomnography (PSG) and is classified into two major categories: obstructive and central.

Obstructive Sleep Apnea

Obstructive sleep apnea (OSA) is potentially life threatening and characterized by repeated episodes of nocturnal breathing cessation. It is caused by occlusion of the upper airway, due to factors such as obesity, and fixed upper airway lesions such as polyps, as well as enlarged tonsils or adenoids or the tongue and blood oxygen (O2) desaturation can occur. Episodes may be caused by obesity or fixed upper airway lesions, enlarged tonsils, amyloidosis, and hypothyroidism. Complications include arrhythmias, hypertension, corpulmonale, and sudden death.

Heavy snoring, severe gas exchange disturbances, respiratory failure, and gasping occur in severe episodes. Patients with OSA usually complain of excessive daytime sleepiness. Other symptoms are morning headache, poor memory, and irritability.

The apneic episode is terminated by a reflex action in response to the fall in blood O2 saturation that causes an arousal with resumed breathing.

Treatment

Goal of Treatment: The goal is alleviate sleep-disordered

It may be alleviated by weight loss, avoidance of sedatives, use of tongue retaining devices, breathing under positive pressure through a mask- CRAP (continuous positive airway pressure), sleep position training

TCAs are sometimes used in sleep apnea in young adults (not in older people).

The newer shorter acting non-benzodiazepine hypnotics seem to be safer in these patients and may be considered in those who snore. Surgery, including pharyngoplasty; may relieve heavy snoring

To date, nasal CRAP remains the initial treatment of choice for moderate to severe sleep apnea; however discontinuation of nasal CRAP even for one night results in complete reversal of the gain made in daytime alertness.

Central Sleep Apnea

- Central sleep apnea (CSA), less frequent than OSA, is characterized by repeated episodes of apnea caused by temporary loss of respiratory effort during sleep. It may be caused by autonomic nervous system lesions, neurologic diseases, high altitudes, opioid use, and congestive heart failure.

Treatment

- PAP with or without supplemental O2 improves CSA.
- Acetazolamide causes metabolic acidosis that stimulates respiratory drive and may be beneficial for high altitude, heart failure, and idiopathic CSA.

Narcolepsy

- Essential features are sleep attacks, cataplexy, hypnagogic and hypnopompic hallucinations, and sleep paralysis. Patients complain of excessive daytime sleepiness, sleep attacks that last up to 30 minutes, fatigue, impaired performance, and disturbed nighttime sleep.
- Cataplexy, which occurs in 70% to 80% of narcoleptics, is sudden bilateral loss of muscle tone with collapse. It is often precipitated by highly emotional situations.
- The hypocretin/orexin neurotransmitter system may play a central role in narcolepsy. An autoimmune process may cause destruction of hypocretin-producing cells.

Treatment

Major goals of treatment of narcolepsy include:
  (a) To improve quality of life.
  (b) To reduce excessive daytime sleepiness (EDS)
  (c) To prevent cataplectic attacks

The major wake promoting medications are:
- Modafinil- Preferred due to efficacy, safety, availability, and low risk of abuse and diversion. Modafinil is FDA approved for EDS treatment. Usual dosing is 200-400 mg each morning.
- Amphetamine and Dextroamphetamine (10 mg morning)
- Methamphetamine (10-20 mg bd)
- Pemoline - carries the rare risk of fatal hepatic toxicity
- Pharmacological treatment of cataplexy, sleep paraoxysm, and hypnagogic hallucination include administration of activating SSRI such as fluoxetine (10-20 mg/d) and TCA such as protriptyline (10- 40 mg/d) and clomipramine (25-50 mg/d)
- Sodium oxybate xyrem, appears to be well tolerated and beneficial for treatment of catalepsy, EDS and inadvertent sleep attacks

References

1. Chesson AL, Anderson WM, Littner M, et al. Practice parameters for the nonpharmacologic treatment of chronic insomnia. Sleep 1999;8:1–6
2. American Psychiatric Association. Sleep disorders. In: Diagnostic and Statistical Manual of Mental Disorders, 4th ed., text revision. Washington, DC: American Psychiatric Press, 2000:597–644.
3. Espie C. Insomnia: Conceptual issues in the development, persistence and treatment of sleep disorders in adults. Annu Rev Psychol 2002;53: 215–243.

CHAPTER - 71

Obsessive-Compulsive Disorder

Introduction to Obsessive Compulsive Disorders (OCD)

OCD is an anxiety disorder in which person is obsessed with a particular thought followed by compusion to do activites due to that obsession.

An obsession is a recurrent, persistent idea, thought, impulse, or image that is experienced as intrusive and inappropriate and produces marked anxiety.

Common obsessions involve thoughts about contamination (e.g., concern with germs or dirt), repeated doubts, and needing to have things in a particular order.

A compulsion is defined as a repetitive behavior or mental act generally performed in response to an obsession. The most common compulsions involve washing and cleaning, counting, checking, and requesting or demanding assurances.

Epidemiology

OCD usually begins early in life, with 20% of cases occurring in childhood, 29% in adolescence, and 49% of cases occurring by age 20. The onset of illness is earlier in men than women.

Etiology

OCD has been characterized as a pediatric autoimmune neuropsychiatric disorder associated with streptococcal infections. In response to streptococcal infection, antibodies are produced in some individuals that temporally precipitate sudden onset or exacerbation of symptoms of OCD

Pathophysiology [1]

- Studies in OCD patients have identified abnormal hyperactivity (when compared with normal controls) in certain frontal lobe and basal ganglia regions, specifically the orbital frontal cortex, cingulate cortex, and head of the caudate nucleus.
- Structural abnormalities have also been identified in OCD, including increased brain cortex and opercular volumes, decreased total white matter volume, and smaller pituitary gland size.

- Specific types of cognitive dysfunction have also been found, including problems with nonverbal memory, visuospatial skills, and visual attention.
- Impairments in memory functioning have been correlated with the aforementioned structural abnormalitiesin OCD.
- In addition to biological factors, twin and family studies support an effect of genetics on risk for OCD. Heredity appears to be most important in early-onset OCD cases (before age 18 years) because familial aggregation has not been observed in OCD cases with a later age at onset. Several studies suggest an association between OCD and specific polymorphisms in the serotonin transporter, 5HT1D$\beta$and 5HT2A receptor genes, but others have failed to replicate these findings.
- Other candidate gene studies have linked OCD with functional polymorphisms in the catechol *O*-methyltransferase, dopamineD4-receptor genes, and a high affinity neuronal/epithelial excitatory amino acid transporter gene.

Clinical Presentation

Obsessions:

Repetitive thoughts (e.g., feeling contaminated after touching an object, doubting whether the stove was turned off)

- Repetitive images (e.g., recurrent sexually explicit pictures)
- Repetitive impulses (e.g., need for symmetry or putting things in specific order,
- impulse to shout out obscenities in a church)

Compulsions

- Repetitive activities (e.g., hand washing, checking, ordering, need to ask, need to
- confess)
- Repetitive mental acts (e.g., counting, repeating words silently, praying)

Diagnosis and Algorithm [2]

Table 70.1 DSM-5 Diagnostic Criteria for Obsessive-Compulsive Disorder.

A. Presence of obsessions, compulsions, or both

Obsessions are defined by (1) and (2):

1. Recurrent and persistent thoughts, urges, or images that are experienced, at some time during disturbance, as intrusive and unwanted, and that in most indivisuals cause marked anxiety or distress.

2. The individual attempts to ignore or suppress such thoughts, urges, or images, or to neutralizw them with some other though of action (i.e., by performing a compulsion)

Compulsions are defined by (1) and (2):

1. Repetitive behaviors (e.g., hand washing, ordering checking) or mental acts (e.g., praying, counting repeating words silently) that the individual feels driven to perform in response t an obsession or according to reules that must be applied rigidly.

Contd...

2. The behaviors or mental acts are aimed at preventing or reducing anxiety or distress, or preventing some dreaded event or situation; however, these behaviors or mental acts are not connected in a realistic way with what they are designed to neutralize or prevent, or are clearly excessive.

   Note: Young children may not be able to articulate the aims of these behaviors or mental acts.

B. The obsessions or compulsions are time-consuming (e.g., take more than 1 hour per day) or cause clinically significant distress or impairment in social, occupational, or other important areas of functioning.

C. The obsessive-compulsive symptoms are not attributable to the physiological effects of a substance (e.g., a drug of abuse, a medication) or another medical condition.

D. The disturbances is not better explained by the symptons of another mental disorder (e.g., excessive worries, as in generalized anxiety disorder, preoccupation with appearance, as in body dysmorphic disorder; difficulty discarding or parting with possessions, as in hoarding disorder, hair pulling, as in trichotillomania [hair-pulling disorder); skin picking, as in excoriation [skin-picking] disorder; stereotypies, as in stereotypic movement disorder; ritualized eating behavior, as in eating disorders; preoccupation with substances or gambling, as in substance-related and addictive disorder; preoccupation with having an illness, as in illness anxiety disorder; sexual urges of fantasies, as in paraphilic disordersl impulse, as in disruptive, impulse-control, and conduct disorders; guilty ruminations, as in major depressive disorder; thought insertion or delusional preoccupations, asn in schizophrenia spectrum and other psychotic disoders, or repetitive patterns of behavior, as in auism spectrum disorder).

Specify if:

With good or fair insight: The individual recognizes that obsessive-compulsive disorder beliefs are definitely or probably not true or that may or may not be true.

With poor insight: The indivual thinks obsessive-compulsive disorder beliefs are probably true.

With absent insight/delusional belief: The indivual completely convinced that obsessive-compulsive disorder beliefd are true.

Specify it:

Tic-related: The invidual has current or past history of a tic disorder.

Treatment

Desired Outcomes

Goals of therapy for OCD include reduction in the frequency of obsessive thoughts and in the time spent performing compulsive acts and reduction in the degree of anxiety.

Treatment algorithm for OCD

1. Confirmed diagnosis of mild OCD- CBT; may add SSRI if patient desires. Symptoms adequately controlled – maintenance therapy
2. Confirmed diagnosis of severe OCD: CBT± SSRI or SSRI alone
3. If inadequate response is seen to
   (a) CBT alone- add SSRI and change CBT approach
   (b) SSRI alone- add CBT. Switch to another SSRI

   (c) CBT+SSRI:
   (i) if partial response is seen-Change CBT approach; switch to another SSRI; add augmentation medication
   (ii) If completely no response is seen to both CBT+SSRI-switch to another SSRI

4. Symptoms are adequately controlled after above respective options-continue for maintenance therapy
5. If still the symptoms are inadequately controlled –use clomipramine after 2-3 failed trials of SSRIs +CBT
6. Symptoms still not controlled consider augmentation or neurosurgery.

Pharmacologic Therapy [3]

Rating scales can be used to measure symptom severity at baseline and during treatment to ascertain the degree of improvement. The Yale-Brown Obsessive-Compulsive Scale (YBOCS) is the most widely used clinicianadministered scale. The Padua Inventory is a useful self-report questionnaire.

The SSRIs are considered to be the drugs of choice in the treatment of OCD. Drug therapy is reserved for patients with moderate to severe symptoms. Antidepressants can be combined with CBT or used alone in adultswith moderate to severe symptoms. An SSRI should be added when there has been no response or partial response to CBT alone.

If one SSRI is ineffective, then another SSRI should be tried. Treatment resistance can be definedas failure to achieve at least a 25% reduction in baseline scores on the YBOCS.

Clomipramine can be selected after two to three failed SSRI trials. Clomipramine can be used to augment an SSRI in partially responsive or nonresponsive patients

Clomipramine

- Clomipramine was the first drug with proven efficacy in treating OCD, and it was considered the standard first-line treatmentfor several years until the SSRIs gained popularity.
- Many large well-controlled studies have documented that clomipramineis far superior to placebo and significantly improve OCDsymptoms in approximately 60% to 70% of patients. Clomipramine is unique among TCAs in its effectiveness for OCD. This distinct property is attributed to its more potent effects on 5-HT reuptake inhibition compared with other TCAs.

Mechanism of action: Clomipramine is often referred to as an SRI (serotonin reuptake inhibitor), not an SSRI, because its major active metabolite, desmethylclomipramine, is a potent inhibitor of norepinephrine reuptake. Clomipramine also blocks adrenergic, histaminergic, and cholinergic receptors similarly to otherTCAs, resulting in an adverse effect profile similar to that of Imipramine. However, clomipramine is less well tolerated than SSRIs, and patients are more likely to discontinue clomipramine treatment because of side effects.

Therefore, clomipramine is currently reserved as asecond-line treatment option for patients who do not respondadequately to SSRI therapy.

Selective Serotonin Reuptake Inhibitors

- SSRIs are the only first-line medication treatments for OCD. Double-blind, placebo-controlled studies have documented the efficacies of fluvoxamine, fluoxetine, paroxetine, and sertraline in the treatment of OCD.
- Citalopram and escitalopram also are effective but there is less evidence to support their use.

Citalopram	Iinitial dose 20mg	dosage range 20-60mg
Clomipramine	Iinitial dose 10mg	dosage range 100-250mg
Fluoxetine	Iinitial dose 20mg	dosage range 20-80mg
Fluvoxamine	Iinitial dose 50mg	dosage range 100-300mg
Paroxetine	Iinitial dose 20mg	dosage range 20-60mg
Sertraline	Iinitial dose 50mg	dosage range 75-200mg

Dosage and Administration

- If there is inadequate response to an average dose, then it should be incrementally increased to the maximum dose within 4 to 9 weeks from the start of treatment.
- If there is an inadequate response after 4 to 6 weeks at the maximum dose, then another SSRI should be tried.
- Eight to thirteen weeks is considered an adequate trial before changing to another drug or augmenting with another agent.
- After patients have responded to the acute phase of treatment, treatment gains are maintained with maintenance-phase strategies.
- Monthly followup visits are recommended for at least 3 to 6 months, and a medication taper can be considered after 1 to 2 years of treatment.
- Medication should not be rapidly discontinued, and booster CBT sessions can reduce the risk of relapse when medication is withdrawn.
- The drug dosage can be decreased by 25%, and then 2 months should lapse before again decreasing the dose, depending on response.
- Long-term or lifelong prophylaxis with pharmacotherapy is recommended after two to four severe relapses or three to four mild relapses.

Nonpharmacologic Treatments

Cognitive-Behavioral Therapies

- CBT is an extremely important component of treatment for OCD and should be incorporated into the initial treatment planwhenever possible.
- CBT alone may be appropriate for mild OCD or in cases in which it is desirable to avoid medication (e.g., pregnancy, medical conditions).
- The combination of CBT and medication is generally superior to either treatment approachused alone. Treatment gains achieved with CBToften are maintained long after its discontinuation, which is an advantage over pharmacotherapy.

- The cognitive therapy component of CBT is aimed toward changing the detrimental thought patterns in OCD and is mosthelpful for obsessions such as scrupulosity, moral guilt, andpathological doubt.
- The behavioral therapy aspect, called exposureplus response prevention, involves exposure to fearedobjects or situations followed by prevention of the usual compulsiveresponse.
- This type of therapy is most beneficial forpatients with contamination fears, hoarding, and rituals involvingsymmetry, counting, or repeating. Because exposure plus response prevention is anxiety provoking and can be very distressing, many patients refuse to participate in it.

Neurosurgery

Neurosurgical treatment of OCD has been practiced sincethe 1950s and is considered an option of last resort in treatment refractory patients. Cingulotomy and capsulotomy are the most commonly used procedures.

References

1. Jenike MA. Obsessive-compulsive disorder. N Engl J Med 2004;350:259–265.
2. American Psychiatric Association. Diagnostic and Statistical Manual of Mental Disorders, Fourth Edition, Text Revision. Washington, DC: American Psychiatric Association, 2000:429–484.
3. American Psychiatric Association. Handbook of Psychiatric Measures. Washington, DC: American Psychiatric Association, 2000:572–576.
4. Jill N fenske et al., Obsessive-Compulsive Disorder: Diagnosis and Management *Am Fam Physician.* 2015 Nov 15;92(10):896-903.